D1030312

Identified Neurons and Behavior of Arthropods

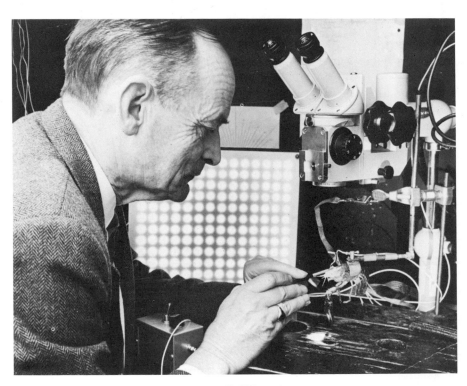

C. A. G. Wiersma

Identified Neurons and Behavior of Arthropods

Edited by
Graham Hoyle
University of Oregon at Eugene

Plenum Press · New York and London

Library of Congress Cataloging in Publication Data

Symposium on Identified Neurons and Behavior of Arthropods, Ojai, Calif., 1976.
  Identified neurons and behavior of arthropods.

  Papers delivered at the Symposium on Identified Neurons and Behavior of Arthropods held at Ojai, Calif. in April 1976 in honor of C. A. G. Wiersma.
  Bibliography: p.
  Includes index.
  1. Arthropoda–Physiology–Congresses. 2. Arthropoda–Behavior–Congresses. 3. Neurons–Congresses. I. Hoyle, Graham. II. Wiersma, Cornelis Adrianus Gerrit, 1905-   III. Title.
QL434.72.S95   595'.2'04188   77-21603
ISBN 0-306-31001-5

© 1977 Plenum Press, New York
A Division of Plenum Publishing Corporation
227 West 17th Street, New York, N.Y. 10011

Printed in the United States of America

Contributors

Hugo Aréchiga, Departamento de Fisiología, Centro de Investigación del IPN, Apartado Postal 14-740, Mexico 14, D.F.

Harold L. Atwood, Department of Zoology, University of Toronto, Toronto M5S 1A1, Ontario, Canada

David Bentley, Department of Zoology, University of California, Berkeley, California 94720

George D. Bittner, Department of Zoology, University of Texas, Austin, Texas 78712

Theodore Holmes Bullock, Department of Neuroscience, University of California, San Diego, California 92037

Malcolm Burrows, Zoology Department, Cambridge University, Downing Street, Cambridge CB2 3EJ, England

Brian M. H. Bush, Department of Physiology, University of Bristol, Park Row, Bristol BS1 5LS, England

François Clarac, C.N.R.S.-I.N.P. 10, 31, Chemin Joseph-Aiguier, 13274 Marseilles, Cedex 2, France

William J. Davis, The Thimann Laboratories, University of California, Santa Cruz, California 95060

John S. Edwards, Department of Zoology, University of Washington, Seattle, Washington 98105

William H. Evoy, Department of Biology, University of Miami, Coral Gables, Florida 33124

Ernst Florey, Fachbereich Biologie, Universitat Konstanz, D775 Konstanz, Germany

Charles R. Fourtner, Division of Biology, State University of New York, Buffalo, New York 14214

Raymon M. Glantz, Department of Biology, Rice University, Houston, Texas 77001

William H. Gordon, Department of Zoology, University of Texas, Austin, Texas 78712

Richard Hirsh, Department of Psychology, McGill University, 1205 McGregor, Montreal H3A 1B1, Quebec, Canada

G. Adrian Horridge, Department of Behavioural Biology, Research School of Biological Sciences, The Australian National University, P.O. Box 475, Canberra, A.C.T. 2601, Australia

Graham Hoyle, Department of Biology, University of Oregon, Eugene, Oregon 97403

Kazuo Ikeda, Division of Neurosciences, City of Hope National Medical Center, Duarte, California 91010

Donald Kennedy, Department of Biology, Stanford University, Stanford, California 94305. Present address: Office of the Commissioner, Food and Drug Administration, 5600 Fishers Lane, Rockville, Maryland

Franklin B. Krasne, Department of Psychology, University of California, Los Angeles, California 90024

James L. Larimer, Department of Zoology, University of Texas, Austin, Texas 78712

R. B. Levine, Department of Biological Sciences, State University of New York, Albany, New York 12222

S. G. Matsumoto, Department of Biological Sciences, State University of New York, Albany, New York 12222

De Forest Mellon, Jr., Department of Biology, University of Virginia, Charlottesville, Virginia 22903

Peter J. Mill, Department of Pure and Applied Zoology, University of Leeds, Leeds LS2 9JT, England

Rodney K. Murphey, Department of Biological Sciences, State University of New York, Albany, New York 12222

Michael O'Shea, Department of Zoology, University of California, Berkeley, California 94720. Present address: Department of Biological Sciences, University of Southern California, Los Angeles, California 90007.

Keir G. Pearson, Department of Physiology, University of Alberta, Edmonton T6G 2E1, Alberta, Canada

C. Hugh Fraser Rowell, Department of Zoology, University of California, Berkeley, California 94720

David C. Sandeman, Department of Neurobiology, Research School of Biological Sciences, Australian National University, Canberra, A.C.T., Australia

Allen I. Selverston, Department of Biology, University of California, San Diego, La Jolla, California 92093

Paul S. G. Stein, Department of Biology, Washington University, St. Louis, Missouri 63130

Peter N. R. Usherwood, Department of Zoology, University of Nottingham, University Park, Nottingham NG7 2RD, England

Talbot H. Waterman, Department of Biology, Yale University, New Haven, Connecticut 06520

Jeffrey J. Wine, Department of Psychology, Stanford University, Stanford, California 94305

Robert S. Zucker, Department of Physiology-Anatomy, University of California, Berkeley, California 94720

Additional Attendees of the Meeting

Professor and Mrs. C. A. G. Wiersma, Department of Biology, California Institute of Technology, Pasadena, California 91109

Joan Roach, Department of Biology, California Institute of Technology, Pasadena, California 91109

Brian Mulloney, Department of Zoology, University of California, Davis, California 95616

Felix Strumwasser, Department of Biology, California Institute of Technology, Pasadena, California 91109

Preface

Identified Neurons and Behavior of Arthropods presents for the larger audience the papers delivered at a symposium of the same title. I organized this symposium so that a few of the many who owe him a great scientific debt could honor Professor C. A. G. (Kees) Wiersma upon his attaining the age of 70 and retiring from the California Institute of Technology.

Every one of the participants publicly acknowledged his debt to Kees Wiersma, but in a sense there was no need to do so, because the research reported spoke for itself. Seldom in a rapidly developing branch of modern science has all of the recent progress so clearly stemmed from the pioneering work of a single figure. But in this subject, the role of identified nerve cells in determining behavior, Wiersma stood virtually alone for 30 years. He it was who first showed that individual nerve cells are recognizable and functionally important and have ''personalities'' of their own.

Eventually the message caught on, and now there is a veritable floodtide of participants in the field, which amounts to nothing less than the cellular analysis of behavior, or neuroethology. Professor Wiersma confined his attention to crustaceans, but his approaches are now being applied also to insects, mollusks, and annelids. To cover all of those classes would have been quite impractical. But the ''crunchies,'' insects and crustaceans, have much in common, including possibly a common ancestor. By leaving out the ''squishies,'' we may have come close to putting together an almost complete state-of-the-art statement on Arthropoda, the phylum that, given man's continuing intransigence, may eventually inherit the earth.

The sequence in Wiersma's research was first a study of motor neurons, the contractions they cause, and the related peripheral synaptic mechanisms. Next, he turned his attention to interneurons and their roles. Finally, he worked, and is still working, on integration of sensory input, especially visual input. This was the path we charted in the conference. For some, the logic of procedure would be reversed; they prefer to start with sensory input and end up with motor output and behavior. For others, the central integrative events are where it's at; for them sensory input is no more than a routine coding process and motor output something that, like muscle itself, can be taken for granted. There is, of course, no ''right'' place to begin, since all are parts of an integrated whole.

For me, muscle has always seemed the starting point rather than the end. Contractility is what distinguishes animals from other forms of life. Nervous sys-

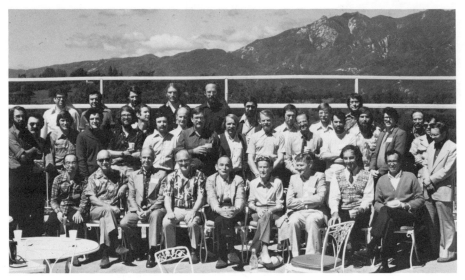

Back row: Hirsh, Fourtner, Bush, Davis, Mulloney, Wine, Burrows, Bentley, Mellon.

Middle row: Evoy, Selverston, Pearson, Clarac, Fraser-Rowell, Atwood, Stein, Mill, Larimer, Murphey, Edwards, Krasne, Usherwood, Strumwasser, Zucker, Glantz, Arechiga, Bittner.

Seated: Ikeda, Bullock, Waterman, Hoyle, Wiersma, Mrs. Wiersma, Florey, Horridge, Kennedy.

tems are there to control and coordinate contractility. The rest is secondary, even though it did, indirectly, produce the mind of man. I know that Kees takes a similar view, so it seemed appropriate in honoring his life's work to follow his own strategy. But the participants are men of vision too, and much of their work does not fall into any simple sequence. Accordingly, while keeping roughly to the original sequence as presented, I have reordered the material somewhat, to make what seems to me the most intellectually reasonable flow. It will be obvious, however, that there is no beginning and no end to the elements involved in determining behavior. The reader may choose to start at any point. From that spot he may progress in circular fashion, either forward (counterclockwise) or backward (clockwise). However, he will not be well advised to dip at random.

Acknowledgments

Financial support for the symposium was generously provided by Grant BMS 75-20538 from the National Science Foundation. Other support was provided by Plenum Press, the California Institute of Technology, The University of Oregon, and a donor who wishes to remain anonymous.

G. Hoyle
Eugene, Oregon

Contents

PART 2
Roles of Interneurons in Behavior

PART 3
Coding and Integration of Sensory Input

Kees Wiersma: An Appreciation

Graham Hoyle

The symposium was held to honor Professor C. A. G. Wiersma, known to most of us as Kees, upon his retirement from the California Institute of Technology, after attaining the age of ultimate wisdom.

I have had the good fortune to share a laboratory bench with him and to enjoy the fruits of many discussions, over a period of more than 20 years. When I met him for the first time, he already seemed like an old acquaintance. This can be the case when a younger scientist meets a peer whose publications are a part of his life and especially so when he has experimentally been asking similar questions.

But such first contacts can be bitterly disappointing. The idol may be aloof, cold, distant, disdainful, distracted, overworked, or just plain ornery. Professor Wiersma was none of these. Instead, I found him charming, warm, interested, attentive, involved, even though he had to put up with a noisy baby in his home for a couple of weeks. Over the years he has changed in none of these respects.

He started his research in 1926, as a student of Jordan in Utrecht after graduating from Leiden. From that time on he became dedicated to exploring physiologically the nervous system of crustaceans, a subject he has embellished for a lifetime. There have been many skirmishings into invertebrate neurobiological research that have been on a hit-and-run basis. These have been aimed at quick returns: a favorable preparation for studying a particular phenomenon or exploitation of a giant cell. Wiersma's extensive studies have been wholly oriented toward what makes crustaceans tick. The whole animal and its behavior have never been far from his mind. In an era when all the plaudits have been bestowed upon ultimate exponents of reductionism, Wiersma has kept returning to the animal itself. It must often have seemed to him that his work was but little appreciated by his contemporaries. Perhaps they were right to want to understand cellular mechanisms first. But Kees may have realized that his time would eventually come, and that time is now very clearly here.

First, he explored peripheral nerves, then neuromuscular transmission, but above all the questions that he addressed were concerned with the way the individual nerve cells of an animal's nervous system operate to achieve behavior. This is the subject that is of greatest interest to a growing band of young, vigorous investigators. Their research forms the emerging discipline of neuroethology.

1

Any one of the many mechanisms Wiersma uncovered might have attracted a biophysical reductionist for a lifetime. But his holism perpetually brought him back to thinking about some other, larger, aspect of his subjects. He has thus illuminated our understanding of nerve cells, neuromuscular transmission, the neural control of muscle, interneuron properties, the functional roles of interneurons, sensory physiology, aspects of visual memory and overt behavior: in other words, the whole spectrum of neuroethology. As much as any other person in the history of behavioral physiology, he has "put it all together."

Arthropods first commanded the attention of physiologists interested in how nervous systems control behavior following a chance discovery. Richet (1879) found that as he gradually increased the strength of faradic electrical stimulus applied to a crayfish claw closer muscle, there came a point where the tension fell abruptly. He considered, correctly, that the fall was due to the threshold for inhibitory nerve action having been exceeded. The phenomenon was subsequently studied by many physiologists, notably the early giant of electrophysiology, Biedermann (1889). He discovered that the antagonist of the claw closer, the opener, can also be inhibited. A need for peripheral inhibition was first shown by Hoffmann (1914), who discovered that a common excitatory nerve supplies the opener and stretcher, so that one must be inhibited if independent contraction of the other is to be achieved.

The control processes should have become much clearer after the young genius Keith Lucas (1907, 1917) deduced that there are separate slow and fast excitatory mechanisms. Wiersma first came into the picture with his paper (Wiersma, 1933) that emphasized the importance of frequency of motor nerve impulses in determining the contraction pattern. The crustacean neuromuscular apparatus at this time also attracted the attention of two other brilliant young men, Carl Pantin (1934) and Bernard Katz (1936). Both emphasized the neuromuscular junction as the site responsible for the peculiar features of integration. Each was thinking in terms of there being an all-or-none law for muscle. Thus the properties of facilitation and summation would need to be explained by *recruitment* of muscle fibers on a statistical basis. The influence of concepts relevant to the vertebrates was paramount in the design of their experiments and interpretation of their results—and they were wrong. What is surprising about the approaches of these distinguished authors was that they did not seem to be able to make speculations in what has turned out to be the right direction. The key to unlocking the mystery of arthropod nerve–muscle systems was a willingness to accept the possibility of graded contraction. This followed logically from polyneuronal innervation and distributed, or multiple, nerve terminals. Both can be detected easily in almost any large crustacean after a few minutes of soaking in methylene blue. Indeed, this had been demonstrated by a number of histologists, and it was even better substantiated for insects. But in neither class of animal was the significance of these observations appreciated. Nor did the authors at any time refer to the published histological data.

Understanding these mechanisms, as significantly different from anything seen up to that time in vertebrates, can clearly be attributed to Wiersma's research. In the

1933 paper he introduced the technique of splitting the nerve bundle. By 1936, in collaboration with his lifetime colleague at Caltech, Anthony van Harreveld, he had refined the method to the point where he was dealing with undoubted single axons. The single fast and slow axons that excite the crayfish claw closer were demonstrated unequivocally in 1936 by van Harreveld and Wiersma (1936). Preparation of the inhibitory axon followed in 1937 (van Harreveld and Wiersma, 1937). Shortly thereafter, in an extremely important paper that seems never to be quoted, Wiersma and van Harreveld (1938b) concluded that both slow and fast axon contractions occur in the same muscle fibers. This paper was published in *Physiological Zoology*. Then as now the subject of zoology was deemed a not quite respectable one by physiologists and biophysicists. Physiological zoology was something you did as a first project, or if you were not quite up to doing cellular biophysics. It never occurred to the majority of physiologists that comparative physiology should serve routinely as the testing ground for all supposed "general" theories. One is reminded of Hallowell Davis's famous quote: "We're down on what we're not up on." The impact of what was truly a major blow, the destruction of one of the few cherished "laws" of physiology, was thereby blunted.

A glance at any modern medical school textbook shows that muscle physiology still suffers from a stubborn reluctance to accept that there is no such thing as an all-or-none phenomenon in physiology.

Wiersma's warning that it is very important to be comparative is also constantly disregarded by the establishment figures of biophysics. Too often they rush to make a generalization that is based on work on a single tissue of but a single species. It is very easy for the "exception ferrets," as Don Kennedy has wittily termed the cautious lovers of diversity, to upset such generalizations—because it seems the latter are almost always produced after the first discovery without recourse to the time-consuming search demanded by the comparative approach.

We owe so much of the expansion of our understanding of the arthropod effector system to Wiersma's insistence on the value of "vergleichende"—comparative—physiology. When I went to work with him at Caltech in 1956, I had just completed a series of studies on neuromuscular transmission and neural control of contraction in the locust. These were the first arthropod studies correlating tension development with intracellularly recorded membrane events of slow and fast axon excitation. Although Ed Furshpan as a Ph.D. student had introduced intracellular electrodes into Wiersma's laboratory, Kees didn't feel happy about working with them. Tension studies correlated with intracellular observations needed to be made during fast and slow axon excitation for a crustacean, and I was hot to "do" them. In the first conversation I had with Professor Wiersma about the proposed collaborative research in the fall of 1956, I gave him the impression, which was true, that I believed that any crustacean preparation would do and that it might just as well be the crayfish claw. This was my first confrontation with a dyed-in-the-wool comparative physiologist, and I got a strong reprimand. "If we only work on the crayfish, you will end up with a distorted and probably incorrect impression as to how it's really done," he said. "We should look at crayfish, certainly, but in the winter first, then again in the spring, when they function differently. Meantime, we should look at the spiny lobster, a crab or two, especially *Blepharipoda,* because that shows the 'paradox'—a lack of correlation between the magnitudes of slow and fast axon electrical events and tension development reported in the claw closer of *Blepharipoda''* (Wiersma and van Harreveld, 1938*b*).

This is exactly what we did, and the experience was a revelation to me. The same species of crayfish was indeed different in the spring, for in an identical saline the ipsp's were depolarizing rather than hyperpolarizing as they had been in the fall. Also, the extents of facilitation required to reach maximum epsp amplitudes were greater in the spring animals.

As we penetrated more and more muscle fibers in each muscle we examined, we became aware of a rich variety of synaptic activity, of which there had been little hint either from the extracellular work or from the itnracellular work of Fatt and Katz (1953*a*,*b*,*c*) on the *Carcinus* closer. The complexity of the detailed patterns of response in different muscle fibers of any given muscle of a particular species astounded both of us. It soon became clear also that each muscle is a law unto itself, both within a single animal and between animals. Until then neuromuscular physiologists had taken it for granted that the fiber composition of muscles was homogeneous. There had long been an assumption, following the suggestion of Katz (1936), that there were differences in facilitation rate at individual junctions, and since Wiersma and I found such differences we were happy to accept them as a primary basis for individual and species differences. We did indeed examine *Blepharipoda,* but our preliminary studies with intracellular electrodes merely confirmed that there was a paradox. We could not explain it. The paradox was eventually explained away by Harold Atwood, working in my laboratory, when he found a deep bundle of slow muscle fibers innervated only by the slow axon (Atwood and Hoyle, 1965).

Seeds of doubt about muscle homogeneity had been sown by Professor Wiersma, and soon Harold Atwood and I were to start a long series of investigations, that are still under way, examining crustacean muscles on a fiber by fiber basis. We now know that there are extraordinary differences between fibers in all measurable parameters, both biophysical and ultrastructural. The permutations are such as to defy any simple classification. The locations of different types of fiber within a muscle are not random, and once a given muscle has been thoroughly examined it is usually possible to locate precisely fibers of each type. Only quite recently have these studies been extended to insects, but already patterns as complex as those found in crustaceans are turning up.

The full significance of all this in adaptive radiation of behavior can scarcely be grasped yet, but is certainly profound. The technical breakthrough of studying the physiological roles of single neurons, introduced by Wiersma, was the starting point for these discoveries.

From efferent axons, Wiersma then moved on to interneurons of the cord and connectives. Suffice it to say that Wiersma's success in this work opened up the science of neuroethology. It was important conceptually as well as technically.

There had been no hint of the underlying simplicity, and therefore single-unit analyzability for arthropods, in any of the previous work on arthropod or indeed any other nervous systems. Everyone had followed the vertebrate tradition of assuming multiple repetition of neural elements, in which the individual neuron is not considered to be significant in determining behavior. The nervous system was still a great mystery box with interpretation colored by shades of vitalism and reticular theory. Wiersma singlehandedly divested arthropod nervous system studies of these confused concepts. He thereby paved the way for a deterministic approach, raising hopes for a full analysis of the cellular bases of behavior. He endowed single neurons not just with identities, but with personalities, individual characteristics by which they may be recognized and their roles in determining behavior examined.

Indirectly, Wiersma's successes have greatly influenced workers on vertebrate nervous systems, although, alas, they are hardly conscious of the debt they owe him. Our symposium will follow in his footsteps. We shall deal with some of the specific anatomical, pharmacological, biophysical, and developmental questions that relate to the special features of arthropod neurons and synapses. But our primary goal, as has been Professor Wiersma's, will be the exhilarating question: How do the nerve cells generate and control behavior?

Career Résumé

WIERSMA, CORNELIS ADRIANUS GERRIT (KEES—affectionately)

Born Naaldwyk, Holland, October 10. 1905: Married 1932.

B.S., Leiden, 1926; M.S., Utrecht, 1929; Ph.D. (comparative physiology), 1933; Dondersfonds Fellow, Cambridge, 1930–1931; Honarary D.Sc., Erasmus University, Rotterdam, November 1976.

Assistant Professor, Comparative Physiology, Utrecht, 1929–1931; Assistant Professor, Medical Physiology, 1932–1934; Assistant Professor, Biology, California Institute Technology, 1934–1937; Associate Professor, 1937–1947; Professor, 1947–1976; Guggenheim Memorial Fellow, 1957; Visiting Professor, Cambridge, 1957–1958.

Member: American Physiological Society; Society for Experimental Biology and Medicine; Society of General Physiology; Corresponding Member Royal Netherlands Academy of Science; Netherlands Royal Zoological Society; IBRO; Society for Neurosciences; AAAS; Society of General Physiology; Sigma Xi.

Part 1

Neural Control of Skeletal Muscle

Crustacean Neuromuscular Systems: Past, Present, and Future

Harold L. Atwood

Past

> We were the first that ever burst
> Into that silent sea.*

Among the early explorers of invertebrate nervous systems, C. A. G. Wiersma and his collaborators made some of the most significant discoveries in their studies on crustacean neuromuscular systems. Their isolation and characterization of the properties of individual excitor and inhibitor axons (reviewed by Wiersma, 1961a) introduced a concept which was later extended to interneurons (INs) and which is still dominant today: individual neurons have distinct or even unique properties and personalities and play well-specified roles in the behavior of the organism. Indeed, it may be that the same concept will be found to apply in some degree to vertebrate nervous systems as well (Bullock, 1975). The more we learn about vertebrate motor neurons (MNs) and interneurons INs, the more individuality they acquire. The Mauthner cells of lower vertebrates are as well known as many identified invertebrate INs, and who today would claim that motor units within a vertebrate muscle or the MNs supplying them (Burke et al., 1971, 1974) are all alike?

Crustaceans and other arthropods get by in life with far fewer neurons than the average vertebrate. Since many arthropods show a complexity of behavior equal or even superior to that of many lower vertebrates, it follows that each arthropod neuron, and even each synapse, contributes more on the average to total function than in lower vertebrates. This is strikingly apparent in crustacean neuromuscular systems, where the number of efferent neurons devoted to muscular control is very small but where a compensatory elaboration of synaptic and postsynaptic control mechanisms has been developed.

Significant themes which have emerged from past work on crustacean neuromuscular systems (Fig. 1) are as follows:

1. Elaboration of antagonistic *excitatory* and *inhibitory* synaptic mechanisms in the muscle itself.

*Samuel Taylor Coleridge, *The Rime of the Ancient Mariner* (1798).

Harold L. Atwood • Department of Zoology, University of Toronto, Toronto M5S 1A1, Ontario, Canada.

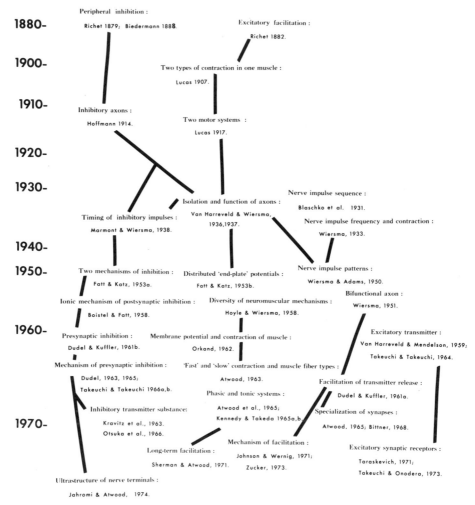

Fig. 1. A short history of work on crustacean neuromuscular systems, showing some of the "main sequence" studies. Inhibitory mechanisms are emphasized on the left-hand side of the chart; excitatory systems and pattern sensitivity of transmission are on the right-hand side.

2. Diversification and specialization of the synapses of individual axons, allowing differential recruitment of postsynaptic elements as well as time-dependent and impulse-pattern-dependent properties of the system.

3. Diversification and specialization of the postsynaptic elements (muscle fibers), giving rise to a final output (muscle response) which is highly dependent on postsynaptic filtering and transformation.

4. Biochemical specialization of individual efferent neurons to provide the necessary transmitter chemicals in appropriate amounts at the peripheral synapses.

Excitatory and Inhibitory Systems

The presence of excitatory and inhibitory systems in crustacean muscles was postulated by several of the early workers (Fig. 1). The idea of two types of excitatory systems within a single muscle was introduced by Lucas (1907, 1917), and the sensitivity of crustacean muscle to incoming impulse patterns was shown by Blaschko *et al.* (1931), who observed that a single extra stimulus introduced into a regular train could trigger a large, sustained increase in muscle tension.

However, all these early studies were done with incomplete isolation of the efferent neurons. It was not until van Harreveld and Wiersma (1936, 1937, 1939) isolated and stimulated individual neurons in crustacean limb nerves that the identities and unique properties of the various excitors and inhibitors could be unambiguously established.

In subsequent physiological work, the focus of attention was shifted from input–output relationships of entire muscles obtained by stimulating the efferent axons to more precise examination of responses of individual postsynaptic elements, and finally to even more precise studies on individual synapses. Concurrently, advances in biochemical, pharmacological, and ultrastructural studies have been made. With each advance in precision of observation, some of the perplexing features arising from earlier studies have been cleared up.

Inhibitory Neurons

The work on inhibitory neurons provides an excellent illustration of the progressive clarification of a confusing system. At present, the cumulative studies on crustacean peripheral inhibitory neurons provide a standard against which work on other neuronal systems can be measured. However, the emergence of this happy situation followed a convoluted and prolonged gestation.

A dual effect of inhibition on crustacean muscles was observed by Marmont and Wiersma (1938): excitatory muscle potentials were drastically reduced in amplitude by inhibitory impulses timed to precede them, but not by impulses arriving late—yet muscle tension was inhibited in both cases. Studies on single muscle fibers with microelectrodes (Fatt and Katz, 1953a) confirmed the timing effect and led to the proposal that the inhibitory transmitter substance could produce two postsynaptic effects: (1) an increased muscle membrane conductance for an ion with an equilibrium potential near the resting membrane potential and (2) a competitive (curarelike) blockade of postsynaptic receptors for the excitatory transmitter substance, seen only with appropriate timing of inhibitory impulses.

Inhibitory increase of muscle membrane chloride conductance was soon shown by Boistel and Fatt (1958), and subsequent work (e.g., Takeuchi and Takeuchi, 1965, 1967, 1969, 1971a,b) has characterized the inhibitory postsynaptic receptors and their ionophores. However, the "curarelike" action of the inhibitory transmitter was illusory, for Dudel and Kuffler (1961a,b,c) showed that correct timing of inhibitory impulses exerted a *presynaptic* effect which reduced the output of the excitatory synaptic transmitter substance.

A morphological basis for presynaptic inhibition has since been established by electron microscopy (Atwood and Jones, 1967; Atwood and Morin, 1970; Jahromi and Atwood, 1974). The ionic mechanism of presynaptic inhibition, involving increased chloride conductance of the presynaptic nerve terminal membrane and consequent depression of the nerve terminal action potential and evoked transmitter release, was worked out by Dudel (1963, 1965a) and by Takeuchi and Takeuchi (1966a,b).

Characterization of the inhibitory transmitter substance as probably γ-aminobutyric acid (GABA) was accomplished after considerable controversy (e.g., Florey and Hoyle, 1961; Florey and Chapman, 1961) through refined biochemical analyses of isolated inhibitory neurons (Kravitz et al., 1963a,b), and by the demonstration of its release from the inhibitory neurons during impulse activity (Otsuka et al., 1966). Further work (e.g., Kravitz et al., 1967) has shown that the biochemical differences between inhibitory and excitatory neurons are attributable to the presence of the enzyme glutamate decarboxylase (which forms GABA) in the former. It is likely that activation or repression of a single gene is sufficient to produce differentiation of excitatory and inhibitory neurons. The problem now becomes a developmental one.

"Fast" and "Slow" Systems

Once the technique of isolating single axons had been developed, it was possible to investigate the responses of muscles to stimulation of individual motor axons. Muscles receiving two motor axons generally showed characteristic differences in speed of response to stimulation of these axons; the axon eliciting the more rapid response was termed the "fast" axon and its partner the "slow" axon. The contractions and excitatory potentials of many different muscles were investigated by Wiersma and his collaborators (reviewed by Wiersma, 1961a). Much diversity was apparent, which was further emphasized by recordings with intracellular electrodes (Hoyle and Wiersma, 1958a,b,c).

Since staining of crustacean muscles with methylene blue had shown parallel branching and distribution of the intramuscular axons, it was originally concluded that each muscle fiber could generate both "fast" and "slow" responses. Moreover, in some muscles the electrical responses evoked by the "fast" axon are larger than those produced by the "slow" axon, but whole muscle tension is less (Wiersma and van Harreveld, 1938a; Hoyle and Wiersma, 1958c). These observations led to the conclusion that "fast" and "slow" neurotransmitters influence excitation–contraction coupling by a mechanism not involving changes in muscle fiber membrane potential.

Refinement of technique enabled Orkand (1962a) to demonstrate that tension in crayfish muscle fibers is directly related to membrane potential. It was then shown that nerve-evoked contractions of single crustacean muscle fibers are generally explainable by changes in membrane potential and that they can be abolished by hyperpolarization while the nerve is still active (Atwood *et al.*, 1965). The latter observation made it clear that the excitatory transmitter cannot produce tension when the muscle fiber membrane potential is more negative than the excitation–contraction coupling threshold.

As work on single muscle fibers continued, it soon became apparent that even within a single muscle the fibers can differ a great deal in their structural, electrical, and mechanical properties (Atwood, 1963; Dorai Raj, 1964; Atwood *et al.*, 1965), Even when electrical responsiveness is similar in two fibers, they may differ in rate of tension development (Fig. 2). In general, the faster-acting muscle fibers tend to have greater electrical responsiveness and shorter sarcomeres (Fig. 2), but the correlation is a loose one when considered over a large sample of different muscles. In swimming muscles of the crab *Portunus*, fibers of different colors have different time courses of contraction in spite of similarity of the sarcomere lengths (Hoyle, 1973). Significant biochemical differences related to mitochondrial content seem to play an important role in this case. Other biochemical differences relating to muscle performance have been described by Hajek *et al.* (1973). Clearly, more work is needed to define the relative importance of biochemical and structural features in determining performance of different crustacean muscles.

Diversity of muscle fiber properties is a key factor in "fast" and "slow" responses. In some of the muscles receiving dual motor supply, there is a differential innervation of the faster-acting, more electrically excitable fibers and the slower-acting, less electrically excitable fibers by the two axons. The "fast" axon tends to innervate the former more heavily, and the "slow" axon supplies the latter more richly, while the majority of muscle fibers get substantial innervation from both axons (Atwood, 1963, 1965). The characteristic differences in "fast" and "slow" mechanical responses seen at low frequencies of stimulation are largely a consequence of the properties of the responding postsynaptic elements; both the electrical and the intrinsic tension-generating features of the muscle fibers play their part.

Muscles which contain exclusively fast-acting or slow-acting fibers rather than a mixture were found by Abbott and Parnas (1965), Kennedy and Takeda (1965*a,b*), and others. It is apparent that much of the diversity seen among crustacean muscles is attributable to postsynaptic properties (Atwood, 1973*b*).

Synaptic Diversity

Crustacean neuromuscular systems are very sensitive to the temporal sequence of nerve impulses (Wiersma and Adams, 1950; Wiersma, 1951; Ripley and Wiersma, 1953). Part of the sensitivity to impulse sequence is attributable to the striking facilitation of transmitter release at the nerve terminals (Dudel and Kuffler, 1961*b*).

The work of Hoyle and Wiersma (1958*a*) provided a strong indication that synapses of both "fast" and "slow" axons have a wide range of response to

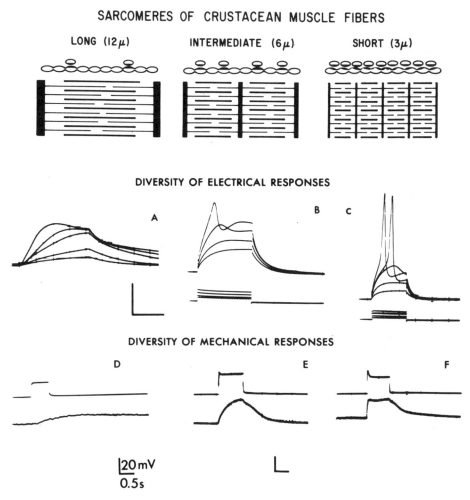

Fig. 2. Diversity of structure, membrane electrical response, and mechanical response in crustacean muscle fibers. Structural diagrams show variation in sarcomere and myofilament lengths and associated differences in the transverse tubular system. Fibers with short sarcomeres have closer spacing of transverse tubules. Electrical responses (A,B,C) are from fibers in the opener muscle of the crab *Chionoecetes* (Atwood, 1965), showing examples of (A) minimal electrical excitability (delayed rectification), (B) graded membrane response, and (C) spike at a discrete threshold. Calibrations: Vertical, 20 mV; horizontal, 400 msec (A), 200 msec (B), 100 msec (C). Mechanical responses (D,E,F, lower traces) are from crab (D) and lobster (E,F) fibers which did not generate electrically excited responses except for a slight amount of rectification (upper traces). Although membrane responses are similar, the tension responses differ for the three fibers. In general, the slower tension responses are produced by fibers with longer sarcomere lengths.

impulse patterns: facilitation and depression are both demonstrable, but the extent of each varies with the axon being stimulated and with intramuscular location. Muscles supplied by a single axon often show a wide range in the amplitude and facilitation properties of excitatory postsynaptic potentials (epsp's) (Fig. 3), attributable to transmitter-releasing properties of the nerve terminals (Atwood, 1967b; Bittner, 1968).

Some of the differences in facilitation between "fast" and "slow" axon terminals to the same muscle fiber have been linked to a faster rate of decay of facilitation in the "fast" axon (Linder, 1973). The mechanisms underlying the variation in facilitation at different terminals are not yet resolved.

Excitatory Transmitter

In crustacean limb muscles, the work of van Harreveld and Mendelson (1959) and of Takeuchi and Takeuchi (1965) has led to the establishment of glutamate as the prime candidate for the excitatory neurotransmitter. Work on the glutamate

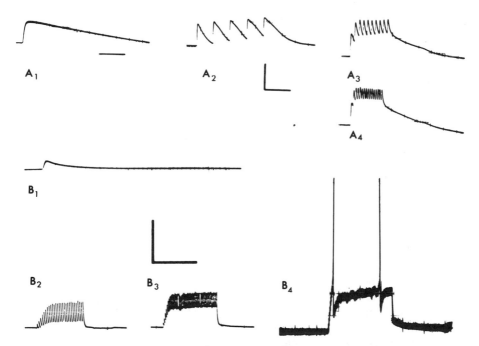

Fig. 3 Epsp's evoked by a single axon in slow-acting (A) and fast-acting (B) muscle fibers of the opener muscle of the crab *Chionoecetes* (Atwood, 1965). The records show a large, poorly facilitating epsp (A) evoked at frequencies of 1 Hz (A_1), 1.4 Hz (A_2), 6 Hz (A_3), and 12 Hz (A_4) and a small, highly facilitating epsp (B) evoked at 1 Hz (B_1), 25 Hz (B_2), 50 Hz (B_3), and 75 Hz (B_4). In B_4, large spikes (accompanied by twitches) are generated in addition to epsp's. Membrane rectification with maintained depolarization contributes to decline in epsp amplitude at higher frequencies in both fibers. Calibrations: vertical, 20 mV; horizontal, 100 msec (A_1), 40 msec (B_1), 1 sec (A_2–A_4, B_2–B_4).

receptors has been carried out by Taraskevich (1971, 1975), Takeuchi and Onodera (1973), Onodera and Takeuchi (1975), and Dudel (1975a,b). It appears that the ionic mechanism of the glutamate response can vary from place to place within the muscle but is mainly sodium dependent.

Acetylcholine has recently been shown to be a probable neurotransmitter in certain crustacean stomach muscles (Marder, 1974).

Present

clearing
their trail of single reason
through a land where geometries are multiple.*

Crustacean neuromuscular systems continue to offer fruitful ground for exploration to those interested in the multiple geometries of the nervous system. Many features of synaptic interaction and synaptic performance seen in central nervous systems appear in simplified and more accessible form in crustacean muscles, where the number of neurons is restricted to a manageable few. The synaptic personalities of individual neurons can be understood and followed through time, thereby providing an opportunity to discover some of the rules which determine the organization, physiological performance, and plasticity of neuronal networks.

Although the properties of crustacean muscle fibers, fruitfully investigated in the past, continue to be of interest (especially in studies dealing with development and trophic effects), synapses have recently taken over center stage.

Receptor kinetics at the synapse have recently been analyzed (e.g. Dudel, 1975a,b), as well as ionic mechanisms (e.g., Takeuchi and Onodera, 1973) and transmitter biochemistry (e.g., Marder, 1974). I will not deal with these aspects here (but see Atwood, 1976). Instead, I will explore the present status of the more "classical" work originating largely from studies by Wiersma and his collaborators, which is aimed at understanding the organization, input–output relationships, and plasticity of crustacean neuromuscular systems.

Organization: Matching

New functionally important features of the organization and matching of pre- and postsynaptic elements in crustacean muscles continue to emerge. The matching of "fast" and "slow" axons with fast-acting and slow-acting muscle fibers, translated functionally into "fast" and "slow" contractions, has already been noted (Fig. 3). In muscles with a single motor axon, another matching effect has been encountered: synapses with high initial output tend to occur on slower-acting muscle fibers, while those with a low initial output and good facilitation (Fig. 3) tend to occur on faster-acting muscle fibers (Atwood, 1965; Sherman and Atwood, 1972). Functionally, this means that the muscle will increase its speed of response at higher

*Margaret Atwood, *The Surveyors* (1968).

impulse frequencies, not only because electrical events in each muscle fiber are larger and faster but also because faster-acting fibers will be recruited (Atwood, 1974).

Two hypotheses to explain matching of pre- and postsynaptic elements are currently available. One of these (Frank, 1973) ascribes matching to the postsynaptic elements. According to this view, synapses are modified according to instructions from the muscle fiber, which is predetermined in its properties. A second hypothesis (Atwood, 1973) implicates the nerve terminals as the primary agents and postulates that the muscle fibers are influenced in their development according to the time at which they become innervated. This view is based on observations of synapses in regenerating limbs, which indicate a temporal sequence of appearance of the different synapses (Govind et al., 1973), coupled with the observation that muscle fibers change morphologically during development and regeneration (Govind et al., 1974). Recent work by Velez and Wyman (1976a,b) on the crayfish slow flexor muscles also supports a neural influence in matching of muscle fibers and synapses. More work will be necessary to decide between the two hypotheses.

Another type of matching has been described for excitatory and inhibitory synapses on the same muscle fiber (Atwood and Bittner, 1971; Wiens and Atwood, 1975). Muscle fibers supplied by excitatory synapses with large initial transmitter output also receive inhibitory synapses with similar properties. Functionally, this allows the inhibitory system to suppress the excitatory effects at a low frequency in some fibers and at a higher frequency in others (Fig. 4).

Organization: Inhibitory Synapses

The arrangement of inhibitory synapses relative to excitatory nerve terminals has turned out to be highly variable, both between muscles and within them.

Some muscles (e.g., those of the crayfish abdomen) do not seem to have any presynaptic inhibition (Kennedy and Evoy, 1966). Among limb muscles, many have it, but some do not (Gainer et al., 1967). The opener and stretcher muscles, with one excitatory axon, often show presynaptic inhibition, especially those parts supplied heavily by innervation from the "slow" axon (Atwood, 1965; Rathmayer and Florey, 1974a,b; Hatt, 1974). It is not clear yet whether "fast" axon terminals receive inhibitory axoaxonal synapses; observations on relative insensitivity of "fast" contractions and electrical responses to inhibition suggest that they do not (Atwood et al., 1967).

Crab stretcher muscles receive a dual inhibitory supply, from a specific inhibitor and from the more widely distributed "common" inhibitor (Wiersma, 1961a). Recent studies of this muscle in several species have shown that both inhibitory axons can produce presynaptic inhibition in the same muscle (Wiens and Atwood, 1975) (Figs. 4 and 5). However, the relative importance of presynaptic inhibition seems to vary from species to species for each of the two axons. In the shore crab Grapsus presynaptic inhibition is strong for the specific inhibitor and weak for the

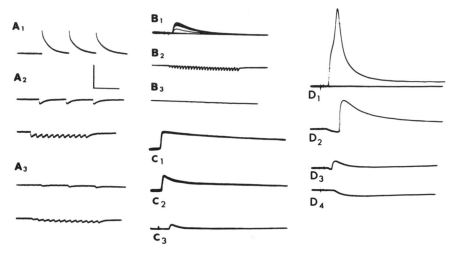

Fig. 4. Inhibition in the stretcher muscle *Grapsus* by specific (SI) and common (CI) inhibitory axons (Wiens and Atwood, 1975). In A, the epsp's of the excitor (E) axon (A_1) and ipsp's of the SI (A_2) and CI (A_3) axons are shown as recorded from a slow-acting muscle fiber; the ipsp's are evoked at frequencies of 1 Hz and 10 Hz. The SI axon produces a larger ipsp with less facilitation. In B, epsp's at 10 Hz (B_1) and ipsp's of the SI (B_2) and CI (B_3) axons at 10 Hz are shown for another muscle fiber with smaller initial epsp; CI's effect is barely detectable, and facilitation is evident in the ipsp of the SI axon, illustrating matching of facilitation between SI and E axon terminals. In C, attenuation of the epsp (C_1) by synchronous (C_2) and optimally timed (C_3) SI impulses illustrates the differences between effects due mainly to postsynaptic inhibition (C_2) and those due to both postsynaptic and presynaptic inhibition (C_3); the time course of the epsp is affected more than the amplitude in C_2, whereas both time course and amplitude are drastically affected in C_3. A further example of these differences is given in D for a fiber in which the epsp evokes a large, graded response (D_1). This is eliminated by an ipsp (D_4) timed to arrive 9 msec earlier (D_2). The epsp is further reduced (D_3) when the ipsp arrives 2 msec earlier than the epsp, corresponding to the optimal timing for presynaptic inhibition. In this fiber, postsynaptic inhibition eliminates the membrane-graded response, while presynaptic inhibition drastically reduces epsp amplitude. Calibrations: voltage, 5 mV (A,B), 20 mV (C), 10 mV (D); time, 1 sec (A, B_2, B_3), 20 msec (B_1, C), 10 msec (D).

common inhibitor, while in the spider crab *Hyas* it is strong for both axons (Wiens and Atwood, 1975) (Fig. 5).

At individual excitatory nerve endings, the presynaptic inhibition can be stronger for either of the two inhibitory axons, even though one of them is more effective over the muscle fiber as a whole (Fig. 5). The records of epsp attenuation obtained with intracellular microelectrodes represent a statistical outcome of variable inhibition at different nerve terminals produced by the two axons.

Additional insight into the physical relationships between inhibitory and excitatory nerve terminals has been generated by ultrastructural studies. Following the identification of axoaxonal synapses in the crayfish opener muscle (Atwood and Jones, 1967; Atwood and Morin, 1970) and further characterization of excitatory and inhibitory nerve endings by selective depletion of synaptic vesicles in 2,4-dinitrophenol (Atwood *et al.*, 1972), it became possible to cut serial sections of long

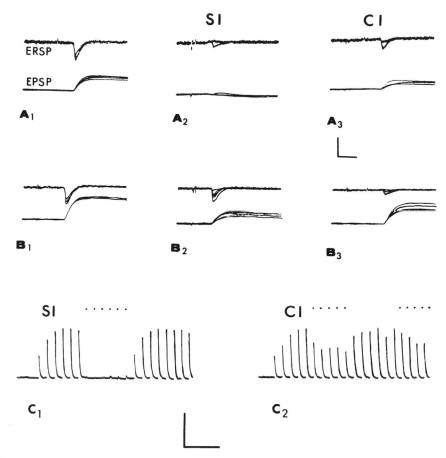

Fig. 5. Effects of SI and CI axons at single excitatory synapses of the same muscle fiber (A,B) and on facilitation of the epsp (C) in the crab *Hyas* (Wiens and Atwood, 1975). In A and B, records of epsp's are accompanied by records of externally recorded synaptic potentials (ersp's) at single synaptic sites. Optimally timed SI stimulation is more effective in reducing epsp amplitude than optimally timed CI stimulation in both A and B. In A, SI stimulation also reduces the ersp more than CI stimulation, but in B, CI's effect on the ersp's is stronger than SI's effect. In C, presynaptic inhibition by SI abolishes facilitation effects in the terminals of the excitatory axon; the facilitation of the epsp recommences when inhibition is turned off. Optimal CI stimulation produces a less complete, gradually developing attenuation of the epsp, with little effect on facilitation. Calibration: vertical, 0.4 mV (A,B, upper traces) and 4 mV (A,B, lower traces, and C); time, 20 msec (A,B) and 4 sec (C).

stretches of the terminal regions and to reconstruct, with some confidence, the excitatory and inhibitory synaptic endings (Jahromi and Atwood, 1974) (Figs. 6 and 7). From these reconstructions, it was possible to measure the sizes of the synapses, count them, and observe their locations.

Inhibitory axoaxonal synapses of the crayfish opener muscle generally occur much less frequently than inhibitory neuromuscular synapses. Many of the inhibitory axoaxonal synapses are stationed at branch points or narrow "bottlenecks" of the excitatory nerve terminals (Figs. 6 and 7). These regions are well known in other systems as points of low safety factor for impulse propagation (Parnas *et al.*, 1969; Parnas, 1972). Thus it seems likely that part of the presynaptic inhibitory effect may be brought about by blockade of impulse propagation into some of the terminal branches.

In some crab fibers, single impulses in the specific inhibitor can abolish transmitter release almost completely (Wiens and Atwood, 1975) (Fig. 5). Facilitatory effects in the excitatory nerve terminal also disappear; the epsp facilitates from its original "starting" amplitude when inhibition is relieved. This effect strongly suggests that electrical activity in excitatory nerve terminals that receive large inhibitory axon synapses is almost completely blocked by inhibition; effective blockade of this sort could be achieved most economically at branch points.

Recently, we have found that some of the inhibitory nerve branches are specialized for presynaptic inhibition, while others are devoted to postsynaptic inhibition (Atwood and Kwan, 1976) (Fig. 7iii). Thus not only do different inhibitory axons vary in pre- and postsynaptic effectiveness, but even within a single muscle fiber the different terminals of a single inhibitory axon can form rather different synaptic connections and become specialized to perform different functions.

Synaptic Diversity

In the past, the physiological diversity of crustacean motor axons and their synapses has been well emphasized. Although the underlying causes of synaptic diversity have yet to be clarified, relevant physiological and morphological evidence has accumulated from a number of recent studies.

Characteristically, many phasic axons generate relatively large (although fatigable) epsp's (Fig. 8). Individual synapses of these axons do not release large amounts of transmitter; quantal contents of 0.5–2 are typically seen at low frequencies of stimulation (Atwood and Johnston, 1968). In keeping with this finding, the contact areas of individual synapses, measured from serial sections cut for electron microscopy, are not different from those of "slow" or tonic axons (Fig. 8C). Sectioning for electron microscopy and probing with external microelectrodes reveal the presence of a large number of synapses on muscle fibers heavily innervated by phasic motor axons. Thus the large epsp's result from simultaneous activation of a comparatively large number of individual synapses.

The mechanisms responsible for variation in output of transmitter from different terminals of tonic motor axons like that of the crayfish opener muscle remain

---

Fig. 6. Axoaxonal synapses in the crayfish opener muscle. A large inhibitory (I) terminal forms two discrete axoaxonal contacts (AA) with a smaller excitatory (E) terminal. Neuromuscular synapses (both E and I) are indicated by arrows. In the enlargement, note that the synaptic vesicles of E and I terminals differ noticeably in size and shape. Scale mark: 1 μm.

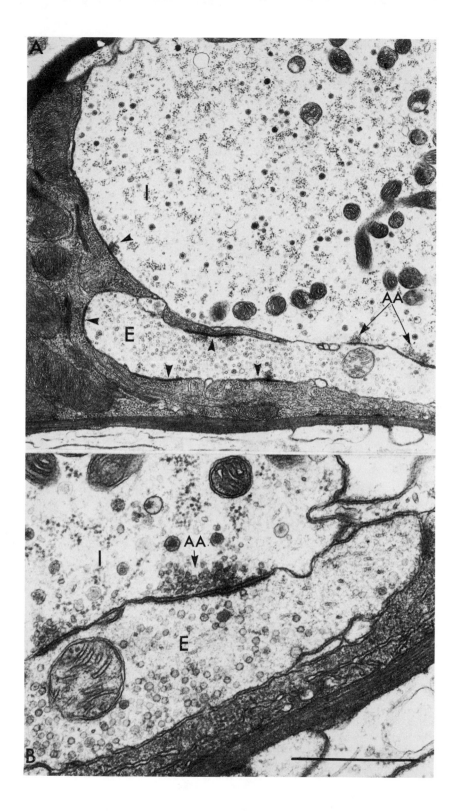

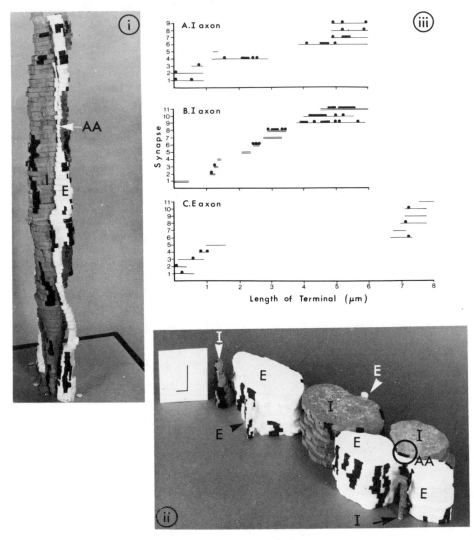

Fig. 7. Three-dimensional models of the excitatory and inhibitory nerve terminals of the crayfish opener muscle (Jahromi and Atwood, 1974). The excitatory (E) terminals are white, the inhibitory (I) terminals are gray, and the synapses are black. Axoaxonal synapses are shown on a bottleneck (i) and at a branch point (ii) of the excitatory innervation. Scale mark: 0.6 μm (vertical), 1 μm (horizontal). In (iii), synaptograms of E and I terminals based on serial sections (Atwood and Kwan, 1976) are presented to show number and distribution of synapses along three nerve terminals. Synaptogenic regions of an E axon terminal (C) and of two different I terminals running parallel in the same region (A,B) are illustrated. Single lines represent neuromuscular synapses; double lines, axoaxonal synapses; dots and bars on the lines, specialized presynaptic dense bodies (possible release points). The length of the lines indicates the length of the synapses. Note that the two inhibitory terminals are specialized for different modes of inhibitory transmission; the terminal shown in (A) has a preponderance of neuromuscular synapses, while that shown in (B) has mainly axoaxonal synapses. Dense bodies (putative release areas) of the I terminals are often relatively large compared to those of the E terminal.

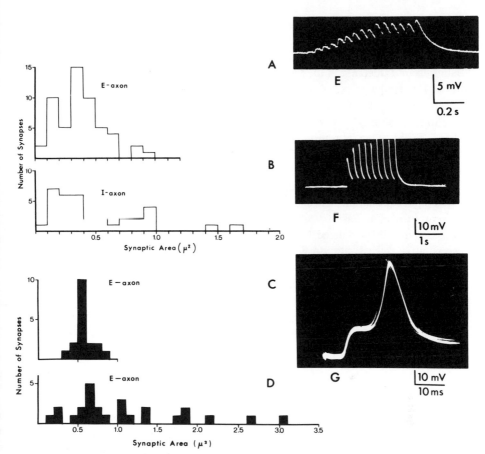

Fig. 8. Histograms to show size distributions for contact areas of synapses in excitatory (A) and inhibitory (B) terminals of crayfish opener muscle (Jahromi and Atwood, 1974), in phasic or "fast" axon synapses of the leg extensor of *Pachygrapsus* (C), and in high-output synapses of a stomach muscle (GM8b) of *Callinectes* (D). Representative electrical records of epsp's in crayfish opener (E), stomach muscle (F), and *Pachygrapsus* "fast" extensor axon (G) are also given to provide a physiological correlate for synaptic morphology.

uncertain. Some possibilities, including differences in rates of transmitter mobilization and in depolarization–secretion coupling, have been rejected as unlikely by Bittner (1968a). Another suggestion, differential invasion of different terminals by the nerve impulse (Atwood, 1967a; Bittner, 1968a; Sherman and Atwood, 1972), was based on observations of Dudel and Kuffler (1961a,b,c), who reported that synaptic terminals in crayfish could not be excited by direct stimulation. However, the demonstration of electrical excitability at facilitating crayfish terminals (Zucker, 1974a) contradicts the earlier findings and renders the differential invasion hypothesis less attractive.

Statistical analyses have shown that synapses with higher quantal content, m, also have higher probability of release, p, of available quantal transmitter units at low impulse frequencies (Johnson and Wernig, 1971). If the action potential characteristics are not different in the various terminals, then what sets the release probability at low frequencies?

Ultrastructural studies suggest an answer. High-output synapses tend to be larger in total area (Fig. 8 A–D) and to have more specialized presynaptic dense bodies (possible sites for transmitter release) than low-output synapses (Kuno *et al.*, 1971; Sherman and Atwood, 1972; Jahromi and Atwood, 1974). Since the presynaptic membrane may be specialized for calcium entry (Katz and Miledi, 1969), it is conceivable that there is more calcium entry at larger synapses. This may contribute to a higher probability of release, p. In addition, if the presynaptic dense bodies represent sites of release for quanta, n (Zucker, 1973), release sites at different synapses may be specialized for release of different numbers of quanta; some of these putative release sites are larger and more complex than others (Fig. 7iii).

It is interesting to note that the total number of discrete synapses is higher in low-output terminals even though average size of synapse is smaller. This could explain the large increase in transmitter output seen with high-frequency stimulation or with drugs: many of these synapses probably are not active except at high frequencies. The crustacean axon may recruit its own synapses as well as the responding muscle fibers.

Synaptic Plasticity

Opportunities for precise study of time-dependent and activity-related changes in synaptic efficacy are provided by crustacean neuromuscular systems. An advantage of these preparations over those provided by CNSs is their accessibility to both intra- and extracellular microelectrodes, which allows for analysis of changes at individual synaptic regions.

Several types of synaptic plasticity have been described and analyzed to at least some degree. Depression of transmission occurs at synapses of phasic motor axons (Hoyle and Wiersma, 1958a), including a long-lasting depression after a single impulse at synapses of the crayfish abdominal giant motor axon (Bruner and Kennedy, 1970) not attributable to transmitter depletion (Zucker and Bruner, 1974).

At synapses of tonic motor axons, short-term facilitation and a more gradually developing and persistent long-term facilitation are strikingly evident. Depression may be superimposed on these phenomena. In general, the synapses with initial high output show less short-term facilitation, less long-term facilitation, and more depression during maintained stimulation than low-output synapses of the same axon.

Short-term facilitation involves an increased probability of transmitter release, but so far it has not been possible to relate this convincingly to a calcium residue left over from previous impulses (as postulated by Katz and Miledi, 1968, for frog neuromuscular synapses), because of the rather low dependence of transmitter release on external calcium (Bracho and Orkand, 1970; Ortiz and Bracho, 1972; Zucker, 1974b). However, it is clear that high-output synapses, with initial high probability for transmitter release, p, are closer to saturation than low-output synapses; i.e., p can increase less with repetitive stimulation.

Long-term facilitation, seen as a progressive increase in epsp's with maintained stimulation, can be distinguished from short-term facilitation on the basis of its different time course of development and its long-lasting aftereffect (Fig. 9). Long-term facilitation may be similar to "potentiation" described at frog neuromuscular synapses by Magleby (1973a,b). A suggested mechanism for the phenomenon, based on observations of Birks and Cohen (1968a,b), is accumulation of sodium ions in the nerve terminals during long-lasting, repetitive stimulation (Sherman and Atwood, 1971h; Atwood et al., 1975).

The action of intracellular sodium ions is probably exerted indirectly through increased intracellular Ca^{2+}, which is either released from mitochondria (Carafoli, 1973) or accumulated through the effect of sodium on nerve membrane transport systems (Baker et al., 1969).

Evidence for sodium accumulation during maintained stimulation includes increased duration and decreased amplitude of nerve terminal potentials and slowing of the axon's conduction velocity (Fig. 9ii,iii). Treatments which increase sodium loading of nerve terminals accentuate long-term facilitation (Atwood et al., 1975), whereas treatments which inhibit entry of calcium into nerve terminals during stimulation do not abolish the aftereffect of long-term facilitation (Swenarchuk and Atwood, 1975). The persistent aftereffect seems to outlast changes in intracellular sodium (Fig. 9ii), suggesting an additional mechanism which produces a very long-lasting or even permanent change in synaptic output.

Central Connections among Motor Elements

The interactions between inhibitory and excitatory neurons at the peripheral synaptic level, manifest as presynaptic inhibition, are not the only ones which take place. As investigations on the central connections of crustacean motor and inhibitory neurons have progressed, evidence for some rather direct central interactions among these neurons has speedily accumulated.

Cross-connections among motor elements are well known in the crustacean stomatogastric ganglion, where they are responsible for much of the patterned output to the gastric and pyloric muscles (Maynard, 1972; Selverston, 1974). Excitatory and inhibitory cross-connections have also been described among MNs controlling crayfish abdominal muscles (Tatton and Sokolove, 1975). Recently, central cross-connections among the MNs controlling the crayfish claw (the classical neurons of Wiersma and van Harreveld) have also been detected by spike-train analysis techniques (Wiens and Gerstein, 1975; cf. Smith, 1972, 1973).

The strongest central effects appear to involve inhibition of the opener excitor by the opener inhibitor, and mutual excitation of the opener inhibitor and its

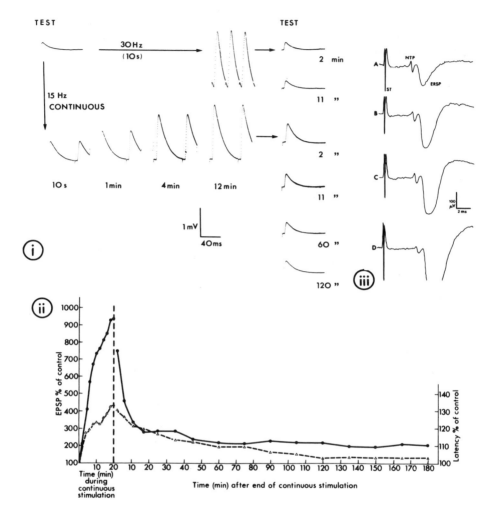

Fig. 9. Long-term facilitation at crayfish (i,ii) and crab (iii) neuromuscular synapses (Atwood *et al.*, 1975). In (i), a distinction between long-term and short-term facilitation is shown. A test response (64 epsp's sampled with signal averaging) was obtained at the start of the experiment; then a short burst of high-frequency stimulation (30 Hz) was delivered, resulting in eightfold growth of the epsp's. After stimulation, test responses obtained at 2 min were of the same amplitude as pretest controls. By contrast, stimulation over 12 min at 15 Hz resulted in a comparable but slower increase in epsp size, but the test response was facilitated even after 2 hr. In (ii), the growth of the epsp during stimulation (solid line) and test response decay following stimulation are compared with the change in conduction of the nerve impulse (dashed line) over the same period. The impulse conduction returned to normal while the epsp was still facilitated, suggesting that continued elevation of axonal sodium ion is not responsible for maintained epsp facilitation. In (iii), external recordings of the synaptic potential (ersp) and nerve terminal potential (NTP) are shown during stimulation (ST) at 1 Hz in ouabain, showing progressive increase in amplitude of ersp (transmitter output) and decline and prolongation of NTP, indicative of sodium loading. Times at which records were obtained: 1 min (A), 7 min (B), 12 min (C), 18 min (D).

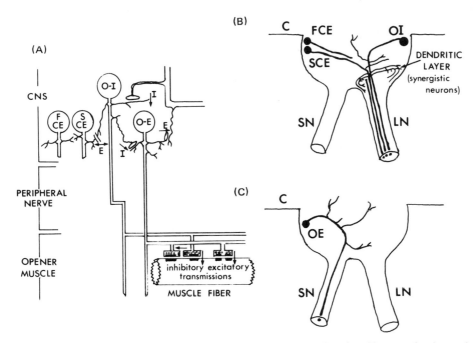

Fig. 10. A: Central connections among efferents controlling the crayfish claw. Note postulated central inhibition of opener excitor (OE) by opener inhibitor (OI) and putative electrical synapse between OI and slow closer excitor (SCE). After Wiens and Gerstein (1975). B,C: Diagrams (from dorsal aspect) of the neurons as seen in cobalt-filled preparations. In B, parallel distribution of major dendrites of the closer synergists is shown. In C, the rather different distribution of the OE dendrites is illustrated from Wiens (unpublished). SN, Small nerve to claw; LN, large nerve to claw; C, connective.

functional synergist, the "slow" closer excitor, through a postulated electrical synapse (Fig. 10).

Pursuing these findings, Wiens (unpublished) has penetrated these neurons in the ganglion with microelectrodes and has obtained direct evidence for some of the connections deduced from spike-train analysis techniques. For example, a well-defined hyperpolarizing inhibitory synaptic potential has been recorded in the opener excitor neuron with activation of the opener inhibitor.

In addition, cobalt fillings of these neurons have shown some interesting features of their dendritic organization. The functional synergists (opener inhibitor and closer excitors) show close parallel distribution of their major dendrites, which form a hoop-shaped lamina near the entrance of the major nerve to the claw (Fig. 10). Simultaneous fillings of all three neurons in the same ganglion have demonstrated the tightness of the dendritic alignment. The opener excitor neuron, by contrast, distributes its dendrites in a plane near the surface of the ganglion. However, meeting places between the dendrites of the opener excitor and the opener inhibitor, where the observed synaptic interactions could occur, are readily apparent in cobalt-filled preparations.

The strategic location of the dendrites of the closer synergists probably enables all three neurons to pick up the same inputs from reflex-generating claw afferents arriving in the major nerve. Intracellular recordings have shown well-defined monosynaptic epsp's generated by sensory fibers in these synergists. The rather different output patterns of these neurons, particularly of the "fast" and "slow" excitors, appear to arise from their different membrane properties: the "fast" neuron has a higher threshold and more rapid accommodation than the "slow" one (see Wright and Adelman, 1954; also Burrows and Horridge, 1974, for a similar case of postsynaptic filtering in locust).

In conclusion, current work on crustacean neuromuscular systems has emphasized the properties of synapses—their organization, physiological performance, ultrastructure, and plasticity. These synapses, unlike the more specialized neuromuscular synapses of vertebrates, seem to retain a strong "central" flavor and provide accessible models for many central operations. It is not surprising that central cross-connections among the motor elements appear to be quite common. These connections probably play a key role in functionally significant exploitation of the organization and pattern-sensitive properties of the peripheral synapses (see Spirito, 1970).

Future

> But more advanc'd, behold with strange surprise
> New distant scenes of endless science rise!*

One hesitates to predict the future course of research on crustacean neuromuscular systems because of the high probability of being proven wrong. Perhaps the key question is: Has research on these systems any future at all? Has the gold already been panned out of the stream?

I venture to think that, although the bulk of future research effort will certainly be directed at the CNS, there is still plenty of interest and promise in crustacean neuromuscular systems, and they will continue to play a major role in research on synaptic mechanisms. The reason for this is that they provide in accessible form small systems of definable, central-type synapses.

In the immediate future, the problems which have motivated present-day research will continue to attract attention. The properties of transmitters and receptors, the basis for physiological differences among synapses, the mechanisms of short-term facilitation and long-term facilitation—all these will attract further attention.

But if the present day belongs to the synapse as we now find it, the future will belong to the developing and altering synapse. I anticipate that future studies will

*Alexander Pope, *An Essay on Criticism* (1711).

exploit the relative simplicity of crustacean neuromuscular systems to define the developmental processes which give rise to the system. How does the system acquire its accurate organization? How responsive is it to alterations in hormonal levels, environmental influences, and activity? Already, several studies of trophic relationships among nerve, muscle, and glial elements have appeared (Bittner, 1973a,b; Bittner et al., 1974), and it is evident that different rules exist for crustacean muscles than for vertebrate muscles (Frank, 1974). Once again, Wiersma was there first: his observation of long-term survival of severed crustacean motor axons led to the more recent work on this topic by Hoy et al. (1967), Hoy (1969), Bittner (1973a), Atwood et al. (1973), and others.

The breadth of these contemporary approaches shows how the ripples of Wiersma's impact continue to spread in ever-widening circles.

ACKNOWLEDGMENTS

Some of the results reported here were from projects supported by grants from the National Research Council of Canada, the Muscular Dystrophy Association of Canada, and the Guggenheim Foundation.

I am indebted to Dr. T. J. Wiens and Dr. R. Wyman for permission to quote some unpublished work and to Mrs. Irene Kwan for help in preparing illustrations.

2

Neuromuscular Transmission in Insects

Peter N. R. Usherwood

Introduction

In his long career as our leading invertebrate neurobiologist, Professor C. A. G. Wiersma has studied a vast array of crustacean preparations, and the many important generalizations and concepts which have emanated from his work will continue to influence neurobiology for many years. The advances in our understanding of nervous systems that resulted from his studies have tended to overshadow those small but significant differences between species that have come to light through his comparative approach. In the fullness of time, such differences will undoubtedly be exploited to good effect, but for the present they serve as a reminder to us all of the dangers of trendy generalization and convenient extrapolation.

Although insect nerve–muscle systems have not received the same attention from invertebrate neurobiologists as have those of crustaceans, there is growing interest in them, especially among applied biologists. There is also evidence that studies of synaptic physiology and pharmacology in insects are having an impact on the vertebrate scene. One cannot fail to be impressed by the incredible numbers and variety of insects which inhabit this planet. Yet comparative insect neurobiology has developed so little that we still tend to refer to studies on *the insect* when we have merely investigated the properties of a single species. This is of course understandable when our information is directed toward ''general'' neurobiologists with little feeling for comparative aspects, but it will be frustrating and misleading for the neurobiologist of the future who is genuinely interested in comparing one insect species with another. In this chapter on the nerve–muscle physiology of insects, I will refer mainly to recent results from locust preparations; these have unquestionably contributed most to the major advances in this field. However, I will endeavor to keep to the spirit of my title by introducing a comparative note wherever possible.

The locust nerve–muscle junction probably has properties basically similar to those of nerve–muscle junctions in many other insects. However, on present evidence, it would be foolish to use this system as a standard, since in doing so we would close our eyes to possible important species differences which could be of special value to applied biologists. Of course, if I were to adopt a completely purist

Peter N. R. Usherwood • Department of Zoology, University of Nottingham, University Park, Nottingham NG7 2RD, England.

approach, it would seem improper for me to refer even to *the locust* nerve–muscle junction. During the past decade, I and my co-workers have restricted our investigations to the desert locust, *Schistocerca gregaria*. Other laboratories have worked on the migratory locust, *Locusta migratoria*. Superficially, one might expect the nerve–muscle properties of these two insect species to be almost identical, but there could be great dangers in extrapolating from one closely related species to another, as Wiersma's work on crustaceans has shown. I am sure that time will show many significant differences between even closely related insects in terms of their nerve–muscle physiology. Even within a single species of locust, there remains the problem of possible variability in different laboratory stocks of that species. I caution myself and others to remain objective about conflicting results of studies on locust nerve–muscle systems obtained from laboratories in, say, Amsterdam, Oregon, California, Kent, Glasgow, and Nottingham. Undoubtedly, differences in experimental approach could account for some of the apparently contradictory discoveries, but there remain unresolved problems concerning the laboratory culture of these insects which could have conceivably contributed to the confusion that has sometimes arisen.

Innervation

The frequent polyneuronal and exclusively multiterminal innervation of insect muscle is well established, although it would come as no surprise to hear of an insect muscle with fibers bearing a single motor nerve (MN) terminal, and with such fibers producing all-or-none action potentials rather than the graded, electrically excited responses that we have come to associate with the extrajunctional membrane of insect muscle.

Osborne (1975) has reviewed the ultrastructural data on insect nerve–muscle junctions, and there is little that I can add to his excellent account. From a comparative viewpoint, these data are rather fragmentary. Even in the locust and cockroach (mainly *Periplaneta* and *Blatta*), where the nerve–muscle systems have been extensively studied, the ultrastructure of the nerve–muscle apparatus is not particularly well understood. Indeed, this is another sad example of structural studies failing to keep pace with developments in physiology. However, at the light microscopic level, the innervation properties of insect muscle still attract considerable attention from behaviorists, synaptic physiologists, and pharmacologists.

Insects have two main types of MNs, excitatory and inhibitory. The synaptic potentials evoked by both types of neurons vary quantitatively; the same neuron may even produce synaptic potentials of different amplitudes in adjacent muscle fibers (Fig. 1). This assists in maintaining the fineness and accuracy of peripheral control of muscle contractions, which is seemingly so important to animals with relatively few MNs at their disposal. Peripheral inhibition of insect muscle by either common or specific inhibitory MNs is usually postsynaptic, although there is evidence for presynaptic inhibition in the phallic neuromuscular system of the cock-

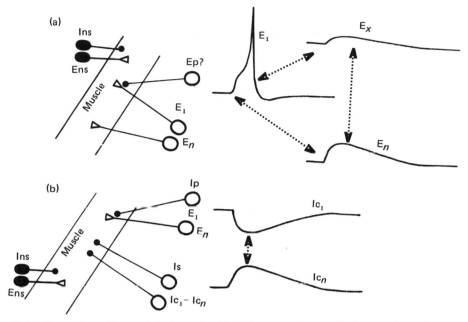

Fig. 1. Innervation of insect skeletal muscle. (a) Excitatory, polyneuronally innervated muscles may receive a number of excitatory axons ($E_1 - E_n$) producing a variety of responses ranging from large epsp's plus graded, electrically excited responses ("fast" axon, E_1) to small epsp's ("slow" axon, E_n). In addition, these axons may each evoke epsp's of different amplitudes in different parts of the same muscle (e.g., $E_1 - E_x$ and $E_n - E_x$). The possible occurrence of presynaptic excitation at some excitatory nerve–muscle junctions is included (Ep?). (b) Inhibitory innervation of some muscles by common (Ic) and specific (Is) inhibitory MNs produces ipsp's ranging from relatively large hyperpolarizations (e.g., Ic_1) to relatively large depolarizations (e.g., Ic_n). In addition, polyneural innervation by either common or specific inhibitors will produce ipsp's with a similar range of amplitudes (not shown), although it remains to be established whether hyperpolarizing and depolarizing ipsp's coexist in the same muscle fiber. Presynaptic inhibition (Ip) may occur at some excitatory nerve–muscle junctions, but one must also consider the possibility of presynaptic inhibition at inhibitory junctions and presynaptic excitation at inhibitory junctions. There is some evidence for innervation of insect skeletal muscles by neurosecretory neurons which have either an inhibitory influence (Ins) or an excitatory influence (Ens). However, it remains to be established whether these neurons generate synaptic potentials in the muscles.

roach *Periplaneta americana* (Parnas and Grossman, 1973). Other instances of presynaptic inhibition in insects will undoubtedly come to light. The discovery by Osborne (1975) of axoaxonal contacts between MN terminals on muscle of *Carausius morosus* suggests some presynaptic interaction. Possibly these contacts represent inhibitory synapses, although one should not exclude the possibility that they are excitatory. Of course, the presence of axoaxonal contacts at this level does not necessarily indicate presynaptic interactions involving neurotransmitters.

Nerves containing neurosecretory granules are known to innervate a variety of tissues in insects, including the skeletal musculature. Osborne *et al.* (1971) found neurosecretory nerve endings in association with the ventral longitudinal muscles of the body wall in *S. gregaria* and *C. morosus*, the neurosecretory endings being distinct from the endings of MNs (Fig. 2). Hoyle *et al.* (1974) have identified neurosecretory fibers in the nerve twigs on the metathoracic extensor tibiae muscle of *Schistocerca*. Osborne *et al.* (1971) concluded that material from neurosecretory neurons is liberated in the vicinity of muscle but not directly onto it. Indeed, there is commonly a connective tissue layer between the sites of release and the membrane of the muscle cell. It seems unlikely, therefore, that secretion of material from such nerve endings is primarily to produce a transient change in membrane potential of the synaptic potential type. A few dense-cored vesicles similar to those associated with neurosecretory neurons are also sometimes found in MN terminals (Osborne *et al.*, 1971; Rees and Usherwood, 1972*b*). Therefore, it may be a mistake to rigidly label insect neurons as either neurosecretory or non-neurosecretory. This danger is underlined by the fact that endings of MNs on the metathoracic retractor unguis muscle of *S. gregaria* become full of dense-cored vesicles after the muscle has been subjected to a prolonged period of tenotomy (Rees and Usherwood, unpublished).

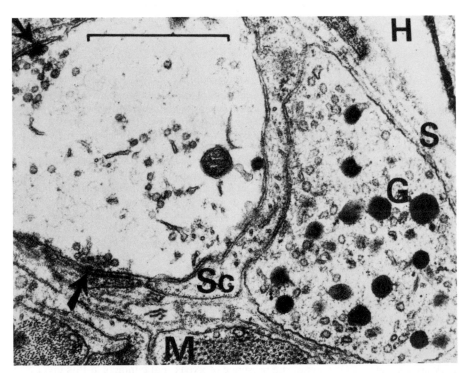

Fig. 2. Transverse section through two nerve processes associated with ventral abdominal longitudinal muscle in *Schistocerca gregaria*. The unsheathed right-hand process shows the characteristic rippled membrane of a neurosecretory nerve ending; the other process is a motor axon and is in synaptic contact (arrows) with the muscle (M). G, Neurosecretory granules; H, hemolymph space; S, stroma; Sc, Schwann cell. Scale: 1μm. From Osborne *et al.* (1971).

According to Scharrer (1968), the function of neurosecretory innervation of muscle tissue is probably to produce a more sustained and widespread stimulation than the normal type of activation by MNs. The recent discovery of rhythmically contracting muscle fibers in the leg muscles of *Schistocerca, Romalea,* and *Locusta* and of the effectiveness of the neurosecretory innervation to the legs of these insects in modifying the activity of these fibers (Hoyle, 1974, 1975*b;* Hoyle and O'Shea, 1974; Hoyle *et al.,* 1974) gives some indication of one possible role of neurosecretory neurons in these insects.

Release of Transmitter from Excitatory MNs

Studies on insects of the release of transmitter from MN terminals have failed to keep pace with those on crustaceans. From the comparative viewpoint, it is unfortunate that they have been mainly restricted to two insect species, *S. gregaria* and *P. americana.*

While recording miniature epsp's (mepsp's) from locust and cockroach leg muscles, I obtained the first indication that the release of transmitter from nerve terminals on insect muscle is a quantal process (Usherwood, 1961, 1963*a*). Later studies (Usherwood, 1972) on the epsp's of leg muscles of *Schistocerca* established that these evoked responses are probably derived from the synchronous release of many quanta of neurotransmitter. In this respect, therefore, the release of transmitter from the terminals of locust MNs follows the classical pattern (Katz, 1966). Nevertheless, when the intervals between the mepsp's were examined statistically, it was found that these potentials do not occur randomly in time as was expected. In addition, the amplitude distributions of *extracellularly* (focally) recorded mepsp's were non-Poisson (Usherwood, 1972). At the classical nerve–muscle junction, the mepsp's occur randomly in time and the amplitude distributions of the *intracellular* epsp's are Poisson in character (Katz, 1966).

My original observations on the interactive nature of the miniature discharge recorded from locust muscle fibers have been confirmed recently by Hodgkiss (1976). Rees (1974) and Washio and Inouye (1975) have observed similar non-Poisson miniature activity in muscles of the cockroaches *P. americana* and *Blaberus giganteus.* According to Washio and Inouye (1975), the mepsp's recorded from depressor muscles isolated from the leg of *Periplaneta* occur basically in a random manner, but this randomness of the discharge is contaminated by short bursts of mepsp's. Rees (1974) recorded mepsp's from the metathoracic retractor unguis muscle of both cockroach species and showed that his data could best be described by the negative binomial theory. He interpreted this as implying some mutual interaction between those processes responsible for the spontaneous release of transmitter from cockroach MN terminals. Rees and I (Rees and Usherwood, 1972*b*; Usherwood and Rees, 1972; Usherwood, 1973) have proposed that the nonrandom distribution of synaptic vesicles in the terminals of locust (and cockroach) MNs and the nonrandom appearance of mepsp's are causally related events.

We must await more information on the role, if any, of synaptic vesicles in transmitter storage and release before this idea can be tested rigorously.

I have pointed out (Usherwood, 1972) that my technique of recording epsp's *extracellularly* from active sites on the retractor unguis muscle of *S. gragaria* did not provide sufficiently unequivocal data to reject completely a Poisson basis for evoked release of transmitter from the retractor unguis MN terminals. It has come as no surprise, therefore, that one of my graduate students, using intracellular recording techniques, has recently obtained a Poisson distribution for the amplitudes of epsp's recorded from fibers of the metathoracic extensor tibiae of *S. gregaria*. When focally recording with extracellular electrodes from active sites on locust leg muscles, the investigator is faced with a number of problems. The nerve terminals on these muscles are often up to 30μm in length, are located some distance from the recording electrode in clefts between muscle fibers, and contain many (30+) synaptic sites (Rees and Usherwood, 1972b). The terminals on the retractor unguis muscle of the cockroach, *P. americana,* have a similar structure (Fig. 3). It is not possible, therefore, to place an extracellular electrode in close juxtaposition to such a nerve terminal. Hodgkiss (1976) has overcome some of these problems by using either the marked miniature technique (Usherwood, 1972) or the calcium electrode technique (Usherwood, 1976), whereby it is possible to study *intracellularly* evoked transmitter release from a single nerve terminal.

It is possible to completely fatigue the excitatory nerve terminals on the white fibers of the metathoracic retractor unguis muscle of *S. gregaria* (Usherwood, 1967; Usherwood and Machili, 1968; Cochrane *et al.,* 1972) by stimulating their motor axons at 20 Hz for 15 min (McKinlay and Usherwood, 1973). This muscle also contains a bundle of red fibers, but the synapses on these fibers are not completely fatigued with the same stimulation. Nevertheless, at the synapses on both sets of fibers, prolonged stimulation for 15 min at 20 Hz leads to changes in the shape, distribution, and population density of synaptic vesicles, and these changes can be correlated with either complete or partial failure of evoked transmitter release and with changes in the mepsp discharge. Fatigue of the neuromuscular junctions on the white muscle fibers is accompanied by changes in the morphological appearance of the glial cells associated with the retractor unguis axon terminals, the normally electron-lucent cytoplasm of these cells becoming markedly electron dense, with dark-staining bodies in the cytoplasm. Possibly these changes in the glial cells are associated with their supposed transmitter sequestration function (Faeder and Salpeter, 1970).

As a result of the need for a more rigorous examination of synaptic events at insect nerve–muscle junctions, the problem of the electrical coupling between adja-

Fig. 3. Low-power electron micrograph of a normal but unidentified motor axon terminal (Ax) making synaptic contact with at least two fibers (MF) of the metathoracic retractor unguis muscle of *Periplaneta americana*. The single terminal possesses 16 release sites (nerve–muscle synapses), of which three are indicated by arrows. Note the extended process (aposynaptic apparatus, Ap) from the muscle fiber which makes contact with the nerve terminal. Scale: 5.0 μm. From Wood and Usherwood (in preparation).

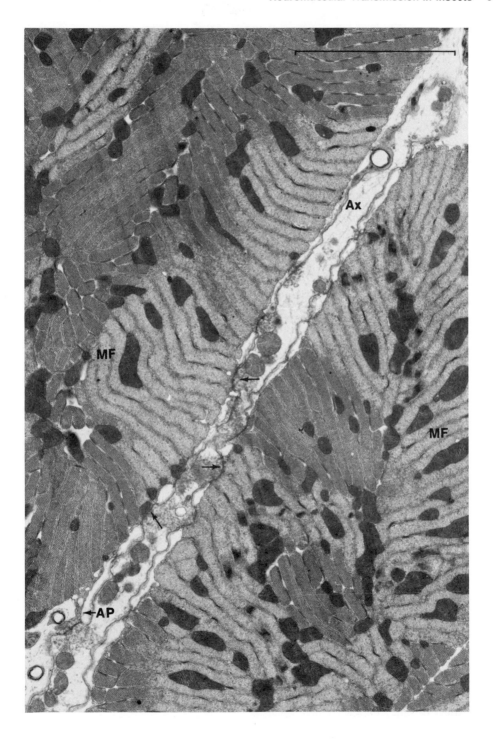

cent muscle fibers which occurs in some muscles requires attention. In the extensor tibiae muscle of adult *S. gregaria,* electrical coupling is restricted mainly to a few fibers in the distal bundles of this muscle and to the tonic fibers (Burns and Usherwood, in preparation) which I consider (Usherwood, 1974) to be responsible for the intrinsic rhythmic contractions of this muscle. Although the tonic fibers of the extensor tibiae are electrically coupled, there is as yet no evidence for protoplasmic bridges between these fibers. However, the fibers are so tightly packed together that extracellular current pathways may be sufficiently restricted to cause the necessary crosstalk between them. One gains the impression that fibers which are electrically coupled are invariably innervated by a "slow" excitatory axon. The occurrence of electrical coupling seemingly represents a lower level of development. It occurs in developing muscles and probably during degeneration of skeletal muscle following axotomy (Usherwood, 1963b; Usherwood and Wood, 1972). Electrical coupling also exists between "muscle fibers" or "subunits" in some crustacean muscles (Reuben, 1960; Parnas and Atwood, 1966). The problems of interpreting results of synaptic events, both spontaneous and evoked, in electrically coupled fibers, obtained by using either intracellular voltage or current recording (voltage clamp) techniques, are obviously considerable. For example, histograms of mepsp amplitudes will be multimodal, the degree of separation of the peaks depending in part on the coupling resistance between the fibers.

Recently there have been reports of miniature events of different decay times recorded from the same fibers either extracellularly or under voltage clamp in *S. gregaria* extensor tibiae (Anderson *et al.,* 1976) and some crustacean *(Maria squinado)* muscles (Crawford and McBurney, 1976). In fact, the first report of such activity in crustacean muscle was made by Atwood and Parnas (1968), who also showed that the epsp's recorded extracellularly from crab muscle fibers sometimes differed in time course from one event to the next. Preliminary studies in this laboratory indicate that the time course of the mepsp's is most variable in those locust muscle fibers with dual excitatory innervation. The mepsp's recorded from such fibers either extracellularly or intracellularly under voltage clamp vary considerably not only in decay time (by a factor of over 100) but also in rise time. There is no clear relationship between rise and decay times. The fact that correlated extracellular mepsp's and intracellular miniature synaptic currents have similar rise and decay time characteristics seemingly excludes the possibility that the variability in time course of these events arises because of electrical coupling between muscle fibers. It also seems unlikely that extracellular mepsp's of different time course result either from differences in postsynaptic properties or from the presence of external structures in extracellular current pathways. It would seem worthwhile to look at the structure of synapses of terminals on the locust extensor tibiae in some detail. There is no reason to suppose that such sites will have exactly the same geometry. If there are differences in cleft width, cleft length, etc., this could cause the observed differences in the duration of action of spontaneously released transmitter at such sites. Another possibility is that local transmitter release follows a variety of time courses.

The width of the synaptic cleft between axon terminal membrane and sarcolemma fibers is quite variable, from 25 nm (Osborne, 1975; Rees and Usherwood, 1972b) to 5 nm (Smith, 1960). Although different fixation techniques could account for some or even all of this apparent variability in cleft width, there is, of course, no reason why nerve–muscle junctions in insects should be standardized in this respect. The cleft width will influence the distribution in space and time of neurotransmitter release from the nerve terminals and as a result will influence the time course and amplitude of the resultant synaptic events. Osborne (1975) also referred to the importance of considering the influence of the material in the synaptic cleft on the time course of the synaptic potential.

It remains to be established whether the factors responsible for mepsp's of variable time course also influence the time course of the epsp. Atwood and Parnas's (1968) observations on crustacean muscle indicate that this is likely to be the case. Nevertheless, we have evidence to support the contention that spontaneous and evoked release of transmitter from locust excitatory MNs could involve different pools of transmitter and that factors which influence one of the release modes do not always influence the other (Usherwood, 1974).

The occurrence of a distinct subpopulation of small mepsp's at some vertebrate nerve–muscle junctions has been a recent talking point among synaptologists. One of my students has recently discovered such events at synapses on the extensor tibiae of S. gregaria (Hodgkiss, 1976). These potentials represent a very small proportion of the total mepsp population at normal nerve–muscle junctions and do not seemingly contribute to the evoked response at these sites. Following MN section, the proportion of small mepsp's increases as the nerve terminals degenerate, until the entire miniature discharge is of this type. As the percentage of small miniatures increases in proportion to the normal-sized mepsp's, the evoked response declines in amplitude; it is not possible to generate an epsp when the normal-sized mepsp's have been completely replaced by the small mepsp's. Perhaps the small ones arise following transmitter release from either small or incompletely filled vesicles which for some reason cannot contribute to the pulse of transmitter released during evoked activity (Fig. 4a). If one accepts the idea of a continuous production of transmitter in MN terminals, then all mepsp's can be viewed as an overspill phenomenon or, in modern Western terms, as nerve terminal "garbage." Of course, this garbage, like any other, has information content which is presumably put to good use by the nerve–muscle system. The release of transmitter from incompletely filled vesicles could be an inevitable consequence of the presence of this overspill system. Presumably, degeneration of the nerve terminals would lead to an increase in the proportion of incompletely filled vesicles in the nerve terminals as a result of the failure of the mechanism producing the neurotransmitter, and this in turn would lead to an increase in the frequency of occurrence of small mepsp's.

There are other possible explanations for the occurrence of small miniatures. For example, they could represent transmitter quanta released from either glial cells or neurosecretory nerve terminals (Fig. 4b,c). However, the similar time courses of the small and normal-sized miniatures seemingly argue against these explanations

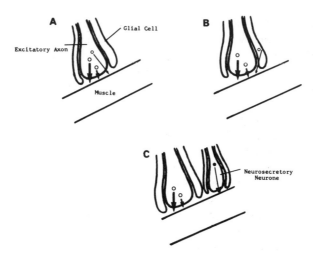

Fig. 4. Possible explanations for the appearance of small mepsp's at synapses on leg muscle fibers of *Schistocerca gregaria*. A: A pool of subnormal-sized vesicles spontaneously releases its transmitter quanta without contributing to the epsp. In this scheme and in B and C, spontaneous transmitter release, which leads to the appearance of normal-sized mepsp's, could arise from a transmitter pool separate from that which gives rise to evoked release of transmitter. B: The small mepsp's are generated as a result of spontaneous release of transmitter (it could be a different substance from that producing the mepsp's) from glial cells. C: A neurosecretory neuron accompanying an excitatory MN terminal releases a substance which produces the small mepsp's. Thin arrows, spontaneous release of transmitter producing small mepsp's; medium arrows, spontaneous release of transmitter producing normal mepsp's; thick arrows, evoked release of transmitter producing epsp's.

since the glial cells and neurosecretory terminals are more distant from the muscle membrane than are the MN terminals.

Chemosensitivity of Locust Leg Muscle

During the past decade or so, a major battle has been fought over the possible role of amino acids as synaptic transmitters in vertebrate and invertebrate CNSs and at neuromuscular junctions in arthropods. There has been reasonable agreement that substances such as γ-aminobutyric acid (GABA) could serve in a neurotransmitter role but much less support for ubiquitous amino acids such as L-glutamate and L-aspartate in such a role. Unfortunately, the combatants in this battle have, at times, assumed postures more suitable to roles in a religious war than to scientific debate.

The possibility that amino acids may function as neurotransmitters in insects was noted by Kerkut *et al.* (1965), Usherwood and Grundfest (1964, 1965), Kerkut and Walker (1966), and Usherwood and Machili (1966). These authors described how GABA and L-glutamate activate muscles in orthopteran insects and proposed that these substances might serve a transmitter role at inhibitory and excitatory junctions, respectively, on these muscles. There was little adverse reaction to the proposal that GABA functions as a peripheral inhibitory transmitter in insects. Presumably, the strong evidence supporting such a role for GABA in crustaceans deterred any such reaction. However, the proposal that L-glutamate may function as the transmitter at excitatory junctions on cockroach and locust leg muscle was much less readily accepted by insect neurobiologists. At that time, there were very good reasons for their reluctance. L-Glutamate is found in high concentrations in insect nervous tissue and does not have the rarity value previously associated with putative neurotransmitters. Furthermore, the concentration of free glutamate in the blood of cockroaches and locusts was believed to be so high that it would inactivate any nerve–muscle synapses which used glutamate as a transmitter.

Over a decade has passed since the initial discoveries of the potent action of certain acidic amino acids on some insect muscles, and there is now growing evidence of a change in attitude toward L-glutamate and its proposed neuro-transmitter role. This change has resulted in part from the discovery that the level of blood glutamate in cockroaches, locusts, and probably other insects would not pose a problem for glutamatergic nerve–muscle junctions. The growing acceptance among vertebrate neurobiologists of the importance of amino acids as central ner-vous transmitters, coupled with the demonstration of glutamatergic nerve–muscle junctions in crustaceans, has also influenced the thinking of insect neurobiologists.

A host of experiments in my laboratory and in other laboratories on leg muscles of *S. gregaria* and on skeletal muscles of other insects have resulted in the following conclusions concerning the role of L-glutamate:

1. L-Glutamate depolarizes the muscles of a number of insect species by reacting with receptors of the postsynaptic membrane of excitatory synapses (e.g., Berànek and Miller, 1968; Usherwood and Machili, 1968; Usherwood, 1969).
2. The reversal value for the gultamate depolarizations and glutamate currents recorded from locust leg muscle fibers is identical with the reversal value for the epsp (Usherwood and Cull-Candy, 1975) and excitatory postsynaptic current (Anwyl and Usherwood, 1974a,b, 1975).
3. The ionic channels in the muscle membrane which are opened during L-glutamate activation have opening times similar to the time constant of decay of the briefest miniature excitatory postsynaptic current recorded from locust muscle (Anderson et al., 1976).
4. Changes in the distribution of glutamate sensitivity on locust leg muscle occur following denervation (Usherwood, 1969). These changes are similar to those observed for acetylcholine on denervated vertebrate muscle.
5. Pharmacological agents which either attenuate or potentiate the responses to glutamate have similar effects on either the epsp or excitatory synaptic current.
6. Uptake of L-glutamate into terminals of excitatory MNs occurs following stimulation of these cells.

7. Extrajunctional receptors for L-glutamate are found on locust muscle fibers (Lea and Usherwood, 1973*a,b;* Cull-Candy and Usherwood, 1973; Usherwood and Cull-Candy, 1974).

This list is by no means exhaustive, but it does clearly establish the claim that L-glutamate is a serious contender for the role of transmitter at excitatory junctions on many insect muscles. For a more complete treatment of the case for and against its proposed neurotransmitter role in insects, the reader is referred to the review by Usherwood and Cull-Candy (1975).

Desensitization and Potentiation at Locust Glutamate Synapses

During prolonged application of high concentrations of putative transmitters to many synaptic sites in many different animals, the resultant potential and conductance changes recorded postsynaptically are often followed by a return of these parameters toward their resting values. This phenomenon is called either "desensitization" (Katz and Thesleff, 1957) or "receptor inactivation" (Nastuk, 1967), and is thought to involve some conformational changes in the receptors for neurotransmitters. Beránek and Miller (1968) and Usherwood and Machili (1968) observed desensitizations at locust excitatory neuromuscular junctions during glutamate application by micropipette, whereas Lea and Usherwood (1973*a*) showed that bath application of GABA to locust inhibitory neuromuscular junctions did not desensitize the GABA receptors at these sites. More recently, Daoud and Usherwood (in preparation) have studied some of the factors which influence desensitization of glutamate receptors at excitatory junctions on *S. gregaria* extensor tibiae fibers. Brief (20 msec, 2 nC) test pulses of glutamate were applied from one barrel of a double-barreled micropipette during application of a long conditioning pulse (6–12 sec, 12–24 nC) from the other barrel. By this means, a relatively precise account of the onset of desensitization and subsequent recovery from this phenomenon at a single nerve–muscle junction (i.e., a single nerve terminal but many synapses) was obtained. In addition, it was possible to gain insight into the phenomenon of potentiation at such a junction.

When the initial depolarization caused by the conditioning pulse of L-glutamate was small (about 1.5 mV), test responses occurring within a period of about 1 sec from the start of the conditioning pulse were potentiated (Fig. 5). With larger-amplitude conditioning pulses, the initial depolarization was increased and potentiation of the test responses was not seen, although a second phase of potentiation of test responses always occurred for a few seconds after termination of the conditioning pulse regardless of the amplitude of the conditioning pulse. With long conditioning pulses, the responses to the test pulses of glutamate inevitably declined with time because of desensitization of the postsynaptic glutamate receptors. If one assumes that the changes seen during the conditioning period reflect changes in the properties of the postjunctional glutamate receptors, then it is possible to develop a model from

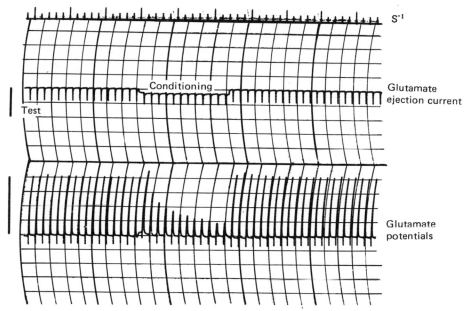

Fig. 5. Intracellular recording (bottom trace) of glutamate potentials generated in a fiber of the extensor tibiae muscle of *Schistocerca gregaria*. The glutamate was ejected from a double-barreled micropipette onto a nerve–muscle junction. A conditioning pulse of glutamate was superimposed on brief test pulses of this amino acid (center trace). Note potentiation of test responses at beginning and immediately after conditioning pulse. Also note rapid decline in amplitude of test response during later stages of conditioning period. See text for further explanation. From Daoud and Usherwood (in preparation).

the results described above to account for desensitization and potentiation at glutamate synapses on locust extensor tibiae fibers:

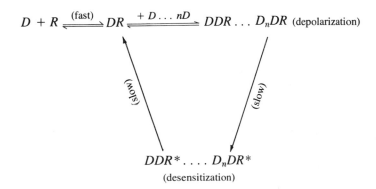

where D is the glutamate concentration, R is the receptor in its original state, DR is the intermediate step in drug–receptor interaction, R^* is the desensitized receptor, and $DDR \rightarrow D_nDR$ indicates that each receptor has at least two binding sites for

L-glutamate (Walther and Usherwood, 1972; Lea and Usherwood, 1973b). In this scheme, opening of the ionophore associated with the glutamate receptor occurs only when at least two molecules of glutamate combine with the receptor. The continued presence of a high concentration of glutamate causes the receptor to revert slowly to a different form in which it can no longer activate its ionophore. During recovery from the desensitized state, the drug–receptor combination reverts to its intermediate form, *DR*.

This model embraces the requirement for a relationship between the rate of recovery from desensitization and the conditioning concentration of L-glutamate which was established in the studies of Daoud and Usherwood (in prepration). It also accounts for conditioning and postconditioning potentiation by virtue of providing a "pool" of *DR* at the beginning of a conditioning pulse of glutamate and again at the end of such a conditioning pulse.

Desensitization of glutamate receptors, junctional and extrajunctional, on locust metathoracic extensor tibiae fibers can be blocked by the tetrameric lectin concanavalin A (Mathers and Usherwood, 1976). When glutamate is iontophoresed from a micropipette onto the extrajunctional membrane of these fibers, a biphasic potential is generated because of the simultaneous activation of two populations of glutamate receptors, designated D-receptors and H-receptors, which are associated with ionophores for cations (D) and ionophores for chloride (H) (Lea and Usherwood, 1970, 1973a,b; Cull-Candy and Usherwood, 1973; Usherwood and Cull-Candy, 1974). With repeated pulses of L-glutamate, this biphasic response quickly wanes to zero, the depolarizing component disappearing before the hyperpolarizing component. In the presence of 10^{-7} M concanavalin A, the depolarizing component of the biphasic extrajunctional response is no longer abolished by repeated pulses of glutamate (Fig. 6c). However, the H-receptors retain their normal rate of inactivation under these conditions. The junctional receptors for glutamate are affected by concanavalin A in a way similar to that of the extrajunctional D-receptors (Fig. 6a,b). From these data, it seems possible that concanavalin A has an affinity for those glutamate receptors associated with cation ionophores. Possibly this lectin prevents desensitization of these receptors by either preventing the inward movement of calcium which accompanies the flow of sodium across the muscle membrane during receptor–transmitter interaction or preventing a conformational change in the glutamate receptor which possibly follows its interaction with glutamate.

Tonic and Phasic Muscle Fibers

Definitive evidence for the occurrence of tonic fibers in insect muscle was first obtained by Hoyle (1961) during studies on locust spiracular muscles, which give only weak contractions and are either electrically inexcitable or weakly excitable. In common with other tonic fibers, they give a sustained contracture during potassium depolarization (Hoyle, 1961; Usherwood, 1967, 1968). Tonic fibers have been

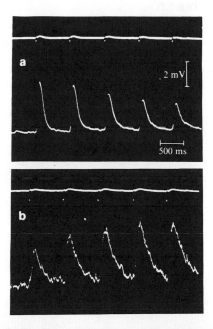

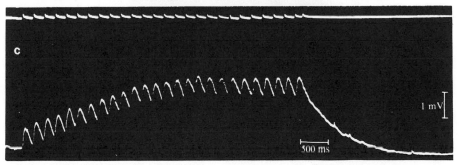

Fig. 6. (a) Iontophoresis of 1 nC glutamate pulses at 720 msec intervals onto an excitatory junction of *Schistocerca gregaria* metathoracic extensor tibiae bathed in 10^{-7} M concanavalin A for 5 hr. Responses showed desensitization at a rate typical of junctional receptors in control fibers. (b) Fiber exposed to 10^{-6} M concanavalin A for 1 hr. Responses now exhibited simultaneous potentiation and summation to 1 nC glutamate pulses delivered at the same frequency as in (a). Note high frequency of spontaneous mepsp's. (c) A prolonged train of 3 nC pulses delivered at intervals of 240 msec evoked a train of D-responses on the extrajunctional membrane. These depolarizations initially showed simultaneous potentiation and summation, leading to the formation of a stable, summated depolarization which decayed rapidly on cessation of glutamate ejection. In the absence of concanavalin A, the D-receptors desensitize very rapidly during repeated application of pulses of L-glutamate even at frequencies of less than 2/sec. From Mathers and Usherwood (1976).

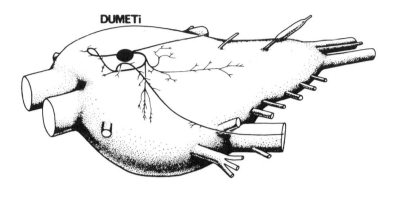

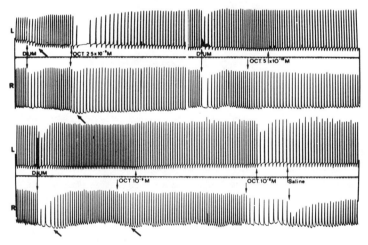

Fig. 7. (a) Reconstruction of DUMETi of metathoracic ganglion of *Schistocerca gregaria* based on projection of serial sections of ganglion after injection of neuron with procion yellow. (b) Threshold effects of DUMETi and octopamine on the intrinsic rhythm (which was slow in this animal) of the left (L) and right (R) extensor tibiae of the Florida grasshopper, *Romalea microptera*. Records are of isometric force and are all from the same preparation. Tension to peak: 1.8 g. A DUM neuron was stimulated extracellularly via an electrode placed above the outside of the dorsal surface of the ganglion, with a short burst of pulses at 20 Hz. Onset of stimulation of the neuron (probably DUMETi, but this was not specifically tested) is indicated by arrows and the letters DUM. Times of introduction of saline drop (approximately 0.01 ml) containing octopamine at concentrations stated are indicated by arrows and the letters OCT. Oblique arrows point to relaxations of tone. Note that some occurred following neural stimulation, others after application of octopamine-containing saline. Several relaxations of tone of the right extensor muscle occurred, but there was only one relaxation of the left muscle—the initial one that followed neural stimulation. The threshold concentration of octopamine which slowed the intrinsic rhythm was below 10^{-9} M. A slightly higher concentration, 2.5×10^{-9} M, also led to attenuation of the intrinsic contractions, which the DUM neurons do too. From Hoyle *et al.* (1974).

found in the retractor muscle of the giant water bug *Lethoceros* (Walcott and Burrows, 1969) and locust metathoracic extensor tibiae (Cochrane *et al.*, 1972). Tonic fibers in the proximal part of ETi exhibit spontaneous rhythmic contractions in *S. gregaria* and *Romalea microptera*. Cochrane *et al.* (1972) described the physiological and ultrastructural features of these fibers, which resemble those of visceral fibers. The ETi intrinsic rhythm is attenuated by the activity of the neurosecretory DUMEti (dorsal unpaired median neuron) (Hoyle, 1974) (Fig. 7). Hoyle (1974) has also shown that whereas the IRC amplitude is more or less immediately reduced by the common inhibitor in a rapidly reversible fashion, impulses in the neurosecretory neuron attenuate the rhythmic activity of the extensor muscle only after a delay of as much as 100 msec, and that this inhibition lasts for periods of 1–88 min after termination of the impulses.

Hoyle and O'Shea (1974) suggested that IRC may promote wakefulness and spontaneous movements of the locust. Another suggestion from these authors is that the rhythm serves to exercise muscle fibers that would otherwise be inactive for long periods. These suggestions and mine (Usherwood, 1974) that the contractions aid hemolymph circulation will undoubtedly be borne in mind during further studies.

The recent studies by Hoyle (1975*b*) on the effects of octopamine and other biogenic amines on the spontaneous contractions promise to provide us with exciting information on the role or roles of neurosecretory innervation of peripheral tissues in insects. Hoyle has found that very low concentrations of octopamine inhibit the rhythmic activity of locust and grasshopper extensor tibiae (Fig. 7b) and has proposed that this substance is released from the DUMETi neuron (Hoyle and Barker, 1975). It may influence a metabolic pump of the IRC generator. It would be of interest to determine whether the tonic fibers still respond to stimulation of the "slow" excitor (SETi) and inhibitor axons which innervate ETi once octopamine treatment has terminated the spontaneous contractions, since it might then be possible to decide whether the site of action of octopamine is either junctional or extrajunctional. The effect of the pentapeptide proctolin (Brown, 1967) on IRC also deserves some attention. Possibly insects have an "autonomic" nervous system which influences many peripheral structures including blood flow through appendages. The substances released by DUMETi, and also possibly excitatory and inhibitory MNs, may, in addition to immediate actions, exert trophic influences on muscle, apodemes, and endoskeleton. Perhaps this would explain why the cuticle of locust legs often softens when the leg muscles are denervated.

Tonic fibers occur also in the prothoracic and mesothoracic extensor tibiae of *S. gregaria* (Burns and Usherwood, in preparation). They develop tension (about 0.02 g) in the absence of neural excitation, but it is steady rather than oscillatory and does not seem to be influenced by their common inhibitory neurons. However, oscillations were found in the baseline tension during SETi excitation at low frequency. The "catch" properties described by Wilson and Larimer (1968) may be localized to tonic fibers.

At present, there is much excitement over recent advances in our understanding of central nervous structure and function in insects. Behavioral studies of the insect nerve–muscle system have, for the moment, taken a back seat. This quiet period will not last for long. The observed close matching of phasic and tonic properties of neurons and the muscle fibers they innervate enables us to anticipate many of the functional properties of locust skeletal muscles merely by studying their neural inputs. However, to fully understand the contribution made by skeletal muscle in framing insect behavior, we must look deeper than this.

3

Synaptic Plasticity at Crayfish Neuromuscular Junctions

Robert S. Zucker

Introduction

Crustacean neuromuscular junctions have provided some very favorable preparations for the study of synaptic plasticity. The crayfish, in particular, has junctions at which facilitation and depression, both rapid and long-lasting varieties, can be studied in great detail. Since the ability of synapses to adjust their strength of transmission as a consequence of previous activity plays a major role in many theories of learning (Mark, 1974), synaptic plasticity has attracted wide interest among neurobiologists. This chapter will summarize attempts to understand synaptic plasticity in terms of underlying cellular processes.

Short-Term Facilitation

Crustacean neuromuscular junctions have been regarded as "plastic" since the pioneering work of Kees Wiersma and his colleagues. Van Harreveld and Wiersma (1936) and Katz and Kuffler (1946) described a facilitation in crayfish in which the successive postsynaptic responses seen in claw opener muscle fibers grew in response to repetitive stimulation of the single excitatory motor neuron (MN) innervating this muscle. Subsequently, Dudel and Kuffler (1961a) showed transmitter release to be quantal at this neuromuscular junction. The number of quanta released by a nerve impulse was a random variable apparently following Poisson statistics. Using a quantal analysis, Dudel and Kuffler (1961b) also demonstrated that facilitation was presynaptic in origin, consisting of an increase in the average number of quanta liberated by an impulse in the MN terminals.

By 1970, considerable evidence had accumulated indicating that the Poisson model for transmitter release did not explain events at crustacean neuromuscular junctions (Bittner and Harrison, 1970). A report by Johnson and Wernig (1971) that transmitter release at the crayfish opener neuromuscular junction could be described

Robert S. Zucker • Department of Physiology-Anatomy, University of California, Berkeley, California 94720.

by binomial statistics clarified the statistical anomalies. The binomial model provided a useful framework in which to study the statistical basis of a change in transmitter release. In this model, the average number of quanta, m, released by a presynaptic impulse is governed by a maximum number of releasable quanta, n, and a probability that such a quantum is released, p. Clearly, changes in m could be due to changes in p or n, or both.

I explored this problem by studying the changes in release statistics using paired responses, or steady stimulation at different frequencies. By recording extracellularly from localized regions of neuromuscular contact on the surface of a muscle fiber, one can observe potentials due to the postsynaptic currents evoked by transmitter action. In a favorable recording condition, the single quanta making up these responses can be distinguished and counted directly (Fig. 1). If the statistical process governing transmitter release is bionomial, p and n can be estimated from the average number of quanta released, m, and the variance of this number, σ^2, by $p = 1 - \sigma^2/m$ and $n = m/p$. When p and n were estimated in this fashion, p increased from less than 0.1 for unfacilitated responses to about 0.3 for moderately facilitated responses. Changes in p were often statistically significant. While n could be measured reliably only for facilitated responses, it ranged between 2 and 5, and seemed to be affected little by changes in the degree of facilitation (Table I). The standard errors for p and n in Table I are computed using the equations of Robinson (1976). They correct a minor error in the previously published values (Zucker, 1973).

How can these statistical changes be interpreted? My initial idea was that n was associated with a presynaptic store of releasable quanta and that p was the probability that such releasable quanta would be liberated by an impulse. This idea has

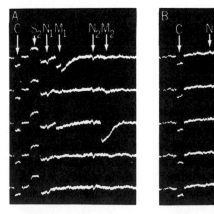

Fig. 1. Extracellular recordings of synaptic currents (M) and nerve terminal potentials (N) from synaptic sites on the claw opener muscle of crayfish. C is a calibration pulse (100μV, 5 msec), while S is a stimulus artifact. A: Five paired responses to two stimuli separated by 40 msec. B: Single responses at a frequency of 5 Hz from another preparation. From Zucker (1973).

Table I. Estimates of Statistical Parameters of Transmitter Release in Different States of Facilitation[a]

Site No.	Responses to	T (msec)	N	$m \pm S.E._{\cdot m}$	$p \pm S.E._{\cdot p}$	$n \pm S.E._{\cdot n}$
I	Stimulus 1		548	0.323 ± 0.029	0.039 ± 0.054	8.33 ± 11.6
	Stimulus 2	40	548	0.540 ± 0.028^b	0.208 ± 0.039^b	2.60 ± 0.47
II	Stimulus 1		736	0.121 ± 0.013	0.007 ± 0.056	16.76 ± 120
	Stimulus 2	30	736	$0.243 + 0.017^b$	0.108 ± 0.035^b	2.25 ± 0.72
	10 Hz		594	0.680 ± 0.027^b	0.357 ± 0.029^b	1.90 ± 0.14
III	Stimulus 1		218	0.486 ± 0.042	0.218 ± 0.059	2.23 ± 0.57
	Stimulus 2	50	218	0.780 ± 0.049^b	0.330 ± 0.053	2.37 ± 0.35
IV	Stimulus 1		500	0.334 ± 0.025	0.081 ± 0.051	4.14 ± 2.59
	Stimulus 2	55	500	0.576 ± 0.031^b	0.165 ± 0.046	3.50 ± 0.95
	5 Hz		710	0.868 ± 0.029^b	0.298 ± 0.032^b	2.91 ± 0.29
V	Stimulus 1		431	0.271 ± 0.026	0.039 ± 0.076	7.02 ± 13.6
	Stimulus 2	40	431	0.499 ± 0.032^b	0.097 ± 0.056	5.16 ± 2.94
VI	Stimulus 1		259	0.224 ± 0.028	0.082 ± 0.065	2.72 ± 2.13
	Stimulus 2	30	259	0.463 ± 0.030^b	0.260 ± 0.048^b	1.78 ± 0.29
	5 Hz		715	1.136 ± 0.033^b	0.332 ± 0.031^b	3.42 ± 0.31

[a] Abbreviations: T, the separation between first and second stimuli in paired stimulus experiments; N, total number of trials; m, average number of quanta released by each stimulus; p, probability that an active zone releases a quantum; n, number of release sites recorded. Parameter estimates are given $\pm$ S.E. Modified from Zucker (1973).
[b] Denotes a significant increase ($P < 0.05$) by t test of this parameter from its value for the unfacilitated first response.

remained popular among many investigators studying the binomial statistical parameters of synaptic transmission at vertebrate neuromuscular junctions and sympathetic ganglia (Bennett and Florin, 1974; McLachlan, 1975b; Miyamoto, 1975; Bennett et al., 1976; Branisteanu et al., 1976). This characterization of n and p suggests that facilitation consists of an increase in the effectiveness of an impulse in releasing quanta available for release, p, and not a mobilization of quanta into a releasable store, n.

However, if n is associated with a releasable store, it must be reduced immediately after an impulse by the amount of the store just released, and then recover before the next impulse. Otherwise, if n did not fully recover we would expect to see synaptic depression and a reduction in n due to a depletion of the releasable store. Such a depression and change in n was never observed in our experiments. My estimates of n (and those of Johnson and Wernig, 1971; Wernig, 1972a,b, 1975) were only about 2–5 at a single extracellular recording site. Clearly, if n were the releasable store it would then drop considerably after the release of a quantum or two, and there is no reason to expect that it would always recover to exactly the same value. Rather, if there were no other restrictions on n, then n should recover randomly to an average value, and fluctuations in n would arise from the statistics of refilling this releasable store from some larger presynaptic depot store. In fact, one would expect the releasable store to recover in a Poisson manner from its depletion due to release. Then n itself would be a temporally fluctuating Poisson random variable. Vere-Jones (1966) showed that if the releasable store recovers in a Poisson manner, release itself will be Poisson. This contradicts our results.

These problems drove me to consider a different formulation for n and p. A binomial process is one in which some constraint fixes the maximum number of quanta that can be released. We have seen that there are difficulties in conceiving of this as some ill-defined releasable store. Perhaps some other presynaptic structure limits the number of releasable quanta. Anatomical studies of neuromuscular junctions show that synaptic vesicles are clustered at discrete release sites or active zones, which appear to be the points of transmitter release. What if each active zone can release only one quantum in response to a nerve impulse? Then if our microelectrode records from a cluster of n active zones, a response could contain at most n quanta. Vere-Jones (1966) showed that such a system leads to a binomial statistical process for m, where n will correspond to the total number of release sites and p will be the probability that one of them releases a quantum.

Ultrastructural work (Atwood and Morin, 1970) showing that there are about 2–5 active zones along a nerve branch within recording distance of an external microelectrode supports this model. Furthermore, Atwood and Parnas (1968) and Atwood and Johnston (1968) reported that at a number of crustacean neuromuscular junctions the evoked and spontaneous quantal units often fell into two or more distinct populations according to size and shape. This again suggests that a microelectrode at a synaptic site records quantal releases from several distinct release sites. Atwood often found that at most one quantum of each type could be released by a nerve impulse. If n is determined by the anatomically defined number of active zones, it is no wonder that only p changes during facilitation.

We may ask how a change in p comes about. If p is the probability that a release site releases a quantum, p would be influenced by both the probability that a release site is occupied by a releasable quantum, p_{occ}, and the probability that a spike is effective in activating a release site, p_{eff}. Vere-Jones (1966) formulated this situation by observing that a fixed number of release sites will be refilled according to a binomial process with parameters n and p_1, where p_1 is the probability that an unoccupied release site becomes filled between stimuli. Now the probability that a site releases a quantum will be the product of the probabilities that it is occupied, p_{occ}, and that it is activated by an impulse, p_{eff} (p_2 in the notation of Zucker, 1973). The probability that a site is occupied at a given moment depends on the probability that it was refilled since the last impulse p_1 and also on the probability that it was available for refilling at the last impulse, i.e., on whether it was emptied by the last impulse, which depends on p_2. In fact, $p_{occ} = p_1/[1-(1-p_1)(1-p_2)]$. Then $p = p_{occ}p_{eff} = p_1p_2/[1-(1-p_1)(1-p_2)]$, and release will be binomial, with $m = pn$.

Another way to formulate this is to consider $m = p_{eff}n_{rel}$, where $n_{rel} = p_{occ}n$ is the average number of occupied release sites or of immediately releasable quanta. This number must be less than n and cannot be estimated from a binomial statistical analysis. It may, however, be estimated from the properties of depression at synapses showing a depression due to depletion (see below). It is interesting that at such synapses the estimate of n_{rel} from depression is less than n measured statistically (Christensen and Martin, 1970).

Is there no way to attribute changes in p to either p_{occ} or p_{eff} from statistical data? Vere-Jones (1966) noted that if release sites are not refilled completely between impulses, then a large release will most likely be followed by a smaller one, and *vice versa*. In fact, an equation for the covariance of successive responses can be solved simultaneously with the above expression for p to get p_1 and p_2. When I measured the covariance of successive responses, it was negligibly different from zero, which means that either p_{occ} or p_{eff} equals 1 and that the other is entirely responsible for facilitation. The absence of depression and the fact that facilitation is maximal immediately after an impulse suggest that p_{eff} is the determining factor, but this is far from proven.

Although we have not explained much about facilitation, the statistical results do suggest some factors that may be at work in limiting quantal release. A necessary requirement for n release sites to generate a binomial with the same parameter n is that each active zone can release only one quantum. Perhaps the rows of vesicles in active zones (Couteaux and Pécot-Dechavassine, 1974) are queuing up for a molecular release site at one point in each zone, or possibly an active zone can accommodate only the membrane surrounding one vesicle (*cf.* Heuser and Reese, 1973). Such possibilities are suggested if we believe that one quantum consists of the release of the contents of one synaptic vesicle. On the other hand, one quantum may consist of the simultaneous release of the contents of those few vesicles attached to the terminal membrane at an active zone. Then variations in quantal effectiveness would be due in part to variations in the number of vesicles contributing to a quantum (Kriebel and Gross, 1974). It is not possible at present to distinguish between these and other intriguing possibilities.

It could also be that our extracellular recordings are made from only one release site. Then n would correspond to the maximum number of quanta releasable from an active zone and might correspond to the number of vesicle attachment sites (Dreyer *et al.*, 1973). However, for the reasons cited above, I think it is unlikely that we are recording from only one release site.

These results differ markedly from those obtained at vertebrate sympathetic ganglia and neuromuscular junctions (Bennett and Florin, 1974; Bennett *et al.*, 1975, 1976; McLachlan, 1975*a*; Branisteanu *et al.*, 1976). There facilitation is frequently accompanied by changes in n, more so than in p. However, crucial differences in method prevent any detailed comparison between crustacean and vertebrate results. The latter analyses all estimated p and n from the variance and mean of the intracellularly recorded epp or epsp amplitude distribution. This method is subject to numerous uncertainties which have not been properly considered in most of these studies.

For example:

1. The quanta composing an epsp sum nonlinearly, but the Martin (1955) correction does not take adequate account of the effect of membrane capacitance on the summation of transient potentials (Martin, 1976).

2. The variance method of statistical analysis must correct the epsp variance for the variance in quantal unit magnitude. It is usually assumed that this can be estimated from the amplitude histogram of mepsp's. However, there is evidence that the evoked quantum and the spontaneously released quantum are not always the same (Highstein and Bennett, 1975), especially under the conditions in which many of the statistical experiments were performed (Dennis and Miledi, 1974; Bennett and Pettigrew, 1975).

3. Souček (1971) has shown that the fluctuations in latency of quantal release times can contribute significantly to the coefficient of variation of an epsp. Considering the known fluctuations in quantal latency, the effective amplitude of noncoincidental summed quanta will be less than 80% of the quantal size. From the theory developed by Williams and Bowen (1974), it can be shown that this leads to a 20% overestimate of p.

4. An intracellular recording from a whole neuromuscular junction is likely to sample from a wider diversity of synaptic sites with different p than an extracellular recording from a single terminal. A spatial nonuniformity in p would result in a serious overestimation of p (Brown et al., 1976). The latter effect could explain, in part, why Wernig's (1975) estimates of p using the variance method were considerably larger than, often double, the estimates based on direct counting of quanta. They may also explain the remarkably large values of p, often approaching unity, that have been reported in vertebrate junctions (Bennett and Florin, 1974; McLachlan, 1975a,b; Bennett et al., 1976).

Actually, a nonuniformity in p is likely to be present even at our extracellular recording sites. The resulting underestimation of n explains the occasional observation of more than n quanta in a response. However, Hatt and Smith (1976b) have shown that a large variance in p is likely to lead to a departure from binomial statistics that is detectable when quanta can be counted directly and n is small. These effects are likely to be exaggerated in intracellular recordings from many terminals, but will be more difficult to detect when m is large (Brown et al., 1976).

Increases in n estimated in vertebrate experiments as a correlate of facilitation, and changes in calcium and magnesium concentrations, have led some authors to doubt that n could be determined by a fixed number of release sites in their experiments. They propose that n reflects a releasable store of transmitter quanta. This implies either that transmitter release at these synapses is not limited by a fixed number of release sites or that an active zone can release a variable number of quanta. However, changes in estimates of n could be caused entirely by changes in factors which confound estimates of n and p. For example, if all values of p were increased by a certain amount at a population of release sites with nonuniform p, a large, spurious increase in the estimate of n would result, even though the actual number of release sites remains constant (Brown et al., 1976). As the estimate of p (also erroneous) approaches unity, apparent changes in n can occur without any further significant changes in the estimate of p. Thus the estimates of n and p

derived from epsp amplitude fluctuations may bear no simple relationship to the actual values of n and p of the underlying binomial statistical process.

These statistical studies prompted a series of experiments to determine what process might be responsible for increasing p during facilitation. Early studies (Dudel and Kuffler, 1961a; Dudel, 1965b) suggested that facilitation might be caused by an increase in the amplitude of the electrotonically conducted presynaptic impulse into inexcitable terminals. However, I (Zucker, 1974a) found that most MN terminals are locally excitable, and that orthdromic nerve terminal potentials contained prominent negative phases indicating that the terminals were actively invaded. When care was taken to avoid artifacts due to nonspecific muscle currents (Katz and Miledi, 1965), muscle movement, and the averaging of nonsynchronous nerve potentials, then no consistent change in nerve terminal potential was seen to accompany facilitation (see also Ortiz, 1972; Lang and Atwood, 1973) (Fig. 2).

Another possibility was that facilitation was caused by an accumulation of intracellular sodium or extracellular potassium during nerve impulses. These ideas were tested by blocking nerve transmission with tetrodotoxin and by eliciting transmitter release by depolarizing a fine nerve branch or a small patch of nerve membrane (Katz and Miledi, 1967a,b). When the parameters of the pulse were adjusted to release as much transmitter as a nerve impulse, it was found that patterns of repeated identical depolarizing pulses caused facilitation of synaptic transmission that was remarkably similar to that caused by similar patterns of repeated nerve impulses (Fig. 3). This confirmed the conclusion that facilitation is not caused by an increase in the presynaptic electrical signal, and also showed that it occurs in the absence of the sodium influx accompanying nerve impulses. That facilitation was not due to an accumulation of extracellular potassium was shown by the fact that increased potassium decreases transmitter release (Zucker, 1974c).

Another hypothesis often put forward to account for synaptic facilitation is that it might be caused by hyperpolarizing afterpotentials in nerve terminals following

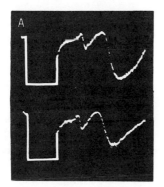
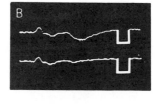

Fig. 2. Facilitation of synaptic transmission with unchanging nerve terminal potentials. Averaged extracellular recordings from two synaptic sites stimulated at 10 Hz (upper traces) and at 5 Hz (lower trace in A) or 1 Hz (lower trace in B). Calibration pulses (retouched): 100 μV, 5 msec (A) or 1 msec (B). From Zucker (1974a).

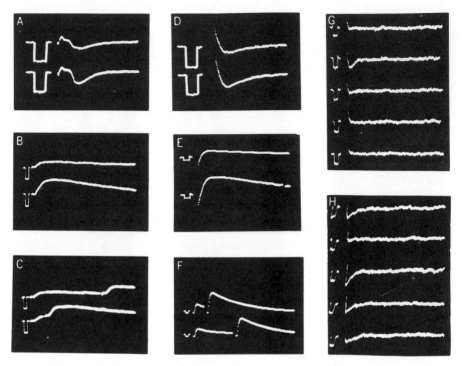

Fig. 3. Facilitated transmitter release evoked by nerve impulses (A–C) and constant nerve-depolarizing pulses (D–H). Averaged responses are recorded extracellularly from a synaptic site in A, D, G, and H, and intracellularly from a muscle fiber in B, C, E, and F. Frequency of stimulation: 2 Hz (upper traces) and 10 Hz (lower traces) in A, B, D, and E. C and F show paired intracellular responses to spikes (C) and pulses (F). On the right is a series of extracellular responses to depolarizing pulses at 1 Hz (G) and 10 Hz (H), showing that the facilitated averaged responses are due to an increase in the average number of quanta released. Calibration pulses: 200 μV, 5 msec. From Zucker (1974a).

stimulation. Dudel (1971) has already shown that artificial hyperpolarization of nerve terminals increased the amount of transmitter released by nerve impulses at claw opener synapses.

Since the state of polarization in nerve can be assessed by measuring its excitation threshold to extracellular currents (Wall, 1958), I set about measuring the postactivation recovery of excitability at MN terminals. To my surprise, the brief refractory period was followed by a period of supernormal excitability corresponding to a depolarizing afterpotential in claw opener terminals (see also Dudel, 1973). This supernormal period was larger following a tetanus, present only in terminals, enhanced by steady nerve hyperpolarization and in potassium-free medium, and abolished by enzymes which digest the connective tissue binding nerve to muscle (Figs. 4 and 5). All these properties are consistent with a depolarizing afterpotential generated by a transient accumulation of potassium ions around nerve terminals (Zucker, 1974c). However, Dudel (1971) showed that depolarization of MN terminals could only decrease the effectiveness of an impulse in releasing transmitter.

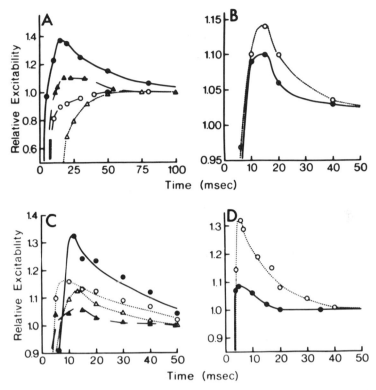

Fig. 4. Postactivation excitability changes in claw opener MN terminals. A: A supernormal excitability is present in all nerve terminals at synaptic sites (●), in some (▲) but not most (○) fine nerve branches, and not in the main axon (△). B: It is larger following a tetanus (○) than one impulse (●). C: It is enhanced in potassium-free medium (●) and reduced in high-potassium medium (▲) compared to normal crayfish saline (○, △). D: It is reduced by proteolytic enzymes (○, before, and ●, after, treatment). From Zucker (1974c).

The hyperpolarization required by the afterpotential hypothesis of facilitation just doesn't seem to be present in crayfish MN terminals.

Next I considered the hypothesis put forward by Katz and Miledi (1968), Rahamimoff (1968), and Miledi and Thies (1971) that facilitation is caused by an intracellular accumulation of calcium or some calcium complex in nerve terminals following stimulation. It is known that calcium enters the nerve terminal during an impulse (Katz and Miledi, 1967a,c) and that calcium injected intracellularly triggers transmitter release (Miledi, 1973). It was also shown that at the frog neuromuscular junction the facilitating effect of an impulse on transmitter release by subsequent impulses was dependent on calcium being present in the medium, and presumably on the calcium influx accompanying an impulse (Katz and Miledi, 1968). Thus one had only to suppose that some of the calcium entering a nerve during a spike

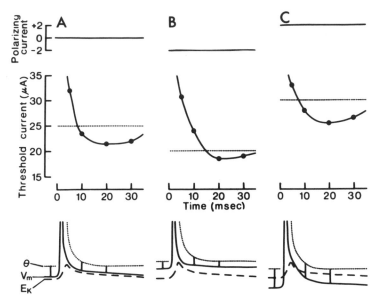

Fig. 5. A: Threshold changes following an impulse in the absence of polarizing current. Depolarization (B) reduces the postactivation period of subnormal threshold; hyperpolarization (C) increases it. Dotted lines on threshold graphs indicate preactivation threshold. Bottom drawings show how a depolarizing afterpotential would affect the extracellular current threshold, which is proportional to the difference between membrane potential (V_m) and the membrane voltage threshold (θ). The afterpotential is probably due to an extracellular potassium accumulation and the consequent change in the potassium equilibrium potential (E_K). From Zucker (1974c).

remained present for a time to deduce that facilitation arises as a natural consequence of the other known properties of synaptic transmission.

Specifically, if each spike is accompanied by an influx of calcium of magnitude A, and if at a given time after previous activity an amount B of "active calcium" remained in the nerve terminal, then the peak amount of active calcium achieved following a new nerve impulse would be $A + B$. Then a facilitated response, R', will bear the following simple relation to an unfacilitated response, R: $R'/R = (A + B)^n/A^n$. Here the exponent n allows for a nonlinear relationship between calcium entry, A, and transmitter release. Since A should be proportional to the external calcium concentration, this fits the finding of a nonlinear (power law) relation between transmitter release and external calcium at frog neuromuscular junctions (Dodge and Rahamimoff, 1967).

In this model, the decay of facilitation following an impulse depends on the decay of residual calcium, B. If n is known from the calcium dependence of transmitter release, the equation allows the prediction of the growth of facilitation during repetitive stimulation, and its subsequent decline from the time course of facilitation following an impulse (Linder, 1973; Younkin, 1974).

In crayfish, a linear relation exists between external calcium concentration and transmitter release (Bracho and Orkand, 1970; Ortiz and Bracho, 1972) even when the calcium is buffered to low levels (Zucker, 1974*b*). With $n = 1$, a linear summation of the facilitating effects of successive impulses is expected. This has not been found (Fig. 6). At highly facilitating synapses, facilitation accumulates more than expected (Zucker, 1974*b*; Linder, 1974; Bittner and Sewell, 1976); however, at synapses showing less facilitation, accumulation is less than linear (Bittner and Sewell, 1976). The latter effect could indicate a saturation of transmitter release at high release levels, as seen before in high calcium concentrations (Rahamimoff, 1968; Zucker, 1974*b*). The former very large growth of facilitation is difficult to explain.

Another difficulty arises from a consideration of the factors which determine the removal of *B*. In one version of the calcium accumulation model (Katz and Miledi, 1968; Miledi and Thies, 1971), *B* is removed by nonlinear rate kinetics. One consequence of this idea is that *B* (and hence facilitation) will decline more rapidly after a tetanus, when *B* is high, than after one spike. This prediction was not confirmed—facilitation declines with the same time course after a tetanus as after one impulse (Zucker, 1974*b*; Linder, 1974). A second consequence of nonlinear *B*

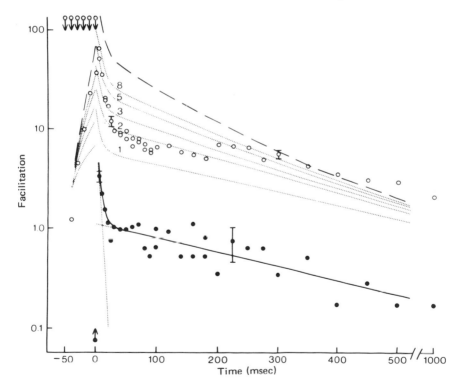

Fig. 6. Time course of facilitation of synaptic transmission following one impulse (●) and during and following a brief tetanus (○). Facilitation is measured as the fractional increase in amplitude of a test response over that of an unfacilitated response. The decay of facilitation can be fitted by a curve which is the sum of two exponentials (note logarithmic ordinate). The dotted lines are the predicted curves for tetanic facilitation and its decay, assuming the values of *n* indicated. The dashed line is the prediction if facilitation is a multiplicative process. From Zucker (1974*b*).

kinetics is that B becomes nearly independent of external calcium, thus accounting for the calcium independence of posttetanic changes in mepp frequency (Miledi and Thies, 1971). But A is dependent on external calcium, and hence so should facilitation be. However, I found facilitation to be calcium independent (Zucker, 1974b), as in the crab (Linder, 1973). These difficulties are not present in a second version of the calcium accumulation model in which B is removed by a series of linear rate processes (Rahamimoff, 1968). Then B and A have the same calcium dependence and facilitation becomes calcium independent (see above equation), and the time course of the removal of B will be independent of the level of facilitation.

Another aspect of the linear summation model is that, as calcium accumulates to cause facilitation, it should also enhance the spontaneous release of transmitter. When a power law governs the calcium dependence of transmitter release, a small residuum of active calcium has little effect on mepp frequency, while its incremental effect on the peak calcium level reached following a spike may cause considerable facilitation (Miledi and Thies, 1971; Barrett and Stevens, 1972). In crayfish, however, a linear calcium dependence of release requires that, if facilitation reaches a level of $R'/R = 5$, then transmitter would be released spontaneously at a rate 4 times greater than the evoked rate of transmitter release for an unfacilitated response! This extraordinary conclusion is emphatically contradicted by the results. Miniature frequency may even deline during facilitation (Dudel and Kuffler, 1961b).

One way out of all these contradictions is to suppose that the linear relation between calcium and transmitter release is misleading. Parnas et $al.$ (1975) have found evidence for a calcium-dependent tonic release of inhibitory transmitter, which acts both pre- and postsynaptically at crab neuromuscular junctions. They found that the calcium dependence of excitatory transmitter release was partially masked by the calcium dependence of tonic presynaptic inhibition. It follows that increasing calcium not only increased excitatory transmitter release evoked by impulses but also increased the level of tonic presynaptic inhibition. When picrotoxin was added to block inhibition, the calcium dependence of excitatory transmission was seen to be quite nonlinear.

It is unlikely that this effect is confounding the crayfish results. Parnas et $al.$ (1975) found that picrotoxin increased the postsynaptic input resistance and the size of ejp's. No such effect was observed at the crayfish junctions (Takeuchi and Takeuchi, 1969). Even if n is greater than 1, there was no value of n which could predict the accumulative properties of facilitation by the above model (Fig. 6). Also, if it is supposed that n calcium ions are needed to form an active complex and that it is this complex, not calcium, which accumulates, then again a linear summation of facilitation is predicted (Magleby, 1973a), which is contrary to what is observed.

Another hypothesis is that calcium acts at a different site to trigger facilitation than the site where calcium entering during an impulse acts to evoke release (Balnave and Gage, 1974; Cooke and Quastel, 1973). Then the cumulative effects of facilitation should be multiplicative. This prediction was also not confirmed by the data (Fig. 6).

We need not abandon entirely the idea that calcium accumulation is responsible for facilitation. It may be that residual calcium neither adds to a constant calcium influx in a spike nor conditions the nerve response to that influx. Rather, residual calcium may affect the magnitude of that influx itself, and this effect could be responsible for facilitation. An increase in calcium influx during successive impulses has been observed in *Aplysia* somata (Stinnakre and Tauc, 1973). It remains to be shown whether this increase is in any way related to the accumulation of calcium or a calcium complex.

Long-Term Facilitation

Another type of facilitation seen at crayfish claw opener and other crustacean neuromuscular junctions has been studied by Atwood and his colleagues. Sherman and Atwood (1971*b*) reported that continuous stimulation of a MN at 5–20 Hz led to a progressive increase in synaptic transmission, growing to many times its short-term facilitated amplitude during the course of an hour. This effect persisted for several hours after cessation of stimulation. This long-term facilitation, which is clearly presynaptic in origin (Atwood *et al.*, 1975), appears parametrically similar to tetanic and posttetanic potentiation at vertebrate neuromuscular junctions (Magleby, 1973*a,b*; Magleby and Zengel, 1975*a,b*).

Long-term facilitation seems to be a consequence of an increase of intracellular sodium during tetanic stimulation. When sodium loading is reduced in low-sodium medium, long-term facilitation is reduced or absent (Sherman and Atwood, 1971*b*; Atwood *et al.*, 1975). Conversely, when sodium loading is enhanced by blocking the sodium pump, long-term facilitation is markedly enhanced and accelerated. None of these effects was observed in vertebrate posttetanic potentiation (Gage and Hubbard, 1966). The latter is highly dependent on calcium entry during a tetanus (Rosenthal, 1969; Weinreich, 1971). In crayfish, long-term facilitation can be elicited in a calcium-free saline or when calcium influx is blocked (Swenarchuk and Atwood, 1975). Thus, unlike vertebrate posttetanic potentiation, crustacean long-term facilitation appears to be due specifically to a sodium accumulation in nerve terminals. It is possible the sodium acts by activating a sodium–calcium exchange pump during the test period (Baker *et al.*, 1969) or by releasing calcium from mitochondria (Alnaes and Rahamimoff, 1975). In that case, the sodium loading may indirectly promote a residual calcium, which may then act in the same manner as in short-term facilitation.

Short-Term Depression

Hatt and Smith (1976*a*) have found a short-lasting depression at walking leg opener junctions of European crayfish *(Astacus leptodactylus)*, using the same sort of stimulus regimen which evokes only long-term facilitation in North American crayfish *(Procambarus clarkii)*. The depression develops only after several minutes of stimulation of 10–20 Hz, but the effect dissipates within a few seconds if stimulation is halted. A similar depression has been observed at neuromuscular junctions onto fast abdominal extensor muscles in lobsters and crayfish (Parnas, 1972).

Recording extracellularly from synaptic sites, Hatt and Smith (1976a) and Parnas (1972) found that failures of transmission were often associated with a sudden loss of the nerve terminal potential. Thus the depression is due, at least in part, to an intermittent presynaptic conduction failure—a block of invasion of MN terminals.

Hatt and Smith (1976a,b) performed a statistical analysis on the postsynaptic responses in *Astacus* and found that binomial statistics usually provided the best description of the results. When they compared the statistics of depressed responses to undepressed (and facilitated) responses, they found that, even for selected responses in which the nerve terminal potential was present, m and p were reduced, and sometimes so was n. They suggest that the reason p was reduced was that responses which follow those containing conduction failures are essentially responses to a lower effective frequency. Thus facilitation will have decayed, reducing p and therefore m. They tested this hypothesis by comparing responses following a transmission failure to those not following a transmission failure. The former group were larger and had a larger m and p. Therefore, depression is due in part to an intermittent presynaptic conduction failure at some MN terminals, and in part to a defacilitation of responses following such failures.

The reduction in n is harder to explain. The results of Brown *et al.* (1976) show that if p is nonuniform, changes in the distribution of p will probably be associated with similar changes in the estimate of n. Hatt and Smith (1976b) have presented evidence for such a nonuniformity in p at this synapse, so the changes in n may be entirely artifactual.

Long-Term Depression

A more persistent form of synaptic depression has been observed at the neuromuscular junctions of the giant MN of crayfish (Kennedy and Takeda, 1965a). These synapses show a long-lasting depression extraordinary for neuromuscular junctions (Bruner and Kennedy, 1970) but comparable to that of central synapses known to be responsible for behavioral habituation (Kandel *et al.*, 1970; Zucker, 1972a). Recently J. Bruner and I have tried to determine the mechanism responsible for this depression.

The usual model put forward to account for synaptic depression is that there is a depletion of the store of transmitter available for release as a consequence of previous release from this store (Liley and North, 1953; Hubbard, 1970). In this model, recovery from depression reflects the mobilization of transmitter into the releasable store from a depot store—or the rate of refilling of unoccupied release sites, p_1. The initial level of depression, measured as the percentage reduction of the response to an impulse immediately following an undepressed response, can be used to estimate the fraction of the releasable store liberated by an impulse (p_2 or p_{eff}). We found that, on the average, a single impulse was followed by a 60–70% depression which recovered exponentially with a time constant of about 4.5 min. The exponential recovery suggests that simple first-order kinetics apply to a refilling of the releasable store. From these parameters, one can predict the time course and steady state of depression expected for any frequency of stimulation. We found that the model predicted depression adequately for stimuli repeated once every 5 min or more, but the data diverged markedly from the predictions at frequencies of 1/min or higher (Fig. 7). Tetanic depression was not nearly as large as expected. The same steady-state level was reached at all frequencies between 1/min and 4 Hz.

One possibility is that during repeated stimulation the rate of mobilization (refilling the releasable store) is increased over that following a single impulse (Kusano and Landau, 1975). In that event, recovery from depression following a tetanus would be faster than following one impulse. However, when we compared

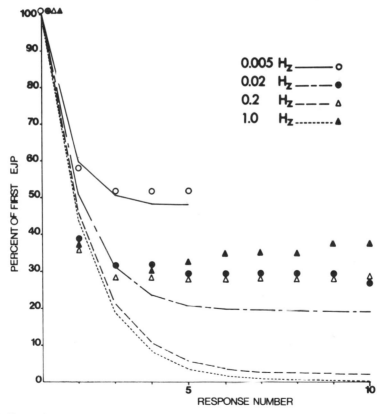

Fig. 7. Successive ejp amplitudes (symbols) in fast flexor muscles to repeated motor giant impulses at the frequencies shown. The lines are predictions of depression based on a depletion model and the recovery from depression following one impulse. From Bruner and Zucker (unpublished).

these recovery rates in a group of seven fibers, we found no difference. We also found that depression immediately following a tetanic response was much less (only 33%) than that following an undepressed response (65%). This result also contradicts the depletion hypothesis.

The hallmark of the depletion hypothesis is that reducing transmitter release alleviates depression by reducing depletion. If the magnesium concentration in the medium is increased sufficiently to reduce transmission to 25%, then the fraction of store released by an impulse should be reduced to one-fourth (Wernig, 1972b), and depression should be similarly reduced. In fact, we found that depression was unaffected by this treatment (Fig. 8). This result stands in stark contrast to the behavior of other examples of synaptic depression (e.g., Thies, 1965; Elmqvist and Quastal, 1965; Betz, 1970; Kusana and Landau, 1975).

It still remained possible that the high-magnesium solution interfered with the mobilization process. Then transmitter would have recovered less between stimuli

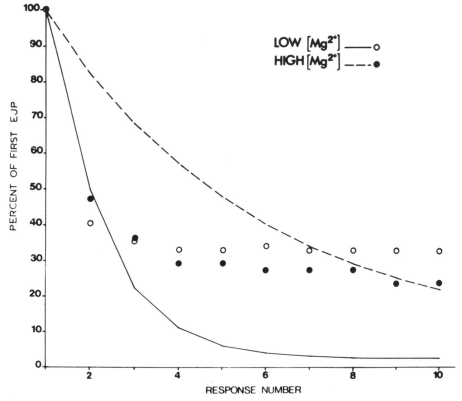

Fig. 8. Successive ejp amplitudes (symbols) to motor giant impulses every 5 sec in high and low magnesium concentrations. The first response in high magnesium was 28% of that in low magnesium. The predictions from the depletion hypothesis are also shown (lines). From Bruner and Zucker (unpublished).

than we had predicted. However, we found no effect of changing the magnesium concentration on the rate of recovery from long-term depression.

In summary, we were unable to confirm any of the predictions of this model and were forced to reject the depletion hypothesis, even in modified form (Betz, 1970; Friesen, 1975), as a satisfactory model for depression at the motor giant neuromuscular junctions. We do not know what may be responsible for this depression. We were unable to record extracellularly from synaptic sites long enough to do a quantal analysis during depression. The absence of distinguishable mjp's in intracellular recordings also precludes a quantal analysis, so we do not even know for sure that the depression arises presynaptically. Clearly, further work is needed to explain this interesting form of synaptic depression.

Other Kinds of Nerve-Induced Modifiability

Besides facilitation and depression, at least two other processes may mediate a modulation of muscle by nerve in crustaceans. Rathmayer and Florey (1974*a,b*) found that ejp's recorded from the closer muscles in a variety of crab species were reduced for several minutes following a brief high-frequency burst of impulses in the inhibitor MN to the muscle. This postinhibitory depression is thought to be presynaptic in origin, because the postsynaptic increase in conductance caused by the inhibitor activity lasted only a few seconds after the inhibitory tetanus.

A very different type of nerve–muscle interaction has been discovered by Evans *et al.* (1975). They have found peripheral neurons in lobster which appear to secrete octopamine into the bloodstream. Searching for an effect of the neurohumor, they observed that octopamine elicits a long-lasting contracture of the lobster leg opener muscle and enhances the tension developed during excitatory nerve stimulation. Octopamine has no effect on muscle membrane potential or on the amplitude of ejp's or ijp's. Apparently, octopamine acts at some other point in the muscle, perhaps modifying the chemical reactions that control muscle contraction.

These examples serve to illustrate the variety and subtlety of the long-term control of muscle by nerve and the plastic nature of the usual neuromuscular interaction. We have a long way to go before these processes are understood in biophysical and biochemical terms. At least we have begun the task.

ACKNOWLEDGMENTS

Much of this work was performed during the author's tenure as a Helen Hay Whitney Fellow in Professor Bernard Katz's laboratory at University College London and in Dr. Lladislav Tauc's C.N.R.S. laboratory in Gif-sur-Yvette, France. Recent work was supported by a U.S.P.H.S. Biomedical Science Grant to the University of California.

4

Crustacean Motor Neurons

William H. Evoy

Introduction

Coordinated movements responsible for the overt behavior of animals all involve specific temporal patterns of activity in motor neurons (MNs). Although considerable summation of excitatory and inhibitory influences is present at the neuromuscular junctions of many invertebrates, particularly arthropods, initiation and control of muscle contraction are due to activity in excitatory and inhibitory MNs. Because MNs convey discrete programs for movement to the muscles, monitoring of their subthreshold and spike discharges during expression of behavior provides for the most convenient analysis of control of locomotion and posture.

Activity of MNs that are involved in a wide variety of behaviors has been examined in different crustaceans under conditions ranging from full constraint to free movement, but generally with the aim of understanding the factors that contribute to the program controlling the movements. There are many studies of changes in MN discharge in response to a variety of experimental manipulations, including selected stimulation of peripheral sources of sensory input (reflexes), central stimulation (command interneurons), and as a result of rhythmic activity in endogenous sources of activity (oscillators). Most of these concepts derived from work by Professor Wiersma and his co-workers over a 15-year period starting about 1950. In a brief summary, Wiersma (1952a) provided the provocative suggestion that complex movements of crustaceans could be controlled by changes in excitability of a single central neuron. Subsequent detailed studies on the sensory, motor, and central nervous integrative aspects of controlled movements in several crustacean species in Wiersma's laboratory and elsewhere have substantiated this idea and incorporated it into an emerging principle that cellular components of the nervous system operate as integrative parts of a complex but remarkably precise system.

We have a general picture of the essential features of crustacean MNs from correlation of the morphological and physiological studies to date. The basic morphology of these neurons has been known from the work of early morphologists such as Bethe (1897a,b), Retzius (1890), and Allen (1894), who stained ganglia with methylene blue. Major features of most MNs include a cell body, usually

William H. Evoy • Department of Biology, University of Miami, Coral Gables, Florida 33124.

located ventrally in the ganglion, and a connection via a fiber process, or neurite, to extensively branched fibers in the central and more dorsal regions of the neuropil. MNs can generally be distinguished from interneurons (INs) by an extension of the fiber processes, the axon, which exits via one of the ganglionic roots of the neuropil. In some cases, the cell body and all of the branches are located on one side of a ganglion; in other cases, the cell body and at least some of the processes are located contralaterally to the side from which the axon exits. Morphological and physiological evidence shows that the cell bodies are devoid of synaptic contacts. No fibers are seen in the region of the cell bodies, and intracellular recordings generally reveal attenuated spikes, usually not more than 5–10 mV in amplitude, that appear to be due to passive electrotonic spread from active regions elsewhere in the cell. Recent studies in which cells of physiological interest are routinely filled with markers such as procion dyes, cobalt ions, or horseradish peroxidase have helped greatly in the identification of the cells and their locations and have added details to the picture of the general morphology. Electron microscopy reveals that the neuropil region is heavily endowed with synaptic contacts between small fiber branches, and it is likely that staining of individual cells by techniques that show up in electron microscopic preparations will reveal significant features of synaptic morphology in identified neurons (Atwood and Pomeranz, 1974). The general picture is that synaptic inputs from INs and perhaps from sensory cells onto the MNs occur at the branching fiber processes in the neuropil. Potential changes evoked by local changes in membrane conductance spread electrotonically to an impulse-initiating zone (IIZ) somewhere along the main fiber process. This crude scheme needs a great deal of testing. Branches of the fibers set up actively propagating impulses that contribute to the final spiking pattern, as discussed in the next section. Some MNs in the stomatogastric ganglion have pacemaker properties that generate rhythmic spike discharges (Maynard and Selverston, 1975). Crustacean and other arthropod MNs clearly possess integrative properties at least as complex as those of vertebrate MNs. Productive investigations in the future will no doubt combine findings on the morphological and functional aspects of integration in the neuropil of arthropod ganglia to develop models of summation at the IIZ similar to those of Rall (1967) and Barrett (1975) for the vertebrate anterior horn cell. Before we can attempt such detailed studies, we must develop better preparations for analysis of the synaptic inputs to certain MNs, and methods for controlling these inputs for experimental study.

This chapter is an attempt to assess some of what is now known about integration by crustacean MNs identified as to function in producing observable movements, particularly those that are involved in posture and locomotion.

Mechanisms of Integration in Identified MNs

The usual morphological and physiological procedures for identifying the location of central processes of motor neurons can be applied successfully to Crustacea.

Antidromic stimulation of peripheral motor axons yields a constant-latency action potential in the neuropil processes or a generally greatly attenuated potential in the soma. It is common to assume that the ability of the intracellularly recorded responses to follow antidromic stimuli at frequencies greater than 100 Hz is an indication that a chemical synapse does not mediate the response, although there is not sufficient information regarding transmission onto MNs from presynaptic cells to assure the validity of this criterion. The waveform of the responses to antidromic stimulation does little to aid in distinguishing between postsynaptic potentials and electronic spike components. Antidromic responses recorded in the soma may have total durations as long as 15 msec, with a rise time considerably shorter than the decay phase, as is typical of epsp's (Treistman and Remler, 1975). If the responses are constant in amplitude, one can be somewhat more confident that they are not epsp's, which normally vary in amplitude because of variations in quantal content, facilitation, or antifacilitation.

It is sometimes possible to evoke spike activity by depolarization in the soma or, more commonly, in a neuropil process, and look for constant-latency spikes in the peripheral motor axon. In several instances, these procedures have been followed by intracellular dye injections; filling of the peripheral motor axons with the dye verifies that the injected soma is indeed that of the MN. In many instances, where relatively intact preparations are used, a much simpler procedure is sufficient to identify intracellularly recorded spike activity as belonging to a particular functional neuromuscular group. Constant phasing of individual intracellular spikes with units recorded from peripheral nerves or muscle indicates identity of a MN with reasonable certainty. By using implanted electromyogram leads, intracellularly recorded activity can be correlated with activity in a moving limb or body segment if the ganglion can be stabilized adequately. Penetration of fibers in the neuropil is likely to produce at least an initial high-frequency injury discharge, and faithful matching of the peripherally recorded responses makes it unlikely that the centrally recorded potentials are in a cell presynaptic to the MN.

Backfilling of MNs with cobalt or procion dyes is extremely useful for general determination of cell locations, although it generally does not produce so detailed a result as intracellular injections. Location of major geometric features of MNs helps enormously in pursuing the physiological approach and leads to useful suggestions about integrative features of the cells. MNs filled from a purely motor branch to the crayfish walking leg depressor muscle are closely grouped together throughout the major fiber processes and in the location of the cell bodies (Fig. 1C). These cells have much the same appearance as insect MNs (Pitman et al., 1972). The major processes course over the dorsal surface of the neuropil with much branching, join the cell body by an extended neurite, and show a marked crook where they exit via the ganglionic root.

A few speculations are possible regarding the grouping of the cell bodies and fiber processes. Cell bodies of the peripheral inhibitors and some of the excitors of crayfish abdominal muscles are closely grouped contralaterally to their axons (Otsuka et al., 1967; Wine, Mittenthal, and Kennedy, 1974; Treistman and Remler,

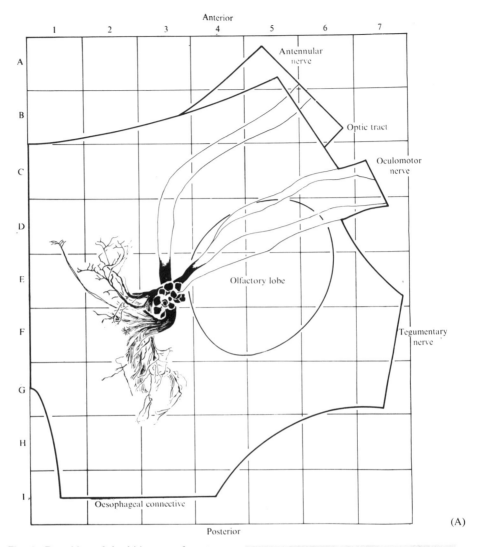

Anterior

| 1 | 2 | 3 | 4 | 5 | 6 | 7 |

A

Antennular
nerve

B

Optic tract

C

Oculomotor
nerve

D

E   Olfactory lobe

F   Tegumentary
                                                     nerve

G

H

I,

Oesophageal connective

Posterior

(A)

Fig. 1. Branching of dendritic trees of crustacean MNs. A: Coincident branching patterns of crab oculomotor neuron dendrites and projections from statocyst thread-hair inputs, as shown by cobalt backfilling of afferent and efferent nerves. Reproduced by permission from Sandeman and Okajima (1973*b*). B: Parallel branching in the dendrites of crayfish tonic abdominal flexor MNs shown by cobalt backfilling of pure motor roots. The dendritic trees of these MNs are bilaterally symmetrical. Reproduced by permission from Wine, Mittenthal, and Kennedy (1974). C: Coincident branching in the dendrites of crayfish walking leg MNs from cobalt backfilling of nerve 2d to the coxopodite depressor muscle. Dendritic branches are ipsilateral to the root of exit and are difficult to distinguish in this photograph because of contiguity. Grid divisions: 250 μm in A, 100 μm in C.

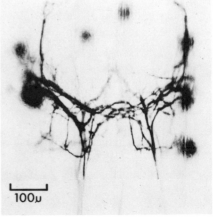

100μ

(B)

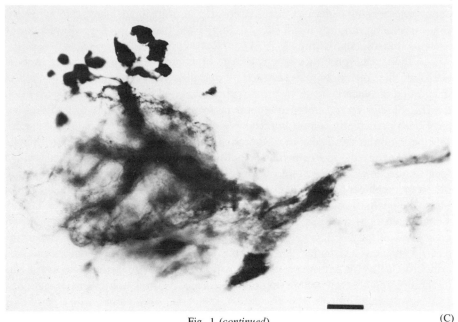

Fig. 1 (*continued*)   (C)

1975), suggestive of common embryological origins of cells that serve similar functions or that innervate the same muscles. Other cell bodies in the abdominal and thoracic ganglia are grouped ipsilaterally. At least some of the MNs that innervate a functional muscle group are likely to share inputs from the same presynaptic cells, and this would be greatly facilitated by a close alliance of the postsynaptic cells in the MN population.

Sandeman (1971) suggests that MNs responsible for eye withdrawal in crabs achieve synchrony of epsp's both from electrical coupling at closely opposed lengths along the axon and by sharing of synapses from common sources at neighboring input regions of the ipsilaterally paired cells. Electrical interactions due to current spread between tightly packed processes may be responsible for some of the phasing between MNs demonstrated by spike-train analysis (Evoy *et al.*, 1967; Tatton and Sokolove, 1975; Wiens and Gerstein, 1975). On the other hand, many of the synaptic contacts from both sensory and interneuronal sources occur at branches of the dendritic trees. Cobalt fills of MNs that control eye movements in nystagmus and simultaneous filling of sensory fibers from the statocysts that provide some of the input to these MNs show that the central projections of the sensory and motor cells in the neuropil are closely coincident (Sandeman and Okajima, 1973*b*) (Fig. 1A). Close phasing of bursts of activity in these MNs is due entirely to the synchronous arrival of the epsp's, presumably at the closely associated dendritic branches in the neuropil. Parallel branching is also typical of other MN populations that form a functional pool to muscles of the abdomen (Wine, Mittenthal, and Kennedy, 1974) and walking legs (Fig. 1B,C). An extension of these ideas on dendritic branching patterns is that functionally separate inputs onto a MN innervate it at morphologically separated sites, as suggested from physiological evidence in insects (Burrows and Horridge, 1974).

Although the processes of crustacean MNs are buried in a complex web of neuropil, their morphology as revealed by dye injections invites a detailed study of integration of synaptic inputs by the fiber branches and summation of the currents at the IIZ. Studies on the crab oculomotor neurons that evoke reflex eye withdrawal have been particularly helpful in providing a beginning of understanding of electrical integration in these cells (Sandeman, 1967, 1969a). These are large cells with peripheral axons 30–50 μm in diameter. Mapping of potentials in these cells with a focal extracellular electrode indicates that the IIZ is removed from the major regions of synaptic contact by about 300 μm. However, in crayfish fast abdominal flexor MNs, the position of the IIZ appears to vary when different presynaptic excitatory sources are stimulated (Takeda and Kennedy, 1964). Synaptic inputs to the neuropilar regions of the fiber evoke electrotonically conducted psp's that spread over the electrically inexcited initial portion of the axon to the IIZ. Thus, spikes initiated orthodromically by excitatory synaptic stimulation fail to actively reinvade the integrating regions where the synapses are located. Correlation of the morphology of dendritic branching from intracellular injections of procion yellow with microelectrode recording of responses to inhibitory and excitatory inputs to the cell provides a general view of the interactions between these inputs that determine the level of depolarization for spike initiation (Sandeman, 1969b). A major part of the summation of depolarization in the integrating segment appears to be due to spikes in side branches in the crab oculomotor cells as well as in the fast flexor MN of the crayfish abdominal ganglia (Takeda and Kennedy, 1964) and in crayfish INs (Takeda and Kennedy, 1965; Calabrese and Kennedy, 1974). The membrane of the integrating segments appears to operate as a low-frequency integrator so that the current reaching the IIZ is smoothed. However, in crab eye movement MNs and nongiant fast flexor MNs of the crayfish abdomen, recordings from the somata also show unitary epsp's (Sandeman and Okajima, 1973b; Takeda and Kennedy, 1964), so there may be additional excitatory inputs that conduct electrotonically to the IIZ as well as to the soma, unaided by dendritic spikes. In neurons of the lobster stomatogastric ganglion, the integrating regions apparently operate as a low-pass filter so that spikes are attenuated far more than psp's in some recordings (Miller, 1975).

Intracellular recording from central fiber processes of MNs of crayfish walking legs shows both epsp's and ipsp's at the same site (Fig. 2). The largest action potentials recorded in the neuropil are about 25 mV, and these become progressively smaller with distance of the recording site from the exiting root. Larger psp's, both inhibitory and excitatory, are found more distant from the root. The study of integration in crayfish leg MNs is just starting, but these appear to be generally similar in physical separation of input and integrating regions and IIZs to other cells. Inhibitory inputs that hyperpolarize the integrating segment decrease the size of the excitatory depolarization, delaying and reducing axonal spike excitability. The inhibitory inputs therefore appear to exert their influences by short-

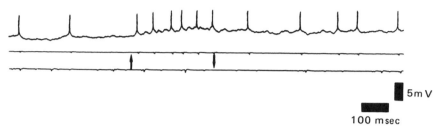

Fig. 2. Intracellularly recorded responses in the dorsal neuropil segment of the slow extensor MN of a crayfish fifth walking leg to imposed movements of the meropodite–carpopodite joint. Flexion of the joint (upward arrow) evokes epsp's, summed depolarization, and increased axonal spike frequency; extension (downward arrow) evokes ipsp's and suppression of spike activity. Traces from top to bottom: intracellular record, extensor myogram, depressor myogram. (Spikes retouched.)

circuiting the summed excitatory inputs from the side branches where they converge at the main integrating segment.

The giant MN to crayfish abdominal fast flexor muscles is unusual in that it lacks extensive branching in the neuropil. Instead, it makes close contact with the four giant INs from which it receives most of its inputs (Kennedy et al., 1969; Selverston and Remler, 1972). Some of the other fast flexor MNs also vary from the general picture in that the soma connects to the main neuropil process by an asymmetrically located neurite, although dendritic trees are often distributed bilaterally. Zucker (1972c) has used an electrical model based on physiological observations of blocking of the orthodromic dendritic spikes in fast flexor nongiant MNs that are evoked by the electrical epsp's set up by presynaptic stimulation of the lateral giant INs. According to this model, the dendritic spikes amplify the synaptic input but are separated from active regions of the axon and soma by points of low safety factor where the dendrites form branches onto the main integrating portion of the cell. Thus, the significance of the very discrete branching patterns of many of these cells is that there are several regions of functionally separated integrative membrane; all make contributions to excitability at the impulse-initiating site and the soma does not contribute to the integrative process (Fig. 3). Eventually this scheme may have to include presynaptic inhibition of excitatory inputs to the MNs such as that found at sensory inputs onto INs in the tail-flip system of crayfish (Kennedy et al., 1974), as well as contributions to impulse generation from electrical junctions. Similar morphologies of the few crustacean MNs studied to date suggest that this model for the integration of synaptic inputs in determining excitability at the IIZ will be generally valid.

The distribution of dendritic branching shows a distinct relation to the type of movement produced by the MNs (Fig. 4). In general, MNs that evoke bilaterally symmetrical movements, such as the slow and fast excitors of the crayfish abdomen and the swimmerets of lobsters, have extensive arborizations in the neuropil of both halves of the ganglion (Davis, 1970; Selverston and Remler, 1972; Wine, Mittenthal, and Kennedy, 1974; Treistman and Remler, 1975). MNs that innervate muscles of appendages that do not show bilaterally coupled movements have dendritic fields

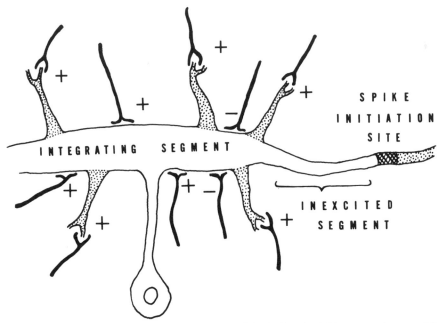

Fig. 3. Generalized model for integration in crustacean MNs. The impulse-initiating zone is removed from the integrating segment by an electrically inexcited segment of axon. At least some of the excitatory inputs sum at the integrating segment from active side-branch spikes. Postsynaptic inhibitory inputs effectively short-circuit the summed depolarization from epsp's and side-branch spikes that contribute to depolarization of the integrating segment. Specific MNs vary in particular respects from parts of this model, and all have more complex architecture than represented here. Stippled areas represent actively propagating membrane of side branches and the axon, clear areas represent the inexcited membrane, and the cross-hatched region represents the impulse-initiating zone of the axon. +, Excitatory synapse; −, inhibitory synapse.

restricted to the neuropil in the half-ganglion from which the axon emerges (Sandeman and Okajima, 1973b; Wilson and Sherman, 1975; Hofmann, 1976).

MN Discharge Patterning

Crustacean MNs vary considerably in the characteristic pattern of discharge that occurs when they are activated by presynaptic inputs or, in a few cases, by pacemaker activity. MNs that are tonically active, or whose levels of discharge are modulated by the inputs to them, provide a wide range of neuromuscular responses but are generally efferent pathways for graded, postural movements. MNs that are normally silent but generate single spikes or short bursts at high stimulation levels are more likely to be involved in rapid movements that are due to activation of twitch-type muscles. Atwood (1973a,b) considered the matching of naturally occurring axonal discharge patterns to neuromuscular and contractile properties and

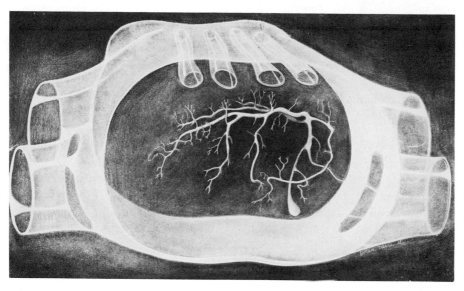

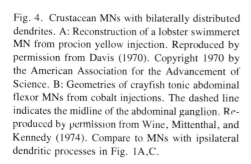

Fig. 4. Crustacean MNs with bilaterally distributed dendrites. A: Reconstruction of a lobster swimmeret MN from procion yellow injection. Reproduced by permission from Davis (1970). Copyright 1970 by the American Association for the Advancement of Science. B: Geometries of crayfish tonic abdominal flexor MNs from cobalt injections. The dashed line indicates the midline of the abdominal ganglion. Reproduced by permission from Wine, Mittenthal, and Kennedy (1974). Compare to MNs with ipsilateral dendritic processes in Fig. 1A,C.

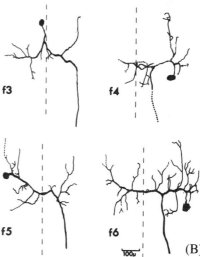

(B)

suggested the term "tonic" for the first type and "phasic" for the second. However, the physiological bases for pattern determination in terms of the relative contributions of inputs to the MNs and membrane properties of the cells themselves have been examined in only a few cases.

Postural adjustments of the crayfish abdomen are controlled by fluctuating levels of activity in the reciprocally active MN populations to two antagonistic sets of tonic muscles, the slow flexors and slow extensors. The central and peripheral components of the slow system for abdominal movements are clearly separated both morphologically and physiologically from the system for rapid movements (Kennedy and Takeda, 1965*a,b;* Parnas and Atwood, 1966). However, in other neuromuscular systems where the MN populations and muscles are not clearly separate, smaller axons are more tonically active and tend to be excited at lower stimulus intensities by both IN and sensory stimulation, whereas larger, more phasic axons require higher stimulus intensities for recruitment. There are not enough quantitative data to validate this idea fully, but the tendency is seen in studies on reflexes in appendages (Bush, 1965*c;* Eckert, 1959; Horridge and Burrows, 1968*a;* Evoy and Cohen, 1969; Vedel and Clarac, 1975; Sandeman, Erber, and Kien, 1975). The order of recruitment from smaller to larger units suggests adherence to the size principle, in which smaller MNs have lower thresholds to comparable presynaptic sources of excitation, due to higher membrane input resistances (Henneman *et al.,* 1965*a,b;* Kernell, 1966; Davis, 1971, 1973*a*). However, the size principle is not followed simplistically in the recruitment of MNs to a given muscle; stimulation of different command INs for tonic abdominal flexion selectively activates different individual MNs (Kennedy *et al.,* 1966; Evoy and Kennedy, 1967).

Gillary and Kennedy (1969*a,b*) found that the largest and least tonic of the crayfish abdominal slow flexor MNs produced pairs (or short bursts) of action potentials due largely to intrinsic properties of the spike-generating mechanism. This pattern was remarkably well adapted to evoke maximal short-term facilitation at the neuromuscular junctions. There is considerable variation in the degree of facilitation at different neuromuscular junctions, but it tends to be more pronounced at terminals of the more tonic MNs (Atwood, 1973*a,b,* and this volume). Thus, bursts with short interspike intervals can favor the buildup of excitation–contraction coupling. In addition to intrinsic membrane properties, various central nervous pathways have different degrees of effectiveness in evoking the patterned discharge in the large flexor MNs as well as tonic discharge in the other MNs to the same muscle (Evoy and Kennedy, 1967). Another tonic MN, the excitor of the claw opener of crayfish, can often be induced to fire paired spikes at its higher average discharge frequencies (Wilson and Davis, 1965). Depolarization of the soma of this cell produces a second spike at a shorter latency than the first (Smith, 1974*b*). The suggestion was made that each spike of the pair could have been generated at an independent initiation site, although it remains to be shown that this cell initiates spikes at separate sites as occurs when the abdominal fast flexor MNs are excited by stimulation of the nerve cord from two different directions (Takeda and Kennedy, 1964).

Smith (1975) pointed out that grouping of spikes into bursts in the opener MN is suitable for recruitment of selected groups of muscle fibers that require high instantaneous frequencies of excitatory input to initiate contraction. He also suggested that rapid bursts could selectively activate the hysteretic properties of tension development of this muscle, in which a high-frequency burst results in a maintained supernormal level of contraction (Wilson and Larimer, 1968; Wilson *et al.,* 1970).

Another approach to characterization of the capabilities of cells for generation of particular impulse patterns is to depolarize the soma or central processes of identified cells with steady currents and examine the resulting spike trains. Not all crustacean MNs generate spikes upon soma depolarization, presumably because of the remoteness of the soma from the IIZ. Depolarization of the soma of nongiant fast flexor MNs generally gives rise to a single spike, although repetitive spikes can be generated in a few cases (Takeda and Kennedy, 1964). Treistman and Remler (1975) encountered difficulty in evoking spike activity in the phasic abdominal extensor MNs by depolarization of the soma; only two of five cells they identified could be driven in this way. Very low-frequency repetition of spiking was observed in these cells when very long depolarizations were applied, but briefer stimuli yielded only single spikes at long latencies. Tonic abdominal MNs, on the other hand, fired repetitively upon soma depolarization (Wine, Mittenthal, and Kennedy, 1974; Treistman and Remler, 1975), although bursts of fixed length were also seen in the slow extensor axons following termination of the stimulus. Tonic spike generation is not restricted to postural MNs. Lobster swimmeret MNs are capable of firing with a variety of discharge patterns depending on the input to them; depolarization of their somata results in repetitive discharges that are steadiest in the smaller cells of the population (Davis, 1971). Preliminary results of direct stimulation of the central fiber processes of crayfish leg MNs indicate that they discharge at frequencies correlated with the intensity of the applied current and that smaller currents than are necessary with soma depolarization are effective (Evoy, in preparation). Wherever technically feasible, depolarization of the integrating region of a MN seems preferable, as it is a closer approximation to normal electrotonic integration than is soma stimulation. No two MNs respond in exactly the same way to similar inputs, nor are any two cells likely to receive precisely the same input. In the final analysis, it is likely that the discharge of a MN is determined by some combination of its synaptic input and its impulse-generating capabilities.

MNs as Components of Functional Systems for Movement

Integration at the level of the MNs themselves in any complex system is likely to include many or all of the features of synaptic interaction that are known today, as well as mechanisms yet to be discovered. In a very restricted network such as the stomatogastric ganglion of the spiny lobster, a variety of connection features are found, including lateral inhibitory synaptic connections, excitatory synaptic inputs, electrotonic coupling, pacemaker activity, and inhibitory synapses that are functional without presynaptic spike activity (see Selverston and Mulloney, 1974b; Selverston, 1976, and this volume). The morphologies, electrical activity, and integrative features of the 23 identified MNs in that system are sufficiently similar to what is known about neurons in less well-understood systems such as those involved in locomotion, ventilation, and eye movements that we can anticipate some common features of network organization. MN populations that supply functionally coordinated muscle groups are often not much larger than in the stomatogastric system, which coordinates the activity of about 40 individual muscles. However, in most of the other systems under study, the sites of input and integration are located in larger central ganglia in association with other functional networks. For this reason, it is unlikely that connectivity in many motor systems will be as readily analyzed as in the small peripheral ganglia. A more productive approach is to try to isolate functional aspects of control involving identifiable MNs and to explore, in a systematic manner, the inputs and outputs at appropriate points in the system.

A control-systems approach to integration of motor function, in some cases, allows predictions of functional sensory pathways to the MNs. Using observed changes in MN activity that are caused by known perturbations of movements, it is possible to predict interactions of the sensory and motor pathways with pattern generators or command signals. The pathways and their interactions cannot always be specified in terms of known neuronal activity and connections. The most conservative catalog of known networks provides several possibilities that could give rise to the same effect. Efforts to establish known interactions between neurons in the more complex ganglia are hampered by a lack of evidence regarding the means by which MN activity is produced for the initiation and maintenance of movement in the face of normal loads encountered during those movements. Monitoring of inputs to one or a few identified cells with intracellular electrodes, combined with selective recording or controlled stimulation of input pathways, may detect at least some of the functional pathways, but is severely restricted in the number of components it can sample at a time.

In spite of the difficulties with both the control system and single-cell approaches, a hybrid or combined approach concentrating on selected MNs and restricted to particular naturally occurring movements is proving to be of value in solving problems of functional neuronal organization. A quantitative description of the theoretical interactions that must take place to support observed MN activities provides a basis for interpretation of known intracellular events. Models of muscular control of vertebrates (Houk, 1972) suggest an approach that is directly applicable to control of decapod crustacean limb muscles. The complexity of interactions of central input and proprioceptive feedback with MN output in the vertebrate models necessitates some knowledge of neuronal connectivity for interpretation. In applying this type of model to crustacean neuromuscular control, we face the difficulty that destruction of portions of the sensory feedback pathways or destruction of portions of the muscles may fail to produce predicted changes in output of the system in unloaded conditions (Evoy and Cohen, 1971; Fourtner and Evoy, 1973), leading to ambiguities in conclusions about the role of sensory elements that were destroyed. However, we are finding it possible to test roles for the sensory components suggested by the control systems by examining the contributions of various parts of the system during controlled perturbations of the movement, as in the experiments outlined below on the meropodite–carpopodite joint of the crayfish cheliped.

Movements of the limbs (pereiopods) of the crayfish and other crustaceans involve motor systems that can be analyzed with respect to their functions in locomotion and in other intended or "voluntary" movements. Walking and other more postural changes in limb positions can be evoked and maintained by stimulation of command pathways in the CNS (Wiersma, 1952*b*; Bowerman and Larimer, 1974*a,b*). However, normal walking movements do not occur unless the legs can contact the surface, indicating that some sensory signal appropriate to the actual movements is fed back to the CNS (Fig. 5). Thus, any system of inherent pattern generation in the central nervous network to coordinate walking is apparently heavily dependent on sensory components for its normal expression. Although patterning is lost, excitation from the command pathways continues to reach the MNs even when the sensory feedback is not relevant to the intended movement (Atwood and Wiersma, 1967).

Stimulation of nerve fibers in interganglionic connectives of partially restrained crayfish that evoke changes in the motor output to the major powerstroke muscles of the walking leg causes definite but not clearly patterned changes in the subthreshold potentials in the neuropil process of these MNs. Summed depolarizations that lead to increased axonal spike frequency do not show individual components (epsp's or branch spikes) that follow the stimulation at constant latencies (Figs. 6A and 7A). Ipsp's also respond to command fiber stimuli at apparently random latencies (Fig. 6B). Thus, the inputs to the MN from these INs do not appear to be via monosynaptic connections as has been suggested on the basis of morphological study of convergence onto dendritic trees in other motor systems (Wine, Mittenthal, and Kennedy, 1974). However, although large individual psp's that apparently are unrelated to the controlled stimulation occur occasionally, the possibility remains that monosynaptic connections from the intersegmental INs occur on remote dendritic branches and that their individual contributions to de-

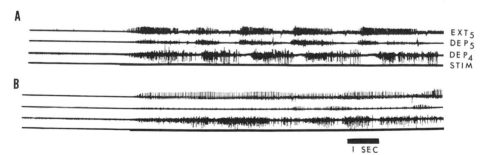

Fig. 5. A: Neuromuscular electrical activity recorded from a crayfish stepping on a freely moving styrofoam disk. The animal was mounted upside down in a bath of physiological solution and small bundles of nerve fibers in the circumesophageal connectives were stimulated at about 75/sec. Recordings were obtained from wires implanted in muscles as indicated. Regularly repeated bursts of activity closely coincide in extensor and depressor muscles of the fifth walking leg and are roughly reciprocal with bursts in the next anterior (fourth) leg upon initiation of the central stimulation. B: The disk was raised so that the legs could no longer contact it and stimuli were applied as in A. The same MNs are excited, but the bursting patterns are absent. Trace labeling Ext_5, record in the meropodite—carpopodite extensor muscle of the fifth leg; DEP_5, record in the anterior depressor muscle of the coxopodite of the fifth leg; DEP_4, record in the anterior depressor muscle of the fourth leg; STIM, monitor of stimuli applied to fibers isolated from the circumesophageal connectives.

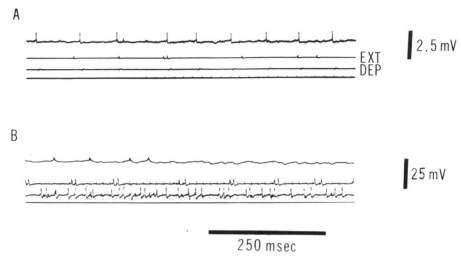

Fig. 6. Excitatory and inhibitory inputs to crayfish walking leg depressor MNs evoked by stimulation of fiber bundles in the circumoesphageal connective. A: Increased discharge frequency following onset of stimulation is accompanied by a slight depolarization of the MN, but no discrete subthreshold potentials can be distinguished. B: Stimulation of inhibitory fiber to a depressor MN in a different preparation suppresses the discharge and evokes distinct hyperpolarizing potentials that are randomly related to the individual stimuli. Traces, top to bottom: intracellular recording, meropodite–carpopodite extensor muscle recording, coxopodite anterior depressor muscle recording, stimulus monitor.

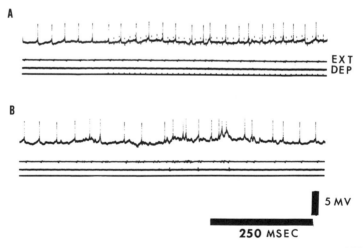

Fig. 7. Central nervous and proprioceptive inputs to a meropodite–carpopodite extensor MN. A: Stimulation of fibers isolated from the circumesophageal connective evokes depolarizations of the MN but without discrete phasic relation to the individual stimuli, resulting in decrease of some interspike intervals. B: Flexion of the meropodite/carpopodite joint evokes reflex recruitment of epsp's to increase spike activity in the same cell. Individual ipsp's are more obvious in B than in A. Traces, top to bottom: intracellular recording, meropodite–carpopodite extensor muscle recording, anterior depressor muscle recording, electrical stimulation of fibers in circumesophageal connective (A only).

polarization in the central integrating segment are not detectable with conventional recording techniques. On the other hand, in several studies based on spike-train analysis of close phasing between spikes in different MNs, the presence of common distributing INs presynaptic to the MNs has been favored (Angaut-Petit and Clarac, 1976; Spirito *et al.,* 1972; Vedel, Angaut, Petit, and Clarac, 1975; Young, 1975). If such presynaptic INs exist, they might integrate inputs from command INs as well as from portions of the sensory input (Field, 1974) (Fig. 7B). Direct physiological and morphological identification of premotor summing neurons would be a major step to analysis of functional organization.

Careful examination of the interactions between central stimulation and proprioceptive feedback in limb movements leads to further suggestions about the nature of the central organization of these motor systems. One important task has been to try to account for the components of proprioceptive information from the many types of mechanoreceptors that interact with the centrally initiated neural driving in intact preparations that are at least partially free to move. Measurement of neuromuscular activity at the meropodite–carpopodite (M-C) joint of the first pereiopod (cheliped) of crayfish during imposed movements combined with move- ment-producing command fiber and sensory stimulation suggests that it is the velocity and perhaps also the force of the imposed movement that provides the most effective feedback interaction with the central pattern generators.

In order to determine the responses of extensor and flexor MNs to imposed movements, the M-C joint of the cheliped was rhythmically flexed and extended through 45° in the midrange of its movement, using a motor geared to produce cycles of 0.38 Hz. Changes in instantaneous frequency were examined as functions of both the position of the joint during the movement and the change in regular velocity. The changes in MN discharge rate closely followed the changes in angular velocity applied to the joint (Fig. 8). However, there was no obvious correlation of the reflex discharge with the position of the joint, although extremes of flexion and extension were avoided in these experiments. The relationship between angular velocity, $d\theta/dt$, of the movement and the instantaneous frequency of motor neuron activity, Y, can be described by the equation for a straight line: $Y = M \times d\theta/dt + B$, where B represents the background level of discharge, or the average discharge rate at zero velocity. Thus, the slope, M, can be taken to represent the gain of the sensory-to-motor neuron pathway (average discharge rate/unit change in velocity).

Stimulation of sensory hair fields on the carapace or of fibers in the cir- cumesophageal connectives thought to be similar to the fibers stimulated by Bow- erman and Larimer (1974*a*) evokes characteristic and repeatable changes in the motor output to the M-C joint flexor and extensor muscles. When these stimuli are applied during the repeated cycles of imposed movements, the linear relationship between MN discharge frequency and angular velocity is maintained, although the strength of the reflex response is altered. The flexor MN responses to imposed extension of the joint increased when flexion-producing stimuli were applied (Fig. 9B), whereas extension-producing stimuli decreased the strength of the same reflex (Fig. 9C). The responses of an extensor MN to imposed joint flexion were precisely

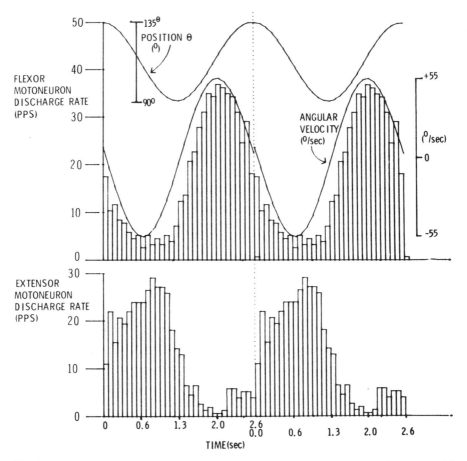

Fig. 8. Responses of crayfish cheliped M-C joint MNs to changes in position and velocity of the joint. The discharge rate of a tonic flexor and a tonic extensor MN to an imposed sinusoidal joint movement was averaged over 19 trials. The discharge rate was found to be proportional to the velocity of the imposed movement.

opposite to those of the flexor MN: attempted extension increased and attempted flexion decreased the responses. The effects on the reflex of sensory hair stimulation that produces intended flexion or extension are summarized in Fig. 10A.

The changes in background discharges of the MNs (Fig. 10C) and their responses to limb movements caused by the various types of stimulation could be interpreted as algebraic summation of excitatory and inhibitory influences at motor or premotor levels. However, analysis of the slope of the relationship between MN excitability and angular velocity permits some further speculation regarding the integration of these several influences. If the sensory hair and central pathways interact only with the proprioceptive feedback by simple summation, the gain or change in MN discharge rate per unit increase in imposed M-C joint velocity should be constant. However, the calculated slopes under different stimulus conditions vary considerably and in a consistent manner (Fig. 10B). Changes of this sort were seen using both sensory hair and central stimulation. Induced active extension resulted in an increased slope of the extensor MN responses and a markedly decreased slope for the flexor MN response. Active flexion produced changes in slope for the antagonistic MNs that were reciprocal with those seen during induced extension.

The availability of measurements of gains of the reflex responses makes it possible to begin to treat the interactions that determine MN excitability as a control system. Modulation of the sensory feedback to the MNs at some premotor level

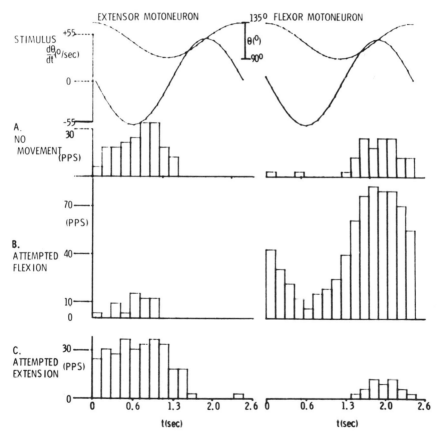

Fig. 9. Discharge rate of crayfish cheliped tonic flexor and extensor MNs to imposed movement plotted vs. time for three different CNS states: A: No attempted movement. B: Attempted flexion (stimulation of sensory hairs on contralateral thorax). C: Attempted extension (stimulation of sensory hairs on ipsilateral thorax). The magnitude of the discharge rate seen in A varies reciprocally between the two antagonist neurons and is directly correlated with the direction of intended movement in B and C.

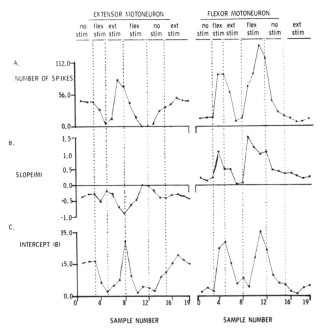

Fig. 10. Three parameters of the discharge rate of crayfish cheliped MNs to imposed movement measured at 2.6-sec intervals during attempted flexion and extension movements evoked as in Fig. 9B,C. A: Number of spikes discharged during a cycle of imposed M-C joint movement. B: Slope of the linear relation between the reflex discharge rate and the velocity of the imposed movement. C: Intercept of the linear relation between the reflex discharge rate and the velocity of the imposed movement. Note that all three parameters vary directly with the direction of the attempted movement.

seems a reasonable possibility for the observed changes in reflex gain for different directions of intended joint movements. In this way, the proprioceptive feedback, usually observed in a quiescent animal as a resistance reflex to oppose the movement, is controlled by a reduction in gain when the intended movement would be retarded by the proprioceptive influences and an increase in gain when the movement would be enhanced. Candidates for receptors that are likely to provide this feedback are discussed by Clarac (this volume).

Another type of central nervous control over the proprioceptive feedback regulating the motor system of the crayfish cheliped M-C joint has been found to occur both spontaneously and as a result of selective stimulation in the circumesophageal connections. Occasionally there is a shift from the familiar resistance reflex pattern, in which effective stretch of a muscle results in contraction to oppose the movement, to a situation in which MNs to the antagonistic muscle are excited. This has the result of aiding the impaired movement, thereby reducing overall joint torque. An example of such an aiding reflex as a result of command fiber stimulation is seen in Fig. 11, in which a flexor MN is excited by joint flexion and an extensor MN by

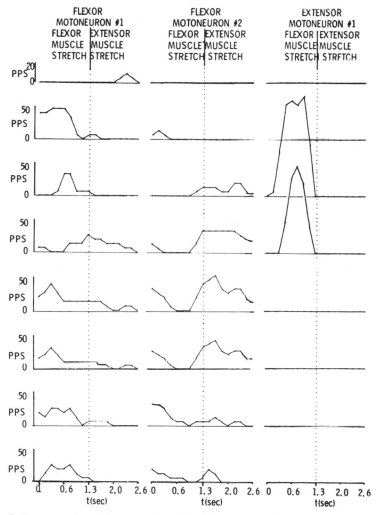

Fig. 11. Reflex properties of three crayfish cheliped MNs upon stimulation of a flexion-producing command fiber. Flexor MN No. 1 fires predominantly during flexor muscle stretch in a resistance reflex pattern. However, flexor MN No. 2 and extensor MN No. 1 fire in an aiding reflex pattern; that is, MNs to a particular muscle fire when that muscle's antagonist is stretched. This tends to aid the applied stretching force.

joint extension, although another flexor MN continues to respond in the resistance reflex pattern. Because this shift in the response to imposed movements has been observed to occur spontaneously, it is unlikely to be an artifact due to the inadvertent stimulation of conflicting central inputs to the motor system. The proprioceptive signals involved in the aiding reflex seem unlikely to be due to the joint angle receptors alone because positive feedback from them would result in unstable oscillations rather than a controlled development of muscle tension and movement. One hypothesis for a peripheral signal to regulate the aiding response involves the assumed but undemonstrated existence of muscle tension receptors in the crayfish M-C joint of the sort described by Clarac and Dando (1973) and by MacMillan and Dando (1972) in other preparations, along with CNS control over their inhibitory input to the MNs. Phasic suppression of motor discharge has been seen when a centrally commanded limb movement is abruptly terminated by a stop (Marrelli and Evoy, in preparation). This is precisely the opposite of the expected result if movements were controlled by resistance reflexes alone and suggests that the proprioceptive signals of changes in joint angle are suppressed in some way. Inhibition of the MNs to a muscle by a tension-sensitive system appears to be a reasonable alternative explanation for this response.

Findings to date on the crayfish limb motor systems indicate that central control of MNs not only involves initiation and maintenance of the motor program but also determines the nature of its sensory modulation through control of reflex gains. By treating these reflex gains in the context of a control system, it is now possible to detect changes in functional elements that are adapted to particular motor patterns for different behaviors.

A great deal more information regarding the actual connections between peripheral and central components of the walking leg and cheliped systems is required before discrete neuronal mechanisms that are responsible for these complex movements can be presented. These mechanisms are far more elaborate and complex than was once thought, but they do show a promising degree of precision and are thus favorable for analysis through careful and diligent experimentation.

ACKNOWLEDGMENTS

The work on cobalt identification of crayfish leg MNs was done in collaboration with Mr. W. P. Hofmann, and the work on the cheliped motor system was done with Dr. J. D. Marrelli. Dr. Marrelli's numerous suggestions and contributions to the preparation of the manuscript are greatly appreciated.

This work was supported by Grant GB 30605 from the National Science Foundation.

5

Morphological and Physiological Properties of Motor Neurons Innervating Insect Leg Muscles

Charles R. Fourtner and Keir G. Pearson

Introduction

In this chapter, we shall first review progress in identifying the patterns of innervation in the muscles of the walking legs of locusts and cockroaches. Second, we shall review recent work on the structure of insect motor neurons (MNs) and describe some of our own unpublished data on the structure of cockroach MNs. Finally, we shall discuss recent studies on the physiological relationships between MNs and their afferent input.

Patterns of Innervation

Excitatory Innervation

In 1939, Pringle established that contraction of a cockroach muscle, as in the muscles of Crustacea (Wiersma, 1961a; Evoy, this volume), is controlled by a very small population of MNs. He clearly demonstrated dual innervation of the cockroach extensor tibiae muscle. He found a "fast" (phasic) MN (a single stimulus to the MN produced a twitch) and a "slow" (tonic) MN (a train of impulses produced a graded contraction). In the past two decades, there have been several studies describing the number and types of MNs innervating specific muscles of the legs of cockroaches and locusts. Results of these studies indicate that the patterns of innervation of the muscles of the distal leg segments and the extensors of the more proximal segments are less complex than the innervation patterns of the flexor muscles of the more proximal leg segments. The muscles of the distal leg segments are innervated by two MNs, one of which is strictly phasic and another which ranges from tonic to phasic according to frequency (Burrows and Hoyle, 1973a); Cochrane *et al.* (1972) have suggested that both of the MNs innervating the retractor

Charles R. Fourtner • Division of Biology, State University of New York, Buffalo, New York 14214.   **Keir G. Pearson** • Department of Physiology,University of Alberta, Edmonton T6G 2E1, Alberta, Canada.

unguis (claw retractor) of the locust should be regarded as phasic. The extensors of the tibia in the locust and the extensors of the tibia and femur in the cockroach are also dually innervated, receiving phasic and tonic MNs. The flexor tibiae of the locust is innervated by at least six excitatory MNs (two phasic, two intermediate, and two tonic); the muscle is composed of two groups, each group receiving a single phasic, intermediate, and slow MN. The flexor of the cockroach femur may be innervated by as many as a dozen MNs, of which there are several phasic and several tonic MNs (Dresden and Nijenhuis, 1958). The complex pattern of innervation of the flexor of the femur suggests that each flexor MN may participate in a specific motor program, whereas the single extensor may participate in a number of different motor programs. Physiological evidence indicates that different flexor MNs are active during different behaviors and the extensor is utilized for several different behaviors (Pearson and Iles, 1970; Pearson, 1972).

Inhibitory Innervation

Although Wiersma and van Harreveld demonstrated in the mid-1930s that peripheral inhibitory MNs innervated several decapod crustacean muscles (Wiersma, 1961a), the existence of peripheral inhibitory MNs in insects was debated until 1965, when Usherwood and Grundfest (1965) demonstrated that the third-largest axon to the extensor tibiae muscle in a locust and a grasshopper (Hoyle, 1955) causes partial inhibition of slow axon-developed tension when stimulated at a high frequency relative to the latter. They had stimulated what subsequently turned out to be a branch of the common inhibitory neuron; that is, it innervates more than one leg muscle. Since Usherwood and Grundfest's original study, common inhibitory MNs innervating several muscles have been described in several insect species (for review, see Pearson, 1973); in fact, some cockroach leg muscles (the extensors and flexors of the femur) are innervated by three inhibitory MNs. Specific inhibitors (inhibitors innervating a single muscle) have been described innervating spiracle muscles in insects (Miller, 1969) but have not been described for muscles of the leg. Two classes of common inhibitors have been suggested: (1) widespread common inhibitors, which innervate muscles in a number of leg segments, and (2) local common inhibitors, which innervate muscles in a specific region of the leg (a single segment) (Pearson and Fourtner, 1973). Flexors and extensors of the cockroach femur receive a branch of the widespread common inhibitor and share two local common inhibitory MNs. Burrows and Horridge (1974) suggested that the flexor tibiae of the locust may also receive triple innervation: by the widespread common inhibitory MN and by two other inhibitory MNs whose branching patterns have not been identified.

MN Structure

There were a few early attempts to identify MN somata and to map their location within the CNS. One such attempt was to sever or injure a nerve and, within a few days, section and stain the ganglion to locate somata undergoing Wallerian degeneration. Using this method, Cohen and Jacklet (1967) and Young (1969) produced maps of MN somata with axons located in specific nerves; however, they could not designate the somata of functionally identified MNs. Since the advent of intracellular staining techniques (procion dyes, Stretton and Kravitz, 1968; Co^{2+}, Pitman et al., 1972), MNs can be physiologically identified and later stained to elucidate the location of their somata and the structure of the neuropilar processes. Another technique, that of placing the cut end of a nerve in either procion dyes or cobalt chloride and driving the ions electrophoretically, or simply allowing the axons to backfill without applying current, has permitted the mapping of MN somata which can be physiologically identified in later experiments (Iles and Mulloney, 1971; Pearson and Fourtner, 1973). These backfilling techniques have proven much more reliable for the mapping of MNs with large axons (greater than 5μm) in the cockroach than the degeneration technique (Pearson and Fourtner, 1973).

Extensive studies on the MNs of the locust metathoracic ganglion have led to the identification and cartography of over 100 MNs in the metathoracic ganglion (for review, see Hoyle, 1975a). In addition to the extensive map of the locust ganglion, there are several detailed accounts of the morphology of the MN processes within the CNS. An exquisite example is shown in Fig. 1. This drawing is the result of the work of Tyrer and Altman (1974) on the flight MNs of the locust. The MN was filled with cobalt, which was intensified in thick sections using a silver staining technique; this allows for identification of very small branches of the neurite. For further information on the structure of locust MNs, see Burrows and Hoyle (1973a), Burrows (1973b, 1975b), and Tyrer and Altman (1974).

Much less is known about the location or the structure of physiologically identified MNs in the cockroach than in the locust. In the cockroach, we have concentrated on the MNs which are active during walking, mapped a number of these MNs, and studied the structure of the neuropilar processes in several of them.

Somata Locations

Using the cobalt staining technique, the locations of 20 functionally identified MNs have been determined in the metathoracic ganglion of the cockroach *Periplaneta americana* (Fig. 2). No uniform scheme has been used to label these somata, and we feel that such a scheme should not be introduced until the somata of the majority of MNs have been identified. Therefore, we have maintained the designations assigned to MNs previously identified physiologically. In addition, we have labeled other MNs according to their specific functions. See Table I for the functions of the identified motor neurons illustrated in Fig. 2.

It is interesting to examine whether there is any functional significance to the location of the somata within the ganglion. We know that, during walking, slow flexor MNs discharge during the swing (protraction) phase of the stepping cycle. The somata of two of the slow flexor MNs (somata 5 and 6, Fig. 2) of the femur are located on the ventral surface of the ganglion just anterior to nerve 3 and are adjacent to each other. These MNs innervate the same muscles and, as far as we can

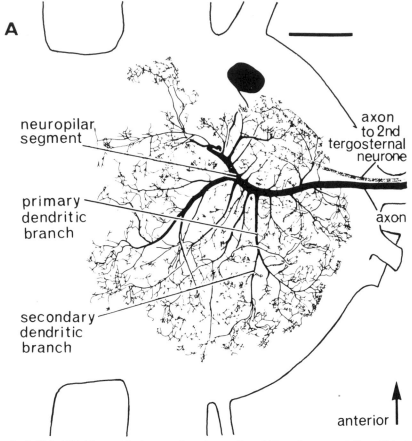

Fig. 1. A flight MN (elevator) in the mesothoracic ganglion of *Chortoicetes terminifera*. This drawing was made from serial sections of the ganglion following Co^{2+} staining and Ag^+ amplification. From Tyrer and Altman (1974).

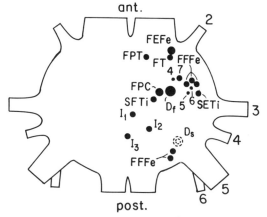

Fig. 2. Identified MN somata in the metathoracic ganglion of cockroach *Periplaneta americana*. Ventral view of the ganglion: only the soma of D_s is located on the dorsal surface. See Table I for somata designations and functions.

Table I. Identified MNs in the Metathoracic Ganglion in the Cockroach

MN	Nerve containing axon	Function	References
D_f $(28)^a$	5r1	Fast extensor of the femur	Pitman et al. (1972)
D_s	5r1	Slow extensor of the femur	Pearson and Fourtner (1973)
I_1 and I_2	5r1–3	Local common inhibitor	Pearson and Fourtner (1973)
I_3	Several	Widespread common inhibitor	Pearson and Fourtner (1973)
4, 5, 6, 7	6Br4	Slow flexor of the femur	Pearson and Fourtner (1975)
FFFe	6Br4	Fast flexor of the femur	—
SETi	3B	Slow extensor of the tibia	—
SFTi	5	Slow flexor of the tibia	—
FPC $(27)^a$	4r2	Fast promotor of the coxa	Young (1972)
FEFe $(18)^a$	4r2	Fast extensor of the femur	Young (1972)
FT	5	Fast flexor of the tarsus	—
FPT	5	Fast flexor of the pretarsus	—

[a] Numbers from Cohen and Jacklet (1967).

tell, have similar responses during walking and reflexly evoked movements (Pearson and Iles, 1970; Pearson, 1972). The only obvious difference is that a flexor MN (6) is consistently recruited after axon 5. The somata of MNs 5 and 6 lie in a group of five, all of which send their axons out nerve 6Br4. We also know that at least one fast MN innervating the flexors of the femur is recruited during walking, and it is quite possible that the soma of this motor neuron lies within the group of five.

MNs 4 and 7 innervate the slow flexors of the femur but do not participate in producing the flexion movement of the femur during walking (Pearson and Iles, 1970; Pearson, 1972). They are probably involved in the tonic control of femur position. The somata of MNs 4 and 7 lie close to each other but medial and anterior to the group of five. This separation of MNs 4 and 7 from the other five flexor MNs can be seen after backfilling the motor axons in nerve 6Br4 (cf. Fig. 7 in Pearson and Fourtner, 1973). Thus there appears to be a slight separation of the somata of MNs having different functions, yet innervating the same muscle (Pearson and Bergman, 1969).

A third but diffuse grouping can be discerned in Fig. 2. The somata of the inhibitory MNs (I_1, I_2, and I_3) are all located medially on the ventral surface just posterior to nerve 3. No excitatory MNs have been found in this region. Since the common inhibitory MN of the locust is also located in the posterior midventral region of the metathoracic ganglion, this region may be a specific locale for inhibitory somata (Burrows, 1973c; Pearson and Fourtner, 1973). Burrows and Horridge (1974) have shown that in the locust the somata of two other inhibitory MNs are also located in this region.

A slow flexor of the tibia (SFTi) is active during the swing phase of the walking cycle, and it bursts simultaneously with the slow flexors of the femur (Pearson and Fourtner, 1975). The soma of SFTi is separated from the somata of 5 and 6 by the somata of at least two extensor MNs (FPC and D_f). Thus, although there appears to be a close association of somata having similar functions and innervating the same muscle, there is no such association for synergistic MNs innervating muscles in different parts of the leg.

Another interesting feature of the somata locations is the positions of the somata of MNs innervating the slow extensor of the tibia (SETi) and the slow extensor of the femur (D_s). These MNs both discharge in bursts during leg extension, yet their somata are widely separated within the ganglion. The soma of D_s is on the dorsal surface, and in insects this is the only MN so far identified with a soma on the dorsal surface; the soma of SETi is located on the ventral lateral surface just anterior to nerve 3. Although these two MNs have similar discharge patterns during walking, it is probable that they have a variety of different functions during standing or locomotion over rough and unpredictable surfaces. In conclusion, excitatory MNs with similar functions and innervating muscles of the same leg segment appear to have their somata close to one another, and all inhibitory MNs thus far identified have their somata in the ventral posterior region of the ganglion.

General Structure of the Neuropilar Processes of Cockroach MNs

The MNs we have identified in the cockroach had the following structural features in common:

1. A single, very fine neurite ($<5\,\mu$m) leaving the soma.
2. An expanded region of the neurite (neuropilar segment, Hoyle, 1970) about $100\,\mu$m in length and 10–$20\,\mu$m in diameter depending on the MN.
3. A significant narrowing of the MN process close to the point of exit from the ganglion.
4. One or more major processes leaving the neuropilar segment.

We made no attempt to determine the structure of all the fine branches of the neuropilar processes as per Tyrer and Altman (1974). The geometry of the processes of D_f and the common inhibitory neurons I_1, I_2, and I_3 have been described earlier (Pitman et al., 1972; Pearson and Fourtner, 1973).

The neuropilar geometry of the slow extensor of the femur, D_s, and the slow flexors of the femur, 5 and 6, have been described elsewhere and are included in Fig. 3a,b (see Pearson and Fourtner, 1975).

Slow Flexor Tibiae MN (SFTi)

Although the soma of the SFTi neuron is some distance from the somata of MNs 5 and 6 (Fig. 2), its neuropilar segment runs very close to that of MNs 5 and 6 in the dorsolateral part of the ganglion (Fig. 3b). The close association of the neuropilar segments of these three MNs may be significant because of their simultaneous burst activity during the protraction phase of walking. The branching from the neuropilar segment of this MN was not extensive, and only a few small pro-

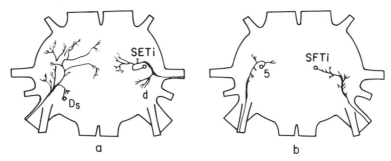

Fig. 3. MNs in the metathoracic ganglion of the cockroach. Whole-mount preparations of MNs injected with Co^{2+}. (a) Slow extensor MNs of the femur (D_s) and the tibia (SETi). (b) Slow flexor MNs of the femur (5) and the tibia (SFTi). Note the greater complexity of the neuropilar processes of the extensor MNs.

cesses were observed. This restricted morphology corresponds well to the relatively simple structure of the slow flexor MNs 5 and 6.

Slow Extensor Tibiae MN (SETi)

The neuropilar processes of the SETi neuron are shown in Fig. 3a. The fine neurite leaving the soma initially runs dorsomedially, then loops around to run laterally on the dorsal surface. The neurite then turns *posterolaterally* and expands into the neuropilar segment. There is a sharp lateral turn in the neuropilar segment before it constricts near nerve 3. A very prominent process leaves the integrating segment at this sharp turn and is directed slightly ventrally. An interesting point is that processes of SETi are not closely associated with those of D_s. This association might have been expected since these two MNs are simultaneously active during the stance (retraction) phase of the stepping cycle. This is to be contrasted with the close association of the neurites of the flexor MNs to tibiae and femoral muscles.

Comparison of the anatomical and functional properties of the flexor and extensor MNs reveals that the flexor MNs, with the single function of producing rapid flexion movements during walking or grooming, have only a few small neuropilar processes. In contrast, the extensor MNs, which function during locomotion, grooming, standing, and postural adjustments, have a number of prominent widespread processes. This obvious correlation between functional diversity and the complexity of neural processes immediately suggests that different processes in the extensor MNs may be involved in different behaviors. For example, the central input to the extensor MNs during walking, standing, and cercal grooming could occur in three different regions of the neuropil, while afferents from various groups of leg receptors (for example, the campaniform sensilla and hair receptors) could terminate on other processes. We have not yet observed the structure of flexor MNs involved in the regulation of posture, but we would predict that these MNs have a more complex neuropilar structure than those that give rapid, short-duration flexion movements. We would also predict that the structure of flexor MNs used for postural control is not as complex as the structure of the slow extensor of the femur since this MN has a greater functional diversity.

In a morphological study of crustacean MNs, Cohen (1970) noticed a similar relationship, in that neurites of the flexor MNs are not as complex as those of the extensor MNs. He suggested the differences in complexity reflect the greater utility of extensors in overall behavior. In Burrows and Hoyle's (1973a) illustrations of the structure of locust MNs (cf. their Fig. 6), it appears that the neuropilar processes of MNs which could be designated flexors (flexors of the tibia, AlFITi, AFFITi; coxa adductor AAdC) are not as complex as those of extensor MNs. Therefore, the occurrence of more complex neuropilar processes in MNs utilized for a number of different behaviors may be a general phenomenon throughtout the arthropods.

Physiological Properties of Cockroach MNs

We have investigated the intracellular activity of MNs by recording primarily from the neuropilar segment of one of the major processes branching from the neuropilar segment. The following are a few of the general physiological characteristics of cockroach MNs.

1. In slow MNs, very few large (>2 mV), discrete postsynaptic potentials were recorded. However, in fast MNs, especially the fast flexors of the femur and tibia, we often recorded quite large (up to 5 mV) hyperpolarizations.

2. In several of the MNs, slow depolarizations or hyperpolarizations occurred. The slow depolarizations could lead to trains of impulses. Such slow waves of activity have also been observed in cricket and locust MNs (Bentley, 1969b; Hoyle and Burrows, 1973b). Hoyle and Burrows attributed these slow waves to the release of neurosecretory products which diffuse throughout the neuropil. We suggest that, in part, these slow polarizations are produced by specific nonspiking interneurons (INs) which synaptically effect specific MNs and MN pools (see Pearson and Fourtner, 1975; Pearson, this volume).

3. From our recordings in various regions of the neuritic processes of the MNs, it is apparent that the impulse spreads decrementally from the axon through the neuritic region and the soma. At no time in our recording from MN processes within the neuropil did we observe an overshooting event. It is clear that the impulse initiation zone is located near the point at which the neurite exits the neuropil (Pearson and Fourtner, 1975) (cf. Fig. 2). Pearson et al. (1976) have recently recorded from the central afferent terminals of the sensory fibers of the trochanteral hairplate of the cockroach. As with MNs, the afferent impulse spreads electrotonically into the neuropil from a site near the border of the ganglion. The amplitude of the afferent spike was variable and never attained the zero level.

4. There is a linear relationship between firing frequency and spontaneous depolarizations in the slow extensor and flexor MNs. Figure 4 illustrates the relationship between firing frequency and membrane potential during spontaneous de-

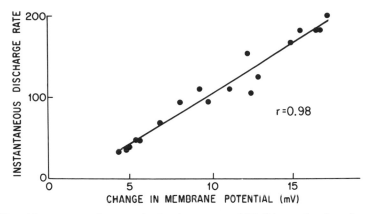

Fig. 4. Plot of instantaneous frequency in the slow extensor MN (D_s) as a function of spontaneous flucuations in the membrane potential of D_s. Note the linear relationship between discharge rate and membrane potential.

polarizations of the slow extensor MN. The exact location of the electrode in neuropilar processes was not known; therefore, one cannot predict the sensitivity of the impulse-initiating zone.

5.   MNs can be activated by current injection into nonspiking INs (Pearson and Fourtner, 1975; Fourtner, 1976; Pearson, this volume). One such nonspiking IN, termed IN1, has an excitatory effect on the slow flexor MNs of the femur and tibia which are activated during walking. Applied depolarizations of IN 1 produce an activation of the flexor MNs such that the smaller MNs are recruited before the larger MNs. In Fig. 5, the firing frequency of the flexor MNs was plotted against the potential change in IN 1 produced by the rising phase of a sinusoidal input to IN 1. Two important characteristics are clear from this graph. First, the MNs are recruited according to size, i.e., according to the diameters of their axonal processes (the flexors are numbered 3, 5, and 6, flexor 3 being the smallest in diameter and 6 being the largest) (cf. Pearson et al., 1973; Pearson and Fourtner, 1975). Note that MN 6 is recruited when MN 5 is firing at approximately 50 Hz; this corresponds with the results of Pearson and Iles (1970), who demonstrated that during spontaneous rhythmic leg movements MN 6 was not recruited until MN 5 was firing at approximately 80 Hz. Second, the slopes of the firing frequency/change in potential of IN 1 for the three MNs differ greatly: MN 3 is 3.5 impulses/mV; MN 5 is 12.5 impulses/mV; MN 6 is 26 impulses/mV. The differences in the slopes could be explained by at least two possible mechanisms. First a nonlinear synaptic relationship may exist between IN 1 and the flexor MNs such that depolarization of IN 1 produces a greater depolarization in the larger MN than in the smaller MN. However, preliminary studies of the cockroach MNs suggest that the depolarizations produced in the flexor MNs during spontaneous rhythmic leg movements are not as great as the depolarizations produced in the slower flexors (5 and 6). Second, the relationship could be explained by a differential sensitivity of the impulse-initiating

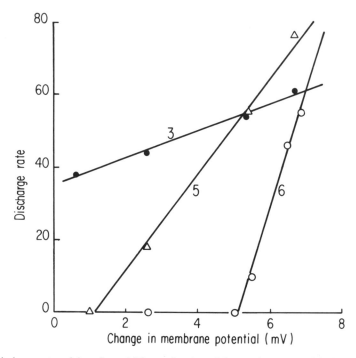

Fig. 5. Discharge rates of three flexor MNs as a function of the membrane potential of nonspiking IN 1 (see Fig. 1, Pearson, this volume). A sinusoidal wave was applied to IN 1 with a rising phase of 400 msec. For MNs 3 and 5, the rising phase of the potential change in IN 1 was divided in four bins of 100 msec each. The average discharge rate in each bin was determined and plotted against the median membrane potential of the bin. For MN 6, bins of 50 msec were used and average discharge rate was plotted against median membrane potential. MNs 5 and 6 are slow flexors of the femur and MN 3 is the widespread common inhibitor.

zone; i.e., the larger MNs may be more sensitive to suprathreshold changes in membrane potential.

Interactions of MNs

For years, the analysis of motor output relied on peripheral recording of impulse trains and bursts from motor axons to specific muscles and examination of the effects on the activity in one MN following antidromic stimulation of a second MN. These analyses led to several models predicting the central connectivity patterns of MNs as well as models of the central control of behavior (Wilson, 1965; Wilson and Waldron, 1968; Pearson and Iles, 1970; Mulloney, 1970). However, quite recently the use of microelectrodes for physiological investigations of insect MNs has produced a tremendous amount of information on the mechanisms underlying patterning of MN activity. These investigations have indicated that there are several possible mechanisms responsible for MN interactions.

Burrows (1973a) has described an IN "delayed excitation" pathway between the MNs innervating the locust flight muscles. An antidromic impulse in a flight MN innervating the wing elevator produces a short series of epsp's in its contralateral homologue, with a delay equal to a single wingbeat, 25–40 msec. A spike in the elevator MN will also produce a group of epsp's in its ipsilateral antagonist, the wing depressor MN. The epsp's occur with a delay of approximately 10 msec and may produce a spike in the depressor MN. The synaptic interactions between these MNs are asymmetrical in that activity in the depressor does not affect the elevator. Another example of delayed excitation has been described in the locust fast extensor tibiae. There is a 20–25 msec delay between an impulse in FETi and an epsp in the slow flexor tibiae. Hoyle and Burrows (1973a) have also described a delayed inhibitory pathway between FETi and the slow extensor tibiae (SETi). There is a 20–25 msec delay between an impulse in FETi and an ipsp in SETi; this pathway is a symmetrical inhibitory pathway since an impulse in SETi will produce a delayed (20–25 msec) ipsp in FETi.

Another example of MN interactions is a short-latency, excitatory connection between FETi and a fast flexor tibiae MN. An impulse in FETi produces an epsp in the fast flexor with a delay of 3–4 msec. Hoyle and Burrows (1973a) suggested that it could be a monosynaptic chemical connection; however, since this response was somewhat labile, it might be mediated by an interposed interneuron.

Monosynaptic electrotonic connections may exist between the flight MNs in locusts and crickets (Kendig, 1968; Bentley, 1969a) since small short-latency depolarizations in one synergistic MN were correlated with spikes in a second MN. However, Burrows, working with the locust flight system, has yet to confirm an electrotonic link between locust flight MNs. In insects, the synaptic organization of the neuropil and the structure of the MNs are such that both input and output must occur central to the axon proper and within the extensive neuritic processes in the neuropil. This raises some interesting questions concerning the functional organization of MN neuropilar processes. In those MNs which do synapse either on INs or perhaps directly on other MNs, are there specific input and output neurites? Or are presynaptic and postsynaptic regions located in nearby neurites or even adjacent synaptic region on the same neurite? Can these presynaptic sites be greatly influenced by postsynaptic potentials generated in their near vicinity? Since subthreshold depolarizations can produce postsynaptic responses in other spiking MN systems (see Maynard and Walton, 1975, on the stomatogastric ganglion), it would be interesting to investigate the input–output relationship of insect MNs to determine whether synaptic inputs subthreshold to the impulse-initiating zone may affect the central output of a MN. Subthreshold effects may well be expected in the central processes of MNs, especially considering that nonspiking INs produce dramatic changes in MN firing rates with only small variations in their membrane potentials (Pearson et al., 1973; Pearson and Fourtner, 1975; Pearson, this volume).

Our investigations on cockroach MNs thus far have been made with microelectrode penetration of single neurons, and therefore we have not performed experiments in which we could test directly the connectivity patterns between MNs. However, in our investigations of the antagonistic MNs, the slow flexors of the femur (5 and 6) and the slow extensor of the femur (D_s), we have not observed synaptic events in the flexors correlated with spike activity in the extensor, nor have we observed synaptic events in the extensor correlated with spike activity in the flexors. In fact, in none of the MNs from which we have recorded have we seen collateral activity associated with spike activity in other MNs. This agrees well with the peripheral recording and stimulating experiments of Pearson and Iles (1970) on the flexor and extensor MNs of the femur. In addition, in our recordings from several nonspiking INs, we have not recorded postsynaptic potentials which correlate with impulses in the femur flexors or extensors. Therefore, at least for the present, we have been unable to demonstrate collaterals from MNs of the walking system to other MNs or INs in the metathoracic ganglion.

Monosynaptic Reflexes in Insects

Reflex activity has been described in a number of insect species, but concrete evidence for the existence of direct afferent input to MNs (monosynaptic reflexes) was lacking until recently. In fact, in their early investigations of locust MNs, Burrows and Horridge (1974) found no evidence of monosynaptic reflexes. They postulated that the lack of afferent MN connections may occur in organisms with few MNs which may not have regions reserved for sensory input, and therefore afferent input would be directed to INs.

Recently, two monosynaptic reflexes in insects have been identified. Burrows (1975a) has described a monosynaptic reflex from wing stretch receptors to wing depressor muscle MNs; there is a short ganglionic delay (approximately 1.0 msec) between the afferent spike and the epsp recorded in the flight MNs. The stretch receptors are activated during wing elevation and therefore play a role in increasing the excitability of the depressor MNs for the next depression cycle. Wilson and Gettrup (1963) originally proposed that the stretch receptors were responsible for maintaining a high level of excitability and thereby produced a higher wingbeat frequency since destruction of the nerve innervating the wing base led to decreased wingbeat frequency. Burrows suggests that the stretch receptors are not responsible for maintaining the frequency of the wingbeat cycle but instead directly amplify the depressor MN output and inhibit elevator output. He proposes that other receptors near the base of the wing may be responsible for the increased central excitable state.

In the cockroach, Wong and Pearson (1976) have discovered a monosynaptic reflex between the trochanteral hairplate afferents and D_s. The hairplates are activated when the femur is flexed. It was proposed that during the stepping cycle the hairplate afferents aid in terminating the flexor activity (swing phase) and exciting the extensors (stance phase). Intracellular recordings from D_s and from the afferent terminals within the neuropil clearly establish a monosynaptically evoked chemical epsp with a delay of 0.4–0.5 msec between the hairplate afferent terminal spike and the epsp's (Pearson et al., 1976).

Burrows (1975*b*) has also suggested that a monosynaptic inhibitory pathway may exist from the stretch receptors to the wing muscles. The delay of the ipsp is 4–5 msec, and could possibly be explained by a stable IN pathway. Such a pathway is postulated in the cockroach for a short-latency (2–4 mesc), stable, inhibitory pathway from the trochanteral hairplates afferent to the slow flexor MNs. Stability would be predicted if a nonspiking IN occurred in the pathway since such a neuron does not need to generate spikes to evoke transmitter release. An afferent impulse would lead to a small potential change in the nonspiking interneuron, which would lead to a postsynaptic response in the MN.

Conclusions

1.   Patterns of innervation of the flexor muscles of the more proximal leg segments in cockroaches and locusts are more complex than those of the extensor muscles. It may be that each flexor MN is utilized for one or two specific motor activities, whereas the extensors must be utilized for several motor activities.

2.   Central processes of the extensor MNs have a much more extensive branching pattern than the flexor MNs. This again correlates with the physiological evidence that the extensors are used for a greater number of motor activities and perhaps play an important role in postural control.

3.   Interneuronal activation of leg MNs in the cockroach is such that the smaller MNs are recruited before the larger ones. Once activated, the firing frequency of the larger MNs is more sensitive to potential changes in the IN than is the firing frequency of the smaller MNs.

4.   There are several examples in the locust of synaptic interactions between MNs; the interactions may be electrotonic, chemically monosynaptic, or via IN pathways.

5.   Two monosynaptic reflexes have now been described in insects, thus demonstrating afferent input directly to MNs.

6.   In summary, MNs are not simply the final common pathway for centrally generated behavior patterns, but because of their physical properties, synaptic input from various receptors, and synaptic circuitry in the CNS they are important as a terminal integrating region for behavioral output.

Acknowledgments

We wish to thank Dr. Charles Kaars for his many comments on the manuscript.
This work was supported in part by NSF Grant B.M.S. 7422818 to C. R. Fourtner.

6

Inhibition in the Center and the Periphery

Donald Kennedy

Introduction

It is a special pleasure to be able to discuss a subject to which Kees Wiersma has made such a remarkable series of pioneering contributions. The phenomenon of peripheral inhibition is now what Kees will not become for another decade, an obstinate octagenarian. It continues to pose questions we cannot answer: What are the functional roles of the pre- and postsynaptic varieties of inhibition? What is the mechanism of the farmer? Why is it used in some places and not in others? Why couldn't arthropods have done without it altogether?

That we do not know more than we do is hardly Wiersma's fault. Although it is easy to slip into the error of believing that he discovered peripheral inhibition, he assures us that Biedermann and Hoffmann were there first. But Wiersma cannot deny that he made it famous. His early explorations of the innervation pattern of crustacean limbs raised the critical questions about its distribution and its use in the control of behavior. And his development with Marmont in 1938 of the limb muscle preparation in which inhibitory and excitatory neurons could be stimulated separately opened the way for the serious analysis of synaptic inhibition. Much of our contemporary knowledge about the mechanism of postsynaptic inhibitory conductance changes, as well as of presynaptic inhibition, has been gained over ground that Wiersma first cleared.

However, the questions I just listed still taunt us. Despite the clear demonstration that presynaptic inhibition involves a reduction in the probability of release of transmitter from excitatory endings, we do not know whether or not the reduction is accomplished by a shunting conductance change, and, if so, whether it is depolarizing, hyperpolarizing, or neither. More awkward still, we don't understand why presynaptic inhibition is a prominent feature of some kinds of peripheral inhibition but not of others—or even why arthropods employ peripheral inhibition when we vertebrates do so nicely without it.

In what follows, I am going to return to these questions and work them over in a frankly speculative way. Those of you who know I have done nothing with

Donald Kennedy • Department of Biology, Stanford University, Stanford, California 94305. Present address: Office of the Commissioner, Food and Drug Administration, 5600 Fishers Lane, Rockville, Maryland.

peripheral inhibition since the middle 1960s will be pardoned for supposing that I am motivated primarily by sentiment in choosing this subject. Actually, I think something new *can* be proposed about peripheral inhibition; the new notions emerge from studies in the central nervous system, not in the periphery, and they have to do both with the mechanism underlying presynaptic inhibition and with the functional role it might play in neuromuscular systems. I will begin with a brief history of these problems as they have developed in the periphery, and then describe some of our recent findings on the electrophysiology of central presynaptic inhibition in crayfish primary afferents. Then I will bring these findings back to the neuromuscular system and try to apply them to peripheral inhibitory processes.

Pre- and Postsynaptic Inhibition in the Periphery: A Brief History

Very early in the game, Wiersma realized that two kinds of inhibition are at work in crustacean muscles. In the first experiment to employ simultaneous mechanical and electrical recording along with selective stimulation of excitatory and inhibitory axons, Marmont and Wiersma (1938) identified a form of inhibition requiring a specific time relationship between inhibitory and excitatory impulses such that if the former arrived at the neuromuscular junction just before the latter, the electrical response of the muscle could be attenuated by about 80% of its uninhibited value. This was called "supplemented" inhibition, to distinguish it from another kind ("simple" inhibition) that could be achieved in the same dually innervated muscle by stimulation of the peripheral inhibitor and the exciter in a random time relation, and appeared not to involve reduction of the excitatory electrical responses. This distinction was noted in other muscles as well (e.g., Wiersma and Ellis, 1942). Kuffler and Katz (1946) continued the differences but changed the terminology for "simple" to β and for "supplemented" to α.

It is clear in retrospect that Marmont and Wiersma had discovered the difference between pre- and postsynaptic inhibition. The only error in the early accounts is a perfectly pardonable one: it is the argument that simple inhibition must be mechanical since it appeared not to have any effect on the electrical response. Because the myograms they took were essentially records of junctional *current,* the shunting effects of postsynaptic conductance changes on membrane voltage changes were missing. This old-fashioned recording method thus actually discriminates much better between pre- and postsynaptic inhibition than does intracellular recording. If one were to change Wiersma's early description only slightly so as to put "simple" inhibition a step earlier, it would cover perfectly our present understanding of the roles of pre- and postsynaptic inhibition.

Fatt and Katz (1953*a*) recognized the error of assuming that inhibition could work directly on the contractile apparatus; they also showed that the inhibitory effect was briefer than the inhibitory junctional potential, and that the conductance change in the muscle fiber membrane could account for only a fraction of it. Like the first workers to observe presynaptic inhibition in the spinal cord (Frank and

Fuortes, 1957), they knew they had something different but could not be certain exactly what it was.

The problem was brilliantly resolved by Dudel and Kuffler (1961c), who showed directly that as a result of inhibitory nerve stimulation in the crayfish opener muscle the probability was reduced that excitatory nerve impulses would release transmitter. This first demonstration of a presynaptic inhibitory mechanism was followed shortly by experiments confirming Frank and Fuortes's conclusion that a presynaptic inhibitory pathway onto afferent terminals also existed in the mammalian spinal cord (Eccles et al., 1961). In the latter case, the inhibition is associated with a depolarization of the primary afferent terminals, which can be recorded as a very small intracellular potential in afferents penetrated near the entry zone, or as a large extracellular potential, the dorsal root potential (for review, see Schmidt, 1971). In neither of these situations is it possible to determine the effect of the presynaptic inhibitory action on the events leading to transmitter release. Excitatory terminals in crustacean neuromuscular systems have not been penetrated with microelectrodes; they are too small to be promising targets, and the sites at which spinal cord afferents may be penetrated are too distant from the synapses to permit any inferences about how primary afferent depolarization affects transmitter release. As a result, we do not know what kind of potential change in crustacean terminals is associated with presynaptic inhibition, nor how *any* kind of potential change actually functions to reduce transmitter output. The *function* of presynaptic inhibition is also equally obscure in the two places.

Central Presynaptic Inhibition

Our studies on presynaptic inhibition in the crayfish CNS were stimulated by the finding by Krasne and Bryan (1973) that the central giant fibers, in addition to activating rapid escape movements, also suppress transmission from afferents that are activated by those movements. Krasne and Bryan showed that the inhibition derived from the escape command functioned to protect the sensory fibers from habituation, and from this reasoned that the site of the inhibition must be presynaptic.

We penetrated these same afferent fibers directly with microelectrodes in the neuropil of the sixth abdominal ganglion, in order to directly examine the electrical correlates of presynaptic inhibition. Before proceeding with an account of the results, I should say a little more about what kind of sensory system we are dealing with. There has been a tendency to think of the hairlike mechanoreceptor sensilla of crustaceans as contact receptors, but in fact they are directionally sensitive detectors of near-field water movements with thresholds very similar to that of the lateral line organs of fish (Wiese, 1976). The hairs are exquisitely sensitive to objects that break the air–water interface and thereby set up traveling surface waves; not surprisingly, these sensilla also respond well to the animal's own movements. The individual receptor hairs are hinged so that they move most readily in a plane parallel to the animal's long axis, and separate sensory axons associated with each hair respond to forward and backward deflection. These axons then make highly selective connections with interneurons (INs) in the CNS such that there are "forward-sensitive" and "backward-sensitive" elements of higher order. Certain INs, however, including some that in turn synapse with the giant fibers and therefore participate in escape responses, are activated by afferents having both forward and backward sensitivity (Wiese *et al.*, 1976).

In our experiments, the largest of these sensory axons (which are *not* those with the lowest thresholds) were penetrated with microelectrodes near the point at which they made synaptic contact with INs. This conclusion is based on the finding, on a number of occasions, that advancing the microelectrode only slightly from the recording site in a sensory neuron impaled an IN whose receptive field included that sensory neuron.

Stimulating either giant fiber resulted in a depolarization of all the sensory neurons; these primary afferent depolarizations (PAD) had amplitudes of up to 15 mV and latencies consistent with a polysynaptic pathway of activation from the giant fibers. Considerable summation and temporal facilitation of giant fiber-evoked PAD occurred, and each depolarization appeared to consist of several all-or-none components. Of greatest functional significance was the observation that the depolarization induced in sensory fibers by giant fiber stimulation not only reduced the baseline-to-peak amplitude of the afferent spikes but also lowered the absolute value of membrane potential reached by the peak. PAD, even though it is sometimes sufficient in amplitude to evoke antidromic spikes in afferents, is therefore nonetheless capable of reducing transmitter release from sensory terminals by decreasing the amplitude of the triggering signal (Kennedy *et al.*, 1974).

It soon became clear that if we were to learn any more about the mechanisms underlying the generation of PAD we needed an easier way of recording it. Ron Calabrese and I did some preliminary experiments in which we were able to record PAD by placing the sensory nerve across a sucrose gap near its point of entry into the ganglion. More recently, in collaboration with Jody McVittie, the relationship between PAD recorded in this way and other events in the ganglion has been explored more fully.

Figure 1 shows PAD that was recorded using the sucrose gap technique. Its identity with the similar potentials recorded intracellularly from single afferents has been demonstrated by experiments in which sucrose gap and intracellular records are made simultaneously. Under these conditions, the potentials are covariant when evoked by a variety of routes, and unitary potentials simultaneously appear and drop out of both records when high-frequency stimuli are used to evoke them.

One of the most interesting similarities between the PAD recorded with the sucrose gap method and that recorded intracellularly involves this component structure. Even though the former technique records a population response from many axons, the PAD is still often seen to consist of a few and sometimes only one component; in fact, it does not differ significantly from the intracellularly recorded response in this regard. We therefore conclude that a small number of INs deliver

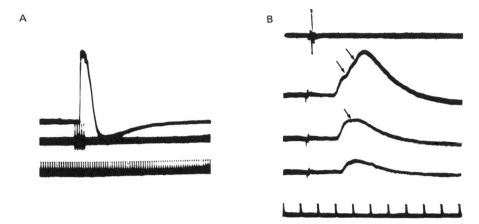

Fig. 1. Sucrose gap records of primary afferent depolarization in the fourth root of the crayfish sixth abdominal ganglion. A: Response to a train of five impulses in the median giant axon at 100 Hz (lower trace). Time mark: 10 msec. B: Responses to single median giant spikes (top trace) during a bout of repetitive stimulation at 10 Hz; the components indicated by arrows dropped out in all-or-none fashion between the sample sweeps shown. Capacitance coupled; time constant: 1 sec.

presynaptic inhibition to the afferents of the fourth root and that each one terminates on most if not all of the sensory neurons.

Elsewhere in this volume, Krasne and Wine report on their analysis of the INs involved. To the limited extent that our work overlaps, the results agree. There are several large INs that are directly activated by the giant fibers; when stimulated, these produce PAD components in our sucrose gap records, but we do not believe that the most prominent of these elements synapse directly on afferents. Some axons that can be isolated from the abdominal connectives do, however, reliably produce unitary PAD upon stimulation. These are relatively slowly conducting cells, the latency with which they activate PAD is short enough to be consistent with a monosynaptic connection, and failure of the spike and the postsynaptic potential at high frequencies of stimulation is always simultaneous.

We have been able to do some experiments in which stimulation of such cells was combined with simultaneous recording of postsynaptic responses from sensory neurons and from INs. PAD was recorded from the sensory root using the sucrose gap method, while intracellular microelectrodes were placed in INs that were activated by that population of afferents. In effect, we were thus recording events on both sides of the same synapses. Under these conditions, hyperpolarizing ipsp's and depolarizing unitary components of PAD had identical latency. Furthermore, in similar experiments where the giant fibers or other polysynaptic pathways were activated, details of the waveform of ipsp's and PAD were often similar, and components were recruited together in response to temporal summation of giant fiber impulses. These results all indicate that the same directly antecedent INs distribute presynaptic inhibition to sensory fibers and postsynaptic inhibition to INs.

This conclusion, of course, raises some questions about the nature of the transmitter involved and the mechanism of the synaptic potential changes that result from its action. William Craelius, Jody McVittie, and I have recently shown that γ-aminobutyric acid (GABA), if iontophoresed from a micropipette in the vicinity of the sensory tract in the sixth ganglion, causes depolarization of the afferents and reduces, presumably by desensitization, the PAD evoked by giant fiber stimulation. In agreement with the conclusions of others that GABA is responsible for the postsynaptic inhibitory conductance change, GABA iontophoresis over a broader area of neuropil dramatically reduces the spontaneous activity of INs. Thus there is good reason to believe that the INs that produce pre- and postsynaptic inhibition in the CNS are like those in the periphery in that they liberate GABA for both purposes. We could not, however, block PAD in the afferents by substituting impermeant anions for chloride in the medium, even though long exposures were used and even though there was dramatic reduction in postsynaptic inhibition. Either a different conductance change is involved in PAD, or some special mechanism is employed to keep extracellular chloride in the vicinity of the afferent fibers unusually low.

The equilibrium potential for the conductance change underlying PAD is between 12 and 20 mV depolarized from the normal resting potential as judged by extrapolation of the reversal potential from current–voltage curves and the maximum depolarizations observed in summated PAD recorded intracellularly; both yield estimates in this range. The upper part of the range should exceed the firing level of some neurons. Under two different circumstances, PAD sometimes yields antidromic spikes: when the cells are penetrated with microelectrodes and thus depolarized through injury; and when summated responses are generated in chloride-deficient media because unusually large compound PADs are produced as a consequence of the elimination of postsynaptic inhibition. We have not been able to produce such discharges under nonpathological conditions, as can be done in the dorsal root response of reflex mammalian sensory neurons subject to presynaptic inhibition.

In summary, our present understanding of presynaptic inhibition in the crustacean CNS is that it is mediated by a small number of GABA-releasing INs that also accomplish postsynaptic inhibition. In these respects, presynaptic inhibition in the center strikingly resembles that in the periphery. We also know that the central kind employs a depolarizing conductance change that shunts the amplitude of the presynaptic spike and thereby reduces its ability to release transmitter; this effect is chloride insensitive. These properties are difficult to compare with the peripheral mechanism since direct measurements of the electrical events associated with inhibition there have not been made.

Possible Functions of Peripheral Presynaptic Inhibition

Our knowledge of inhibition in the CNS of crustaceans has thus leaped ahead of our understanding of its role in the periphery. We still do not have a functional explanation, for example, of why certain muscles have peripheral inhibitors while others lack them, or why there is a presynaptic component of peripheral inhibition in some neuromuscular systems and not in others. Neither do we have any idea what kind of membrane events are involved in peripheral presynaptic inhibition. The facts I have just recited about central inhibition suggest some new notions to test about the peripheral kind. The idea that inhibition functions to "protect" synapses against effects of repetitive action might, for example, find some application in peripheral neuromuscular systems, and the data on membrane conductance changes in afferents support the notion that presynaptic inhibitory conductance increases might block or shunt excitatory impulses at critical points in the subterminal arborization, as suggested by Wiens and Atwood (1975). The use of the central inhibitors as functional models for the peripheral ones is encouraged by the basic similarities between the two systems.

The first test that any functional proposals about peripheral presynaptic inhibition must survive is that they be consistent with the facts about its distribution. Since its discovery in crustaceans in the last century, peripheral inhibition has been studied primarily in the distal limb muscles of decapods. Only in the past 15 years has the analysis been extended to a wider range of muscle types and taxa. Early work on innervation patterns of crustacean limbs by Wiersma showed that essentially every muscle received a peripheral inhibitory axon, and that—with the exception of specific inhibitors known to supply the opener or the stretcher muscle of the dactyl in different crustacean groups—these had innervation fields that included different muscles, often with antagonistic functions (Wiersma, 1941; Wiersma and Ripley, 1952). The discovery of "common" inhibitors presented a paradox so durable that Wiersma's description of it 35 years ago can hardly be improved on: "Thus reflex movements in which only one of these muscles is involved can only be performed with simultaneous inhibition of the other. Why such a strange mechanism should have developed in all these decapods is a mystery; it is certainly not clear what advantage this mechanism has over that of a simple arrangement of one motor fiber for each muscle and no obligatory inhibition" (Wiersma, 1941).

Inhibitors in other places, too, have turned out typically to have much broader innervation fields than exciters: this is true of the fast abdominal flexor muscles in the crayfish (Kennedy and Takeda, 1965a), as well as the fast extensors (Parnas and Atwood, 1966); the slow abdominal flexors, which we originally thought did not all receive innervation from the inhibitory axon (Kennedy and Takeda, 1965b), now turn out to do so (Evoy and Beranck, 1972). In insects, a large number of common inhibitory axons are now known; they resemble those in crustacean limbs but can have even wider fields of innervation (e.g., Pearson and Bergman, 1969).

The question of how the task of peripheral inhibition is divided between pre- and postsynaptic mechanisms had not been approached until relatively recently. Virtually all of the studies on mechanisms of crustacean neuromuscular transmission until the early 1960s had been carried out using the opener (abductor) of the dactyl in chelipeds or the walking legs in decapods, especially the crayfish. This monomania is a tribute to Wiersma's skill at preparation founding, and also to a fortunate accident: the opener is one of the few crustacean muscles in which the effective input persistence is high enough to permit the recording of miniature junctional potentials. Dudel and Kuffler (1961c) used this property in showing that properly timed inhibitory impulses reduce the quantal content of ejp's. Atwood and his colleagues later found that axoaxonic endings were associated with the ability to accomplish this presynaptic effect (Atwood and Morin, 1970) and demonstrated by selective depletion that the presynaptic members were inhibitory (Atwood et al., 1972).

Shortly after the presynaptic component of inhibition in the claw opener was discovered, it was realized that the motor programs for activating this muscle are unusual. In most natural opening movements, the specific inhibitory axon to the opener is *coactivated* along with the exciter (Bush, 1962a; Wilson and Davis, 1965). This situation explains the utility of the presynaptic component of inhibition, although it leaves Wiersma's more general paradox unanswered. In other muscles, however, central motor programs were found in which fairly strict reciprocity was observed between excitatory and inhibitory neurons; this is true in the slow abdominal flexor system (Kennedy and Takeda, 1965b; Larimer and Eggleston, 1971). This difference led us to devise a test for the presence of presynaptic inhibition (Kennedy and Evoy, 1966). Figure 2 shows a comparison between critical-interval dependence in the claw opener and in the slow abdominal flexors. In the latter case, artificial "coactivation" was achieved by electrical stimulation of the inhibitory axon, but in the former it occurred naturally. It is obvious that, in the claw, critically timed inhibitory impulses nearly abolish the ejp's, whereas in the slow flexors, despite a substantial postsynaptic conductance increase (indicated by the obvious

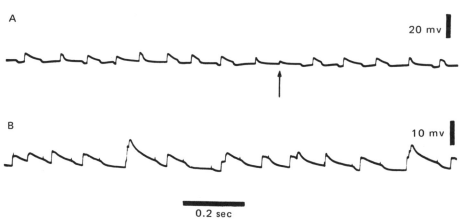

Fig. 2. Excitatory and inhibitory junctional events recorded intracellularly in the crayfish claw opener (A) and a slow abdominal flexor (B). In A, a segment of record has been chosen to show a range of phase separations between spontaneous excitatory and inhibitory impulses; the arrow marks the inhibition of an ejp at optimal interval. In B, the ijp's were produced by electrical stimulation of the inhibitory neuron at 10 Hz (artifacts). Two different spontaneously active excitatory neurons produce ejp's of two different amplitudes, but at no I-E interval is there a reduction comparable to that in A. From Evoy and Kennedy (1967).

ijp's), similar intervals produce no such dramatic reduction. This is already a strong indication that presynaptic inhibition is present in the former case but not in the latter. The more stringent test is to pass a depolarizing current through a second intracellular electrode in the muscle fiber with a waveform similar to that of an ejp; the influence of preceding inhibitory impulses on this depolarization is compared, at various intervals, with their effect on the similar depolarizations evoked by stimulating the MN. If any component of the inhibition is presynaptic, it will be revealed as a differential effect on the "natural" as compared with the "artificial" junctional potential. As expected, such tests showed that the inhibitor to the slow abdominal flexors lacked a presynaptic component (Fig. 3).

Extensions of this approach, some of them involving the latter test and some only an examination of postjunctional responses for critical-interval sensitivity, make possible further generalizations about the distribution of pre- and postsynaptic inhibition in the periphery. Specific inhibitors to various distal limb muscles in crustaceans all appear to exert presynaptic inhibition (Atwood, 1967a; Spirito, 1970) as well as postsynaptic inhibition. More recently, it has been found that some fibers in crab closer muscles also have a presynaptic inhibitory mechanism (Rathmeyer and Florey, 1974b; Parnas et al., 1975). These findings demonstrated for the first time that common inhibitors can have the presynaptic component and that it can be allocated selectively to different fibers in the same muscle. Wiens and Atwood (1975) have now studied the situation in crab stretcher muscles, which receive both a common and a specific inhibitor. They find that in all cases both components of inhibition can be demonstrated for each axon, thus providing the first demonstration of convergent presynaptic inhibition. Comparisons between species reveal that in some the common inhibitor has the higher ratio of pre- to postsynaptic inhibitory effectiveness, whereas in others it is the specific inhibitor.

The situation in insects has been less fully investigated, but an important clue is found in the analysis of a common inhibitory neuron by Pearson and Bergman (1969). This neuron, which is found in both cockroaches and locusts, was previously studied by Usherwood and Grundfest (1965) and Hoyle (1966), although before Pearson and Bergman's work it was not realized that inhibition was supplied the extensor tibiae and the anterior coxal abductor muscles by branches of this same neuron. The earlier workers had shown a tendency of the inhibitory neuron to innervate muscle fibers that also received slow excitatory innervation, and Pearson and Bergman demonstrated that a particular slow axon supplying the posterior coxal levator muscle is selectively accompanied by the common inhibitor. Their measurements of critical interval for inhibition in paired interactions between these neurons are strongly suggestive of presynaptic inhibition, although at the time the authors concluded that only postsynaptic inhibition was at work. Admittedly, the matter requires further testing, but at this writing it appears that common inhibitors *always* exert a presynaptic effect on at least some of their peripheral targets.

There is, furthermore, the much older set of observations indicating that inhibitors (especially common inhibitors) tend to affect selectively those excitatory axons mediating "slow" contractions. This generalization was first made in explicit

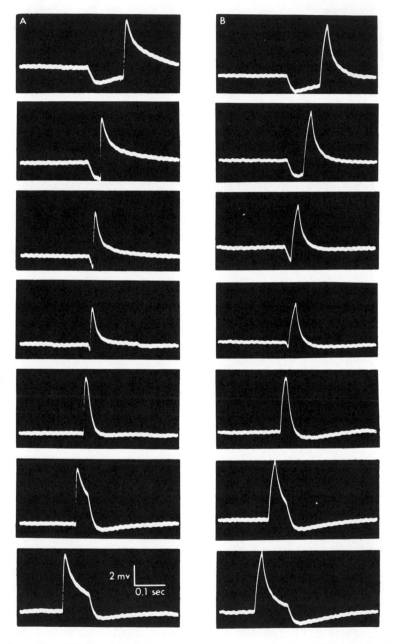

Fig. 3. Interaction of inhibitory stimulation with ejp's (column A) and with depolarizations produced by current pulse delivered through a second, citrate-filled microelectrode (column B) in lobster slow flexor muscles. From Evoy and Kennedy (1967).

form by Wiersma and Ellis (1942) and extended by later work from Wiersma's laboratory. In a series of elegant investigations, however, Atwood and his collaborators have shown that much of this differentiation can be accounted for by subpopulations of muscle fibers that receive selective innervation by the inhibitory axon (for review, see Atwood, 1967a, 1973b). As a result, there has been a tendency to view the selective inhibitory effect as resulting simply from specialization of muscle fibers and their connections. Just because this can account for the observations in some muscles, however, does not mean that it accounts for all. There are suggestions (e.g., Pearson and Bergman, 1969) that inhibitors ending on a polyneuronally innervated muscle fiber can exert a strong effect on one of the excitatory axons and little or none on another. Inhibitory axons can also produce presynaptic inhibition in one part of the innervation field but not in another (Parnas et al., 1975). It is therefore likely that the presynaptic inhibitory mechanism can be employed selectively so as to inhibit some forms of excitatory action but not others. This could be accomplished in the simplest case by a branching pattern that allowed the inhibitor to "track" a particular exciter and make axoaxonic contacts on it but not on others. A still more specific mechanism is suggested by the ability of single excitatory axons to make different types of endings on similar fibers within the same muscle (Bittner, 1968a). Some endings have very high facilitation requirements, while others have much lower ones. This differentiation is paralleled by the inhibitory terminals that accompany the excitatory ones (Atwood and Bittner, 1971). In principle, the inhibitor could make presynaptic contacts on one kind of excitatory terminal but not on the other.

What functional sense would such an arrangement make? For an answer, I think we have to return to the use made of peripheral inhibitory neurons by the animal during normal behavior. We know less than we would like about these patterns, but a few general conclusions seem secure enough. First, the inhibitory neurons that clearly lack presynaptic inhibition at any of their branches are employed reciprocally in motor programs (Kennedy and Takeda, 1965b; Larimer and Eggleston, 1971; Sokolove, 1973); it is thus hardly surprising that they operate only postsynaptically, since a presynaptic mechanism would be useless in such a motor program. Second, coactivation of exciters and inhibitors is common wherever presynaptic inhibition occurs (Bush, 1962a; Wilson and Davis, 1965; Smith, 1975) or where there is strong reason to suspect it (Hoyle, 1966; Pearson and Bergman, 1969); there is even evidence in some cases that the central program for coactivation can supply the cross-channel intervals appropriate for inhibition at the optimal interval (Spirito, 1970). Finally, strong excitation is provided in such situations after inhibitory discharge is stopped. The remarkable record shown in Fig. 4 was made by Marmont and Wiersma (1938) using a Matthews oscillograph. In record B, the bundle containing the inhibitory nerve was stimulated with an inductorium timed to give optimal intervals for "supplemented" (read: presynaptic) inhibition, i.e., just before the excitatory shocks. The largest mechanical and electrical responses follow the cessation of inhibitory stimulation. Marmont and Wiersma wrote:

> The fact that the action currents, after a period of prolonged supplemented inhibition, can rebound to a size they could not have attained otherwise, must result from a prevention of fatigue during their reduction . . . . Since the height of the action currents must largely be determined by the interaction between their facilitation and their fatigue, it is clear that the more efficient the reduction caused by inhibition is, the more effective the facilitation process will be. (Marmont and Wiersma, 1938, p. 191)

Paul Fuchs and I recently repeated this old experiment on the opener muscle of the crayfish claw with a few minor embellishments. As Marmont and Wiersma suspected, facilitation of ejp's can occur despite the dramatic reduction in their electrical signs during the period in which facilitation is taking place. Put another way, presynaptic inhibition—even optimally timed and highly effective—cannot destroy facilitation in these muscle fibers. In other muscles in which the excitatory junctions have a much lower facilitation requirement, there are indications that the sparing of facilitation during presynaptic inhibition is variable, but is more prominent when there is a higher facilitation ratio (Atwood, 1973a; Wiens and Atwood, 1975). It is also likely that the degree of inhibition is important. Terminals appear to control facilitation and momentary transmitter release by quite separate processes. A reduction in presynaptic spike amplitude sufficient to reduce transmitter release dramatically thus may not affect facilitation at all, and a further small decrease might eliminate facilitation while adding only a little more inhibition. These proposals are illustrated in Fig. 5. The slopes of the relationships could, of course, differ among terminals.

The preservation of facilitation during relatively complete inhibition in the crayfish opener muscle means that, after inhibitory discharge stops, unusually rapid activation of the muscle takes place. Our results show that an additional contribution is provided by a protection effect of some kind, due presumably to presynaptic

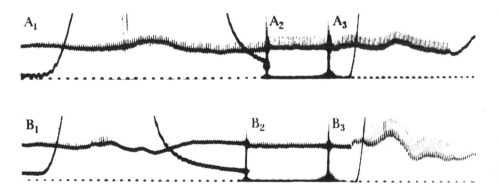

Fig. 4. Contractions evoked in crayfish opener muscle following combined inhibitory and excitatory stimulation. A: The phase relationship between I and E was allowed to vary. B: I preceded E by the optimal time interval for "supplemented" inhibition. Inhibitory stimulation was begun in A_1 and B_1, A_2 and B_2 show the heights of the junctional potentials 1 min afterward, and in A_3 and B_3 inhibitory stimulation was stopped. Note the height of the facilitated junctional potentials in B_3. The lower trace, often not visible, recorded tension. Time marks: 100 msec. From Marmont and Wiersma (1938).

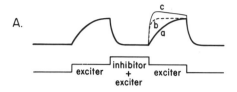

A.

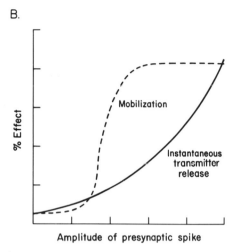

B.

Fig. 5. A: possible roles for presynaptic peripheral inhibition. Curve *a* represents the postinhibitory response expected when facilitation is removed by inhibition, curve *b* when facilitation is spared, and curve *c* when facilitation is spared and there is also protection from depression. The graph below (B) is a hypothetical relationship between the amplitude of a presynaptic spike and two different processes that depend on it, instantaneous transmitter release and mobilization. The postulated relationship for mobilization (dotted curve) is steep, allowing a degree of presynaptic inhibition that nearly abolishes transmitter release to spare the facilitation process.

inhibition. If inhibition is stopped just before (say) the twentieth excitatory nerve impulse, the ejp it produces has an amplitude greater than that of the twentieth ejp in an uninhibited train of the same frequency. Presumably this occurs because the amplitude in the latter case represents a balance between facilitation and some kind of depression process in the first 19 ejp's. The kind of "protection" observed here, however, may not depend (as it apparently does in the CNS) on blocking transmitter depletion.

Still another possibility, not yet fully evaluated in our own experiments but suggested by the results of others, is that certain regimes of stimulation applied to the inhibitory axon *alone* can generate increases in the amplitude of ejp's quite apart from their role in permitting "protected" facilitation to occur in the simultaneously active exciter. Such an action is hinted at by the effect of inhibitory discharge in "conditioning" subsequent excitatory responses in insects (Hoyle, 1966). It is raised in even more tantalizing fashion by a result reported by Pearson and Bergman (1969). In studying the optimal interval for inhibition by the cockroach common inhibitor neuron, they found a deep inhibitory trough at short pairing intervals, followed by a period during which the amplitude of the following ejp was increased by about 30% (Fig. 6). They attribute the enhancement to the displacement of membrane potential by the tail of the hyperpolarizing ijp; after the inhibitory con-ductance change is over, the long time-constant of the muscle fiber membrane holds the membrane potential away from the resting value, and during this time the ejp should be larger because it is farther from the equilibrium potential. The logic of this argument is impeccable, but the authors did not measure the conductance change, and they assumed that the inhibitory effects were all presynaptic—an assumption (see above) that does not appear justified. Moreover, this effect seems quantitatively quite inadequate to account for the large amplitude increases observed. At a point where the ejp was displaced by less than 5 mV from an equilibrium potential presumed to lie about 50 mV below resting potential, the amplitude of the depolari-zation was nearly a third larger. This increase is much greater than would be expected from the small change in driving force.

These considerations suggest that Pearson and Bergman may have discovered a *bona fide* case of heterosynaptic facilitation involving the presynaptic effects of a nominally inhibitory neuron. There are situations in which presynaptic inhibition

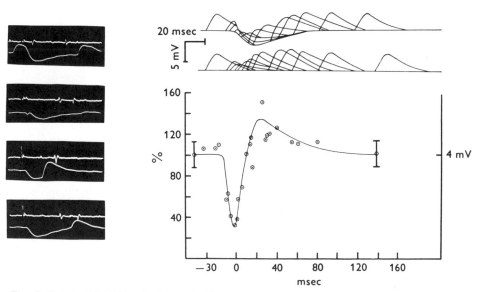

Fig. 6. Peripheral inhibition in the coxal adductor muscle of the cockroach. The interval was varied between an impulse in the common inhibitor and one of the excitatory axons; the curve gives the percent reduction in the ejp, measured from intracellular recordings shown in the sample sweeps at left. Above the curve are tracings of the ejp's, uncorrected (top) and corrected (bottom) for changes in baseline due to the hyperpolarization of the ijp. From Pearson and Bergman (1969).

can turn to excitation: chloride-deficient solutions apparently make the presynaptic inhibitory potential so depolarizing that it can discharge the excitatory terminals and produce excitation of the muscle (Hironaka, 1975). Suppose, by analogy with afferent endings in the CNS, that MN terminals are normally subjected to depolarization by presynaptic inhibitory action. Following inhibitory nerve stimulation, the depolarization might outlast the shunting conductance change and actually add to the transmitter-releasing effect of the impulse—especially if the latter does not fully invade the excitatory terminals.

There are thus several ways in which presynaptic inhibitory action, preceding or coactive, could enhance excitation. Most simply it could, by masking facilitation *and failing to abolish it,* generate unusually rapid movements in relatively slow, facilitation-requiring muscles by postinhibitory rebound (Atwood, 1973a). Also, it could confer a protection effect on the excitatory terminals during long bouts of joint activity, an effect that resembles the role of presynaptic inhibition in the CNS. Finally, it might under some circumstances yield a genuine kind of heterosynaptic facilitation of excitation, a proposition that still needs to be tested adequately. Support for these roles comes from the normal form of activity of many inhibitors, especially those that possess the presynaptic mechanism. Not only is coactivation common in insects (Hoyle, 1966; Pearson and Bergman, 1969) as well as in crustaceans (Bush, 1962a; Wilson and Davis, 1965; Spirito, 1970), but also patterns of activation are common in which the inhibitor is discharged rapidly before and during an initial excitor burst, and then stopped while the excitor continues to discharge at lower frequency (Smith, 1975). The contraction rates following such motor programs are unusually fast, and they presumably benefit from at least the first two of the mechanisms just mentioned.

7

Role of Peripheral Inhibition in the Control of Arthropod Muscle

Ernst Florey

Introduction

Peripheral inhibition, i.e., the suppression of excitatory phenomena of effector organs by the action of inhibitory nerve fibers, is a feature common to many animal phyla including vertebrates, mollusks, and arthropods. In the vertebrates, peripheral inhibition is restricted to the action of neurons belonging to the autonomic division of the nervous system; in mollusks, as far as is known at the present time, peripheral inhibition is restricted to the heart and the gut. In arthropods, however, inhibition involves also—and predominantly—the skeletal muscles, and inhibitory neurons are part of the regular efferent innervation of striated skeletal muscle. This was first recognized by Biedermann in 1888 and later confirmed by Mangold (1905) and Hoffmann (1914), working on crayfish. Since then some alternative hypotheses have been proposed which explain inhibitory effects of nerves on muscles in a different way, ascribing the inhibition of contraction to an effect of the motorneurons (MNs) themselves ("overexcitation," "Wedensky inhibition": Fröhlich, 1907; Fraenkel-Conrat, 1933; Segaar, 1929).

It was the work of Wiersma (1933) which convincingly demonstrated the "reality" of peripheral inhibitory axons in the muscle innervation of a variety of crustacean species, and the now classical papers of Wiersma and van Harreveld (1936) and van Harreveld and Wiersma (1937, 1939, and many others) described in more detail effects and distribution of inhibitory axons innervating several muscles of several crustacean species, notably of crayfish. The papers represent the first physiological experiments involving selective stimulation of single efferent axons.

The presence and functional importance of inhibitory neurons have also been demonstrated for other arthropod groups: insects (Usherwood, 1968), *Xiphosura* Parnas *et al.*, 1968), and Chelicerata (Brenner, 1972). Crustacean preparations, however, have been studied most extensively and have provided the most detailed information about the mechanism of action of inhibitory neurons on muscle. This preoccupation with the *mechanism* of inhibitory action has almost obscured the

Ernst Florey • Fachbereich Biologie, Universitat Konstanz, D775 Konstanz, Germany.

biologically fundamental question about the functional significance of this inhibitory innervation. Most investigations have been concerned with the electrophysiological aspects of the problem and have restricted their attention to single muscle fibers.

The biological significance of peripheral inhibition can become obvious, however, only when the experimental animals are considered as neuromuscular machines and when the significance of the inhibitory innervation is investigated in the light of the operation of these machines: the role of peripheral inhibition must be understood in the context of movement control. In the arthropods, particularly in the well-studied decapod crustaceans, each skeletal muscle is innervated by only a few motor axons; in fact, some muscles such as the opener muscle of the walking legs receive only one motor axon. Many or even all muscle fibers of a given skeletal muscle are innervated by branches of one and the same MN. Therefore, movement resulting from a particular activity of this neuron is the result of the combined action of all the innervated muscle fibers. The movements of the animal are the result of the total power output of each of its muscles. The role of peripheral inhibition must therefore be sought in its effect on this total power output.

For these reasons, it is absolutely necessary to study the contractile responses of an entire muscle, not just the electrical (and contractile) events of single fibers. Arthropod muscles are composed of structurally and functionally differing muscle fibers, and the contractile behavior of the whole muscle must be the result of the integration of the differing functional properties of its component fibers. Through very few (in some cases, only one) MNs, the CNS sends out a temporal pattern of nerve impulses to the muscle, and it is this pattern, combined with the particular responsiveness of the innervated muscle fibers, that yields the power output that results in movement.

The resulting movement therefore is determined by two factors: the centrally produced motor program and the peripheral responsiveness. The term "peripheral responsiveness" includes such parameters as membrane potential, amplitude and time course of postsynaptic potential, facilitation of transmitter output, excitation–contraction coupling, velocity of contraction and relaxation, and the contractile process itself.

The same motor program can produce different movements when the responsiveness of the muscle fibers is altered. It is also possible that, by an appropriate adjustment of the responsiveness of the periphery, different motor outputs can elicit the same movement.

Movement control can thus be accomplished at two levels: in the CNS by altering the motor program, and in the periphery by altering the responsiveness to the motor program.

Central regulation of the motor program can be achieved by sensory feedback and must involve both excitatory and inhibitory inputs to the MNs. Peripheral regulation can be achieved by activation of inhibitory neurons which innervate the muscle fibers and change their responsiveness to the motor input.

Specific and Common Inhibitory Neurons

As early as 1941, Wiersma showed that in the crab *Cancer anthonyi* the muscle fibers of the opener muscle (the abductor of the dactylopodite) of the walking legs are innervated by branches of two inhibitory neurons and that one of these, termed the "common inhibitor," innervates no less than five different muscles of the same leg. Most leg muscles, in fact, receive only the innervation of this common inhibitor, while others receive a separate inhibitory innervation by what has been termed a "true" (or specific) inhibitory neuron.

Double inhibitory innervation has also been described for the abdominal flexor (Kennedy and Takeda, 1965*b*) and extensor muscles (Parnas and Atwood, 1966) of crayfish *Procambarus* and the rock lobster *Panulirus*.

It is well worth examining the innervation scheme for the distal muscles in the thoracic limbs of the four tribes of the Decapoda Reptantia, as presented by Wiersma and Ripley in 1952 (Fig. 1). It can be seen that in the Brachyura and Anomura the stretcher as well as the opener receives a dual inhibitory innervation. Only in the Anomura and Astacura does the opener muscle receive an exclusive "true" inhibitory innervation; in the Brachyura, one of the opener inhibitors is the "common" inhibitor; the other axon branches and also innervates the flexor muscle. In the Palinura, the opener muscle receives innervation only from the "common" inhibitor, and in these animals it appears that only the stretcher receives an independent, "true" inhibitory innervation. It has since been suggested that in the Astacura* all but the opener muscle receive branches of the common inhibitor and the branching point lies proximal to the pattern represented by the diagram (Fig. 1d).

If that is so, the branching pattern of the common inhibitor is similar in three of the four tribes, the Brachyura, the Anomura, and the Astacura, and one wonders whether the Palinura will be found to follow the same pattern: as far as Wiersma and Ripley (1952) were able to ascertain, the stretcher is the only muscle receiving an independent inhibitory axon; all other muscles, including the opener, are innervated by the "common" inhibitor—and only by this neuron!

Regardless of the way this question is finally resolved, it is clear that the functional role of peripheral inhibition in crustaceans cannot be simply that of reciprocal activation and inactivation of antagonistic muscles: in the Palinura both opener and closer muscle are innervated by a common inhibitory axon, and in Anomura and Palinura both flexor and extensor are innervated by the same ("common") inhibitory neuron. The original hypothesis of Biedermann (1888)—that the inhibitory innervation is part of the reciprocal activation and inactivation of antagonist muscles—can hold true only for those cases where truly independent inhibitory innervation occurs. These are opener and closer of Brachyura, Anomura, and

---

*As pointed out by Wiersma and Ripley (1952), "It is possible, and indeed from a functional point of view seems probable, that all but the opener inhibitor are branches of a single axon."

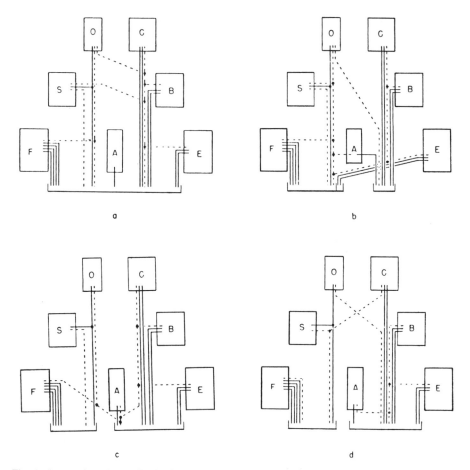

Fig. 1. Innervation schemes for the distal muscles in the thoracic limbs of the four tribes of the Decapoda Reptantia. (a) Brachyura; (b) Anomura; (c) Palinura; (d) Astacura. A, Accessory flexor; B, bender; C, closer; E, extensor F, main flexor; O, opener; S, stretcher. A, E, and F are the muscles of the meropodite that move the carpopodite, S and B are the muscles of the carpopodite that move the propodite, and O and C are the muscles of the propodite that move the dactylopodite. Solid lines represent single motor axons; broken lines represent single inhibitory axons. In the Brachyura and Palinura only the stretcher and in Anomura only the opener and stretcher receive an independent inhibitory innervation. In the Astacura this is true for the opener and flexor muscles. From Wiersma and Ripley (1952).

Astacura (but not Palinura); stretcher and bender of Brachyura, Anomura, and Astacura; and flexor and extensor of Brachyura and Astacura.

Experiments on Crayfish (e.g., *Procambarus*, Wiens and Gerstein, 1975) have indeed shown that the motor axon to the closer muscle fires at the same time as the opener inhibitor and that activity of the opener MN coincides with activity in the closer inhibitor. In the fiddler crab *Uca*, Spirito (1970) noted that the stretcher inhibitor and the opener inhibitor are independently activated during reflex opening and stretching, respectively.

The role of the common inhibitor, however, remains an enigma both in crustaceans and in insects, and in a way this must be said with regard to the brachyuran opener inhibitor, which also supplies the flexor muscle, and for the astacuran closer inhibitor, which also inhibits the stretcher muscle.

The fact that several muscles are innervated by endings of one and the same inhibitory neuron does not imply that all these muscles are affected in the same way and to the same degree by a particular firing pattern of the inhibitory neuron. In isolated nerve–muscle preparations of the opener muscle of crayfish, Marmont and Wiersma (1938) showed that when the MN and the inhibitory neuron are stimulated at the same frequency, the relative times of arrival of excitatory and inhibitory nerve impulses determine the extent of inhibition of the excitatory junctional potential. The authors showed, however, that even when the inhibitory impulses were timed to arrive several milliseconds after the motor impulses, so that no effect on the ejp's was noticeable, there was still complete suppression of contraction. Therefore, they considered the electrical signs of inhibition (suppression of the ejp's) as a supplemental feature not essential for the inhibition of the mechanical effects of motor stimulation and called this "supplemental inhibition." Later, in 1946, Kuffler and Katz, working with the opener muscle of crayfish *Euastacus* and crabs *Portunus* and *Leptograpsus* found that this inhibition of the ejp's did reduce the contractile response: mechanical inhibition was stronger when the inhibitory impulses were timed to arrive shortly before the motor impulses.

Spirito (1970), working with *Uca,* was able to show that the intact animal makes use of such optimal phase coupling of exciter and inhibitor discharge in reflex movements of the limbs: in these animals, as in other crabs, both the opener and the stretcher muscle are activated by branches of the same motor axon, E, but each of these muscles receives an independent inhibitory innervation by an opener inhibitor (OI) and a stretcher inhibitor (SI) neuron. When reflex opening of the claw occurs, E discharges are coupled with SI discharges to give optimal inhibition of the stretcher. When reflex stretching occurs, the coupling is switched so that E and OI fire together. Spirito also demonstrated that the effectiveness of mechanical inhibition is critically determined by the relative arrival times of E and I pulses when both neurons fire at the same frequency. Depending on the E-I interval, mechanical tension development may be maximally suppressed somewhere between 50% and 100%!

This example can serve as a model for other types of muscle innervation: when an inhibitory neuron supplies two muscles that receive separate motor inputs, selective inhibition of only one of the muscles may result if the I-neuron fires in phase with one of the MNs but out of phase with the other.

The great variety of possible limb movements makes it unlikely that the coupling of E and I neurons is fixed or permanent. The results published by Spirito (1970) show that such coupling, or phase locking, is transient, and investigations of several other investigators have demonstrated that E and I neurons can fire independently (e.g., Bush, 1963; Smith, 1975). On the other hand, the experiments published by Wiens and Gerstein (1975, 1976) provide proof of presumably electrotonic coupling between the MN supplying the closer and the inhibitor of the opener muscle of *Procambarus*.

The role of the peripheral inhibition becomes more significant when it is viewed in the context of proprioceptive feedback control of movement and of reflex-induced movement. When the CNS sends out a motor program to the muscles, it must, at the same time, prevent proprioceptive reflexes from antagonizing the "intended" movements. As was shown by Spirito *et al.* (1972) and Barnes *et al.* (1972) for the crab *Cardisoma,* the motor output patterns associated with walking are quite different from those occurring during resistance reflexes. This was also shown by Vedel and Clarac (1975) for the antennae of an anomuran crustacean, *Palinurus*: the flexor and extensor muscles that operate the flagellum of these powerful appendages receive innervation by a common inhibitory neuron. The efferent output, involving both motor and inhibitor units, induced by imposed movement (causing opposition to that movement) differs from that which occurs during "spontaneous" movements. If nothing else, such findings demonstrate that the peripheral inhibitory neurons are employed in well-defined but different combinations with the MNs.

Still, there is the problem of the common inhibitory neuron that supplies several, if not all, muscles of a leg or other appendage. When such a neuron fires, all the innervated muscles become affected. And if all muscles of a leg are involved in movement and posture, then the firing pattern of this common inhibitory neuron must, somehow, affect the performance and motor control of all these muscles simultaneously. Here it is not the question of whether or not the common inhibitor is activated when a particular movement occurs (whether as the result of a resistance reflex or as the result of a centrally elaborated command) but how a given impulse pattern in this neuron affects the responsiveness of all the innervated muscles to their respective motor inputs.

The common inhibitors may well function as "scaling factors," i.e., as agents that permit a graded reduction of the effectiveness of any tonic activation via specific MNs.

Presynaptic vs. Postsynaptic Inhibitory Action

It is now recognized that the terminals of inhibitory axons may make synaptic contact not only with skeletal muscle but also with motor terminals. While postsynaptic inhibition involves a conductance increase to Cl^- of the inhibitory postsynaptic membrane, the presynaptic mechanism of action of inhibitory neurons involves depolarization of the MN terminal associated with increased membrane conductance, presumably to Na^+, and/or reduced invasion of the presynaptic MN terminal by the presynaptic impulse. Presynaptic inhibition thus involves a reduced transmitter output, while postsynaptic inhibition does not. Postsynaptic inhibition, on the other hand, reduces the effectiveness of the transmitter substance released by the excitory nerve fiber.

Pre- and postsynaptic inhibition are differentially distributed. While postsynaptic inhibition appears to be always present wherever inhibitory innervation of muscle occurs, presynaptic inhibition occurs only in certain muscles and sometimes only in certain muscle fibers of a given muscle.

With the exception of the truly "fast" neuromuscular systems in which single motor impulses give rise to conducted muscle action potentials, the nerve–muscle systems of crustaceans are generally subject to pronounced facilitation of both transmitter release and contractile response during repetitive activation of the motor synapses. Where inhibition is predominantly postsynaptic, the action of the inhibitory neuron does not interfere with the facilitation of transmitter release. When both excitatory and inhibitory neurons are fired at the same time or over the same time interval, contraction may be inhibited, but facilitation of excitatory transmitter output continues; as soon as the train of inhibitory pulses stops, the continuing motor impulses can set up facilitated contraction because the maximal (facilitated) transmitter output can now become immediately effective. This has already been shown by Marmont and Wiersma (1938) and by Kuffler and Katz (1946) for the crayfish opener muscle.

When presynaptic inhibition is prominent, facilitation of transmitter output by the MN terminal is stopped, and when the inhibitory impulses cease the continuing motor pulses must now start the facilitation process anew. This has been seen in crab muscles by Wiersma and Helfer (1941) and Wiersma and Ellis (1942), and has been analyzed in detail by Wiens and Atwood (1975).

In their important paper of 1941, Wiersma and Helfer showed that the effects of the two inhibitory neurons that innervate the opener muscle of the crab *Cancer anthonyi*, the "true" inhibitor and the "common" inhibitor, are fundamentally different in that the one causes a pronounced reduction of the ejp's while the other fails to do so; both inhibitory neurons, however, are able to achieve similar mechanical inhibition. The differences show only in the way these two inhibitory neurons affect the facilitation of the ejp's and the contraction development immediately after the release from inhibition. Today, we can ascribe the difference of the effects of the two inhibitory neurons to their differing ability (or failure) to achieve presynaptic inhibition. A modern analysis of this has been presented by Wiens and Atwood (1975), who have studied the stretcher muscle of three species of crabs, *Hyas, Grapsus,* and *Gecarcinus*. In crabs, this muscle, like the opener muscle, receives a dual inhibitory innervation (see Fig. 1). Both axons had pre- as well as postsynaptic effects, but which effect predominated depended on the species, as is shown in Table I.

The inhibition by a neuron that causes only postsynaptic inhibition permits a type of motor control that may not be possible when presynaptic inhibition is effective: simultaneous activity in the inhibitory neuron can suppress the mechanical

Table I. Relative Effectiveness of the Specific Inhibitory Neuron (SI) and the Common Inhibitory Neuron (CI) Supplying the Stretcher Muscle of Walking Legs of Three Species of Crabs Causing Pre- and Postsynaptic Inhibition[a]

Species		Presynaptic	Postsynaptic
Hyas araneas	SI	+++	++
	CI	+++	+
Grapsus grapsus	SI	++	+
	CI	+	++
Gecarcinus lateralis	SI	++	++
	CI	+	+

[a]According to Wiens and Atwood (1975).

response to MN activity without preventing facilitation of motor transmitter output. The MN terminals are thus primed for maximal effectiveness once the firing of the inhibitory neuron is terminated. The same motor axon can now achieve a fast contraction that otherwise would initiate a contraction that develops very slowly. Figure 2 illustrates contraction patterns and underlying neuronal and synaptic activities resulting from the interaction of a MN with two types of inhibitory neuron, one giving rise to postsynaptic inhibition only, the other causing presynaptic inhibition as well. In the latter case, presynaptic inhibition prevents facilitation of transmitter release; when inhibition terminates, contraction develops slowly because facilitation of ejp's begins only after ijp's have stopped.

Wiersma and Helfer (1941) have already shown that the same inhibitory neuron (CI) may cause postsynaptic inhibition only in one muscle (the closer) and presynaptic inhibition as well in the opener muscle of the same leg of the same crab. This is an important example of the fact that a common inhibitory neuron need not affect all the muscles it innervates in the same way and that phase locking of inhibitory and excitatory impulses (with different phase angles) may be very effective in one muscle and more or less inconsequential in another muscle.

The two types of effect of inhibitory neurons on subsequent tension development of the innervated muscle exemplified in Fig. 2 are not the only possibilities of motor–inhibitor interaction. Marmont and Wiersma (1938) described a conspicuous "postinhibitory rebound" of the ejp's recorded from the opener muscle of *Procambarus*. The rebound was accompanied by an enhanced contraction and was stronger when the impulses of MNs and inhibitory neurons were timed for maximal presynaptic (supplemented) inhibition. The magnitude of this rebound phenomenon was proportional to the duration of the preceding period of inhibition. The phenomenon is represented in Fig. 3.

The investigations of Dudel and Kuffler (1961c) and subsequent studies (Dudel 1965b) have clearly shown that the "supplemented" inhibition of Marmont and

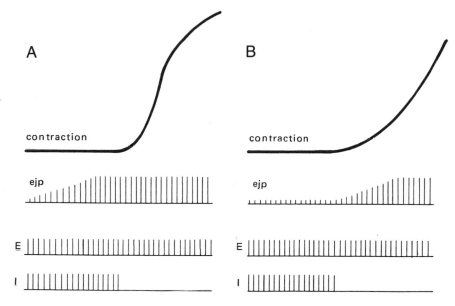

Fig. 2. Schematic diagrams of the time course of tension development in certain crustacean limb muscles after release from inhibition. Heavy lines show the tension developed (plotted against time). Below the tension records are the ejp amplitudes (transmitter output) and the firing pattern of the motor (E) and the inhibitory (I) axon supplying the same muscle. A: Inhibition is purely postsynaptic; facilitation of transmitter release and of ejp's is not impeded. B: Inhibition is presynaptic as well as postsynaptic. Ejp's are depressed and start facilitating only after release from (presynaptic) inhibition.

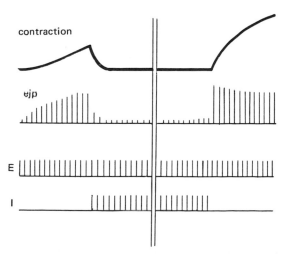

Fig. 3. Postinhibitory rebound of ejp amplitude and of contractile response. During ongoing train of motor impulses (E), firing of the inhibitory neuron (I) causes presynaptic as well as postsynaptic inhibition. Ejp's are suppressed during inhibition but show enhanced amplitude immediately after end of inhibitory action.

Wiersma (1938) is a presynaptic effect which results in reduced transmitter output from the inhibited terminals. The observed rebound demonstrates that the processes underlying facilitation are not inhibited even though the inhibition reduces the transmitter output. An obvious possible explanation of the postinhibitory rebound is that the nerve impulses that arrive at the MN terminals induce accelerated transmitter synthesis. In the noninhibited terminal, this would lead to larger and larger amounts of transmitter available for release by subsequent nerve impulses. During (presynaptic) inhibition the release of motor transmitter is reduced even though transmitter synthesis is enhanced. The net effect is an accumulation of releasable transmitter in the terminal. When inhibition stops, the next motor impulse can release a large proportion of the accumulated transmitter; at the same time, this and later motor impulses will stimulate further transmitter synthesis. Thus transmitter output may continue at a high level.

The molecular and ionic mechanism of nerve impulse-induced transmitter synthesis may well be similar to the one proposed by Birks (1963) in connection with his investigations of transmitter synthesis and release from nerve terminals in the superior cervical ganglion of the cat. Birks's results suggested that the Na^+ ions that enter the terminal at the time of the invading action potential are inducing transmitter synthesis and that the rate of transmitter synthesis is proportional to the momentary concentration of Na^+ in the terminal.

Inhibition of transmitter release without interference with enhanced transmitter synthesis represents another case of a "priming" function of peripheral inhibition.

The possibilities of movement control by patterned activation of slow and fast motor axons innervating a whole spectrum of functionally (and structurally) different muscle fibers are enormous, but the variety of movement control permitted by the additional availability of peripheral inhibitory neurons is truly staggering. The question now is if and how these possibilities are actually utilized by the animal.

Unfortunately for the physiologist, the game of designing neuronal circuit diagrams is singularly inadequate in this context. Not only are the activity patterns of the efferent neurons unstable and variable depending on the conditions of the CNS and its sensory input, but even the peripheral system of efferent nerves, muscles, and neuromuscular synapses is inconstant and subject to as yet unpredictable variation.

The effects of MN and of inhibitory neuron activity vary from one individual to another. Wiersma and Helfer (1941) pointed to this diversity of responses. They noted that in some preparations the optimal "supplemented" (presynaptic) inhibition was very pronounced, while in others (same species, same muscle) it was very slight. It was found, however, that "as a rule, the results of each preparation are uniform." Similar variations have been described in other papers and by other authors. In fact, it appears that even the differentiation of the muscle fibers of a given anatomical kind of muscle (e.g., the closer or the opener) into functionally different units (e.g., "fast"- or "slow"-type muscle fibers) is subject to individual variation. Observations of this type are contained in an important paper by Atwood *et al.* (1965) in which the electrical and mechanical responses of single muscle fibers are considered. It is not known whether these individual differences are the result of genetic variation or phenotypic expression, nor has anyone yet attempted to study effects of hormonal agents on the performance of peripheral nerve–muscle mechanisms. Here lies a rich field for physiological exploration. In this context, the reported release of synapse-affecting substances such as 5-hydroxytryptamine, substance X, and octopamine by neurosecretory cells and their terminals within neurohemal organs (Cooke, 1967; Kravitz *et al.*, 1976) of crustaceans offers a particular challenge, suggesting deliberate employment by the animal of hormones for the purpose of modifying the effects of the peripheral innervation and performance of the skeletal musculature.

Such variations of the effectiveness of inhibitory neurons (and of excitatory neurons) are a peripheral phenomenon. It would be interesting to know if the efferent output from the CNS can be modified to compensate for changes in the performance of the periphery.

Control of Relaxation

Excitation–contraction (E-C) coupling in crustacean (as in vertebrate) muscle appears to be strictly dependent on membrane potential, as was convincingly demonstrated by Orkand (1962*a,b*). Contraction is induced whenever the membrane potential is reduced beyond a threshold level. Ejp's depolarize the muscle fiber membrane, and contraction is proportional to this depolarization. In many cases, this membrane potential is so critically poised that depolarizations of less than 1 mV may induce contraction. Atwood *et al.* (1965) called these "supersensitive fibers."

If it is true that tension development is strictly dependent on membrane potential (once this is smaller than E-C threshold), it must also be true that inhibitory neurons may cause contraction in supersensitive muscle fibers if the ijp's are depolarizing. That this is indeed the case has been shown by Zachar *et al.* (1964) for crayfish muscle, by Usherwood (1968) for locust muscle, and by Florey and Rathmayer (1972) for crab muscle: the normally hyperpolarizing ijp's were inverted to become depolarizing by the simple expedient of reducing the external (Cl⁻) concentration and thus lowering the chloride equilibrium potential (the inhibitory transmitter increases the Cl⁻ conductance of the inhibitory sybsynaptic membrane and thus shifts the membrane potential of the muscle fiber toward the Cl equilibrium potential).

Numerous studies have revealed that the normal ijp's of crustacean muscle are depolarizing. In this connection, it is of interest that Hoyle and Wiersma (1958*b*) noted that, contrary to what one might expect, the electrical sign of the ijp's is independent of the resting membrane potential: even fibers of low membrane potential showed depolarizing ijp's. The direction of the ijp's was, however, found to be correlated with the season: the fibers of the opener muscle of "spring" crayfish *(Procambarus)* were found to exhibit predominantly depolarizing ijp's, while hyperpolarizing ijp's were found to predominate at other times. In no case, however, were depolarizing ijp's found to cause contraction; obviously they did not reach E-C threshold, and muscle fibers with normally low resting potentials must have had an even lower E-C threshold potential. In some insect muscles, naturally occurring depolarizing ijp's do cause contraction (Hoyle, 1968, and in preparation). So far, there has been no report that depolarizing ijp's cause contraction in normal crustacean muscle, but there is a definite possibility that this sometimes occurs. It is important to emphasize that effective mechanical inhibition is achieved only by a high frequency of inhibitory axon discharge relative to excitatory axon frequency in both crustaceans and insects.

The fact that the inhibitory transmitter shifts the membrane potential toward the Cl^- equilibrium potential (which is usually close to the resting potential of the muscle fibers) may have important consequences. Even at a high frequency of firing, the inhibitory neuron can never shift the membrane potential beyond this equilibrium potential. Should muscle fibers exist whose E-C threshold potential is larger than the Cl^- equilibrium potential, tension would still be developed when the membrane potential is set at the Cl^- equilibrium potential, but the tension would now be held at this precise level. The inhibitor neuron would, in effect, achieve a tension clamp. This has already been discussed in another context (Florey, 1975).

As has been shown by Hoyle (1968, and in preparation) there are muscles that exhibit a resting tension even when they are not activated by MNs. A striking example is the levator muscle of the eyestalk of the Hawaiian crab *Podophthalmus*. Its resting tension (which keeps the eyestalks raised) is abolished by ijp's which polarize the membrane potential, resulting in "uncoupling" of the contractile apparatus and relaxation.

This is an extreme case of a more general phenomenon: inhibitory neurons, when they exert a polarizing action on the membrane potential, speed up relaxation. If appropriately timed, a burst of impulses in an inhibitory neuron can lead to a quicker relaxation of contraction than occurs simply after termination of excitation. That this possibility of sequential firing of MNs and inhibitory neurons is actually utilized in movement control has been demonstrated by Kennedy and Takeda (1965*a,b*) and Kennedy and Evoy (1966) in their studies on the slow abdominal flexor muscles of *Procambarus*: the inhibitory neuron was found always to fire in alternation with the firing of the MNs that innervate the same muscle. It was concluded that this "reciprocal firing" can change a tonic system into a more phasic one by quickly abolishing residual tension. The authors were quick to point out that "it is, however, not clear why this particular system of muscle fibers employs this reflex mechanism . . .": the slow flexors are delicate muscles which are capable of subtly adjusting abdominal posture and movement. The quick tail flips result from contractions of the powerful fast flexors.

We are still far from the goal of understanding animal behavior in terms of efferent control of the numerous muscles that participate in those movements which are part of specific behavior patterns. Results obtained with one muscle cannot be applied to another muscle, and what is true for one species may not be true for another. This is probably the reason for the apparently contradictory results obtained by Bush (1962*a*), Smith (1975), and Wiens and Gerstein (1975)—all working with the opener and the closer muscle, but of different species of crustaceans!

Spontaneous Transmitter Release

Intracellular recording from crustacean and insect muscle often reveals that MN terminals spontaneously release transmitter even in the absence of nerve impulses. The resulting miniature excitatory junctional potentials (mejp's) may well affect the excitability of the muscle fiber and, in some cases, may even cause tension development. Firing of inhibitory neurons can abolish the effect of the mejp's.

On the other hand, there is evidence that inhibitory nerve terminals also release transmitter, causing the appearance of miniature ijp's (mijp's). Again, this spontaneous transmitter release can be expected to affect excitability. Where muscle fibers tend to develop a resting tension, such inhibitory transmitter output may not only counteract this tension but also be utilized in delicate tension control if there are peripheral mechanisms such as hormonal agents that control the spontaneous transmitter output from the terminals. Inhibitory neurons may thus be effective not only when they are firing but even when they are electrically silent.

Temperature Adaptation

In their important paper of 1953, Fatt and Katz (1953*c*) described the effects of temperature on the electrical properties of muscle fibers of the extensor muscle of the carpopodite of the crabs *Portunas* and *Carcinus*. They noted a drastic change of membrane resistance and of membrane potential: as the temperature was raised from 2°C to 17°C, the mean membrane resistance decreased from 194 to 52 $\Omega \cdot cm^2$ and the mean membrane potential rose from 64 to 80 mV. Florey and Hoyle (1976) studied the effects of temperature on tension development and ejp's of the closer muscle of the crab *Ocypode*. It was found that amplitude and time course of both slow and fast ejp's change profoundly, as does the tension development. Experiments on closer muscles of the crayfish *Astacus* (Harri and Florey, 1977) also revealed major effects of temperature.

Crustaceans are poikilothermic animals that may encounter different temperatures in the course of the seasons and even in the course of a day. Because of the enormous changes in peripheral responses (synaptic events and tension development), the same motor output must have profoundly different effects when the animal becomes exposed to different temperatures.

As yet, we know nothing about the temperature dependence of the effectiveness of the peripheral inhibitory synapses. It would be most interesting to find out if inhibitory neurons are employed—and how—in the regulation of the peripheral responsiveness to the motor program sent out over the MNs. Perhaps here is the key to the significance of the common inhibitory neurons that innervate whole sets of muscles.

Summary

Peripheral inhibitory neurons can have the following functions:

1. Rapid termination of contraction (accelerated relaxation): inhibitory neuron fires immediately after termination of a burst of activity of the MN.
2. Reciprocal inhibition: inhibitory neuron to antagonist fires while MN to agonist fires. This is possible only where the antagonistic muscles receive independent inhibitory innervation.
3. Graded reduction of muscle response to given motor output: inhibitory neuron fires in predetermined phase relation to motor impulses. Requires presynaptic inhibition and optimal timing to be maximally effective.
4. General reduction of responses of several muscles to given motor output program: common inhibitor fires tonically.
5. Shifting the effectivenes of given motor program to new response pattern: tonic firing of common inhibitory neuron whose "inhibitory strength" varies from muscle to muscle in a characteristic manner, resulting in a new and predetermined response pattern.
6. Speeding up of tension development: simultaneous firing of MN and inhibitory neuron innervating same muscle prior to "intended" movement which occurs when inhibitory neuron stops firing and activity of MN continues. May be the result of post- as well as presynaptic inhibition.
7. Depression of contractile response to given motor input: inhibitory neuron fires repetitively before onset of train of motor impulses. Depends on presynaptic mechanism of inhibition.
8. Reduction of resting tension: hyperpolarizing action of inhibitory neuron abolishes or reduces excitation–contraction coupling. Permits graded relaxation in accordance with frequency of discharge of inhibitory neuron.
9. Reduction of effect of spontaneously released transmitter of MN terminals: effect of excitatory miniature potentials on membrane potential and membrane resistance of muscle fibers is reduced by effect of inhibitory transmitter released either spontaneously or in response to nerve impulses from inhibitory terminals.
10. Compensation of temperature effects on motor synapses and muscle performance: requires direct or indirect temperature effect on discharge pattern of inhibitory neurons.

Clearly, this is a formidable repertoire and suggests an almost incredible degree of sophistication of the nervous control of muscular movement. The evolution of a peripheral inhibitory innervation obviously compensates for the possible limitation imposed by a muscle innervation that consists of only few (often only one) motor axons per muscle and in some cases involves even a sharing of the same motor axon by two separate muscles.

8

Compensatory Eye Movements in Crabs

David C. Sandeman

Introduction

The eye movement control system of the crab provides opportunities for the study of a wide range of basic neurophysiological phenomena extending from receptor dynamics through central nervous integration to motor control. It is an almost unique preparation in that we can now make careful quantitative behavioral mea surements simultaneously with electrophysiological sampling of the system at five different identifiable levels: the retinula cells, the lamina ganglion cells, higher-order neurons, motor neurons (MNs), and eye muscles. It is inevitable with such a system that many detailed observations obscure the main threads which run through the endeavors of different investigators over a period of more than a decade. It is the purpose of this chapter to review the progress made in this field since our first studies on the crab eye movements were made in 1961 (Sandeman, 1964; Horridge and Sandeman, 1964). I have attempted to present here what has been firmly established about the most relevant aspects of the system, and therefore much has been left out. All the information is readily available in the original publications.

Crabs have eyes which are movable in relation to their bodies. In an alert animal, the eyes appear to maintain a fixed direction of gaze: when the animal moves, the eyes move together, maintaining a strict positional relationship to each other and to the environment (Barnes and Horridge, 1969). The conjugate eye movements and their compensatory action during movements of the animal are the most striking features of the behavior, and there are remarkable similarities between the eye movement control systems of crabs and vertebrates which lead to the impression that there are some basic and common factors in the control of movable eyes.

There are several ways in which the compensatory eye movements in the horizontal plane can be produced, but all result in eye movements which tend to keep the eye stationary with respect to the environment. The most natural expression of the behavior is found in an animal which turns itself about its vertical axis. The eyes move slowly in the direction opposite to the rotation of the body, thus maintaining their position relative to a point in the environment. At a certain point,

David C. Sandeman • Department of Neurobiology, Research School of Biological Sciences, Australian National University, Canberra, A.C.T., Australia.

when it appears that they can rotate no farther in their sockets, they will very quickly flick in the direction of body movement and then begin again the same slow compensatory movement. These slow and fast eye movements have been collectively called nystagmus, and the two components are called the slow and fast phases of nystagmus.

Nystagmus can be evoked in more convenient ways than waiting for the animal to turn itself. It will occur if the animal is kept stationary and a vertically striped drum is rotated around the animal (the optokinetic response), or it can be produced by rotating a blinded animal about the vertical axis (the statocyst-induced response).

The optokinetic response, produced by the surrounding striped drum, has been exploited as a means to determine the acuity of the visual system (Clark, 1935) and its sensitivity to color contrast (Schlieper, 1927; von Buddenbrock and Friedrich, 1933). Experiments have also been done to determine the size of the visual field necessary for nystagmus to occur. Our own work, however, started with the question of the control of the eye movements, and this required a careful examination of the physiology and anatomy of the eye muscles, a quantification of the behavioral response, and a physiological and anatomical study of the neural elements involved. Both the visual and the statocyst inputs have been used, the first to ask questions about the control of eye position and the second to examine the generation of patterned discharges in the MNs which produce the nystagmus.

In addition to the compensatory movements in the horizontal plane, crab eyes will alter their position with respect to gravity if the animal is tilted about the transverse or longitudinal axis (pitch or roll). These geotactic responses are not considered here.

The Eye Assembly

The eye assembly consists of several skeletal portions (Fig. 1). A centrally located plate bears two laterally projecting eyestalks (the proximal joints), which in turn carry the eyecups (the distal joints). The eyecups bear the retinae and contain the optic ganglia. The central plate and eyestalks of *Carcinus* are enclosed by the rostral projection of the carapace but are nevertheless still able to rotate about their longitudinal axis. This rotation has the effect of altering the position of the eyecups about the transverse axis of the animal (pitch). The control of the eystalk rotation, effected by a set of medial muscles, is unique among the eye movement systems studied so far in that proprioceptive information plays an important role (Steinacker, 1975). The eyecups project from sockets in the carapace, and they are, within the limits set by the edges of the sockets, able to move around both the vertical and transverse axes.

Two nerve bundles contain axons running to and from the eyecup. The optic nerve contains interneurons (INs) linking the optic ganglia with the cerebral ganglion and, in *Carcinus* and *Scylla,* two large MNs responsible for the protective withdrawal of the eye. The oculomotor nerve contains the axons of the MNs of the

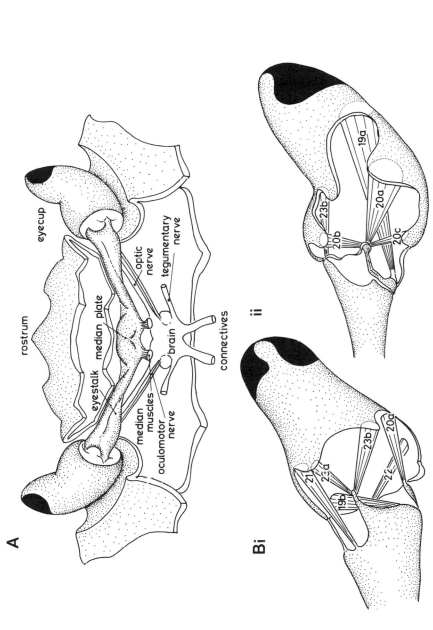

Fig. 1. A: Eye assembly of the crab revealed by dissecting away part of the dorsal carapace. The eyestalks unite in the median plate. The median muscles act on this and roll the eyestalks around their longitudinal axes. The eyecups are borne on the distal ends of the eyestalks and are free to move within the limits of the eye sockets. After Horridge and Sandeman (1964). B: Eye muscles of the crab *Carcinus*. (i) The right eye from above; (ii) the right eye from the side. Muscles 21, 19b, and 20a are the prime movers for horizontal eye movements. After Burrows and Horridge (1968a).

eye muscles and axons from mechanoreceptive hairs of the eyestalk. On no occasion could a proprioceptive function be demonstrated for these receptors. Electrical recordings show instead only phasic discharges to tactile stimuli applied to the eyecup or to gross movements of the eyecup (Horridge and Sandeman, 1964).

Functional Anatomy of the Eye Muscles

The eye muscles of the portunid *Callinectes sapidus* have been described by Cochran (1935); and the anatomy of the eye muscles of *Carcinus* is essentially the same (Fig. 1B). The function of the various muscles was not known until careful studies were made of both extracellular and intracellular responses of all the eye muscles of *Carcinus* during compensatory eye movements for pitch, roll, and yaw (Burrows and Horridge, 1968a,b).

The eyecup has no condylic articulation with the eyestalk, and apart from three small sclerites embedded in the arthrodial membrane which serve to stiffen it, the eyecup is suspended only by its nine muscles, which are responsible for all movements and for the maintenance of its postural attitude. Recordings from the various muscles reveal considerable functional overlap, and a picture emerges in which any eye movements are the result of nearly all the eye muscles acting in concert. It is nevertheless possible to assign a major function to several muscles. Thus the large muscle at the base of the eye, 19a, is active only during the rapid withdrawal of the eye. The much smaller muscle, 23a, is centrally inhibited during eye retraction but is vigorously active during reextension of the eye. Its sensitivity to movements of the animal about the transverse axis leads one to assign to it the role of controlling vertical eye position. It is assisted, however, by 18 (not an eyecup muscle but one which rolls the distal end of the eyestalk), 20b, and to a lesser extent 23b.

During movements of the eye in the horizontal plane, several muscles can be assigned the function of prime eye movers by virtue of the correlation between the frequency of their action potentials and the position of the eye.

The action of all the muscles in horizontal eye movements is summarized in Fig. 2, which shows that for a slow movement of the eye toward the midline, units in 19b and 21 increase their frequency. During movements away from the midline, these muscles are nearly or completely silent, and units in 20a show a significant increase. No other muscles show responses that can so clearly be related to eye position. There are further complications within 19b, 21, and 20a, because they comprise mixed motor units. For descriptive convenience, these have been divided into "tonic" if they show a maintained discharge and "phasic" if they are silent until a certain point has been reached in the traverse of the eye across the socket. In measurements of eye torque coupled with muscle recordings from 21, it was found that the phasic and tonic systems complemented each other, so that initially all the eye torque was produced by the first or tonic system, but at a certain point, when the tonic system had reached its peak frequency and therefore peak torque output, the

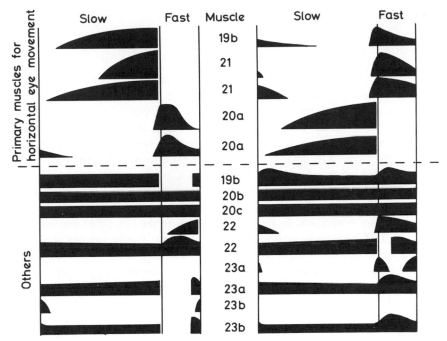

Fig. 2. Activity of the eye muscles during nystagmus. The relative firing frequencies during the slow and fast phases are shown during a slow phase and a subsequent fast phase. The time scale for the fast phase has been expanded. The first two columns represent a slow phase toward and a fast phase away from the midline. The second two columns represent the opposite case. Note the different activities of different parts of the individual muscle blocks. After Burrows and Horridge (1968a).

second or phasic system was recruited to produce a further increase in eye torque. The two systems may operate in parallel, the phasic (late) one being excited when the input to the velocity detection system of the eye exceeds a certain value and excites a "fast" movement perception system, the tonic (early) one being operated by a "slow" movement perception system (Horridge and Burrows, 1968a), or both may be driven by the same movement perception system but have different thresholds (Sandeman, et al., 1975a). The outcome, regardless of mechanism, is that the crab is able to extend the functional range of its eye movement system beyond the constraints associated with either type of muscle alone.

The activity, recorded within the eye muscles during the slow and fast phases of nystagmus, is the same regardless of whether the eye is clamped or free to move. In both cases, the frequency of discharge to the muscles of one set increases up to a certain point during the slow phase and then abruptly declines, while a burst of activity corresponding with the fast phase occurs in the antagonists. The intracellular recordings from the muscles of the clamped eye show (1) that the onset of the fast phase is not controlled by the position of the eye in its socket and (2) that there is no peripheral inhibition in any eyecup muscles (Burrows and Horridge, 1968b).

Behavioral Phenomena

The Visual Feedback Control System

The usual way to evoke optokinetic eye movements in crabs is to fasten the animal, with its legs bound or completely removed, at the center of a drum with vertical black and white stripes having a spatial wavelength of about 20°. The upper edge of the drum should subtend an angle at the eye of more than 20° from the horizontal, and the lower edge one of more than 5° below the horizontal. With drums narrower than this, the stimulus becomes less effective (Kunze, 1963, 1964). Smooth rotation of the drum in either direction produces the eye movements. Patterns with spatial wavelengths of between 10° and 40° all give the same response curves for a wide range of velocities of drum movement (Sandeman *et al.*, 1975a).

A lightweight wand can be fastened to the top of the eyecup so that it projects over the back of the animal and does not occlude vision. The excursions of the wand can be detected in various ways (Horridge and Burrows, 1968a; Sandeman, 1968) and yield an accurate measure of the angular excursion of the eye. When this is related to the angular excursion of the drum, it is found that the freely moving eye lags behind the movement of the drum by a small amount. Thus if the angular excursion of the eye is plotted against that of the drum, which is moving at a constant velocity of about 1.0°/sec, the result will be similar to that shown in Fig. 3. It can be seen that for a drum movement of 1.0° the eye movement is only 0.9°; for a drum movement of 10° the eye movement is 9°. From this it follows that the effective

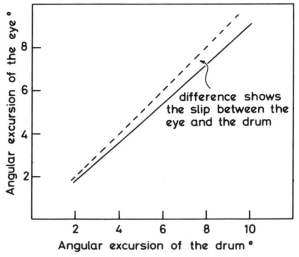

Fig. 3. Angular excursion of the eye compared with the angular excursion of the striped drum to show the "slip" between the eye and the drum. The dotted line represents the plot which would be obtained if the angular excursions of the eye and the drum were both exactly the same. The solid line shows what actually happens.

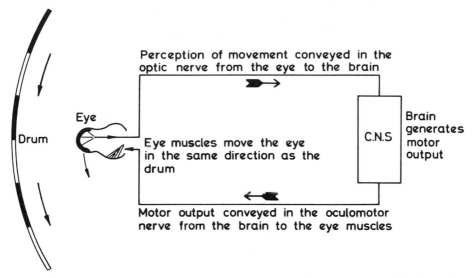

Fig. 4. Feedback control system of the crab eye. Movements of the eye in the same direction as the stimulus act to lessen the stimulus. By prevention of eye movement, the feedback loop is opened.

stimulus, which produces the optokinetic response, is the difference in the relative velocities of the drum and the eye, or the "slip."

The ways in which this so-called slip produces the optokinetic response can be demonstrated in another way, by keeping the visual field stationary and gently moving the eye. The success of this demonstration relies on the link between the two eyes which results in conjugate eye movements even if one eye is blinded. In the experiment, one eye is blinded by painting or capping it and its movements are monitored. The seeing eye is then gently forced to move while viewing a stationary pattern of stripes. The blind eye now moves as though the visual field had moved in a direction opposite to that in which the seeing eye is pushed, exactly as expected. If both eyes are blinded, there is no transferred movement; if both are allowed to see, the unforced eye begins to move in the appropriate direction, past the stationary visual field, and then stops abruptly. The inference which can be drawn from these experiments is that movements of the visual world relative to the eye, whether produced by actual movement of the visual field *or of the eye*, produce an optokinetic response which will diminish the difference in velocities between the eye and the world. The receptors are carried on the eyecup, and the system is a negative feedback loop (Fig. 4).

The finding that the movement of the eye will generate an optokinetic response in itself is basic to the concept of the visual control of the position of the eyes, and it can be demonstrated in many ways. If, for example, an eye is gently pushed to a new position in the dark and then confronted with a stationary striped pattern, it will keep its new position. Small drifts of the eye back to its original position are immediately corrected. The same result is obtained if a crab is made to move its eyes through only half a normal slow phase and then the drum is stopped. Another demonstration of the effect of the visual feedback on eye position is provided by the amount by which the eyes drift. When *Pachygrapsus* was surrounded by a striped drum in which the light intensity was 12.5 lux, the eye position was almost perfectly maintained, whereas in the dark the eye drifted about this position by up to 5° (Fig. 5). Thus, while it is possible to build a good case for the visual control of the eye movements, it has been impossible to show any effect on eye movements which could be attributed to proprioceptors.

The optokinetic eye movements clearly reduce the effective stimulus of a moving visual field because they are in the same direction. This feedback loop can be opened by the simple procedure of restraining the eye so that the drum velocity is now the same as the "slip" velocity. The response of the open-loop system to different velocities can be determined either by measuring the movements of the other eye, which is blinded but free to move, or by using a torque meter, which allows so little movement of the eye that the feedback is effectively broken. The open-loop response of the system is shown in Fig. 6. It is clearly nonlinear, and a calculation of the system's gain (i.e., output/input) shows that it is highly sensitive to movements of very low velocities. This characteristic of the system is demonstrated by responses of crabs to the movement of shadows cast by the sun. These shadows moved past the animal at about 0.007°/sec, which is well above the known threshold of about 0.002°/sec (Horridge, 1966b).

Voluntary Eye Movements

Like most positional control systems, the eye control system is overridden by "voluntary" movements of the animal (Horridge and Burrows, 1968c). A good example is the extension of the crab eye after a reflexive withdrawal. If a crab is facing a stationary striped pattern and is made to withdraw the eye on one side, when it reextends its eye the eye returns nearly to its original position, although to do this it must sweep past the contrasting visual field. By blinding the contralateral

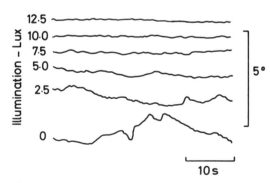

Fig. 5. Drift of the eye of *Pachygrapsus* at different light intensities, showing the stabilizing effect of the visual feedback control system.

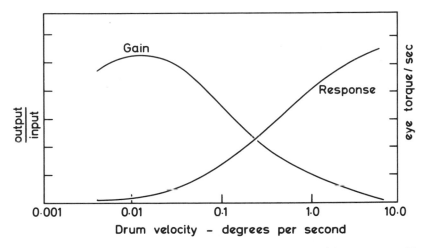

Fig. 6. Open-loop optokinetic response of *Carcinus* to different velocities of drum movement. The gain curve shows that the system is highly sensitive to velocities of about 0.01° sec. After Sandeman, Erber, and Kien (1975).

eye and measuring its movement, it can be shown that the movement of the reextending eye generates *no* optokinetic effect on the system. However, it can also be shown that the visual input to the system is not blocked, because small oscillations of the target *are* perceived and transmitted to the blinded eye. It may seem that this is a beautiful example of efference copy, but the simple test of preventing the reextension of the seeing eye with a mechanical stop (so that the compensatory efference copy signal, if it exists, should produce a movement in the blinded eye) shows that the blinded eye makes no movement, so an efference copy mechanism cannot be operating. One is left to suppose that the animal has other cues which allow it to distinguish between visual field movements caused by eye extension and those of the visual field itself. An analogy can be drawn here with leg resistance reflexes, so well known in many arthropods. Forced movements of the eye are resisted via the visual feedback loop, as are forced movements of legs via their proprioceptive systems. In both cases, these feedback systems are disregarded during voluntary movements.

Optokinetic Memory

One of the most remarkable phenomena associated with the crab optokinetic system is the so-called optokinetic memory (Horridge and Shepheard, 1966; Horridge, 1966a). This occurs if an animal is allowed to view a stationary target of stripes, or even a single light, for some time. The target is then occluded (by a screen or by darkness) and moved by a few degrees around the horizontal plane. After some time (from seconds to 10 min), the animal is allowed to see the target again, and it responds by moving its eyes in the direction the target moved, apparently attempting to reestablish the original alignment of the eyes with the target. This pehenomenon has been well studied by Wiersma and Hirsh (1974, 1975a,b) and is the subject of a separate chapter in this book. However, it can perhaps be said here that the term "memory" applied to this phenomenon may be a little misleading. The phenomenon is much more likely to be only one aspect of the animal's perception and response to movement and may be better compared with the well-known ϕ phenomenon, i.e., apparent movement generated when two images appear in different positions separated by a short dark period. The crab, known to be very sensitive to very slowly moving targets, may have a movement perception system sensitive to ϕ phenomena well beyond the range of humans, who use real memory to detect the different positions of the two objects which appear at different times in space and which are then not perceived as *movement*.

Statocyst-Induced Responses

Blinded crabs, if rotated on a turntable, will move their eyes in the direction opposite to the imposed rotation (Bethe, 1897a,b; Dijkgraaf, 1956a). An acceleration from a stationary start to some constant velocity usually results in one or two slow and fast phases, after which the eyes come to rest in their normal position. If the turntable is now abruptly arrested, the eyes move slowly in the direction the turntable was moving and undergo one or two fast phases in the opposite direction (Dijkgraaf, 1956b). The behavior is precisely like that found in vertebrate animals, which detect imposed angular accelerations with the fluid-filled canals of the vestibular system. Although it is not practical to produce a large number of consecutive slow and fast phases in crabs using the statocyst input, the slow-phase system can be studied by sinusoidally oscillating the animal about its vertical axis (Silvey and Sandeman 1976a,b,c; Silvey et al., 1976). The gain of the system is now high for high angular velocities and low for low angular velocities, unlike its response when driven by the optokinetic input (Fig. 7).

A single slow phase and the subsequent fast phase of nystagmus can be artificially evoked in crabs by opening the statocysts and allowing saline to flow gently through them. The advantage of this technique is that it can be used to produce nystagmus in semi-isolated eye/brain preparations in which access to the somata of the oculomotor neurons is possible (see below).

Neuronal Systems

Anatomy

The neural systems concerned with the production of the compensatory eye movements are contained in the optic and cerebral ganglia. The optic ganglion in crabs consists of the retina, lamina, and external, internal, and terminal medulla

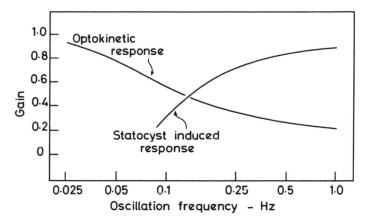

Fig. 7. Comparison of the gains of the optokinetic and statocyst-induced compensatory eye movements. The optokinetic response is produced by oscillating a striped drum around the animal; the statocyst-induced response is obtained when a blinded animal is oscillated on a torsion swing. After Silvey and Sandeman (1976a).

neuropils. The optic nerves, containing about 20,000 axons (Nunnemacher *et al*; 1962), link the optic ganglia with the brain. The fibers contained in the optic lobe are by no means only those associated with vision but range from axons from mechanoreceptive hairs on the eyecup through MNs to the eye-withdrawal muscles and to visual and multimodal INs which carry information to or from the brain or between the two optic ganglia (Wiersma, 1967).

The response characteristics of a number of optic nerve neurons are known (see below), but no single neuron which responds to a visual input has been fully described anatomically and physiologically.

The oculomotor neurons are better known. They have their somata located laterally between the deutocerebral neuropils and the olfactory lobes. The axons and axon arborizations of these cells are all ipsilateral as revealed by reverse filling of the cells with cobalt sulfide. The central synaptic fields of the oculomotor neurons and the thread-hair receptor axons from the statocyst occupy the same areas of the deutocerebrum.

Sensory Input from the Eye

Many of the fibers in the optic nerve which respond to visual cues have not been tested with optokinetic stimuli, or do not show an obvious response to moving patterns. However, all types are reported here because their presence is now well established not only for crabs but for other decapod crustaceans as well (Wiersma, 1967; Wiersma and Yamaguchi, 1966, 1967a,b; Wiersma and Yanagisawa, 1971).

Sustaining Fibers

Sustaining fibers appear to be the simplest type of fiber. They have large axons and so are relatively easily found in the optic nerve by a prospecting extracellular microelectrode. Two types, with different latencies, are reported for *Podophthalmus* (Waterman *et al.*, 1964) and *Carcinus* (Wiersma, 1970). The *Carcinus* responses, which are similar to those described for crayfish and rock lobsters, consist of a burst of spikes at the beginning of a light-on stimulus, followed by a maintained train of impulses at a lower frequency. The frequency of the maintained discharge is roughly proportional to the light intensity (Wiersma, 1970). The fibers invariably have wide visual fields, covering many ommatidia. Sustaining fibers are multimodal in that the frequency of a sustaining fiber is increased if the light-on stimulus is paired with mechanical stimulation or occurs simultaneously with voluntary leg movements. This phenomenon, i.e., an increased activity of a neuron's specific response produced by nonspecific inputs which alone produce no reaction, is a characteristic of several neurons in the eye movement system. This is discussed at greater length in connection with MN discharges (see below).

Multimodality is found in a variety of INs in the optic nerve. The most common type respond to either visual or mechanoreceptive inputs, but the most remarkable example of multimodality is found in some sustaining fibers which exhibit a property that has been called "space constancy" (Wiersma, 1966). Essentially, it is an interaction between the animal's position with respect to gravity and the visual field size of the sustaining fiber. A unit with a 90° visual field, for example, will increase the size of its visual field to 180° if the animal is rolled on its side with the eye pointing upward. The unit becomes unresponsive (blind) if the animal is rolled so that the eye points downwards.

Dimming Fibers

Dimming fibers complement the sustaining fibers in that they increase their rate of firing with decreasing levels of light intensity.

Movement Fibers

Barely responsive to changes in intensity in *Podophthalmus,* movement fibers react when an object is moved with respect to the background. Several classes can be distinguished by differences in their habituation to repeated stimuli and sensitivity to different velocities. "Slow" movement fibers respond to 0.016°/sec or less, and faster units respond with less habituation to velocities of 0.016°/sec to 1.6°/sec. They show some directional selectivity in *Podophthalmus* (Waterman *et al.*, 1964) and in hermit crabs (Glantz, 1973*b*). In *Carcinus,* the movement-sensitive fibers respond with prolonged activity if the target is moved erratically, hence the term "jittery movement fibers" for these neurons. Significantly, these fibers do not respond at all to the movement of a striped drum (Wiersma, 1970).

Optokinetic Fibers

In *Carcinus,* axons from directionally selective units which respond to movements of a striped pattern run between the internal medulla and external medulla. The units can be arranged into three classes depending on their response to velocity, direction of selectivity, binocular or monocular input, etc. (Sandeman *et al.,* 1975*b*). Two classes (1 and 2) of units respond to drum movements over velocities from about 0.005°/sec to 10°/sec. The third class (3) responds to velocities from 1.0°/sec to above 10°/sec. Class 1 has a high frequency of spontaneous discharge in the absence of movement in the visual field; this is unchanged when the striped drum is moved in the nonpreferred direction. Class 2 units are inhibited by drum movements in the nonpreferred direction.

Simultaneous measurements of eye torque and optokinetic IN discharges show a close correlation between neuron frequency and eye torque, so that even small irregularities of the neuron's frequency are reflected in the eye torque (Fig. 8A).

Sensory Input from the Statocyst

While the mechanism of the visual perception of movement is not yet known, the detection of angular acceleration by the crab statocyst is now quite well understood. Basically, the crab statocyst resembles the vertebrate vestibular system in that it is fashioned into a system of circular canals. The compensatory movements of the eyes in the horizontal plane are caused by the fluid in the horizontal canals being displaced by angular accelerations about the yaw axis (Sandeman and Okajima, 1972). The fine thread hairs, which extend across the canal, can alone produce compensatory eye movements when the sensory nerves from all other receptor hairs

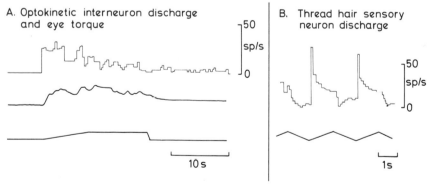

Fig. 8. A: Correlation between the firing frequency of an optokinetic IN (top trace) and the eye torque (center trace). The bottom trace indicates the changes in drum velocity. B: Responses of a thread-hair sensory neuron (upper trace) of an intact crab statocyst rotated at constant velocity first in one direction and then the other. The lower trace indicates changes in position. A after Sandeman, Kien, and Erber (1975); B after Silvey *et al.* (1976).

in the statocyst are cut (Silvey *et al.,* 1976). Recordings from the thread-hair sensory nerve of intact statocysts show that there are two populations of neurons, each sensitive to fluid flow in one direction or the other. Acceleration from zero to a constant velocity results in a phasic burst, which adapts within about 1 sec to a new maintained level of discharge. This ceases abruptly if the direction of angular rotation is reversed (Fig. 8B). The information about the direction and the magnitude of the angular velocity of the crab is all represented in the two classes of thread-hair neurons. If these are correctly addressed to the appropriate MNs of the eye, there would seem to be no need for any complex integrative IN circuits, at least as far as the slow-phase movements of nystagmus are concerned.

The Oculomotor Neurons

Recordings from the axons of the oculomotor neurons during optokinetic nystagmus reveal little more than do recordings from the eye muscles themselves and do not have the advantage of the latter method of being able to make positive identifications. No one has yet succeeded in obtaining intracellular recordings from the MNs during optokinetic nystagmus, but this has been possible in semi-isolated eye/brain preparations using the statocyst input to drive the MNs into nystagmus. This method requires that the statocyst be opened and the horizontal canal gently irrigated with saline. A maintained flow of saline produces a slow and a fast phase in the appropriate MNs and eye muscles, and a small-amplitude oscillatory flow produces slow-phase movements of the eyes first in one direction and then the other (Sandeman and Okajima, 1973a; Silvey and Sandeman, 1976a). Positive identification of the MNs, which can be seen but cannot be visually identified as belonging to particular eye muscles, relies on backfiring of their axons with an extracellular stimulus applied at a known eye muscle and recording of the antidromic spike in the cell soma. Two problems have been explored using this technique: the first relates to the integrative action of the CNS in transforming the thread-hair nerve discharge into slow-phase eye movements, and the second is concerned with the onset of the fast phase of nystagmus, known for some time to be centrally initiated (Horridge and Sandeman, 1964; Horridge and Burrows, 1968b).

Slow-Phase Movements

Frequencies of discharge of MNs supplying muscles 20a and 21, which move the eye away from and toward the midline, respectively, show a close relationship with the discharge frequency of the thread-hair sensory nerve, suggestive of a direct and possibly monosynaptic link between the two (Silvey and Sandeman, 1976a). Electrical stimulation of the thread-hair nerve evokes an epsp in the MN which, with carefully controlled increases in stimulus intensity, increases in a smooth and graded way. Step increments, suggesting that the recruitment of single sensory axons resulted in recordable unitary epsp's in the MN, have never been seen. The synaptic delays between the sensory nerve and the MN are about 1.3–1.4 msec, and perfusing the preparation with high magnesium results in a gradual loss of epsp amplitude rather than a sudden failure such as would occur if the epsp depended on the integrity of an IN pathway. The thread-hair neurons of different directionalities therefore appear to be connected in such a way that the oculomotor neurons are driven directly and simply by them. The intracellular recordings, however, provide evidence of an additional IN input to the MNs (Silvey and Sandeman, 1976b). A single sensory neuron from the statocyst, as has been pointed out above, does not produce recordable unitary epsp's in the MNs, but unitary epsp's nevertheless frequently appear in the somata of MNs supplying muscle 21. These increase in frequency, although spikes result only erratically when other nonspecific inputs such as the tegumentary nerve are stimulated. The epsp's will elicit spikes if the membrane of the MN is smoothly depolarized by the action of the thread-hair neurons following statocyst irrigation. It would appear that the specific response of the MNs to the statocyst signal is gated by nonspecific inputs from other sources. The model suggested for this system is one in which the direct path from the sensory to the MNs is paralleled by a multimodal gating IN (Fig. 9). The phenomenon of increased activity of the MNs and visual fibers, caused by nonspecific mechanoreceptive inputs, has been noted several times in the eye movement system (Wiersma, 1967; Aréchiga and Wiersma, 1969a; Wiersma and Fiore, 1971a,b). It is

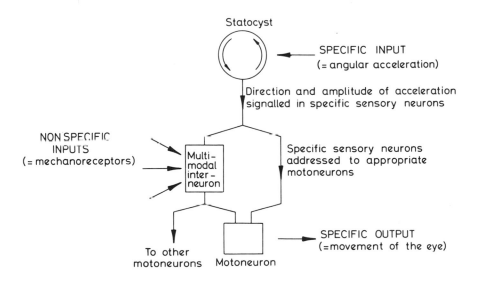

Fig. 9. Parallel-gating circuit proposed for the statocyst-induced eye movements. The specific sensory neurons send branches directly to appropriate MNs as well as to the multimodal gating IN. This IN also receives other nonspecific inputs; its action is to raise the probability that certain muscle systems will react to their specific inputs.

conceivable that such a relatively simple neuronal network is fairly widespread and probably not only in the crab eye movement system.

The Fast Phase

The mechanism of generation of the fast phase is still not known, but there are several well-established points. Early experiments showed that there was no relationship between position of the eye and the onset of the fast phase of nystagmus. The demonstration that fast phases can be generated in oculomotor neurons with the eye completely removed establishes conclusively the central origin of the behavior (Sandeman and Okajima, 1973b). Furthermore, in both optokinetic and statocyst-induced nystagmus the fast phase has never been seen to occur without the precursive slow phase, although in freely moving animals a fast flick of the eyes in the direction of turning is sometimes the first eye movement observed.

Several models for the fast-phase system of both vertebrates and invertebrates have been proposed. All depend on a central "fast-phase generator" which, once its threshold has been overcome by some measure of slow-phase activity, abruptly inhibits the slow-phase muscle system and briefly excites the antagonists. Intracellular recordings from the oculomotor neurons show that they are certainly strongly hyperpolarized during the fast phase (Sandeman and Okajima, 1973b), but direct depolarization of single MNs never triggered a fast phase, nor did hyperpolarization prevent a fast phase. It seemed that the fast-phase generator was not triggered by MN activity. However, recent measurements of eye torque and eye muscle activity in *Carcinus* lead to the conclusion that fast phases of the eye away from the midline will occur only if the late-firing system of muscle 21 has been activated; the fast-phase generator could be linked with this system, but the connection between the two is gated by the activity of the early-firing muscle system (Sandeman et al., 1975a).

One of the difficulties with the original model is that a transient inhibition delivered to only the MNs would not explain how the whole system becomes reset, nor why it does not rebound to the same level it held before the inhibition. Here, too, recent work sheds some light: the optokinetic INs in *Carcinus* are clearly partially inhibited during the fast phase and then gradually increase their discharge frequency again during the next slow phase. The implication is that the transient inhibition during the fast phase is delivered to all levels in the system, thus effectively resetting it.

Conclusion

The study of the neural control of crab eye movements has yielded a great deal of information, some of which may be of general applicability and some of which is appropriate only to the crab eye. Some aspects of the control system are beginning to be understood, but as a preparation the crab eye has only now reached its most interesting stage, because research has begun on the activity of the neural elements of the optic ganglia. Recordings have been made from retinula cells, lamina cells, and higher-order neurons in the ganglia during the presentation of visual stimuli (Erber and Sandeman, in preparation). We hope that in the future the crab studies will provide some understanding of the general features of the visual detection of movement.

9

Central and Peripheral Features of Crayfish Oculomotor Organization

De Forest Mellon, Jr.

Introduction

Animals which see utilize a number of reflex movements tending to stabilize on the retina those features of the visual environment which have immediate selective value. The movements may themselves be evoked by visual events, as in optomotor or optokinetic reactions, and compensatory behavior can involve the head or even the entire body. In vertebrates, some mollusks, and a number of crustaceans, however, the retinal surfaces are mounted on paired platforms which are capable of movement relative to the head proper. In these animals, many visual stabilization reflexes are the sole domain of an independent oculomotor system.

Oculomotor control of the stalked compound eyes of decapod crustaceans is of interest for a number of reasons. The eyes serve as an attractive model system to study ballistic activation of muscles. In addition to the visually evoked tracking movements, the eyes adopt reproducible angular deviations from their usual rest position when the animal is rotated in the dark about the longitudinal or transverse body axis. Since these eye movements do not of themselves result in corrective changes of body position by the animal, and as there is reason to believe that proprioceptive input is not an important feature of the eyestalk muscle system, the final position of the eyes in response to body rotation must be precisely "read in" to the motor command in all its detail from information gleaned entirely by other sensory systems.

Optokinetic control also exhibits the intriguing property of memory (e.g., Wiersma and Hirsh, 1974). In a suitably contrasty environment, the compound eyes will adopt a mean rest position. If the visual environment undergoes translational shifts during a period of total darkness, then upon subsequent reillumination the position of the eyes will change so that the visual surround once again corresponds to its former rest state. It is apparent that the animal remembers salient features of the original surround, since reillumination triggers accurate corrective movements of the eyes following a dark period of up to 10 min in duration (Horridge, 1966a).

De Forest Mellon, Jr. • Department of Biology, University of Virginia, Charlottesville, Virginia 22903.

The precision of oculomotor reflexes suggests a high degree of functional organization in the neural apparatus which provides for their control. We wished to examine the anatomical and physiological features of this organization and chose the crayfish *Procambarus clarkii* for a number of reasons. The neurobiology of this animal has been more extensively studied than that of any other crustacean and perhaps—with the possible exception of the locust—any other arthropod. More important, this animal provides a unique and intriguing opportunity to investigate at first hand the evolutionary changes which can occur in the form and operation of neuronal systems. Individual species of at least three separate crayfish genera are found in the subterranean cave environment throughout the southeastern and south midwestern United States (Hobbs and Means, 1971; Hobbs and Barr, 1960, 1972). The conditions of total darkness within which these animals have evolved have led to degenerative changes in the sensory structure of the compound eyes. Where these changes are severe, the animals are blind, and it is relevant to ask whether that part of the nervous system which is concerned with visual stabilization reflexes has itself undergone alterations.

As with the visual sensory structures themselves, one should expect a deterioration in the oculomotor apparatus, if from no other mechanism than through the maintenance of random mutational changes which no longer are eliminated from the genome by acute selective pressures. The form which these degenerative changes take can possibly establish a hierarchy of organization features in terms of evolutionary stability. In other words, following a reduction of the selective pressures which maintain a part of the nervous system in a pristine condition, it would be interesting to know which features of its functional organization will be the first to change and which will resist mutational change through an inherent genetic stability. It is possible that answers to these questions can point to general processes through which evolutionary change in nervous structure and function comes about.

Spatial Organization of Oculomotor Neurons

The structure of the crayfish oculomotor system has not been previously described. We have used a combination of fine dissection, electrophysiology, axonal backfilling with cobalt chloride, and electron microscopy to examine the organization of the eye muscles and the oculomotor neurons in *P. clarkii*.

General Anatomy

A diagram of the crayfish brain is provided in Fig. 1, along with a photograph of a cleared preparation in which the oculomotor neurons of the right side have been visualized by the cobalt technique. The somata of the oculomotor neurons on each side exist within three separate groups (Mellon *et al.*, 1976; Mellon, 1977*b*): (1) an anterior cluster of nine cells (AMC), (2) a giant cell cluster with three somata (GC), and (3) a lateral cluster (LC) containing 18–24 small cell bodies. Axons of all the oculomotor

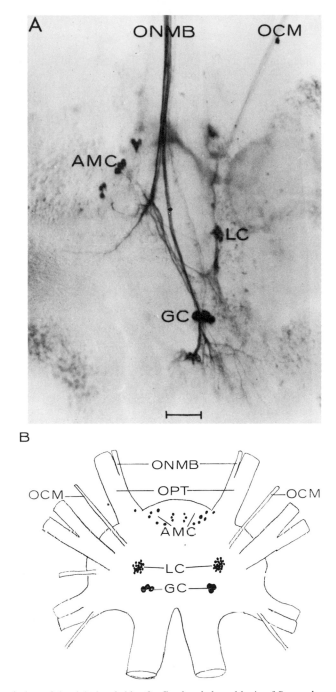

Fig. 1. A: Dorsal view of the right-hand side of a fixed and cleared brain of *Procambarus clarkii*. All oculomotor neurons have been backfilled with cobalt chloride via their peripherally transected axons. AMC, Anterior MN cluster; LC, lateral MN cluster; GC, giant cell cluster; ONMB, optic nerve motor bundle; OCM, oculomotor nerve. B: Diagram of the crayfish brain showing the relative disposition of the various neuron somata of the oculomotor system.

neurons exit the brain within one of two separate nerves, and in this respect the brain of the crayfish shares organizational features with that of crabs (Bethe, 1897a; Sandeman, 1964; Burrows and Horridge, 1968b). Axons of both the AMC and the GC run first within the optic nerve and then in a separate nerve branch, the optic nerve motor bundle (ONMB). In contrast, axons of the neurons in the LC supply the eyestalk by a distinct oculomotor nerve (OCM) which emerges from the dorsal surface of the brain just posterior and lateral to the optic nerve. While neurons in each of the two motor pathways supply only selected muscles of the eye, their separation seems to be based more on functional than on anatomical ground, because some eyecup muscles receive the terminations of axons from both sources. Before the physiological differences reflecting this separation in the efferent supply are discussed, it will be appropriate to examine an anatomical question which excited our interest early in this study (Mellon et al., 1976).

Statistical Analysis of AMC Distribution

The technique of axonal backfilling with cobalt ions works very reliably with the AMC in the crayfish oculomotor system, and it became apparent that the high success rate justified the expenditure of some time in quantifying positional variability in the spatial location of the individual neurons. We chose cell body position in the study, because the soma is the most easily identified landmark of the entire cell, often the only portion of the cell that is visible in the cleared preparations. The techniques we used in our study do not depend on knowing the location of the soma per se, however, and they have general applicability not only to other identifiable regions of neurons but to other neuronal systems as well.

Our efforts to establish a numerical basis for soma position presented two problems. The first was that of coordinate normalization. The dimensions and boundary features of different brains always differ to some extent, and, without some means of establishing a system of generalized coordinates having a fixed point of reference in relation to the brain, spatial variability between neuron homologues would be lost in the noise created by real differences among individual brains. Our solution involved a standardized set of so-called local coordinates, to which photographic projections of two different views of a cleared brain could be roughly fitted (Fig. 2). The local coordinates in this system of each of the nine AMC somata on one side of a brain were recorded and used to determine a center of population density for that AMC. This point became the origin of a new "absolute" coordinate system, the dimensions of which were scaled in each preparation after comparing the distance between the population centers on the two sides with an arbitrary value. Finally, in order to simplify the computational procedures, the right-hand AMC coordinates were inverted to their mirror image and translated so that the coordinate origins of the two sides were superimposed. Thus further processing of the data was accomplished using 100 individual "left-hand" sides.

Generation of the absolute coordinate system left unsolved the second major problem, namely, the difficulty in providing accurate identifications of each cell type in every preparation. Some consistent visual cues such as differences in soma

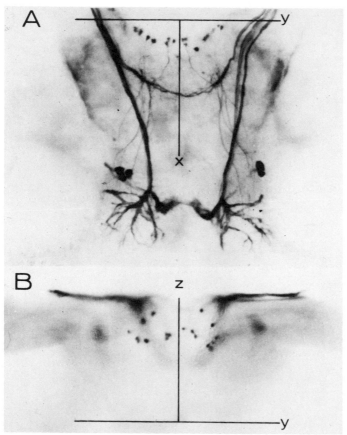

Fig. 2. Fixed and cleared crayfish brain seen from a dorsal (A) and an anterior (B) view. Both photographs are shown superimposed on the axes of the local coordinate system. AMC and GC somata have been visualized by the cobalt backfilling technique.

size, cell groupings, and relative position within the brain allowed positive identification to be made of four out of the nine cells in each half brain. In others, however, close groupings and similar cell size precluded an absolute identification, and there was often confusion as to which cell was which. In the establishment of ideal positions for each soma type, misnaming of cells in some preparations would be expected to produce errors in the final mean coordinates. We therefore sought an independent means of verifying the ideal positions calculated from individual cell identification. The technique chosen is one designated by Sneath and Sokal (1973) as complete linkage clustering; it provides a way to group entities which have affinities with one another. We wished to determine whether this technique would place the 900 cell positions into coherent clusters having arithmetic centers similar to those obtained by the technique of assigning a particular designation to each cell in a preparation. This clustering technique was performed twice; in each case, the 100 data sets (half brains) were grouped into ten lots. All 90 cell positions in a lot were run through the clustering routine by computer, and the results were plotted as

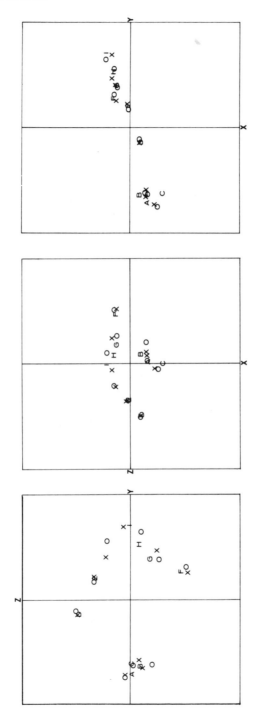

Fig. 3. Views down the three axes of the absolute coordinate system showing the positions of the means for each of the nine AMC somata (A–I) obtained by visual analysis and those of the cluster centers obtained by the two complete runs of the linkage analysis (X, O). There is close correspondence between the two methods for cells D, E, F, and G.

projections upon the absolute coordinate system. We restructured each plot by eliminating the most poorly defined clusters and reassigning the resulting uncommitted cell positions to the nearest cluster. New cluster center locations were then calculated. When this had been done for all ten lots, the 90 resultant cluster centers were themselves submitted to the clustering routine to obtain the centers of the nine "best" clusters.

Views down the three axes of the absolute coordinate system are illustrated in Fig. 3. In each projection, the ideal positions for each of the nine AMC somata obtained by individual cell identifications are shown by the block letters A through I. Centers of the nine best clusters obtained in each of the two complete linkage procedures are shown as points marked with an X and an O. It is clear that there is excellent agreement between the two methods with regard to cells D, E, F, and G. This result gave us sufficient confidence in the accuracy of the mean positions of these four cells to pose a question regarding the development of bilateral symmetry in the brain. We simply asked whether the variability in the position from the mean of an individual cell would be greater between left–right pairs of homologous neurons from different brains compared to pairs across the same brain. Put another way, we wished to find out if an accurate prediction of the position of a cell could be made by knowing the absolute coordinates of its opposite homologue in the same brain. A t test was performed on the difference in the position of pairs of cells D, E, F, and G from the same animal and those randomly selected from opposite sides of different animals. The results of these calculations are shown in Table I. No significance can be attributed to the difference between cell pairs from the same brain as opposed to those between pairs from opposite sides of different brains. These somewhat startling findings allow us to draw the following conclusion: bilaterally homologous cells from the same animal do not possess identical spatial orientation within the absolute coordinate system even though they carry an identical genome. Variation in individual cell position from the ideal value cannot therefore be under direct genetic control.

Table I

Cell name	Pairing mode	Mean cross-brain difference	S.E.	t
D	Same-animal	33.844	2.124	0.226
	Different-	38.150	2.828	
E	Same-animal	30.406	2.042	0.160
	Different-	34.460	2.004	
F	Same-animal	37.100	2.983	0.293
	Different-	41.698	3.168	
G	Same-animal	36.472	2.724	0.657
	Different-	38.220	2.833	

It is now generally assumed that the amount of specific genetic information available to the developing metazoan is not sufficient to account directly for the finished details of nervous system fine structure (e.g., Horridge, 1968). This generality appears to be supported by the oculomotor neuron positional data. Since neurons on each side of the brain themselves possess, and are derived from cells which bear, an identical set of genetic instructions, differences in the adult homologues must arise from discrepancies occurring during the reading out of the genetic instructions. Thus, insofar as precise anatomical detail is concerned, the findings of bilateral independence of position would appear to support a permissive rather than an instructive mode of control by the genetic information store.

Functional Segregation of Oculomotor Neurons

The dual supraesophageal pathways to the muscles of the crayfish eye reflect a segregation in function as first suggested by Wiersma and Oberjat (1968); different reflex or centrally generated behaviors are mediated through different efferent pathways (Mellon and Lorton, 1977). Even though some eyecup muscles receive axon terminations from neurons of different divisions, the sensory modalities which drive different eyestalk movements are well specified. The three divisions will be arbitrarily named the "cuticular division," the "peduncular division," and the "optokinetic division."

The Cuticular Division

Axons of the cuticular division supply the muscles of the eye via the ONMB. They mediate three distinct kinds of reflex behavior:

1. Motor neurons (MNs) of the AMC supply muscles which retract the eyecups during protective withdrawal following tactile stimulation of the head region. Rapid withdrawal appears to be driven aditionally by activity in the three giant MNs (GC), two of which supply the largest muscle in the eyestalk, muscle 15. The targets of the third axon are muscles 16, 17, and 18 (Mellon, 1977b). The largest impulses which can be discerned in extracellular records obtained from ONMB following intense tactile stimulation of the cephalothorax, those of the giant cell axons, are correlated with excitatory junctional potentials (ejp's) in muscle 15. Other neurons of the ONMB are excited by the stimulus as well, and axons of these cells innervate both fast phasic and slow tonic fibers of other muscles of the eyecup.

2. Rotation of the crayfish about the longitudinal or transverse body axis in the dark elicits eyestalk movements which are driven by afferent input originating in the statocysts. Figure 4 illustrates simultaneous electrical activity in both ONMBs of an animal during oscillatory rotations about the longitudinal body axis. During imposed roll to the right, impulse activity in the ipsilateral ONMB is increased over levels obtaining when the animal is in the horizontal attitude. Activity in the contralateral ONMB is simultaneously reduced. These findings are in agreement with

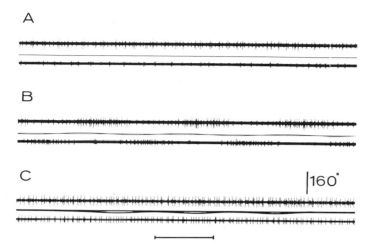

Fig. 4. Simultaneous extracellular records (top and bottom traces) from both ONMBs of a crayfish resting in normal posture (A) and during oscillatory roll about the animal's longitudinal axis (B). The middle trace in each frame monitors movement. C: Conditions similar to those in B, but records obtained from both oculomotor nerves (OCM) of another preparation. Time: 1 sec.

the behavioral studies on *Procambarus* by Fay (1973, 1975). Axons of the ONMB primarily supply those muscles (11, 12, 13a, 14a) which act as a suspensory system for the eyecup (Mellon and Lorton, 1977), and compensatory counterrotation of the intereyestalk axis which occurs during an imposed roll must result from an increase in the activity of those muscles on the depressed side of the animal and a simultaneous decrease in activity of those muscles on the elevated side. Recent evidence (Mellon and Lorton, 1977) suggests that additional AMC neurons assist the latter.

    3.   When a crayfish is held horizontally by means of a carapace clamp, the position of its legs relative to the body provides information which is used to control the attitude of the eyecups (Fay, 1973). This behavior is mediated mainly by axons of the cuticular system, as illustrated in the records of Fig. 5. An animal was

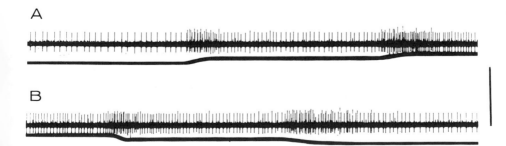

Fig. 5. A,B: Continuous extracellular recordings (upper traces) from the right-hand ONMB during roll (lower traces) imparted to the platform supporting the animal's walking legs. Upward movement of the lower trace indicates a roll of the platform to the left. Calibration: 120° and 1 sec.

suspended in air by a clamp around the cephalothorax, while the legs rested in normal posture on a flat polyurethane cushion. Roll imparted to the leg platform produced steady changes in the frequency of impulses recorded from the right-hand ONMB: a roll of the platform toward the right was followed by a reduction in impulse frequency, while roll in the opposite direction increased average impulse frequency. This reflex control of efferent activity thus cooperates with that evoked by statocyst input, since induced roll of a freely moving animal toward the right, for example, would generate reflex output in the ONMB both from the statocysts (*cf.* Fig. 4) and from flexion of the legs of the right-hand side. Fay's (1973) behavioral observations in fact showed that the two effects were additive, and the final position attained by the eyes during induced roll of the animal was less extreme if the platform on which the legs rested was rolled in congruence with the animal itself. When the leg platform was rotated in a sense opposite to that of the animal, the magnitude of the response to the roll was even further reduced.

The Peduncular Division

Roll impressed upon a crayfish when the ambient illumination originates from directly overhead generates a counterrotation of the eyecups which is quantitatively greater than that resulting from the same degree of roll under conditions of absolute darkness (Fay, 1973). This dorsal light response must originate from an unbalanced illumination of the compound eyes, and it is effected, at least partly, through MNs of the peduncular division. This reflex action is shown graphically in Fig. 6. An animal was fixed in its normal posture in a dissecting dish and a black light-tight mask was fitted over the right-hand eye. Suction recording electrodes were then

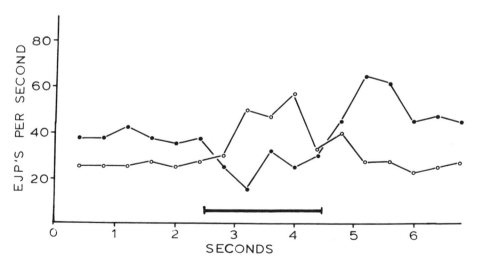

Fig. 6. Changes in the frequency of tonic ejp's in muscle 12 on the two sides of an animal during brief illumination of the left eye. ●, Records from the ipsilateral muscle; ○, contralateral records. Illumination period indicated by the horizontal bar.

placed on the dorsal surface of the main suspensory muscle in each eye, muscle 12, and after several minutes' adaptation in total darkness a light was directed on the seeing left-hand eye. This stimulus had the effect of causing an increase in frequency of ongoing ejp's in muscle 12 of the blind eye and simultaneously decreasing ejp frequency in muscle 12 of the seeing eye. These experimental conditions, while extreme, reflect the more subtle changes in relative excitation of muscle 12 on the two sides when a freely moving sky-lit animal rolls about its longitudinal axis. The reflex acts in such a way as to maintain the horizontal disposition of the intereye axis, and its effects are additive with those generated by input from the statocysts.

Surgical isolation of the eye from the supraesophageal ganglion (SOG) by transecting the OCM and ONMB allows one to eliminate possible visual reflexes which cross over from the opposite side, or which are mediated by pathways within the SOG. Recent electrophysiological data, supported by studies employing axonal backfilling with cobalt, indicate that a pair of MNs supplying muscle 12 originate within the most proximal ganglion of the optic peduncle, the medulla terminalis. At least one of these tonically active MNs responds to illumination of the retina by a reduction in the frequency of impulse output. Additional work will be necessary to determine to what extent the observation of Fig. 6 can be explained on the basis of activity in this pair of peduncular MNs.

The Optokinetic Division

The optokinetic division consists of neurons from the lateral cluster. Axons of these cells travel within the OCM and probably supply a majority of the 11 muscles of the eye. However, details of the anatomical organization of this division are not well understood at the present time. The optokinetic division provides the major control for movement of the eyes in the horizontal plane, and reflexes involving these translational movements are driven by two major sources of sensory input.

1.   A crayfish fixed in the usual posture by a carapace clamp, but whose legs rest on the center of a level circular platform, will move its eyes toward the direction of imposed rotation of the platform. It is demonstrated in Fig. 7b not only that impulse activity occurs in the right-hand oculomotor nerve in response to platform rotation, but also that such activity is direction specific: rotation to the right produces an increase in the discharge frequency of at least one small unit and inhibits ongoing activity in a larger unit. The opposite effect occurs in response to leftward rotation of the platform.

Several sources of proprioceptive input to the oculomotor system could be responsible for this reflex drive (e.g., Evoy and Cohen, 1971), but the most favorable candidate is the muscle receptor organ which spans the thoracicocoxal joint at the base of each walking leg (Alexandrowicz and Whitear, 1957; Whitear, 1965). Platform rotation will produce a torque at this point similar to that generated during voluntary movement of the legs in effecting a body turn in the same direction. I shall return to this point later on.

2.   Translational movement of the visual environment causes the crayfish to perform tracking movements with its eyes, the well-known optokinetic nystagmus

which has been examined extensively in crabs (Horridge, 1966*a*,*b*,*c*,*d*; Horridge and Sandeman, 1964; Burrows and Horridge, 1968*a*,*b*,*c*; Horridge and Burrows, 1968*a*,*b*,*c*). This reflex, which must assist in retinal image stabilization, can be examined by clamping an animal in the center of a drum having alternating black and white vertical stripes painted on its inside surface. Rotation of the drum will generate movement of the eyes in the same direction. The neuronal basis of this behavioral reflex can be illustrated by electrical records from the oculomotor nerve, as shown in Fig. 7A. As with the leg rotation, impulse activity in the right oculomotor nerve is highly specific for the direction of drum movement. In fact, when the two reflexes are examined in the same preparation, it is apparent that the same axons are utilized to control the respective movements of the eye, since the same direction of rotation of either the leg platform or the visual surround excites the identical neurons (Fig. 7B).

According to behavioral observations (Dijkgraaf, 1955, 1956*a*; Olivo, personal communication), freely moving crustaceans will signal a change in direction by moving their eyes toward the side on which the turn occurs. The functional significance of this behavior is not immediately apparent; its discovery in fact confounds the assumption that reflex eye movements provide exclusively for visual stabilization. Nonetheless, the presence of the response to leg rotation provides a possible mechanism through which these anticipatory eye movements may be controlled.

The thoracicocoxal muscle receptor organs previously mentioned are anatomically arranged in parallel with the coxal promotor muscle in each walking leg (Alexandrowicz and Whitear, 1957; Whitear, 1965). The promotor muscle provides the power stroke to the legs during an ipsilateral turn—the animal, in effect, walks backward, with the legs on the inside of the turn. Now, rotation of the substrate will passively stretch the coxal muscle receptors on the side toward which rotation occurs, so that this mode of stimulation can thus provide appropriate sensory input to excite the oculomotor neurons. If all or part of the motor supply to the inside promotor muscle is shared with that of the coxal receptor muscle, an anticipated or executed turn by the animal would increase receptor tension and reflexly move the eyes in the same direction. Although experimental evidence is lacking for the involvement of the thoracicocoxal receptors in either substrate-driven or anticipa-

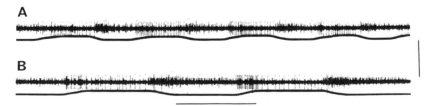

Fig. 7. Extracellular records from the right-hand oculomotor nerve during rotation of a vertically striped drum around the animal (A) and during rotation of the platform supporting the legs (B). Downward movement of the lower trace indicates platform rotation to the right. Calibration: 2 sec.

tory eye movements, the proposed mechanism is presently the simplest explanation which will account for both the behavioral and anatomical observations. The functional significance of the oculomotor reflex to passive torsion of the legs during platform rotation, whether or not controlled by thoracicocoxal proprioceptors, remains largely a point of conjecture. One can speculate that this movement constitutes a primitive efference copy mechanism. When a crayfish makes a voluntary turn—say, to the right—its eyes will perceive a relative motion of the visual environment *to the left*. The usual visually induced optokinetic reflex ought to drive both eyes to the left under these circumstances, but this does not happen. Instead, the eyes actually move in the opposite direction, possibly as a result of proprioceptive feedback, as discussed above. If one assumes that a net leftward movement of the eyes during a right turn by the body is disadvantageous in a selective sense, proprioceptive influences may have evolved by counteracting this effect of visual reafference.

Anatomical Comparisons between Epigean and Troglobitic Species

A major reason for undertaking the study of the crayfish oculomotor system was to provide anatomical and functional templates for comparison between surface-dwelling and cave-dwelling forms. It will therefore be appropriate to conclude this chapter with a brief account of the comparative studies so far completed.

We chose to examine *Procambarus erythrops*, a newly described troglobitic species found in limestone caves and associated sinkholes in northern Florida (Relyea and Sutton, 1975) and having largely degenerate visual structures.

The eyecups of *P. erythrops* are much reduced in size compared to those of *P. clarkii*. While the corneal surface of the eyecups in the latter species occupies the terminal half of the eyecup, that in *P. erythrops* is reduced to a small apical region which, in the living animal, can be delineated by a red subcuticular pigmentation. All traces of corneal faceting—prominent in the epigean species—are lacking in *P. erythrops* (Fig. 8).

Microscopic examination of the retina and visual ganglia in the eyes of *P. erythrops* indicates that these structures are anatomically degenerate (Fig. 9). Ommatidia in the cave form are sparse, and their structure appears to be abnormal. The well-defined laminar organization of the three most distal eyecup ganglia in *P. clarkii* is clearly lacking in *P. erythrops*. Finally, attempts to obtain electroretinograms from the intact corneal surface of the living *P. erythrops* have yielded only negative results. We have been forced to conclude that these animals are functionally blind.

A careful examination of the muscular anatomy in the reduced eyes of *P. erythrops* has shown that all 11 muscles described for the surface-dwelling species are present (Mellon, 1977*a*). Nonetheless, the individual muscles are all very much smaller in the troglobitic form, in some cases containing only a very few fibers. We

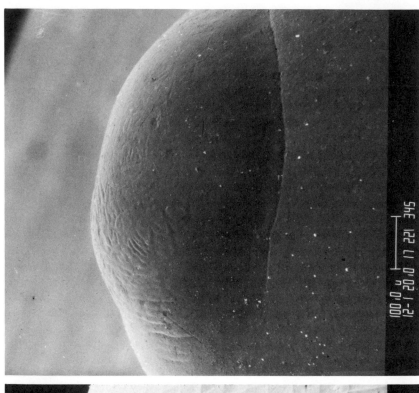

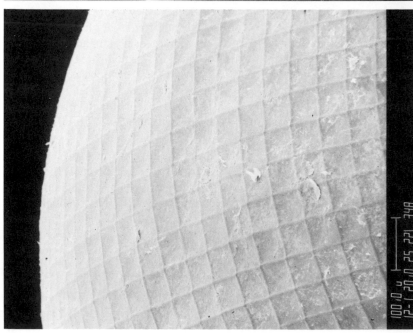

Fig. 8. Scanning electron micrographs of the eyes of *Procambarus clarkii* (A) and of *Procambarus erythrops* (B). Markings at bottom: 100 μm.

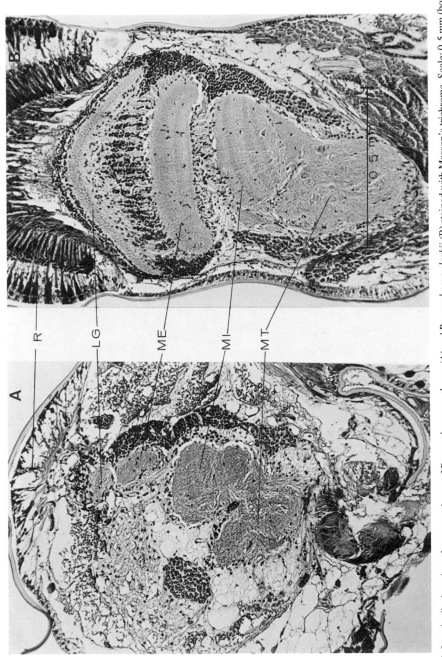

Fig. 9. Longitudinal section of compound eyes of *Procambarus erythrops* (A) and *Procambarus clarkii* (B) stained with Masson's trichrome. Scale: 0.5 mm (both micrographs). R, Retina; LG, lamina ganglionaris; ME, medulla externa; MI, medulla interna; MT, medulla terminalis.

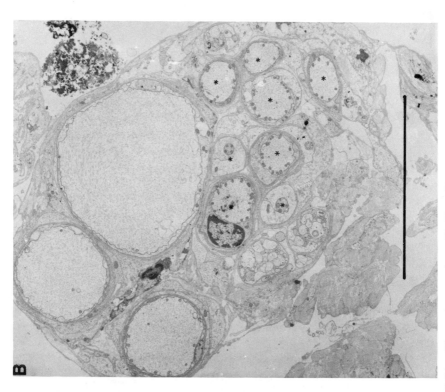

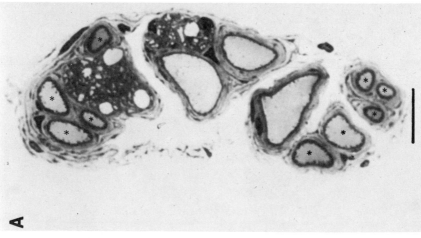

Fig. 10. Transverse sections of the ONMB of *Procambarus clarkii* (A) and *Procambarus erythrops* (B). Three GC axon profiles are seen in both nerves but there appear to be only eight AMC axon profiles (asterisks) in the section from *P. erythrops*. Calibration bars: 20 μm.

are now beginning fine-structural comparative studies of these muscles to determine to what extent phasic/tonic fiber ratios have been altered in the cave animals, and whether or not a reduction in innvervation has accompanied the loss of size.

As a first step in the search for anatomical changes in the oculomotor system of *P. erythrops,* we are attempting to obtain counts of motor axon profiles in thick open sections of the ONMB. Figure 10A is a toluidine blue-stained 1-μm section of the ONMB from *P. clarkii.* Twelve large profiles are present, three of them probably belonging to the axons of the giant cells. The remaining nine are presumably those of the AMC axons.

Thin sections of the ONMB in *P. erythrops* reflect the generalized anatomical reduction in the oculomotor system of this species (Fig. 10B). Not only are the individual axons smaller in diameter, but also careful examination of cross-sections with the electron microscope supports the conclusion that the total number of motor axons in this division has been reduced by at least one member. Such studies are not easy to confirm because of the presence of numerous small sensory axon profiles. Moreover, there is always the possibility that branching of individual axons will generate spurious total axon counts. Nevertheless, we are confident that examination of additional animals will eventually provide us with a conclusive figure.

Conclusions

Organizational features of the crayfish oculomotor system make this a useful entity for the examination of a number of questions having interest to neurobiologists. The study of AMC somata distribution has pointed out problem areas in our very imperfect knowledge of the way in which the details of nervous anatomy come about during development. For instance, albeit that the precise location of somata may not be especially important to the functioning of arthropod neurons, there are regions of these nervous systems where an extremely high degree of structural (and thereby spatial) integrity is developed and maintained. In these regions, is there a specific control of spatial position (of cellular processes) by the genome, or can principles similar to those controlling soma position, but operating within a different environmental framework, account for the apparent disparate quality of the two situations?

The presence of a functional segregation in the motor supply to the eye muscles provides a fortuitous, peripherally accessible organizational framework within which the effects of evolutionary modifications in cave-dwelling species can be examined. The ONMB is principally concerned with either rapid retraction of the eyecups or nonvisually controlled movement of the eyes in a vertical plane, while the OCM axons generally control precise movements in the horizontal plane. Visually controlled movements of the eyes within the vertical plane are, at least partially, under the influence of MNs which originate from the optic peduncle itself. To a large extent, therefore, the functions of different parts of the oculomotor system have been conveniently subdissected by nature. We hope to use this advantage in our attempts to generalize the mechanisms through which evolutionary change is being effected in cave-dwelling species.

ACKNOWLEDGMENTS

I am grateful to Mr. Gene Lorton, whose efforts and technical skill are largely responsible for the data presented in this chapter. Robin Pool kindly cut thick and thin sections for electron microscopy. I also wish to thank Dr. Kenneth Relyea of Jacksonville University, who very kindly arranged for the collection of cave crayfish. This research was supported by a grant from the Division of Academic Computing, University of Virginia, and by Research Grant NS 04989 from the United States Public Health Service.

10

Motor Coordination in Crustacean Limbs

François Clarac

Introduction

Over the past decade, it has become generally accepted that the cyclic patterns of motor neuron (MN) discharge which underlie rhythmic behavior can be generated in the absence of sensory feedback (Evarts, 1971; Grillner, 1975; Kennedy and Davis, 1976; Selverston *et al.*, 1976). Nevertheless, the motor output observed in behaving animals is quite variable and capable of considerable adaptive response. Clearly, central oscillators are under the control of command systems (Hughes and Wiersma, 1960*a,b*; Ikeda and Wiersma, 1964; Davis and Kennedy, 1972*a,b*; Bowerman and Larimer, 1974*a,b*). The question of how central oscillators interact with the mechanical systems which they control has received much less attention (Kennedy and Davis, 1976). Here I shall review the role of proprioceptive feedback in the modulation of posture and locomotory behavior in decapod crustaceans. Crustaceans offer several technical advantages in the study of central peripheral interactions: First, the behavior of crustacean limbs is easily quantifiable in terms of joint position, movements, and tension and is interestingly variable. Second, the crustacean limb is controlled by a restricted number of identifiable motor units (Wiersma, 1961; Atwood, 1967*a*, 1973*a*). Third, crustacean appendages possess a rich complement of discrete receptor organs, each of which is sensitive to a limited range of inputs and can be studied in isolation (Alexandrowicz and Whitear, 1957; Whitear, 1962; Bullock and Horridge, 1965; Wales *et al.*, 1970). Last, altered sensory feedback can cause major changes in the output of the central oscillators, and these phenomena can presumably be explained in terms of interactions between the different neuronal components.

Comparative Study of Different Decapod Walking Legs

The joint of the crustacean walking leg can be operated essentially in two perpendicular planes: the movement of some joints occurs in the roll plane, i.e.,

François Clarac • C.N.R.S.-I.N.P. 10, 31, Chemin Joseph-Aiguier, 13274 Marseilles, Cedex 2, France.

perpendicular to the axis of the body, and other joints move in the yaw plane and produce movement from front to rear.

In different decapod groups, the walking legs have become quite specialized: comparisons among *Homarus, Palinurus, Eupagurus,* and *Carcinus* demonstrate the anatomical diversity present in four main decapod groups. The *Homarus* leg is evolutionarily the most primitive. In this species, one finds all the basic leg segments, but the joints moving the leg from front to back have a larger range of movements or greater degrees of freedom than the joint moving in a perpendicular plane. By contrast, the "dorsoventral" joints are much more developed in the crab (see Table I). This presumably reflects the fact that crabs walk sideways for the most part. In this regard, in the crabs, not only has the basi-ischiopodite become fused into one leg segment but also the I-M joint is rarely used.

Many receptors have been described in some species only, and their presence seems doubtful in others. The tension receptors on the apodemes of the muscles, for example, have been observed only in the Brachyura; their presence in the other group has never been confirmed (MacMillan and Dando, 1972). The different groups also present a wide range of exteroceptors, e.g., the campaniform organ (Shelton and Laverack, 1968) on the dactylopodite of the crab and *Homarus,* the hydrodynamic receptors (Vedel and Clarac, 1976), and the *hairpeg* or *hairfan* organs (Laverack, 1962).

Chordotonal Organ

Chordotonal organs are composed of a connective support in which are inserted uniterminal neurons ending in pairs in scolopidial structures (Whitear, 1962; Mill and Lowe, 1973; Moulins, 1976). In primitive decapods, one or two chordotonal organs are present in every joint (Fig. 1). In more specialized forms where a joint is missing or fused with another, the chordotonal has been lost. At the T-C joint, *Homarus* possesses a chordotonal structure in parallel with the TRO receptor, but this is missing in the other groups. Structurally, the receptors can be divided into two forms in *Carcinus:* sheet chordotonal organs occur in IM, MC1, and CP1, but strand organs are found in CB, MC2, CP2, and PD. In *Homarus, Palinurus,* or *Eupagurus,* the organization is much more variable (Fig. 2). Although IM, MC1,

Table I. Range of Movement at the Joints of Walking Legs

	T-C	C-B	B-I	I-M	M-C	C-P	P-D
Lobster	135°	95°	15°	45°	145°	135°	65°
Crab	90°	135°	—	18°	150°	70°	140°
	130°	155°	—				

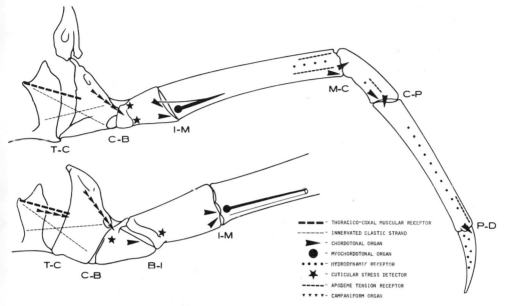

Fig. 1. Lateral view of a crustacean walking leg illustrating the different proprioceptors. Top drawing: Walking leg of reptantian decapods, where the basipodite and the ischiopodite are fused. Bottom drawing: Proximal region of a *Homarus* leg.

and CP are similar in structure to those of the crab, MC2 and CP2 which cross the joint differ in their attachments. In general, it appears that where the receptors form flat sheets the articulation of the joint is looser [e.g., CP2 of the walking legs; see Fig. 2(4)]. The sheet may represent an early stage in strand development, having been formed by a condensation of a more diffuse system of cells and connective tissue fibers.

External Structures Associated with Chordotonal Organs

It has been demonstrated that *hairplate* structure plays an important role in insect walking (Wendler, 1974). Similar structures have been found in crustaceans, Distal to the I-M, M-C, and C-P joints of the walking legs, groups of sensilla are readily observed on the surface of the limb. They lie close to the endings of internally placed chordotonal organs (MC2 and CP2) or myochordotonal organ (MCO at the I-M joint). The sensilla are small spines situated in pits at the end of canals through the cuticle, and they have been named as cuticular articulated pegs. Laverack proposed naming them *hairplates*. The groups of these sensilla lie in such a position as to be touched by the cuticular membrane during extreme movements of the joint. Because of the difficulties in recording from their sensory afferents, their role is not yet known. There has been a reduction of these structures in reptantian forms compared with natantians.

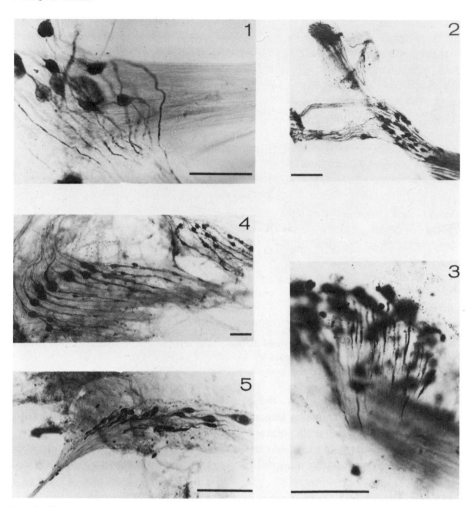

Fig. 2. Photomicrographs of methylene blue-stained preparations of myochordotonal organs: *1, Astacus leptodactylus; 2, Palinurus vulgaris; 3, Carcinus mediterraneus;* and of chordotonal organs: *4,* CP2 of *Palinurus vulgaris; 5,* IM1 of *Carcinus mediterraneus.* Horizontal bars: $100\,\mu$ m for *1,3,* and *4;* $250\,\mu$m for *2* and *5.*

Myochordotonal Organ (MCO)

The myochordotonal organ, a sensory structure, is associated with the M-C accessory flexor muscle and is composed of two parts, one flat and distal, the other spindle shaped and proximal (Barth, 1934; Clarac and Masson, 1969; Alexandrowicz, 1972). In the different species, the MCO differ in several anatomical details (muscular organization, connective membrane attachments from the muscle to the cuticle, connections with the hairplate sensilla when they exist, etc.) (Fig.

2,*1–3*). The MCO, for example, is composed of two receptors in *Palinurus*, *Eupagurus*, and crabs but only one in *Homarus*. In this last form, the 30 bipolar cells are embedded in a support. The pathway of the dendritic process is different for the proximal cells than for the distal one. In *Palinurus vulgaris*, all the bipolar cells (about 50) are clustered together. The number of distal dendritic processes in each scolopidium varies: sometimes there is only one; sometimes there are two or even three (Lombardo and Moulins, in preparation). As in *Eupagurus*, they are embedded in the same support, with two sorts of cells (50 μm diameter for the larger one, 10 μm for the smaller). In *Carcinus*, the receptor is composed of a greater number of cells which can be divided into two cellular groups (Barth, 1934; Clarac, 1968*a*), one proximal and one laterally disposed from the muscle, the main organ (Fig. 2,*3*). There have been several conflicting reports of the structure of this organ (Barth, 1934; Cohen, 1963, 1965; Finlayson, 1968). It appears evident following Barth (1934) that MCO has to be considered as composed of bipolar cells in series with the proximal head of the accessory flexor muscle, which is itself in parallel with the main flexor muscle.

In *Palinurus, Eupagurus,* and *Carcinus*, there is a second receptor (MCO2) situated in the ischiopodite. It is connected by an elastic strand to the proximal head of the accessory flexor (AccFl). It is sensitive to M-C joint movement (Cohen, 1963; Clarac, 1968*b*) but also to AccFl contraction (Cohan, 1965). In the Astacura, a chordotonal receptor (IMa) is disposed in an identical region but without connection with the AccFl. It is sensitive to movement at the I-M joint (Clarac, 1970). Ultrastructural study reveals that this IMa chordotonal organ possesses a scolopidium with one dendrite similar to MCO2 of *Cancer pagurus* (Mill, personal communication). This provides strong evidence that it is this receptor which has been associated with the AccFl in the other species.

In the Astacura, the I-M joint possesses two chordotonal organs, whereas the M-C joint is innervated by two chordotonal organs and one MCO structure. In the other groups, the sensory structures recording I-M movements are reduced, there is only one small chordotonal structure, and the M-C joint has two myochordotonal receptors in addition to joint chordotonal organs.

Cuticular Stress Detectors (CSD)

The cuticular stress detectors in crustaceans (CSD1 and CSD2) can be compared to the campaniform sensilla of insects. CSD1 and CSD2 do not cross a limb joint, nor are they attached to a muscle or a tendon; they are associated with a region of soft external cuticle. CSD1 lies dorsally in the basipodite, proximal and parallel to the preformed breakage plane when it exists. The CSD1 strand is innervated by more than 40 bipolar cells: its central attachment lies close to the distal end of the CB chordotonal organ. Some minor anatomical differences are visible between the species (Wales *et al.*, 1971). However, CSD2 is a larger structure in the Astacura. Ventrally disposed in the ischiopodite, distal to the B-I joint, it is composed of two strands, one of which forms a spiral half turn. It is innervated by 60 bipolar cells. This receptor is smaller in size in *Carcinus,* where there is a general reduction of the basi-ischiopodite region.

It is interesting to compare the sensory organization of a walking leg with that of an appendage having a similar structure but that is not involved in posture and locomotion (the third maxilliped). This appendage in *Homarus* has no chordotonal structure at the T-C joint; it has two IM chordotonal organs (IM_1 and IM_2), one MC, and one CP. The chordotonal organs of the M-C and C-P joints correspond to CP2 and MC2 because of their association with external sensilla. CP1 and MC1, more closely connected with muscle, are missing, but CSD1 and CSD2 are present. The major difference with a walking leg is nevertheless the absence of a myochordotonal organ. This lack is correlated with the lack of AccFl. One may draw the conclusion that the structures associated with exteroceptor organs are retained in the maxilliped, whereas pure proprioceptive structures are reduced.

Anatomically, it appears that the evolutionary transition in decapod walking legs has been from primitive limbs, exemplified by those of *Homarus,* to the much more organized ones found in *Carcinus.* This evolutionary trend is accompanied by structurally significant modifications of the proprioceptors; external structures become reduced, while the muscle receptor organization is enhanced.

Receptors Used during Walking

Movements of joints such as those underlying walking produce characteristic response in the different walking leg receptors.

Chordotonal Organs (ChOs)

Chordotonal organs detect both the position and rate of movement of the joint. Since Wiersma (1959) and Wiersma and Boettiger (1959), it has been repeatedly confirmed that there are four types of sensory units: two indicating the stretched or released position of the strand and two indicating the rate of movement of the strand in two directions. A first group of chordotonal organs possess these four types (PD: Burke, 1954; Wiersma and Boettiger, 1959; Hartman and Boettiger, 1967; CB: Bush, 1965b). MC1 and CP1 differ slightly: they respond more strongly to movements in one direction than the other; e.g., MC1 possesses more "extension units" than "flexor units" (Bush, 1965a). A second group of ChOs is composed of those in BI (when it exists), IM, CP2, and MC2 (Bush, 1965a; Clarac, 1970); in these receptors, only one direction of movement elicits a discharge of sensory units and only one type of position units is present. The response is therefore completely asymmetrical and concerns only the release of the strand. IMa of *Astacus* is an exception; it responds to stretch of the strand but it is atypical, and in the other group becomes MCO2 by its connection with AccFl. The response characteristics of these receptors are quite similar in the different decapod groups (Wales *et al.,* 1970).

Nevertheless, some differences exist; e.g., Field (1974) demonstrated that CP2 in *Eupagurus* responds to both CP and PD movements.

Because of their anatomical position, ChOs could conceivably respond to muscle tension. The discovery of tension sensibility of some leg receptors in crabs (MacMillan and Dando, 1972) poses questions concerning the different physiological modality of the chordotonal and MCO receptors. It has been difficult to get a clear answer to this question. In experimental procedures used by previous authors, the receptors were stimulated by passive movements of the appropriate joint, not by active movements produced by muscular contraction. To answer this question, we compared the MC1 discharge when the joint was moved passively or moved by stimulation of the given muscles with the joint unrestrained to the situation with the joint held in a fixed position. Stimulating the Fl or AccFl motor nerve when the joint is unrestrained elicits flexor unit discharge. When the stimulation ceases and the meropodite returns to the extended position, a discharge occurs in extension units (Fig. 3A). When the joint is restrained, similar stimulation elicits a comparatively poor sensory response (Fig. 3B). At the onset of the Fl contraction, a very small

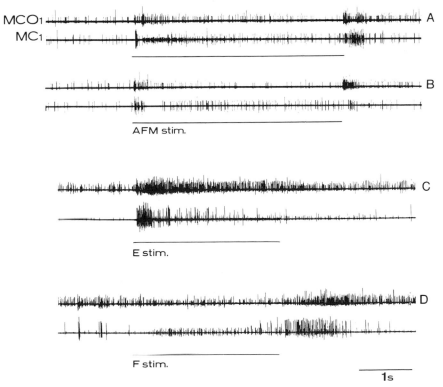

Fig. 3. Myochordotonal (MCO1) and chordotonal (MC1) responses to the stimulation of the accessory flexor motor nerve in walking legs of *Palinurus vulgaris*. A: M-C joint unrestrained. B: M-C joint restrained at 90°. C: Stimulation of the extensor motor nerve. D: Stimulation of the main flexor nerve. In C and D, M-C joint is unrestrained.

number of units are activated; furthermore, when the muscle relaxes no sensory MC1 response occurs. These results clearly indicate that, even though MC1 is closely related to the two different flexor muscles by its connective attachments, it is unlikely that to be specifically involved in recording their increasing tension.

Apodeme Tension Receptors

Little activity is recorded in either of the apodeme sensory nerves when a joint is moved passively in the relevant major muscles, but if the motor nerve of the muscle is stimulated at the same time the response is stronger (MacMillan and Dando, 1972). These receptor discharges are correlated with an increasing tension.

MCO Afferents

We have studied MCO1 in *Astacus, Palinurus,* and *Carcinus* (Clarac, 1968*b*, 1970; Clarac and Vedel, 1971). MCO2 was studied in *Cancer magister* (Cohen, 1963) and *Carcinus* (Clarac, 1968*b*). It can be summarized that MCO1 and MCO2 are both sensitive to M-C joint movement and AF muscle contraction. Concerning MCO2, in some species it seems sensitive not only to M-C joint movement but also to I-M movement (Clarac, unpublished).

Alexandrowicz (1972) suggested from anatomical consideration that the AccFl may produce movements of the M-C joint. In *Palinarus,* we have demonstrated this point by electrical stimulation (Fig. 3A). M-C movements elicit tonic and phasic units of MCO1; there are more extensor phasic units than flexor ones (this is visible in Fig. 3C,D where the joint movement is elicited by contraction of the extensor or flexor muscle). A stimulation at high frequency (100–200 cycles/sec) of AccFl causes it to contract and elicits MCO discharge. If the joint is unrestrained, one burst occurs at the onset of the AccFl contraction and another at the AccFl relaxation. If the same stimulus is applied when the M-C joint is restrained, MCO bursts appearing at the initiation and at the cessation are reduced.

The discharge of extension units is increased by AccFl stimulation (Fig. 4). If the M-C joint is moved passively, responding extension units can be characterized (Fig. 4B,C). If at the same time AccFl contracts, the extension units are facilitated. For flexion units, the contraction seems to depress their discharge. This means that an AccFl contraction dissociates the MC1 and MCO1 responses. A slight AccFl flexion excites MC1 flexion units and MCO1 extension units. For that reason, understanding the role of MCO may come through the modulation of AccFl command in relation to the discharges of the motor nerves to the two main muscles, E and F.

CSD Response

The CSD discharge is elicited by several modes of stimulation (not considering the problem of autotomy with which CSD1 seems closely associated; see Clarac, 1976). Pressure applied to the basi-ischiopodite produces a great response in CSD1

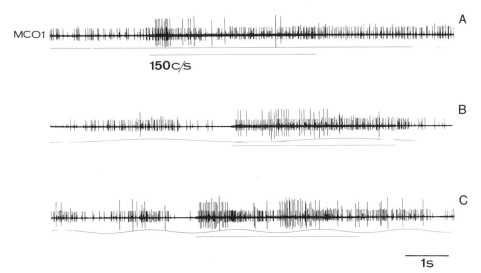

Fig. 4. Myochordotonal (MCO1) response in a walking leg of *Palinarus vulgaris* to AccFl motor nerve stimulation (A) and to combined AccFl stimulation and passive movement at different frequencies in B and C, extension is upward.

and CSD2; the degree of receptor activity is dependent on the magnitude of the force applied. Clarac *et al.* (1971) stimulated the discrete soft cuticle area and found "on" and "off" sensory units. They observed that these as well as other units can respond to increased tension in the coxobasipodite joint muscles and to C-B or B-I movements. Nevertheless, in this latter case the threshold is relatively high. Also sensitive to cuticle distortion, the campaniform organs of the dactyl are adequate to record the position of the leg with respect to the ground. They can differentiate specifically when there is or is not contact with the substrate.

Reflex Elicited by Proprioceptors

Stimulation of many of the proprioceptors can elicit MN discharge in quiescent animals. We shall first describe the reflex effect of each proprioceptor and then examine the interactions of several sensory actions.

Reflex Effects of Proprioceptor Organs

Chordotonal organs elicit resistance reflexes in every joint of the leg where they exist (Bush, 1965*c*) (see Fig. 5A,B). Recently, we have discovered a new class of reflexes: a chordotonal organ can modify the motor output of muscles of other leg joints; stretching CB in the stationary limbs excites a single extensor motor unit and releasing CB inhibits it. Sometimes this unit discharges tonically at a frequency which depends partly on the degree of flexion of the M-C joint. For any given M-C

176   François Clarac

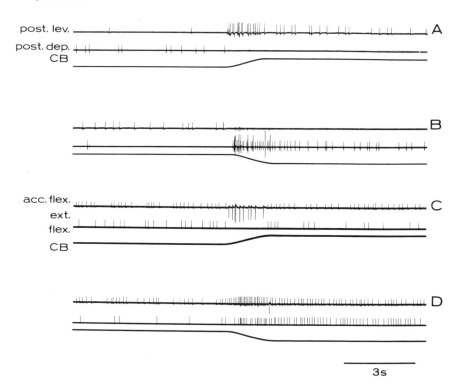

Fig. 5. Muscle activity induced by mechanical CB chordotonal stimulation in walking leg of *Palinurus vulgaris*. A,B: Posterior elevator and posterior depressor muscle responses. C,D: Accessory flexor, extensor, and flexor muscle responses. CB is stretched (upward) and released (downward) in a range of 2 mm.

position, this tonic discharge is generally somewhat greater when CB is held stretched than when it is at a shorter length. Both flexor muscles (Fl and AccFl) are excited by releasing CB and inhibited by CB stretching. The AF discharge does not seem to vary consistently with the resting position of the M-C joint. It appears to depend on factors which affect the degree of central excitability. In the resting position, CB position influences much more the Fl activity than the AccFl (Fig. 5C,D).

The MCO receptor also evokes a reflex to M-C muscles: in crayfish (Vedel, Clarac, and Bush, 1975), it stimulates the flexor muscle when it is stretched and the extensor when it is relaxed. It also has influence on its specific AccFl muscle, facilitating it during stretching. Cohen (1965) and Evoy and Cohen (1969) established in *Cancer magister* that MCO acts on E and Fl motor command as do the other chordotonal organs, but on its proper muscle, the AccFl, the action is facilitatory according to a central reference; it depends on the initial length of the AccFl muscle fibers.

Electrical stimulation of the apodeme sensory nerve at very low voltage effectively inhibits any spontaneous motor activity of the muscle where the nerve is inserted. In contrast, it seems that it excites the discharge of the antagonistic muscle (Clarac and Dando, 1973).

CSD1 activation leads to strong contraction of C-B muscles, mainly the posterior elevator but also the depressor, and to weak contraction of the anterior levator (Clarac and Wales, 1970). A pressure applied to the CSD2 soft cuticle in several decapods (*Astacus leptodactylus, Palinurus,* and crabs) evokes a response in both tonic MNs of Fl and AccFl; the frequency of Fl discharge is always higher than that of the AccFl. In the extensor nerve, the tonic unit is not noticeably modified. Stimulation of CSD1 also facilitates the AF1 and Fl activity. There receptors appear to influence both opener and closer activity (Clarac, unpublished). C-B, M-C, and P-D, i.e., all the joints which move the leg dorsoventrally are under the control of the CSD.

Interaction of Effects

These reflexes loops in normal behavior are integrated with other influences; particularly the different receptors can have combined effects. In the literature, a principal question in recent years has been the role of the resistance reflex during a motor sequence. Barnes *et al.* (1972) showed that, during normal locomotion, resistance reflexes do not occur. We have confirmed this point in both antennal movement of the rock lobster (Vedel and Clarac, 1975) and leg movement of *Astacus leptodactylus* (Vedel, Angaut-Petit, and Clarac, 1975). During a centrally driven flexion movement, the response of the flexor MNs to passive joint extension is strongly increased, whereas the response of the extensor MNs to imposed flexion is decreased or completely inhibited. In fact, the whole organization is arranged to facilitate the centrally programmed movement, the opposing neuronal action being depressed.

In the M-C walking leg joint, there is a close connection between chordotonal and myochordotonal activity: a very peculiar action occurs on AccFl. We have confirmed by means of electrophysiological methods the early anatomophysiological work of Wiersma and Ripley (1952) that the same inhibitory MN was innervating the extensor and the AccFl muscle (Fig. 6). Therefore, it appears that the two motor axons to AccFl, the excitatory and the inhibitory, fire during the same sequences. This means that at the AccFl muscle fibers an excitation could be prevented (Fig. 6C). There is a close relationship between MC1-MC2 and MCO reflexes. If centrally driven flexion occurs by means of Fl and AccFl excitatory units as of E-AccFl inhibitory impulses, the AccFl muscle contracts much more slowly than Fl muscle. The AccFl being released passively, the MCO sensory response is composed mainly of flexion units, like the sensory chordotonal response; reflexes elicited by these two sorts of receptors stimulate the extensor muscle. If, by contrast, the centrally driven flexion is composed of only excitatory output, AccFl must

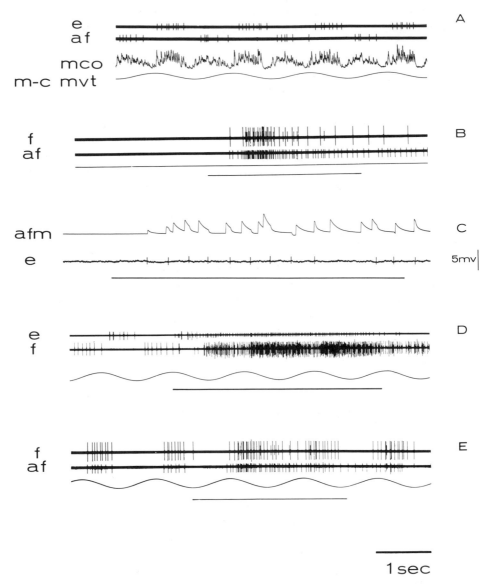

Fig. 6. Reflex responses in the chelae of *Astacus leptodactylus* of extensor motor nerve (e), accessory flexor motor nerve (af), accessory flexor muscle fiber (afm), and flexor motor nerve (f) to M-C movements (M-C mvt in A, D, and E) and to centrally driven flexion (indicated by horizontal bar under the traces) elicited by mechanical stimulation of pleopods. In A, M-C movement elicits a MCO sensory response and elicits resistance reflexes in the M-C motor nerves. Because of a common inhibitor to E and AF, a centrally driven flexion elicits ejp's and ijp's synchronously in the AF muscle fiber.

contract as well as Fl. This evokes a flexion response of the chordotonal organs and stimulates the MCO "extension units." In this case, the reflexes elicited by the two sorts of receptors are different. Unfortunately, we have no information for the moment concerning reflexes elicited by MCO following AccFl contraction; all previous studies have been made passively moving the AccFl tendon (Evoy and Cohen, 1969; Vedel, Angaut-Petit, and Clarac, 1975). It is suggested that, in view of the complexity of AccFl motor command, MCO must elicit reflexes analogous to those evoked by the chordotonal organ, as well as other sorts of reflexes. The CB influence on the AccFl excitatory MN also confirms a chordotonal action to MCO which enchances the complexity of this system.

Stimulation of the apodeme sensory nerve (tension receptor) reduces or even inhibits the chordotonal resistance reflexes elicited by M-C movements. This effect depends on the intensity of the stimulus voltage. The extensor apodeme sensory nerve inhibits the extensor discharge and the flexor apodeme sensory nerve inhibits the flexor discharge. That the apodeme sensory input which is dependent on muscle tension can profoundly modify the resistance reflexes due to the chordotonal organs may explain the inhibition or reduction of resistance reflexes during walking, although an entirely central inhibition would seem a more adequate mechanism. These receptors seem important in that they appear able, by negative feedback, to prevent too strong a contraction, according to variety of behavior and reflex loop.

The CSD receptors influence the resistance reflexes in the same way as in a quiescent animal: they facilitate C-B, M-C, and P-D MN discharge. CSDs may modify the chordotonal influence as well as the myochordotonal effect because of their action on AccFl. This very complex system is able to amplify or diminish the motor discharge, producing an active movement.

Ayers (1976) reached a similar conclusion for *Homarus*. He detected several sorts of reflexes initiated by passive movement of the different joints, detected by recording electromyographically. Since the initial description of the resistance reflex, our knowledge has increased. These reflexes are able both to activate the appropriate ongoing movement and to inhibit the antagonistic muscle which is at rest.

Sideways Walking in *Carcinus maenas*

To examine the role of proprioceptive loops during locomotion, we have performed experiments on freely behaving animals as well as ones with joints immobilized and tendons cut.

Normal Sideways Walking

We have simultaneously measured the angles of the C-B, M-C, and P-D joints by film analysis (Clarac and Coulmance, 1971). During normal locomotion on the trailing side (Fig. 7), the C-B joint elevates to 50°. Depression lasts longer, starting rapidly and finishing slowly. Flexion starts before the leg is off the ground (the M-C angle decreases to 60°); when the cephalothorax is pushed by the leg, the M-C angle extends to 160°. The P-D joint is quickly closed and opens just before touching the ground; the joint stays nearly closed until the end of the extension, when it opens quickly. During the return stroke, elevation is synchronous with flexion and closing. During the power stroke the leg depresses, extends, and "opens"; this phase is generally longer than the return stroke. On the leading side, the leg does not elevate as on the trailing side. The amplitude of the movement is smaller. During slow walking, the leg depresses regularly. During fast walking, the depression is faster at the onset and stays longer. Elevation occurs synchronously with extension (the M-C angle reaches 100–130°): it is the return stroke which corresponds also to P-D joint closing. The propulsive forces of lateral leading are provided by cyclic depression, flexion, and opening movements; those of lateral trailing are provided by cyclic depression, extension, and opening movements. In the C-B and P-D joints, the same muscles drive the power stroke or the return stroke; in the M-C joint, muscles are uni- or bifunctional depending on the direction of walking; e.g., the extensor is a power stroke muscle on the trailing side and a return stroke muscle on the leading side.

To define the speed of this rhythmic behavior, elevation seems the more appropriate movement. Taking it as a reference, we studied the M-C cyclic movement (Fig. 8). In lateral leading, the onset of the elevation corresponds to the onset of the extension with very slight variation (one or two frames of the film, i.e., 20–40 msec); on the trailing side, elevation starts with flexion, with the same slight delay. By contrast, the elevation always stops before the following movement of the M-C joint (the difference could reach 100 msec); depression starts before extension for lateral trailing or before flexion for lateral leading. Nevertheless, the changing direction of the M-C joint occurs before the leg returns to the ground. The M-C cyclic activity is thus not linked with this contact.

During lateral walking, crabs therefore exhibit two models of coordination: the "lateral leading mode" and the "lateral trailing mode." Ayers (1976) studied tethered lobsters walking on a treadmill. In this experimental situation, animals are able to walk in four directions against the direction of belt movement: forward, backward, lateral leading, and lateral trailing. In forward and backward walking, the main operating joints are C-B and T-C. Ayers found that the protractor and the retractor muscles present analogous linkage with C-B muscles as do the M-C muscles during lateral walking; the T-C muscles are bifunctional depending on the forward or backward direction as the M-C muscles depend on the leading or trailing direction.

Modifications during Locomotion

We have fixed the C-B and M-C joints of one leg at an extreme angle in the two different lateral situations and found that maintaining C-B in full elevation modified

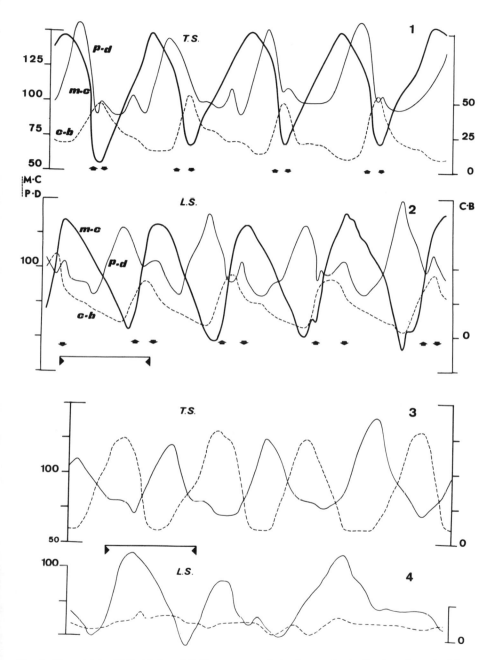

Fig. 7. Normal joint (C-B, M-C, and P-D) movements during locomotion in *Carcinus* determined by motion pictures (50 frames/sec). *1*, T.S.; trailing side; *2*, L.S., leading side. When M-C joint is blocked at an angle of 180° *(3* and *4)*, C-B elevation is enhanced on the trailing side *(3)* and depressed on the leading side *(4)*. Horizontal bars = 1 sec.

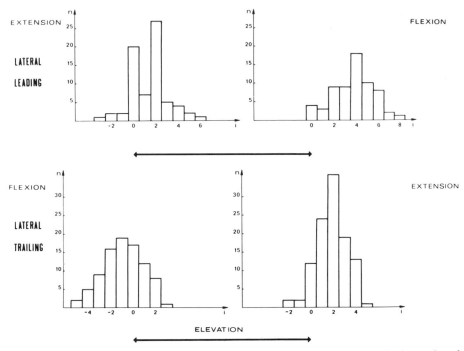

Fig. 8. Correlation between elevation and onset of flexion and extension movements for the two lateral directions of walking. Joint angle has been measured from single motion-picture frames (50 frames/sec). Each column of the histogram corresponds to 20 msec.

the M-C cyclic movement while maintaining M-C in complete extension or flexion changed the C-B pattern.

C-B in Complete Elevation

The M-C joint is much more flexed than in a normal situation during lateral trailing. The fifth pereiopod stays completely flexed at about 50° without rhythmic activity. Nevertheless, the rhythmic activity persists for the other legs but in a flexed angular range (30–75°). The P-D joint seems more normal, but the amplitude of its angular range is also smaller. For a lateral leading leg, large-amplitude extension/flexion movements occur. The rhythmic movements appear to be enhanced (M-C joint angle reaching 100°).

M-C Joint in Complete Extension

On the trailing side, elevation is increased in amplitude; the duration of the phase on the ground is restricted (Fig. 7,3). The P-D joint movement is also modified, being much more closed (70–130°), but its rhythmic bursts are normal (elevation synchronous with closing and depression synchronous with opening).

On the leading side, where M-C stays in complete extension, the leg does not elevate (Fig. 7,4). The dactylopodite drags and leans upon all small perturbations of the ground, staying closed. If a T-C movement occurs, it induces very small elevation movements and rhythmic P-D movement. It is possible that a forward/backward walking is superimposed on the lateral one. Thus a dynamic interaction exists between the M-C and C-B joints which depends on the direction of the walking.

M-C in Complete Flexion

Although complete flexion of M-C proves to be a mechanical hindrance because the leg may drag on the ground, during lateral trailing the C-B joint does not elevate completely. In lateral leading the cyclic elevation persists.

The tendon of M-C muscles has been cut to confirm the importance of the proprioceptors in this C-B control. If the apodeme of the extensor muscle was cut and the flexor was intact during a complete M-C extension, the previous effects observed with blocking were not changed. Section of the flexor muscles (Fl and AccFl), on the other hand, greatly modified the effects of complete M-C extension. When the leg was in its lateral trailing situation, the elevation was reduced; in a lateral leading situation, the elevation of the leg was exaggerated but the rhythmic cycle was perturbed, the leg being elevated three or four steps with irregular movements. P-D also made irregular movements and stayed closed when C-B was elevated. Fl and AccFl, whose contractions excite the chordotonal organs and MCO, seems necessary for these C-B modifications to occur.

Proprioceptive Coordination during Sideways Walking

It is now well established that the sensory information is not able to generate the walking pattern but can modify by inhibition or facilitation each step of a given sequence (Kennedy, 1973; Evoy and Cohen, 1971; Davis and Ayers, 1972; Evoy and Fourtner, 1973b; MacMillan, 1975). Recent studies have provided a general model for a control of oscillatory behavior. This consists of segmental oscillators, controlled by intersegmental fibers, which excite or inhibit MNs (P.S.G. Stein, 1974; Pearson and Iles, 1973; Selverston, 1974; Maynard and Selverston, 1975). It has been demonstrated in crayfish that one fiber can control backward or forward walking (Bowerman and Larimer, 1974a,b); presumably others elicit lateral leading or lateral trailing. The mechanisms of intersegmental coordination are not as well understood in the walking system.

What evidence have we that bears on the question of separate central oscillators controlling locomotion of each leg? Two pieces of indirect evidence suggest that CB elevator/depressor antagonist pairs or their central antecedents comprise the segmental oscillators. First, similar elevation/depression cycles underlie walking in all four directions. Second, the periodicity of discharge in the elevators most accurately predicts the periodicity of discharge in all other leg muscles during rapid variation in period (Ayers, 1976). It appears that the muscles of the other joints are selectively coupled to the C-B system. Each joint movement evokes several feedbacks. For a given movement, there are several parallel feedback systems so that a great deal of redundancy occurs. For example, the flexor muscle of the walking leg is under the control of MC1, MC2, and CB chordotonal organs MCO1 and MCO2, a tension receptor, and the CSDs. Thus it can be understood that one receptor ablation does not greatly disturb the walking behavior. The importance of these reflexes in walking is likely to be in facilitating the ongoing movements and regulating the random events which occur during behavior. Good evidence concerning the effectiveness of the reflex loop has recently been given. Studying different reflexes, Ayers (1976) showed that the maximum efficiency of a reflex appears at a speed movement which corresponds to the normal velocities during walking.

If we summarize our data, it appears that there is a very close linkage between the C-B and M-C joints. Two types of reflexes are present during lateral trailing (see Fig. 9B). One concerns the loops that increase elevation; for example, the CB chordotonal organ increases the flexor burst during the elevation. The CSD discharge elicited by elevation stimulates the elevator MN and also Fl and AccFl. During the power stroke, CB stretching, which occurs during depression, must facilitate extension. CSD could increase at the same time the depressor muscle discharges. The tension receptors of the M-C muscle apparently regulate the flexor or the extensor burst similarly to vertebrate tendon organs. Second, resistance reflexes may possibly strengthen the coupling between sequential bursts in antagonist muscles, as demonstrated in the swimmeret system (Davis, 1973b). We have pointed out that an extended position increases the elevation while a flexed position increases the depression. In contrast to resistance reflexes, these loops appear directly linked with and specific to the direction of locomotion. These influences may be elicited by chordotonal and myochordotonal pathways onto the elevator and depressor muscles, as has been confirmed by experimentally cutting their tendons.

Proprioceptive support of lateral leading (Fig. 9A) seems, in the present state of our knowledge, weaker. The CSD control could be important during the power stroke for depression and flexion movements. If CSD is involved in supporting the body weight, it can exert a good control of the ongoing depression and flexion. In addition to the resistance reflexes, there is some coupling between sequential bursts because of the facilitation of depression movements associated with an extended position and of the elevation associated with a flexed position.

A comparison of the angular range of each joint seems significant between lateral leading and lateral trailing; e.g., the M-C joint often reaches 160° during lateral trailing. By contrast, it is much more flexed (50°) during lateral leading; this corresponds to a maximum of activity for MC1, MC2, and MCO1 in the first case and to a maximum for MC1 and MCO2 in the second case. The effectiveness of the proprioceptive loop must be different for each side. Once the direction of walking

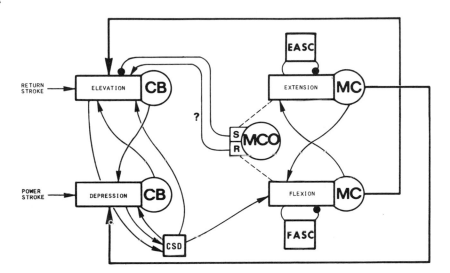

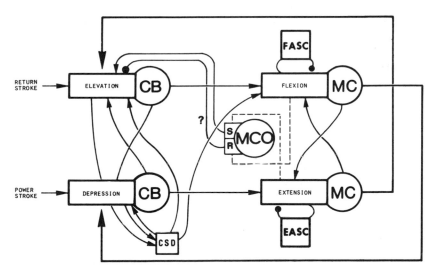

Fig. 9. Summary of the proprioceptive loops between C-B and M-C joints which can be used in the two lateral directions of walking. A: Lateral leading. B: Lateral trailing. CB and MC represent chordotonal inputs. MCO represents the myochordotonal afferents which depend on the stretch or the released position of the AF muscle (dashed lines represent mechanical linkage between the main M-C muscles and the AF muscle). FASC and EASC represent the flexor and extensor apodeme sensory nerves which can strongly inhibit the discharge of the muscle where they are situated. Black arrows indicate an excitation, black dots an inhibition. Refer to text for details.

has been determined, these afferent feedbacks could be able to maintain its laterality.

Is there a predominance during lateral walking of the trailing side or of the leading one—i.e., is the animal pulled or pushed? Considering the different decapods which walk laterally, it seems that a great variability occurs. In *Homarus,* Ayers (1976) did not find major differences between each side, but in the ghost crab *Ocypode* during rapid running the extensors and flexors alternate only on the trailing side (Burrows and Hoyle, 1973*b*). On the leading side, they frequently show a reduced activity which maintains only the muscle tonus. In *Carcinus,* the burst of MN discharge appears greater in duration and in frequency to that for muscles of the trailing side. This could increase the differences between the two sensory regulating pathways presented. Another question may be raised concerning these pathways: do they act mainly positively, turning on the system, or do the inhibitory loops become more significant, turning off some part of the network and modifying duration and frequency of other bursts? In our model, we have more evidence of positive influences than of negative ones. If we try now to give a generalized model of walking, it must be compatible with the data of Ayers (1976). In forward/backward walking, the M-C joint moves very slightly as in the T-C joint during lateral leading/lateral trailing. This does not mean that the muscles are not bursting. Preliminary data on freely walking *Palinurus vulgaris* showed that during forward/backward walking a coactivation of the two antagonistic M-C muscles occurred, even though there was an alternated predominance that determined the cyclic behavior (Ayers and Clarac, in preparation).

The neural organization determining the central patterns responsible for walking has not yet been studied experimentally, nor have the different elements which compose the network been determined. By contrast, the sensory pathways now seem deciphered: these feedbacks suggest that the walking leg proprioceptors can control the MN discharge and even modulate the C-B activity, i.e., the cyclic burst in closest relationship with the central oscillator. This means that they regulate the frequency of discharge of the main return stroke/power stroke muscles. The reflexes are in fact necessary and appropriate to regulate the ongoing cyclic movements. Locomotion in Crustacea is a good system in which to examine the role of sensory feedback in the adaptive regulation and generation of cyclic motor program.

Acknowledgments

I thank Drs. J. P. Vedel, M. Moulins, and D. Angaut-Petit for collaboration in many experiments presented in this chapter. I also thank N. Dusticier for technical assistance and for making the illustrations. I would like to acknowledge the help of J. Ayers for discussion and editorial assistance during the preparation of the manuscript.

11

Ventilation Motor Mechanisms in the Dragonfly and Other Insects

Peter J. Mill

Introduction

Ventilation in arthropods is achieved in one of two ways. Either movements of the gills or other appendages produce the ventilatory current, or movements of parts of the body wall produce volume and thus pressure changes in the body, and such changes in pressure produce the ventilatory current. It is this latter mechanism which will be considered here. In insects with an open tracheal system, these movements result in air passing in and out of the spiracles, while in the aquatic larvae of anisopteran dragonflies, which have a closed tracheal system and gills enclosed in a modified region of the hindgut, they result in water passing in and out of the rectum (Mill, 1972, 1974).

Description of Ventilatory Movements

In all insects which ventilate using body wall movements, the normal, relaxed rest position of the animal during apnea is the fully inspired position, and hence expiration is always the first phase of normal ventilation.

In many insects, ventilatory movements are restricted to the abdomen; in others, one or more thoracic segments are also involved. In dragonflies, locusts, cockroaches, and mantids, dorsoventral movements of the abdominal sterna produce the ventilatory current: upward movements increase the internal abdominal pressure, causing the outward movement of water from the branchial chamber or air from the tracheae (expiration), and downward movements have the reverse effect (inspiration). These dorsoventral movements of the abdominal sterna are aided by similar movements of the mesothoracic sterna in *Sphodromantis lineola* and of the metathoracic sterna in *Melolontha melolontha,* and by longitudinal telescoping movements of the abdomen in some prionine beetles (Miller, 1971). Furthermore, under certain conditions, auxiliary ventilatory mechanisms are brought into play.

Peter J. Mill • Department of Pure and Applied Zoology, University of Leeds, Leeds LS2 9JT, England.

Although this "normal" ventilation is generally styled as rhythmic activity, the degree of rhythmicity varies in different animals. Thus dragonfly larvae and adult locusts often ventilate continuously for long periods of time, but the former at least may also exhibit long periods of apnea (Tonner, 1936; Miller, 1960a; Hughes and Mill, 1966). Furthermore, in resting cockroaches such as *Byrsotria* and *Blaberus* ventilation is only intermittent, with small groups of ventilatory cycles separated by periods of apnea (Myers and Fisk, 1962; Myers and Retzlaff, 1963; Miller, 1973). *Periplaneta* shows even less rhythmicity and normally tends to ventilate only when agitated or after a period of activity (Schreuder and de Wilde, 1952). Also, some prionine beetles usually ventilate only during and after periods of activity, but may continue at a lower rate when at rest (Miller, 1965).

The various components of ventilation will be described separately.

The Primary Ventilatory Rhythm

In aeshnid dragonfly larvae, the upward, expiratory phase is elicited primarily by the segmental respiratory dorsoventral muscles (RDVs), which are heavily tracheated and well endowed with mitochondria (Mill and Lowe, 1971a) and which are differentiated from the general dorsoventral musculature in abdominal segments 5–9 (Whedon, 1919; Mill, 1965) (Fig. 1). In libellulid dragonfly larvae, the oblique tergopleural muscle is probably also an expiratory muscle (Mill, 1970). The anterior dorsoventral muscles (ADVs) may assist in this phase. Inspiration is achieved by the contraction of two large transverse muscles, the diaphragm and the subintestinal muscle, which pull the sides of the terga inward in the middle region of the abdomen and hence force the sterna downward (Fig. 1). This is aided by the natural elasticity of the sclerites (Mill and Hughes, 1966). Similarly, in locusts both phases are active, but in cockroaches only expiratory muscles are present and inspiration is effected entirely by natural elasticity (Farley *et al.*, 1967). In locusts ventilation is complicated at lower frequencies by a pause during the expiratory phase (Miller, 1965).

Apart from the muscles directly concerned with the production of ventilatory movements, others are involved which ensure that the ventilatory movements have the desired effect. Thus the pressure increase produced during sternal lifting in the dragonfly larva must be transmitted to the branchial chamber to effect expiration and the energy not dissipated through abdominal extension. Hence most of the longitudinal muscles receive rhythmic innervation synchronized with expiration; this presumably raises their tension during expiration so as to prevent longitudinal extension of the abdomen (Mill, 1970; Pickard and Mill, 1975).

In all ventilatory systems, the expiratory phase of normal ventilation commences with the onset of sternal lifting and ceases when the sterna are fully raised; conversely, the inspiratory phase starts when the sterna start to fall and finishes when the rest position is resumed (Fig. 2).

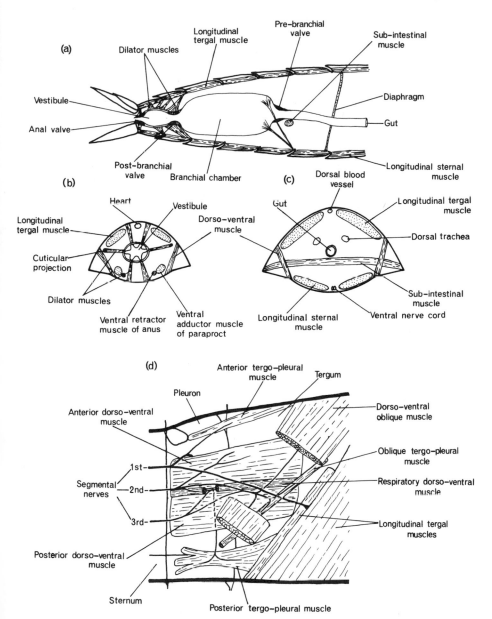

Fig. 1. Morphology of the ventilatory system in an aeshnid dragonfly larva. (a) Longitudinal section. (b) Transverse section through the region of the vestibule. (c) Transverse section through the region of the subintestinal muscle. (d) Tergopleural region of the right side of the fifth abdominal segment showing the motor branches of the second and third lateral nerves to the muscles in this region. (a,c) After Mill and Pickard (1972b); (b) after Hughes and Mill (1956); (d) after Mill (1965).

Activity Coupled with the Primary Ventilatory Rhythm

Superimposed on the basic ventilatory rhythm is the control system for organizing the fine details of the flow of water (in and out of the branchial chamber) or air (in and out of the tracheae).

In dragonfly larvae, movements of the branchial chamber, the muscular vestibule, and the anal and postbranchial valves are coupled with the dorsoventral movements of the abdomen (Fig. 2). Thus during expiration the anal valve opens to about one-third of its maximum extent, while the pressure in the branchial chamber caused by the rising sterna is enhanced by its own contraction, reaching about 4 cm H_2O in a large larva. Hence exhaled water is forced some distance from the animal. During inspiration, a negative pressure of about 0.5 cm H $_2$O has been recorded from the branchial chamber, resulting from the lowering of the sterna and expansion of the vestibule (Hughes and Mill, 1966). The anal valve is fully opened (Mill and Pickard, 1972b), and water is thus drawn into the branchial chamber.

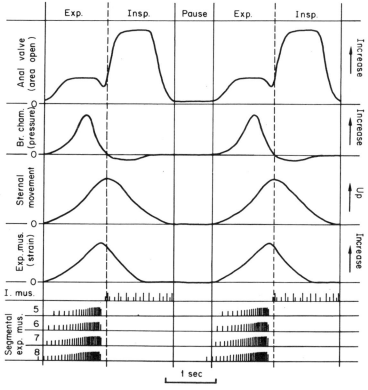

Fig. 2. Sequence of events which occur in normal ventilation in an aeshnid larva. From Mill (1972), after Mill and Pickard (1972b).

In air-breathing insects, the spiracles are each controlled by a closer muscle and, in many cases, also by an opener muscle. In some insects (e.g., certain dragonflies, Miller, 1962), the spiracles tend to remain open most of the time and hence a tidal flow occurs; in others (e.g., other dragonflies and locusts), a unidirectional air flow occurs in the main tracheal trunks due to some spiracles opening during expiration and others during inspiration, a pattern which may vary under different conditions.

Auxiliary Mechanisms

Under conditions of stress, such as high carbon dioxide tension, auxiliary pumping mechanisms may be utilized, and these typically involve longitudinal movements which produce telescoping of the segments. Instances of this include the longitudinal pumping movements of the abdomen, prothorax, and head in *Schistocerca gregaria* and the prothoracic pumping of *M. melolontha* (Miller, 1960a, 1974a).

Other Forms of Ventilation

Apart from normal, rhythmic ventilation, some animals may exhibit alternative patterns. Thus in dragonfly larvae the rhythmic sequence of normal ventilation may be periodically interrupted by "gulping" ventilation, in which the branchial chamber is "pumped up" by a series of contractions of the water-filled vestibule (inspiration), expiration being achieved in the same way as in normal ventilation (Pickard and Mill, 1974a).

Locomotion

Certain locomotory movements, which of course require rapid expenditure of energy, subserve ventilation. In the jet-propulsive swimming of aeshnid dragonfly larvae, longitudinal telescoping of the abdominal segments occurs, in addition to rapid dorsoventral movements. The combined effect of rapid sternal lifting and abdominal shortening is to produce pressures of up to 40 cm H_2O in the branchial chamber (Hughes and Mill, 1966). Coupled with a fairly narrow anal aperture, the net effect is not only to propel the animal forward during the "expiratory" phase but also to produce very rapid water changes in the branchial chamber. Similarly, in locust flight the movements of the pterothorax producing wing movements also serve as an efficient ventilatory pumping mechanism.

Control of Ventilation

It follows from the above that the ventilatory process is divisible into certain basic categories, and it is both useful and convenient to deal with these separately.

Ventilatory MNs

Expiratory MNs

The cyclical, expiratory sternal lifting of normal ventilation is undoubtedly the basic underlying rhythm of the ventilatory process insofar as it is *always* the initial phase of each ventilatory cycle and it is always an active process. It involves the obligatory activation of certain muscles whose primary role is expiratory, together with those muscles which may aid the expiratory movement and those which prevent, for example, longitudinal abdominal extension during expiration.

In aeshnid larvae, the main expiratory muscles are the paired RDVs which are innervated by the second segmental nerves. The available evidence indicates innervation by only a single expiratory motor unit whose firing frequency normally increases during a burst and then ceases more or less abruptly (Figs. 2 and 3). The frequency increase is apparently accompanied by facilitation of the muscle potentials (Fig. 3b). In a few instances, this unit has been seen to fire occasionally between expiratory bursts. The individual pulses in the bursts of the motor units on either side of one segment may or may not be precisely synchronized, although the overall burst duration is about the same (Mill and Hughes, 1966; Mill, 1970), which indicates that there is probably a common interneuronal (IN) input.

The expiratory motor neurons (MNs) in the eighth abdominal ganglion fire first and are followed sequentially by those in more anterior ganglia (as far forward as the fifth), with an interganglion delay time averaging about 50 msec (Mill and Hughes, 1966). Occasionally a ganglion may fire out of turn. In spite of the delays in starting time, all of the expiratory bursts end together and hence the duration of the bursts decreases from posterior to anterior (Figs. 2 and 3). It can be seen from Fig. 3c that activity in these expiratory units ceases before the sterna reach their fully raised position, whereas the strain developed in a single RDV reaches a peak at the end of the burst (Fig. 2). This can be explained by assuming either that there are two stable positions of the sterna (fully inspired and fully expired) so that once the fulcrum has been passed during sternal lifting the sterna will carry on moving upward, or, alternatively, that the inertial effect of water passing out of the branchial chamber is sufficient to cause the movement to continue (Mill and Pickard, 1972b; Pickard and Mill, 1972). At the peak of sternal movement, the pressure in the branchial chamber has fallen to zero and water flow out of the branchial chamber has ceased (Fig. 2).

In contrast, in the locust the expiratory bursts start anteriorly and have a mean intersegmental delay of 10–12 msec. However, there is considerable variation in the timing between the onset of bursts in the different segments, and it is not unusual for the expiratory MNs of one ganglion to fire after those in the next most posterior ganglion (Lewis *et al.*, 1973). In teneral aeshnid dragonflies, there is also considerable variability in the timing of the onset of the expiratory bursts in different abdominal segments. Furthermore, the patterning within the expiratory bursts in the second segmental nerves is less precise than in the larva, and expiratory bursts are

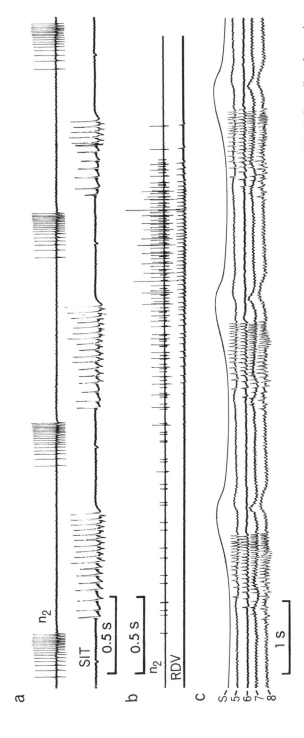

Fig. 3. (a) Alternation of expiratory bursts in a second lateral nerve (n₂) and inspiratory bursts in the subintestinal transverse muscle (SIT). (b) Recording of an expiratory burst from a second lateral nerve (n₂) and from the respiratory dorsoventral muscle which it innervates (RDV). Note the 1:1 relationship between the action potentials of one of the MNs and the muscle potentials. (c) Expiratory bursts in the respiratory dorsoventral muscles of four consecutive abdominal segments (5–8). s, Sternal movements of abdominal segments 4–6 with upward movement indicating sternal lifting (expiration). The muscle recordings are extracellular. Some spikes have been retouched. Larvae of (a) *Aeshna* and (b,c) *Anax*. (a,b) From Mill (1970); (c) from Pickard and Mill (1972).

always present in the third segmental nerves (Mill and Hulme, unpublished observations) (Fig. 4a).

Other motor units which are synchronized with the expiratory bursts to the RDV in the dragonfly larva are present in the second nerves, and at least two such units have been recorded in *Anax* (Fig. 3). This nerve innervates only three other muscles: the anterior dorsoventral muscle (ADV) and two oblique muscles. Electromyograms have shown that the ADV is often involved in aiding expiration (and may be concerned with strong ventilation) and that the (main) unit innervating it tends to start firing before that innervating the RDV but does not reach such a high frequency (Fig. 5a).

Methylene blue staining has revealed only four motor axons in each second lateral nerve (one to the RDV, two to the ADV, and one shared by both oblique muscles) (Mill and Parker, unpublished observations), but back-staining of axons with cobalt chloride suggests that there may be five to seven of them. However, this is still less than the number of larger axons seen in sections of the nerve (about 30 larger than 1 μm diameter) (Mill and Hulme, unpublished observations), which implies either that some MNs have remained unstained by the other techniques or that there are a number of large sensory axons.

The longitudinal musculature (tergal and sternal) is innervated by the first nerves, and a considerable number of motor axons are involved. Few, however, are activated during expiration. Figure 5b shows an electromyogram from a second longitudinal tergal muscle (LT$_2$), in which only a few spikes occur during each expiratory cycle, while in Fig. 5c an electromyogram from a first longitudinal tergal muscle (LT$_1$) reveals a unit which often fires during inspiration also but at a lower frequency than during expiration. This latter unit tends to reach its peak firing frequency near the onset of expiration. Since in dissected preparations these muscles are not seen to contract during expiration and since there is no abdominal shortening during normal ventilation in intact larvae, it is assumed that the function of these motor units is to prevent elongation of the abdominal segments by increasing the tension in the longitudinal muscles during expiration. In teneral aeshnid dragonflies, motor activity in the first segmental nerves consists of inspiratory as well as (often) expiratory bursts (Fig. 4b), and details of the destination of individual units are being determined (Mill and Hulme, unpublished observations).

There are thus basically three types of expiratory MNs: (1) a MN in which the overall firing rate during expiration tends to be fairly high and which fires in a similar pattern at all depths and rates of ventilation (the MN innervating the RDV); (2) MNs which do not fire, or which only spike a few times during each expiratory phase, at low ventilatory rates, but whose frequency increases as the ventilatory rate goes up (probably the MN innervating the ADV); and (3) MNs which fire just a few times during each expiratory burst and which may increase in frequency slightly at higher ventilatory rates (the MNs innervating the longitudinal musculature). Any of these may fire occasionally during inspiration.

Less is known about the details of the units innervating individual expiratory muscles in other insects, but in general a number of units occur in each expiratory

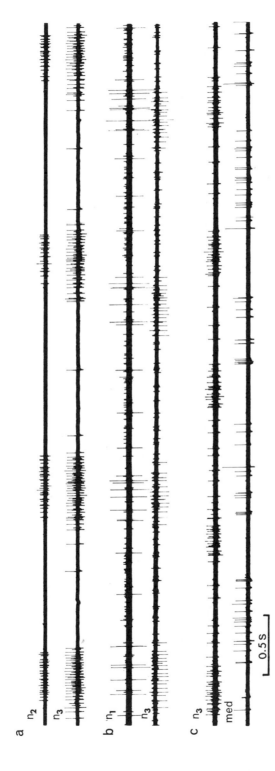

Fig. 4. Motor activity in teneral aeshnid dragonflies (a) In second (n_2) and third (n_3) lateral nerves of *Aeshna*. (b) In first (n_1) and third (n_3) lateral nerves of *Anax*. (c) In a third lateral (n_3) and a median (med) nerve of *Anax*. From Mill and Hulme (unpublished observations).

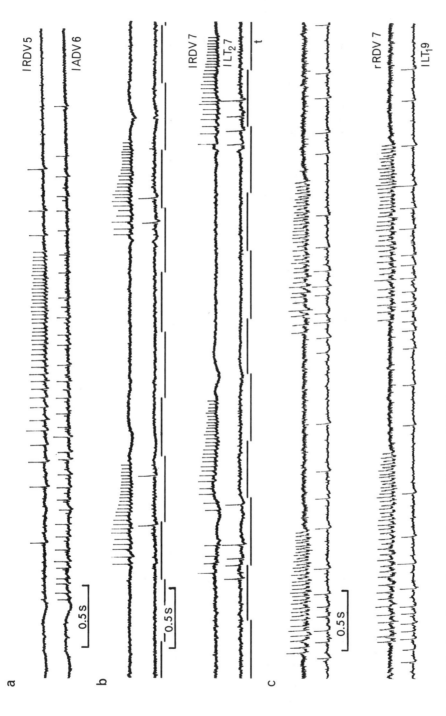

Fig. 5. Activity in respiratory dorsoventral muscles (l RDV5, l RDV7, r RDV7) compared with that in (a) anterior dorsoventral muscles (l ADV6) and (b,c) longitudinal tergal muscles (l LT$_2$7, l LT$_1$9) during normal ventilation in aeshnid larvae l, Left; r, right; numeral indicates abdominal segment. From Pickard and Mill (1975).

burst. In the locust *Schistocerca,* Burrows (1974) has recorded intracellularly from the cell bodies of a number of expiratory MNs. It is not yet possible to compare this work in detail with peripheral data from the same animal, but of particular interest in the present context is the marked similarity of the firing pattern of many of the MNs he described to those present in dragonfly larvae, although no MN with the precise firing pattern of the expiratory MN to the RDV has been described in the locust. However, ventilatory MNs with a similar buildup in frequency have been described in *Limulus* (Wyse, 1972).

Figure 6a shows a unit which fires thoughout expiration, but not during inspiration. Since it has the highest firing frequency recorded from any expiratory MN in the locust, it is suggested here that this is the unit which corresponds functionally to the expiratory MN innervating the RDV in the dragonfly larva; i.e., it innervates an obligatory expiratory muscle. It receives an excitatory input during the latter stages of inspiration, the epsp's reaching a maximum frequency at the start of the burst. The frequency steadily declines and ultimately stops at the end of expiration. Hence this unit stops firing as a result of the removal of excitatory input.

A second type of unit described fires continuously but at a decreased frequency during inspiration. The high expiratory frequency is initiated and maintained by excitatory input, while the lower inspiratory frequency is initiated by inhibitory input. A similar unit apparently receives both excitatory and inhibitory inputs

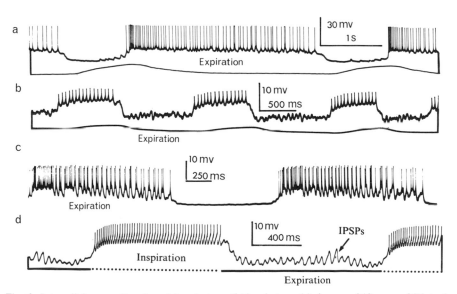

Fig. 6. Intracellular recordings from (a) expiratory, (b) inspiratory, (c) closer, and (d) opener MNs in the metathoracic ganglion of the locust. Lower trace in (a) and (b) shows dorsoventral movements of the first abdominal segment, with downward indicating expiration. Ipsp's, inhibiting postsynaptic potentials. (a–c) From Burrows (1974); (d) from Burrows (1975*c*).

throughout the ventilatory cycle, the former dominating during expiration and the latter during inspiration (Burrows, 1974). In some cases, two peaks of firing frequency occur, one at the start and the other at the end of expiration, and this can probably be correlated with the expiratory pause observed by Miller (1965).

Expiratory MNs have also been described which fire with just a few spikes during expiration, or which have a patterned, rhythmic input, but which have not been seen to spike at all. At least one of this type remains silent at low ventilatory frequencies but starts to fire with just a few spikes during expiration at higher ventilatory frequencies and is somewhat reminiscent of the unit innervating the ADV in dragonfly larvae. It receives an excitatory input during expiration, as well as an inhibitory input throughout the cycle, but at a higher frequency during inspiration. Conversely, there is one unusual unit reported in *Schistocerca* which produces fewer spikes with increase in ventilatory frequency (Burrows, 1974). Bentley (1969*a*) has described an expiratory MN in *Gryllus* which produces only a few spikes, and this receives excitation during expiration and inhibition during inspiration. In dragonfly larvae, a unit has been observed which shows a depolarization and fires during expiration, with occasional spikes during inspiration. However, this could be an IN (Mill and Hulme, unpublished observations).

Another unit described by Burrows fires sporadically at low ventilatory frequencies, but as the ventilatory frequency increases the spikes occur only during expiration (but with excitatory and inhibitory inputs both occurring throughout the cycle). At still higher frequencies, spikes occur during inspiration also, but at a lower frequency. This unit may correspond with those innervating the longitudinal musculature in dragonfly larvae. The MN types in aeshnid dragonfly larvae and the locust are summarized in Figs. 7 and 8.

Inspiratory MNs

In dragonfly larvae, inspiration is effected by the two large inspiratory muscles, the diaphragm and the subintestinal muscle, both of which are innervated by

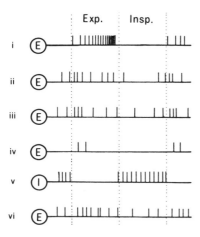

Fig. 7. Types of ventilatory MNs recorded from the abdominal nerves of aeshnid larvae. (E, expiratory; I, inspiratory). (i) The expiratory MN to the respiratory dorsoventral muscle, (ii) An expiratory MN to the anterior dorsoventral muscle. (iii,iv) Expiratory MNs to the longitudinal tergal musculature. (v) An inspiratory MN to the subintestinal muscle (or diaphragm). (vi) An expiratory MN to one of the accessory muscles of the branchial/vestibular apparatus. The expiratory (Exp.) and inspiratory (Insp.) phases are indicated.

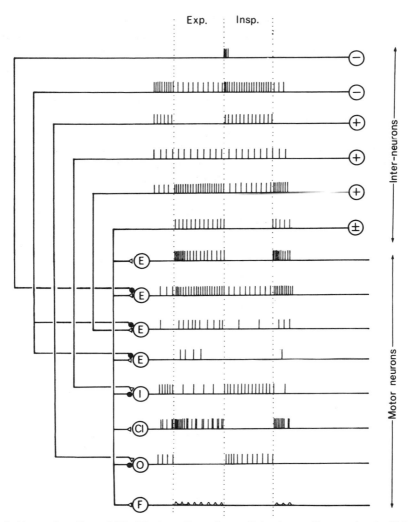

Fig. 8. Types of ventilatory MNs (Cl, closer; E, expiratory; I, inspiratory; O, opener) and a flight MN (F) recorded from the metathoracic ganglion of the locust, and the possible types of "command" INs which synapse on them. The INs, shown at the top, are indicated as excitatory (+), inhibitory (−), or both (±). The IN indicated by (±) is one of the pair of INs described in the text as synapsing bilaterally with the MNs. All records read from left to right. The expiratory (Exp.) and inspiratory (Insp.) phases are indicated. Based on data in Burrows (1974, 1975c).

median nerves. Records have been obtained which indicate two inspiratory MNs firing almost in phase and fairly regularly throughout the burst (Fig. 3a). There is good evidence from methylene blue staining (Zawarzin, 1924a; Mill, unpublished observations) and from back-staining with cobalt chloride (Mill and Hulme, unpublished observations) that the axons of these inspiratory MNs branch, as indeed they do in other insects, sending one branch to either side. This is supported by the 1:1 relationship observed between muscle potentials recorded in the subintestinal muscle from opposite sides of the animal (Mill and Hughes, 1966). The course of the motor axons is unusual since, while the cell bodies are in the ganglion anterior to the median nerve from which their axons emanate, the axons first run backward to the next posterior ganglion (where they do not appear to give off any collaterals) before entering the median nerve. The destination of these axons in segments other than those concerned with the two transverse inspiratory muscles has not yet been determined, but it is of interest to note that these could well be the same motor neurons which innervate the spiracle closer muscles in adults. Activity in the median nerves is variable in teneral aeshnid dragonflies and is often continuous. Although modulation generally occurs, with increase in frequency during inspiration (Fig. 4c), expiratory bursting has been observed occasionally (Mill and Hulme, unpublished observations).

Inspiration in the locust is achieved by dorsoventral muscles which are also innervated by two MNs (Lewis et al., 1973) that show similar activity to those in dragonfly larvae. Burrows (1974) has recorded intracellularly from these (Fig. 6b) and shown that the inspiratory burst is terminated by an inhibitory input which persists throughout expiration, while excitatory input continues throughout the cycle. However, the inhibition is not always sufficient to completely inhibit firing during expiration. Although the two inspiratory MNs in the locust are not always so closely phase-locked as in the dragonfly larva, there is some indication that they receive the same synaptic input.

MNs of Coupled Activities

Little is known about the MNs associated with the branchial chamber, vestibule, and their valves and with the anal appendages in the dragonfly larva, except that both segmental and median nerves are involved. In the fifth segmental nerves, bursts coupled with both expiration and inspiration occur, the former including one very large unit which also fires occasionally during inspiration. The last median nerve contains at least one expiratory MN (Mill, 1963, 1970).

In adult dragonflies and other insects, the spiracle closer muscles are innervated by the median nerves; the opener muscles are innervated by median nerves, segmental nerves, or both. In resting *S. gregaria,* spiracles 1 and 2 close during expiration and open during inspiration, spiracle 3 remaining closed. When flight commences, spiracle 1 maintains the same pattern, but spiracles 2 and 3 remain fully open. Later in flight, spiracles 2 and 3 start to close slightly during inspiration, and immediately after flight they close and resume opening movements during inspiration (Miller, 1960b). Hence, unlike the MNs innervating the expiratory and inspiratory muscles of the abdomen, the closers and openers can be linked to either expiration or inspiration and the role of the muscles concerned with a single spiracle may change.

In *Sphodromantis*, the ventilatory air flow may completely reverse direction, with spiracle 1, which normally closes during expiration, closing instead during inspiration (Miller, 1974*a*).

Closer MNs

In the resting adult dragonfly, the paired MNs to the spiracle closers of the first two pairs of spiracles both fire at a steady rate (Miller, 1962). This is rarely observed in the locust but may be initiated if the nerve cord is cut between the meso- and methathoracic ganglia. This pattern, called "free running" by Miller (1965), is normally overridden by a ventilatory pattern. In the intact locust, the closer MNs of the first two pairs of spiracles fire with a high-frequency burst during expiration. Although the individual spikes are synchronized between the members of each pair of MNs, there is no such synchronization between the MNs of spiracle 1 and those of spiracle 2. At all except the highest frequencies of ventilation, this burst of activity is generally followed by a lower firing rate in which not only are the members of each pair synchronized but also those of spiracle 1 are synchronized with those of spiracle 2. Furthermore, each MN may fire impulses in pairs. Other variations may occur, including an increase in frequency at the end of the expiratory phase (Miller, 1965, 1967).

Burrows (1974) has recorded from the cell bodies of the above MNs to spiracle 2 and also from those to spiracles 3 and 4, which behave similarly. Each burst starts with a high firing frequency which gradually declines; the spikes tend to occur in doublets or, occasionally, triplets, a phenomenon which is particularly noticeable after the initial high-frequency phase (Fig. 6c). At low, but not higher, frequencies of ventilation, these MNs fire occasionally during inspiration. A declining excitatory input occurs throughout expiration, and the burst is terminated by lack of excitatory input rather than by inhibition. The synaptic input to the motor neurons of both spiracles is similar and thus they are probably driven by the same presynaptic inputs (Burrows, 1974, 1975c).

Opener MNs

At higher frequencies of ventilation, the two opener MNs in the median nerve to the first pair of spiracles of the locust fire only during *expiration*. They are still able to aid spiracular opening during inspiration because they have a slower conduction time than the closer MNs and because tension in the opener muscle decays more slowly than in the closer muscle after cessation of input. At lower ventilatory frequencies, firing of these MNs extends into inspiration. The third (mesothoracic) opener MN fires throughout the ventilatory cycle with a higher frequency during inspiration but not at low ventilatory frequencies (Miller, 1965).

Intracellular recordings have been obtained (Burrows, 1975c) from an opener MN of spiracle 4 which fires only during inspiration. It has a fairly high firing rate, showing a slight decline throughout the burst. The burst is terminated by an inhibitory input which lasts throughout expiration (Fig. 6d).

MNs Associated with Other Forms of Ventilation

Various alternative forms of ventilation have been described. In dragonfly larvae, for example, gulping breathing is characterized by intermittent bursts of activity in the RDVs. Another, similar, type of ventilation also occurs periodically in this animal, in which the sterna are raised as in normal ventilation but their descent is interrupted by brief lifting movements caused by rapid bursts of activity in the MNs innervating each RDV. The overall firing frequency tends to fall off after the first two or three of these bursts (Pickard and Mill, 1972).

Locomotory MNs

In the dragonfly larva, jet-propulsive locomotion is an exaggerated ventilatory movement and hence, apart from producing rapid movements of the animal, also serves to exchange the contents of the branchial chamber several times faster than in normal ventilation.

The RDV is of importance in raising the sterna, and the MN innervating this muscle fires a short, high-frequency burst of impulses rather than the patterned burst of normal ventilation (Fig. 9a). The muscle potentials are considerably larger than those occurring in normal ventilation, but whether a second MN is activated is uncertain. The changeover from normal ventilation to swimming is often very abrupt, since jet propulsion is used as an escape mechanism, but may be more gradual as in Fig. 9a. A very similar burst of activity coinciding with that in the RDV has been observed in electromyograms of the ADV (Fig. 9b); also the PDV, a muscle which is innervated by the third segmental nerve (Fig. 1d) and has not been observed to be active in normal ventilation, is activated during the propulsive (expiratory) phase of swimming (Mill and Pickard, 1972a, 1975) (Fig. 9c).

Apart from sternal lifting, active contraction of some, at least, of the longitudinal tergal and sternal muscles occurs (Fig. 9d,e), and also of the oblique dorsoventral muscles on both sides (Mill and Pickard, 1975). The anal appendages are adducted during each expiratory thrust, and activity synchronous with that in the RDVs has been recorded from the ventral adductor muscles of the paraprocts. Similarly, the legs are retracted during swimming and hence the leg MNs must receive synchronous information.

The recovery (inspiratory) phase involves activity in the sub-intestinal muscle at least, and electromyograms from this muscle indicate that synchronous firing of the pair of inspiratory MNs is occurring.

It has been shown (Burrows, 1975c) that in the locust many flight MNs receive some of the same excitatory synaptic inputs that go to the abdominal expiratory MNs, the closer MNs of the thoracic spiracles (acting in an expiratory capacity), and certain expiratory MNs involved in auxiliary head pumping. Furthermore, the abdominal inspiratory MNs, thoracic spiracular opener MNs, and certain inspiratory MNs involved in head pumping receive simultaneous inhibitory input. In some instances, it has been possible to match epsp's in one cell with epsp's or ipsp's in another, and this has led Burrows to postulate a single IN on each side synapsing bilaterally with each of these MNs (Fig. 8). This is by no means an uncommon situation since synchronization of the ventilatory rhythm with the stridulatory rhythm in crickets has been reported by Huber (1960a), Kutsch (1968), and Bentley (1969b). Stridulation occurs at a higher frequency than ventilation, and so modulation of the slower rhythm by the faster one occurs in this case (Bentley, 1969a).

Sensory Control of Ventilation

Little is known about the involvement of sense organs in the control of ventilation, although they are likely to play a smaller part than in waking, where substrate irregularities need to be compensated for.

Nevertheless, we do know something about the receptors likely to be stimulated by ventilatory movements. In aeshnid larvae, on each side of the mid and hind abdominal segments there are three proprioceptors, all innervated by the first segmental nerve: the longitudinal and vertical stretch receptors and the ventrolateral chordotonal organ. Both stretch receptors are phasotonic, and, with the possible exception of the longitudinal ones in abdominal segments 6 and 7 which are obliquely oriented, it is unlikely that they are stimulated by normal ventilation. Nevertheless, they will be affected by jet-propulsive swimming, since this alters the length of the abdominal segments. The chordotonal organs, on the other hand, will undergo length changes during inspiration and expiration (Finlayson and Lowenstein, 1958; Lowenstein and Finlayson, 1960; Mill, 1963, 1965). They contain three sensory cells, each with its own associated scolopidium (Mill, 1965; Mill and Pill, unpublished observations). There is also a large ventral type II neuron, innervated by the second segmental nerve, on each side of these abdominal segments, the dendrite of which lies across the sternopleural suture, and this may also be affected by ventilatory movements (Mill, 1965). Orchard (1975) has shown that the ventrolateral chordotonal organ of Carausius is purely phasic, responding to vibrational stimuli, and Finlayson (1976) suggests that it may monitor ventilation.

In Periplaneta, sensory feedback occurs during ventilation, and two sensory units appear to be involved. Brief lowering of the abdominal sterna (in headless animals at least) elicits a delay in the onset of the next expiratory burst. Electrical stimulation of the segmental nerve containing the motor units similarly causes a delay, but in this case it may be due to antidromic stimulation. Rhythmic stimulation of either type, applied at a frequency similar to and below that occurring, causes the ventilatory rhythm to lock into the new rhythm (Farley and Case, 1968).

Conversely, in dragonfly larvae electrical stimulation of a first segmental nerve (which does not contain the motor units innervating the main expiratory muscle) between expiratory bursts can elicit an expiratory burst and hence reset the rhythm,

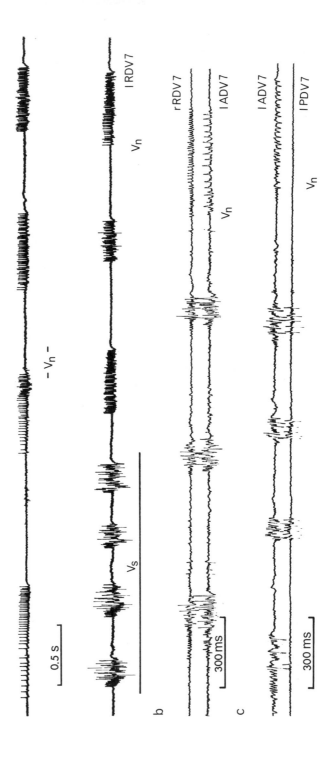

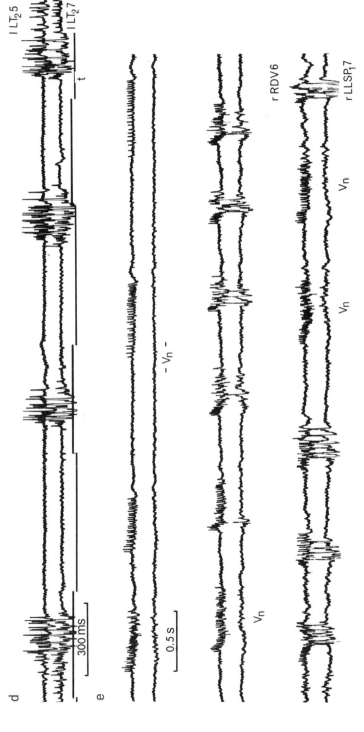

Fig. 9. Extracellular muscle recordings from unrestrained aeshnid larvae. Activity in (a) a respiratory dorsoventral muscle illustrating the transition from normal ventilation to jet-propulsive locomotion and back again, (b) respiratory (r RDV7) and anterior (l ADV7) dorsoventral muscles during jet-propulsive locomotion compared with one cycle of normal ventilation, (c) anterior (l ADV7) and posterior l PDV7) dorsoventral muscles during jet-propulsive locomotion compared with one cycle of normal ventilation, (d) two longitudinal tergal muscles (l LT_25, l LT_27) during jet-propulsive locomotion, and (e) respiratory dorsoventral (r RDV6) and longitudinal sternopleural (r $LLSP_17$) muscles during normal ventilation and jet-propulsive locomotion. l, Left; r, right; numeral indicates abdominal segment. From Mill and Pickard (1975).

while stimulation during expiration has no effect on the rhythm. Consecutive stimuli delivered at a rate slightly higher than that of the ventilatory rhythm can thus increase the ventilatory rate (Mill and Hughes, 1966; Mill, 1970). A similar response to electrical stimulation has been observed in mantids (Miller, 1971). The spikes in one expiratory MN in *Schistocerca* are inhibited by tactile stimulation.

In many insects, carbon dioxide acts on centers in the head and thoracic ganglia, with increase in pCO_2 having the general effect of increasing the overall frequency of ventilation as well as tending to increase activity in the spiracular opener MNs and decrease that in the spiracular closer MNs (Miller, 1974a). Burrows (1975c) observed a decrease in the number of spikes in one expiratory MN in *Schistocerca,* but carbon dioxide has little or no such effect on others. Adult dragonflies differ somewhat in that the effect on the spiracular closer MNs is produced by decrease in pO_2 more readily than by increase in pCO_2 (Miller, 1964). In aeshnid larvae, an increase in pCO_2 may or may not effect a slight increase in the ventilatory rate before the rhythm starts to break down (Pickard and Mill, 1974b).

Hoyle (1960) has shown that carbon dioxide acts directly on the closer muscle of spiracle 2 of *Schistocerca*. Increase in pCO_2 reduces tension in the muscle, thereby reducing the effect of its motor input. Hence the spiracle tends to flutter open as a result of cuticular elasticity.

Central Control of Ventilation

In various insects, isolated ganglia are capable of producing a rhythm resembling that of ventilation, but in the intact animal the rhythm is obviously coordinated (e.g., Farley *et al.,* 1967). In an earlier section, it has been mentioned that dragonfly larvae have a posterior–anterior abdominal rhythm, while the locust rhythm emanates from the metathoracic ganglion and shows a tendency to be directed anteroposteriorly, particularly during strong ventilation.

The idea of the occurrence of command INs which drive such activity is well established and the existence of multiple command INs, some of which are excitatory, others inhibitory, was demonstrated by Wiersma and Ikeda (1964) who electrically stimulated INs in the crayfish nerve cord to determine their effect on swimmeret beating. In *Periplaneta* and *Schistocerca*, rhythmic activity in the ventral nerve cord suggests that, in intact ventilatory systems, some at least of the command INs have a rhythmic firing pattern (Farley *et al.,* 1967; Miller, 1974a). Furthermore, in *Schistocerca,* the expiratory MNs studied by Burrows (1974) all receive rhythmic excitatory input and, in some, rhythmic inhibitory input also. The inspiratory MNs tend to receive a rhythmic inhibitory input as well as a fairly steady excitatory input lasting throughout the ventilatory cycle. The spiracular closer MNs, which are linked with expiration, receive only rhythmic excitatory input, while the spiracular opener MNs, linked with inspiration, receive rhythmic excitation and inhibition. In many cases, there is good evidence for at least two excitatory inputs.

There is also evidence for a common IN input to most or all of the ventilatory MNs as well as a number of flight MNs (Burrows, 1975c) (Fig. 8).

Burrows (1974) has demonstrated the effects of stimulating a whole pro-mesothoracic connective. Apart from producing epsp's in various MNs which follow the stimulation with a 1:1 ratio, the effect on inspiratory MNs is of particular interest. During expiration, a brief burst of stimuli has no effect on the rhythm. However, if applied during the inspiratory phase, the inspiratory burst is terminated, and thus if the stimuli are applied repetitively this can result in a slight speeding up of the rhythm. Stimulation early in the inspiratory phase has the effect of considerably shortening the delay before the onset of the next inspiration. Although Burrows suggests that these effects are the result of IN stimulation, they are similar in many respects to those produced in aeshnid larvae by first segmental nerve stimulation (Mill and Hughes, 1966; Mill, 1970), and sensory axons do not run along the connectives between segmental ganglia (Mill, 1964), a phenomenon not restricted to the insects (e.g., Wiersma and Mill, 1965). Conversely, peripheral root stimulation may act via INs.

There is good evidence for central control via intersegmental command INs which selectively elicit responses in the various MNs associated with ventilation depending on the needs of the animal, and this may be all that is required for the system to function. However, it is difficult, on this basis alone, to explain certain intersegmental interplays such as the anteriorly directed ventilatory rhythm of aeshnid larvae, and it is possible that more localized INs are present in the system (Fig. 10).

Figure 10 shows a simplified plan for the possible intersegmental control of ventilation in aeshnid larvae and *Schistocerca*. In the latter, both the anteriorly and posteriorly directed pathways from the segmental INs (S) are of equal importance, and all such neurons have similar threshold levels. There will thus be a tendency for the rhythm to run anteroposteriorly since the information flow in the command IN is in this direction. In aeshnid larvae, the segmental INs, or the expiratory INs (E) themselves, exhibit decreasing sensitivity from behind forward, and the importance of the posteriorly directed flow of information from the segmental INs is negligible compared to the anteriorly directed flow. It is further postulated that the expiratory

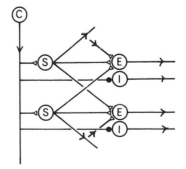

Fig. 10. Possible interconnections of a command IN (C), segmental INs (S), and ventilatory MNs (E, expiratory; I, inspiratory). For further explanation, see text.

MNs in each ganglion require the additional input from the next posterior segment before they reach their firing level. This would explain the anteriorly directed rhythm and the marked intersegmental delay.

It is possible to produce numerous wiring diagrams to explain various aspects of ventilation. However, as yet, we know little of the internal connections between INs and MNs and hence I feel that it is perhaps best to refrain from the temptation. Suffice it to add that despite the great progress that has been made in our attempts to understand the control of ventilation there is still much to be learned, and the promise of the next few years is considerable.

12

Mechanisms for the Production of Rhythmic Behavior in Crustaceans

Allen I. Selverston

Introduction

It is from some of the original work of Wiersma that the concept of identified neurons emerged. The idea that a single unique neuron could be repeatedly studied in different preparations was a milestone in the development of invertebrate neurophysiology and has resulted in extensive usage of invertebrate systems as models for studying vertebrate integrative mechanisms.

The question of whether or not these simple systems as models will provide us with rules which can be generalized to more complex systems is still unanswered. My own bias is, of course, that they will. I cannot argue that the circuits and neuronal properties will be identical; given the limited number of cells available, single invertebrate neurons may have to perform more complex integrative functions. However, what the analysis of invertebrate motor circuits can provide are ideas which can serve as a more rational basis for the study of vertebrate systems. The convergence of recent work on cat locomotion and invertebrate central pattern generation is to me a remarkable validation of this hoped-for goal.

Recent experimental evidence (Egger and Wyman, 1969; Grillner and Zangger, 1974) has convincingly demonstrated that the mechanisms for the production of cyclical motor output in vertebrates are located entirely within the spinal cord. These mechanisms, termed "central pattern generators," must not only be turned on and off by higher centers but also be continuously modulated so as to adapt movements to any particular environmental situation. We stand very little chance at present of describing these vertebrate motor systems in terms of all their component neuronal interactions. Although recordable neurons are "identifiable," they are not "identified"—and in addition there are just too many of them.

In this chapter, I would like to use the lobster stomatogastric nervous system as a model network by which oscillatory motor output can be studied in great detail. We will begin first with the behavior, then consider the neural circuitry underlying that behavior, the mechanisms involved at both the circuit and the cellular level, and finally some anatomical correlates related to the functional studies.

Allen I. Selverston • Department of Biology, University of California, San Diego, La Jolla, California 92093.

Stomatogastric System

The stomatogastric nervous system of the spiny lobster not only has a very limited number of nerve cells but also contains cells which show considerable integrative activity. This means that not only can the behavior of the system be studied but also the all-important questions of neuronal circuitry and of cellular properties underlying the behavior. The first intracellular study of this network was undertaken by Maynard (1966). For the past 7 years, we have extended his original work to the point where this system is one of the best-described networks currently under investigation. Since certain aspects of this system are remarkably similar to the functional properties of cat locomotion, I will emphasize these similarities wherever possible.

The stomach of the lobster may not seem to be an ideal place for an examination of arthropod behavior since its location within the thorax precludes casual observation. But if behavior is operationally defined to be patterned muscular contractions, then the stomach does behave, for, instead of being an intrinsically controlled sac like our own stomachs, it is a complex structure containing "teeth" and a filtering system, all movements of which are caused by striated muscles under neuronal control. The muscles are typically arthropodan, each being innervated by from one to four motor axons originating in the stomatogastric ganglion. The arrangement of the muscles is basically antagonistic so that, except for an absence of peripheral inhibition, the system is quite similar to an arthropod limb.

What makes this system particularly advantageous, however, is that the approximately 30 neurons in the ganglion reveal subthreshold integrative activity when intracellular recordings are made from their somata. The ganglion can also be easily studied in the completely deafferented state or with various sources of input connected to it.

The output consists of two separate rhythms, one operating the teeth of the gastric mill and the other controlling the pyloric filtering region. Motor neurons (MNs) in the ganglion are identified by matching soma spikes with extracellularly recorded spikes in the peripheral nerves. When recordings are made from the nerves in an isolated preparation, two different rhythms can be clearly seen.

The faster rhythm is the pyloric one, which is produced by a system of 14 neurons. The slower rhythm is that of the gastric mill, which is produced by a network of 12 neurons. The behavior, as interpreted by Hartline and Maynard (1975), consists basically of an opening and closing of two lateral teeth and a power and return stroke of the single medial tooth. All three teeth function smoothly to chew food which is stored in the cardiac sac region. The pyloric region is less complicated, and its behavior consists only of alternating dilation and constriction.

The antagonistic bursts recorded from isolated stomatogastric ganglia exhibit temporal patterns of discharge similar to those which underlie both vertebrate and invertebrate locomotion. In the cat, as the speed of locomotion increases, there is an increase in the number of steps per second. The shortened cycle duration, however, is due mainly to a decrease in the extension phase, i.e., that portion of the cycle in which the foot is on the ground, with the flexion or swing phase remaining constant

(Goslow *et al.*, 1973). Such organization, characteristic of relaxation oscillators, is observed in many invertebrate locomotory systems as well (Kristan *et al.*, 1974; Ayers, 1976; Pearson and Iles, 1970).

The dynamic substructures of both the stomatogastric rhythms exhibit similar forms (Ayers, unpublished). In the pyloric system, the PD bursts remain relatively constant, while those of the PD antagonists, such as LP, vary linearly with burst period. In the gastric system, the LG motor neuron exhibits bursts of constant duration while its antagonists, the LPGNs, vary linearly with burst period, with a regression slope of approximately 1. Thus in the gastric system we can attribute all variation in period to variation in the duration of LPGN activity.

Circuitry

By intracellular recording from pairs of cells during ongoing activity, the synaptic relationships underlying the rhythms have been almost completely established (Mulloney and Selverston, 1974*a*; Selverston and Mulloney, 1974*a,b*; Maynard and Selverston, 1975) (Fig. 1). Our criterion for a monosynaptic connection has been a fixed-latency unitary postsynaptic potential following a spike in the presynaptic cell. In most cases, the reversal potentials can be demonstrated. Electrotonically coupled

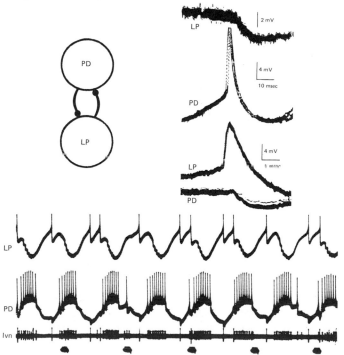

Fig. 1. Synaptic circuitry for the LP-PD neurons of the pyloric cycle. The two cells are reciprocally inhibitory and show unitary, fixed-latency ipsp's. During spontaneous activity (lower), the intracellular spikes can be matched with extracellular ones in the LVN nerve. Time marks: 1/sec.

cells could be identified by the passage of direct current between somata. The results of the synaptic analysis are shown in Fig. 2 as a circuit diagram.

There are a total of 153 chemical synapses between MNs and the two interneurons (INs) of the ganglion. The synapses are predominantly inhibitory, mostly reciprocal between neurons innervating antagonistic muscles, and probably heavily influenced by the large number of electrotonic junctions. Our analysis to date has not included a description of the dynamic nonlinear properties of each synapse, nor has it accurately determined their functional strengths.

Mechanisms of Burst Production

There appear to be two basically different mechanisms responsible for the stomatogastric rhythms. The pyloric rhythm, as Maynard originally suggested, relies on a group of three electrotonically coupled endogenous bursters—the two PDs and the AB. The synaptic circuitry among the other MNs is responsible for the production of bursts and their proper phase relationships among the pyloric group. The gastric mill rhythm, on the other hand, appears to be produced entirely as a consequence of the synaptic connections, with no single cell or group of cells acting as a "godfather" to the rest.

Pyloric Rhythm

There are several lines of evidence which suggest that the PD-AB group consists of endogenous bursters.

1. Hyperpolarization of the PD-AB group stops bursting in all other pyloric rhythm cells. Hyperpolarization of any of the pyloric cells except PD-AX can affect the burst rate but will not prevent bursting in the PD-AB group.
2. After uncoupling of the network with high-magnesium, low-calcium saline, it is only the PD-AB group which continues to burst.
3. In detailed studies using voltage clamping, various pharmacological agents, and ionic alterations, it is clear that the PD-AB cells behave in a way similar to endogenously bursty cells of mollusks. These studies will be discussed in more detail in a later section.
4. Intracellular injection of current alters the bursting of the PD and AB cells at a rate proportional to the amount of polarization.

Examination of the pyloric circuit shows that it is made up entirely of inhibitory connections (Fig. 2). If we make some assumptions about synaptic properties, it is possible to suggest how the pyloric pattern is produced. We start with the fact that the PD-AB group consists of endogenous bursters and that all the other pyloric cells will fire spontaneously if not inhibited. Examination of the extracellular burst pattern shows that when the PD-AB group fires (causing dilation of the

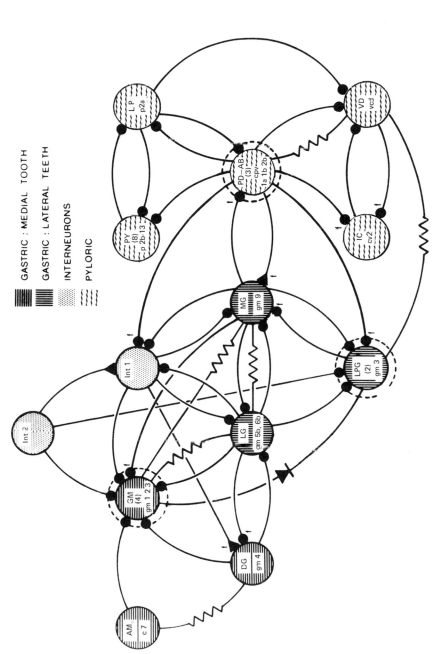

GASTRIC : MEDIAL TOOTH

GASTRIC : LATERAL TEETH

INTERNEURONS

PYLORIC

Fig. 2. Stomatogastric neural circuitry. Black dots represent inhibitory synapses. Black triangles represent excitatory synapses. Resistors indicate nonrectifying electrical junctions; the diode indicates a rectifying electrical synapse. The letter "f" near some synapses indicates a functional connection.

pyloric region of the stomach) all the other cells are inhibited. When the PD-AB burst is terminated, the other cells fire in order LP-IC, VD, and PY (causing a wavelike constriction of the pyloric region). To explain the sequence, we must assume three classes of synapses (Fig. 3):

> Class 1: From the PD-AB group, so that when these cells burst all other cells are inhibited. When the burst terminates, LP and IC are disinhibited and can fire.
>
> Class 2: From the LP and IC to the VD; keeps VD inhibited so that its firing is delayed.
>
> Class 3: From LP to PY; stronger than the VD synapse so that PY fires last.

The VD and PY bursts are normally terminated by a fresh burst in the PD-AB group, but how are the LP and IC bursts stopped? In the case of the LP, this probably results from reciprocal inhibition by the eight PY cells. There is a further role for the other reciprocal inhibitory pairs:

1. LP helps keep the PD-AB pair shut off, as well as the PY group.
2. VD helps shut off the IC.
3. IC delays the start of VD.

The role of the electrotonic coupling between VD and PD is more difficult to ascertain but is probably responsible for the wide variations in phase we see in the VD pattern-firing ranging from in phase with the PD-AB group to 180° out of phase with it.

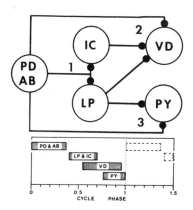

Fig. 3. Simplified pyloric circuit in which black dots represent inhibitory synapses. The PD-AB cells are electrically coupled to one another and are endogenous bursters. The most common phase relationships between activity in the different units are shown below the circuit. The numbers 1, 2, and 3 refer to classes of synapses described in the text.

Gastric Mill

Before examining the ionic mechanisms responsible for the endogenous bursting, we should consider the circuit mechanisms responsible for the gastric mill cycle. There are a large number of interactions possible in this network, and it is probably useful to attempt to simplify it somewhat. We start with the premise that no cells in this group have the property of endogenous bursting; at least that we have been able to demonstrate by all the criteria which were applied to the pyloric group—intracellular current injection, TTX, and high-Mg^{2+}, low-Ca^{2+} saline. All gastric rhythm cells, if not influenced by any of the others, either fire spontaneously (not in bursts) or are silent resting potentials below threshold). It is our feeling at present that the properly phased bursts generated by this network are a result of the connectivity itself—a so-called emergent property. The probable basis for the alternating bursts is the extensive number of reciprocal inhibitory connections, but to understand the whole pattern we must break the circuit down into its component parts.

In Fig. 4, we see that there are alternating bursts between the LG-MG group, which closes the lateral teeth, and the LPG-IN 1 group. IN 1 is one of two INs in the ganglion, while the LPGs are MNs which open the lateral teeth and therefore fire out of phase with the LG-MG pair. We also see in Fig. 2 that this lateral tooth network is composed basically of reciprocally inhibitory connections between the antognists. Such networks have been shown by the use of neuromimes (Wilson and Waldron, 1968) and digital computer simulations (Perkel and Mulloney, 1974) to be able to produce rhythmic alternating bursts. In this pair, the LPG and IN 1 normally fire if not inhibited by other inputs. LG and MG are normally silent. Apparently,

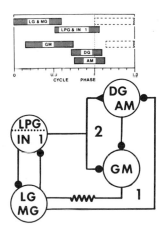

Fig. 4. Synaptic and electrotonic connections between lateral and medial teeth subgroups which could account for the mechanism of the total gastric mill pattern shown above. The black triangle represents a chemical excitatory synapse and the resistor represents an electrotonic junction. Note that the class 1 connections active when the LG and MG burst excite the GMs and inhibit their antagonists, DG and AM. When LPG and IN 1 fire (class 2), the DG and AM are excited and GMs are inhibited.

when inputs to this group raise the general excitability of the pair, the system undergoes a transition from a nonbursting state to alternating burst production. If we examine Fig. 4, we see no such reciprocal inhibition between the GM neurons (medial tooth power stroke) and the DG-AM pair (medial tooth return stroke). This means this group cannot work in isolation but must receive both phasic excitatory and inhibitory inputs from other cells in order to burst reciprocally.

By incorporating these two subgroups into one simplified circuit, however, a mechanism for both alternating pairs emerges. We see that the alternation between the LG-MG and the IN 1–LPG group could provide the driving force for the GM and DGN-AMN pair. LG-MG firing not only inhibits the IN 1 and LPG pair but also starts the GMs and stops the DGN.

The other synapses and electrotonic connections probably serve to greatly increase the dynamic range of possible behaviors, but these are mainly an elaboration of the basic mechanism just described.

Inputs to the Stomatogastric Ganglion

Like all central pattern generators, those which produce the gastric and pyloric rhythms are modulated by higher centers: in this case, these centers are located in the commissural and esophageal ganglia. Although the isolated stomatogastric ganglion can burst spontaneously, the gastric mill almost never cycles, and the pyloric burst rate is greatly reduced without these inputs. The effects of the descending afference has been investigated by Russell (1976). Taking advantage of the fact that all descending input is via the stomatogastric nerve, Russel has used a sucrose gap around the nerve to reversibly block traffic to and from the ganglion. When the pathway is open both rhythms occur reliably, but during blockage the gastric rhythm disappears entirely and the pyloric is reduced by about one half.

The total number of inputs affecting the stomatogastric rhythms is not known, but several of them have been partially characterized by Russell. It was known that two key neurons of each cycle, the AB cell and IN 1, send axons up the stomatogastric nerve to the commissural ganglia. Their apparent function is to send phasic information about each rhythm to cells outside the ganglion. These other cells then actually become part of the circuit because they in turn send phasic excitatory information back to the stomatogastric ganglion. In combined preparations, i.e., those with the commissural and esophageal ganglia left intact, the effects of this "extended" gastric mill circuit can be seen clearly by shutting off parts of the network (Russell, unpublished). During spontaneous bursting in a combined preparation, we have the following events occurring:

1. IN 1 and LPG are alternating with LG and MG to produce reciprocal bursts.
2. IN 1 activity modulates cells in the commissural ganglia (E cells). From their activity, as seen in the stomatogastric nerve, we know they are phasically inhibited.

3. When E cells fire, their bursts correspond temporally to GM bursts, suggesting an excitatory pathway to these cells.

Since what appears to be involved is a phasic excitatory loop, stopping the LG and MG should interrupt the loop. Such an experiment is shown in Fig. 5. During the time LG and MG are hyperpolarized, IN 1 fires tonically and the E cells receive no phasic inhibition and so also stop bursting. The entire gastric mill system is arrested and resumes only when the LG and MG are released from inhibition. Note that this experiment also strongly supports the idea that bursting in the gastric mill system is an emergent property of the network.

Intracellular recording from gastric mill neurons reveals that E-cell afferent spikes can be correlated with epsp's in the GM, ,LPG, LG, and MG neurons (Russell,

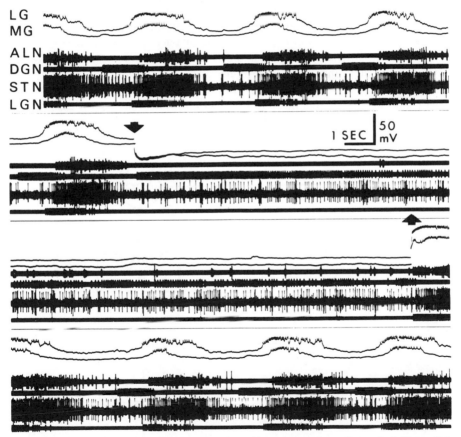

Fig. 5. LG/MG shutoff experiment in a preparation with commissural ganglia attached. Extracellular recordings show the GMs on the ALN trace, DG on the DGN trace, E cells on the STN trace, and LG on the LGN trace. LG and MG were both hyperpolarized at the downward arrow. Gastric units fired tonically while LG and MG were off. Cycling resumed after release of LG + MG (upward arrow). Courtesy of D. Russell.

1976). Since some of these cells normally fire antagonistically to one another, the most probable role for the E-cell inputs is to provide a generalized but phasic form of excitation. Building this into the simplified gastric network shown in Fig. 4 leads to the slightly more complex structure shown in Fig. 6. In this latter figure, we see that the periodic firing of IN 1 produces phasic bursting of the E cell by inhibition. The E cell then acts to turn on the GMs directly and turn off the DG–AM antagonists indirectly via the LG-MG pair. Its concomitant activation of LPG must also mean that it can act to raise the overall excitability to the system.

Why has such an extended loop arisen in this system? Several explanations are possible. There are other bursty rhythms present in the foregut which operate the esophagus and cardiac sac. These oscillatory centers are located in the commissural and esophageal ganglia (Selverston *et al.*, 1976) and are coordinated with the rhythms produced by the stomatogastric ganglion. The E cells may serve as the interface for these coordinating mechanisms. A further possibility is that most sensory input from the wall of the stomach does not act directly on the stomatogastric ganglion but instead enters the commissurals. For example, the DPON nerves lead directly to the commissurals and probably contain many primary sensory INs. When stimulated, they can turn on the gastric mill (Fig. 7). We have not found direct connections from this nerve to the gastric mill neurons, and it is likely that such effects are via E cells or similar INs.

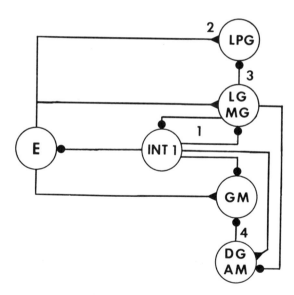

Fig. 6. Postulated mechanism for production of reliable gastric mill bursting: (1) Reciprocal inhibitory network between LG-MG and IN 1 causes periodic inhibition of the E cells. (2) The E cells deliver phasic excitation to LPG, LG, MG, and GM timed by the gastric cycle, increasing the overall excitability of the network. (3) Inhibition from LG/MG to LPG is stronger than the excitatory input from the E cell. (4) Inhibition from DG/AM onto the GM ensures alternate firing of these two cells.

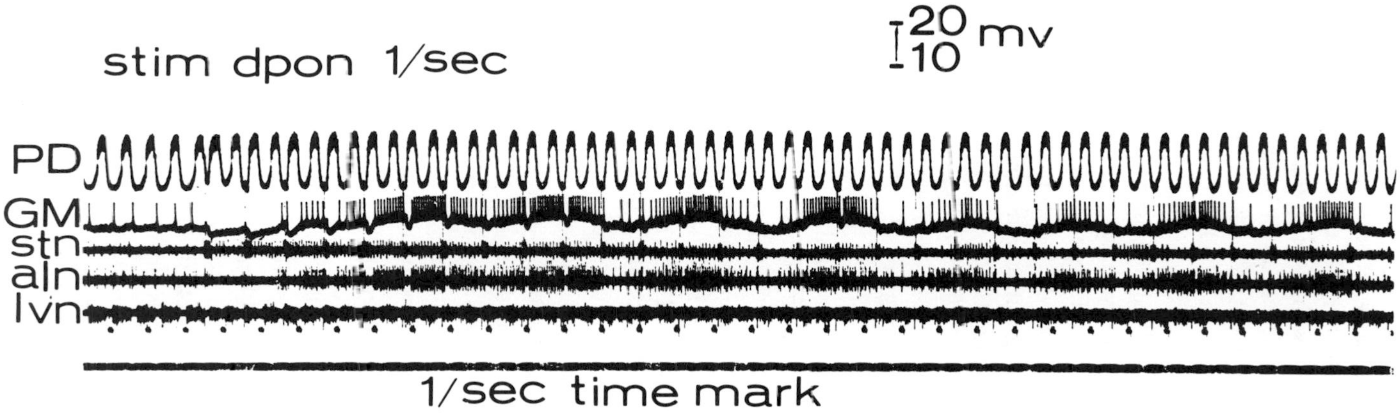

Fig. 7. Stimulation of DPON, a nerve attached to the commissural ganglion, at 1/sec turns on the gastric mill as shown in the intracellular and extracellular traces. Note the slight increase in frequency of the PD cell of the pyloric rhythm. The DPON contains many sensory fibers, so the effect is probably the result of mixed inputs to the system.

There is a remarkable similarity between the extended networks described here and those found in the cat spinal cord. In the cat, we know that the central pattern generator is located exclusively within the spinal cord because a spinalized animal which has been completely deafferented can be shown to be capable of producing rhythmic locomotory discharge if dorsal roots are tonically stimulated or the cord is treated with pharmacological agents which mimic descending input (Grillner and Zangger, 1974). The efferent phasic information carried to the commissural ganglia by IN 1 and the AB cells is entirely analogous to ascending phasic efference seen in the ventral spinocerebellar tract (Arshavsky *et al.*, 1974). Phasic input to the stomatogastric networks carried by E-type neurons would seem quite analogous to the descending phasic information which occurs in the rubrospinal, reticulospinal, and vestibulospinal tracts during cat locomotion (Orlovsky, 1970) and which is modulated by the locomotor rhythm.

Endogenous Burst Mechanisms

If our hypothesis about burst production in the gastric mill system is correct, we must learn much more about the nonlinear properties of each synapse in order to understand how the whole system works. Such a network could eventually be usefully modeled with computer simulations using experimental data. Such modeling studies should be able to suggest minimal networks and the effects of perturbing these networks; these findings could then be confirmed in wet preparations.

If we are correct about the pyloric rhythm being generated by a group of endogenously bursty cells, then it is of some interest to know the mechanisms which produce the membrane potential oscillations in the AB and PD neurons. Such endogenous bursters have been studied in great detail in mollusks, where the site of slow wave production is very near the soma. This makes voltage clamp analysis possible so that even though the functional role of these cells is usually not known, a good deal about their burst-generating mechanism is. Although the basic structure of crustacean and molluscan cells is similar, the somata of crustacean cells are not electrogenic, and the slow potentials monitored from this point are actually being generated at some distal point in the neuropil.

In preliminary experiments with Maurice Gola, some details of the slow-wave-generating mechanism are begining to emerge. Despite the fact that the slow-wave-initiating zones of the PD-AB cells are located distal to the soma, voltage clamping of the soma does provide some useful information about the currents involved. Unlike a voltage-clamped *Aplysia* neuron with endogenous burst characteristics, the PD and AB cells do not show a steady current but rather an inwardly directed one that oscillates slowly, corresponding to the slow potential waves. The frequency and time course of this slow, transient, inward current are dependent on the membrane potential (Fig. 8); the frequency and rate of development of inward current amplitude decrease with depolarization so that the apparent reversal potential (about 40 mV) is positive with respect to the midpoint of the slow

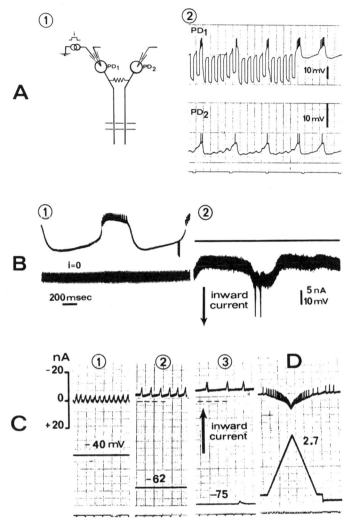

Fig. 8. Slow conductance changes in PD cells in current and voltage clamp conditions. A1: Diagram showing experimental arrangement. PD_1 penetrated with a double-barreled microelectrode for recording membrane potential and current injection. PD_2, electrically coupled to PD_1 (resistor), penetrated by a single microelectrode. A2: Short pulses of inward current are passed into PD_1 and can be seen after electrotonic attenuation in PD_2. Note the increase in size of the electrically coupled potential in PD_2, indicating an increasing coupling factor during the slow depolarization phase. B1: Spontaneous burst of activity in PD cell under zero current injection. B2: Voltage clamp condition. The membrane potential (upper trace) is maintained constant at the level shown in B1. Lower trace: Resulting spontaneous, slow, transient inward current. The two fast inward phases correspond to axonal spikes from unclamed region. C1,C2,C3: Spontaneous, slow, transient inward currents for different command potential levels. Note the decrease in frequency and the increase in amplitude of the slow, transient inward current. D: Membrane activation, under voltage clamp conditions, with a symmetrical triangular ramp pulse (slope ±2.7 mV sec^{-1}). The spontaneous inward current increases in frequency and decreases in amplitude upon depolarization. Time marks: 1/sec, when not indicated otherwise.

potential wave. Although these results do not provide direct proof, they strongly suggest that the slow-wave-generating mechanism is a voltage-dependent phenomenon rather than an oscillating electrogenic pump.

This conclusion is also supported by the fact that when the ganglion is perfused with zero-potassium saline the slow wave persists for more than ½ hr, and following a return to normal saline shows no hyperpolarization (Fig. 9A). These results would not be expected if the slow wave were due to a pump mechanism.

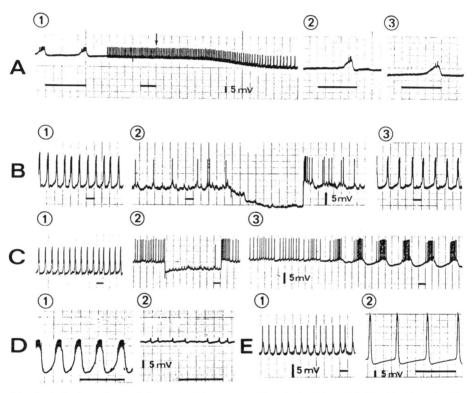

Fig. 9. Ionic dependency of slow potential waves in PD cell. A: Effect of 0 K^+: A1, Control; A2, immediate hyperpolarization and frequency decrease following change to K = 0 saline (arrow); A3,A4, spontaneous slow wave after 6 and 30 min of 0 K^+. Time base: 1 sec. B: Effect of TTX:B1, Control; B2, irregular firing after 4 min in 6×10^{-10} TTX. A hyperpolarizing current pulse indicated by bar fails to restore slow waving. A tendency toward slow waving appears following the current pulse. B3, Return of normal burst production after 2 min in normal saline. C: Effect of 0 Ca^{2+}: C1, Control; C2, continuous firing and depolarization after 3 min in 0 Ca^{2+} saline. The slow wave does not reappear upon hyperpolarization (indicated by bar) of the membrane to the original level. C3, During the recovery from 0 Ca^{2+}, the cell repolarizes and the slow waving resumes but at a lower frequency and greater duration. After 4 min, the bursts look like the original control. D: Effect of replacing Ca^{2+} with Co^{2+}: D1, Control; D2, after 4 min in Co^{2+} saline the bursts stop and the potential stabilizes at a level corresponding to the top of the control slow waves (the effect of Co^{2+} is reversible after a 10-min washing). E: Effect of replacing Ca^{2+} with Ba^{2+}: E1, Control; E2, 2 min 20 sec in Ba^{2+} saline. The cell generates slow potential waves at a greater amplitude. Note change in calibration between E1 and E2. Horizontal bars: 1 sec, if not otherwise noted.

We also have evidence that there are conductance changes during the slow wave. We have taken advantage of the fact that electrotonic junctions between PD cells are probably located electrotonically close to the slow wave generation site. Passage of hyperpolarizing current pulses through the soma and recording of the resultant potential change in the same soma show no measurable change in the input resistance of the cell during slow waves. However, the potential change in the other PD cell is due to current crossing the electrotonic junctions. A decrease in conductance of up to 50% is observed during the slow depolarization preceding the burst (Fig. 8). Since the reversal potential for K^+ is negative to the resting potential, the conductance decrease may be due to a decrease in gK^+ of a type that has been described in *Aplysia* (Brodwick and Junge, 1973; Chalazonitis, 1963).

Another result of the 0 K^+ experiment is that although the soma potential is increased by 7 mV (by increasing the K^+ differential) the burst period is increased from 1 to 2 sec. To get an equivalent slowing of the bursting by passage of current through the soma requires a hyperpolarization of 21 mV, indicating that there is an attenuation factor of about 3 for voltages between the soma and the slow-wave-initiation zone.

When the Na^+ is totally removed from the solution by replacement with tris or sucrose, the slow wave is reduced by about one-half. Replacement with ½N or ¼ N Na^+ gives the same result as 0 Na^+, which means that not only do the Na^+ currents not depend on the highest Na^+ concentrations but also there must be another inward charge carrier. As further proof for a Na^+ role, TTX (6×10^{-10} M) also reduces the inward currents and the amplitude of the slow potential wave, whereas the same concentration completely blocks axonal spikes (Fig. 9B).

Experiments substituting Ba^{2+} or Co^{2+} for Ca^{2+} in the saline strongly suggest Ca^{2+} as the other inward charge carrier. Barium is known to have a greater conductance than Ca^{2+} in normal Ca^{2+} channels. We have found that Ba^{2+} greatly increases the slow wave amplitude in a graded fashion (Fig. 9E). We know this is not an exaggeration of the Na^+ conductance because the same increase in amplitude can be observed in the presence of TTX. Cobalt, which is known to block Ca^{2+} channels in mollusks (Geduldig and Junge, 1968) and crustacean muscle (Hagiwara and Takahashi, 1967), completely blocks slow waving of the PD cells. It is interesting that the final effect of Co^{2+} on the cell is to depolarize it, possibly through blockage of K^+ channels (Meech and Standen, 1975). When the cell stops firing, it does so in this depolarized state (Fig. 9D). When the K^+ channels are blocked with TEA, the slow wave is elongated. Blockage by Co^{2+} in the depolarized state and the effect of TEA are indirect evidence that the outward current during the slow wave could be due to K^+ activation, as proposed by Meech and Standen (1975) for molluscan neurons.

In sum, the slow depolarization preceding the burst is probably due to a slow decrease in gK. The inward current associated with the burst appears to be carried by Na^+ and Ca^+. Repolarization following the burst is apparently due to a K^+ activation, but our evidence for this is incomplete at this time. These mechanisms appear to be entirely analogous to those underlying slow waving in *Aplysia* neurons (Gola, 1976).

Neuronal Anatomy

It has been possible to examine the branching patterns of identified nerve cells by using intracellular dye injections. To quantify these measurements, we have developed a technique of computerized reconstruction (Selverston *et al.,* 1976). If branching patterns between identifiable cells are compared, it is at once obvious that there are considerable differences in both topology and topography. Functional interactions between identifiable cells occur, however, with a minimum of variation from preparation to preparation. To understand these seemingly contradictory statements, King (1976) examined the ultrastructure of the ganglion in some detail. From extrapolation of sample counts of synaptic contacts in the stomatogastric neuropil, there appear to be on the order of 1 million chemical synapses. Counting

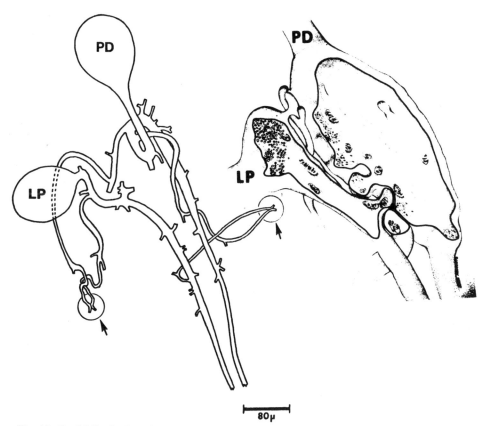

Fig. 10. Spatial distribution of the PD-LP synapse. The sketch shows a partial reconstruction from serial sections of identified PD and LP neurons including two sites of synaptic contact (arrows). At the right is a sketch based on several serial sections through short segments of two dendrites. These dendrites were traced from identified cell bodies of a PD neuron and LP neuron. Note that synaptic vesicles and membrane specializations are restricted to localized swellings on each dendrite. Courtesy of D. King.

the number of functional synaptic connections from the circuit diagram and estimating the number of descending synaptic inputs from counts of fibers in the stomatogastric nerve, we are off by several orders of magnitude if we assume each functional synapse has only one anatomical correlate.

Serial section electron microscopy through parts of identified cells revealed several important anatomical correlates:

1. Synapses are located only on the terminal branches, i.e., those processes which are free of glial sheathing.
2. Synapses occur on bulblike swellings of the processes in a bidirectional manner; i.e., the bulb both transmits and receives information (Fig. 10).
3. Synapses from one identified cell onto another are multiterminal so that presynaptic terminals are distributed widely over the branching processes of the postsynaptic cell (Fig. 10)

We have no way of knowing how many of the anatomical contacts are actually functional, but it is probably safe to assume that, like multiterminal neuromuscular synapses, they all are. What the spike-initiating zone sees is the integrated results of a cloud of synaptic input coming in from the terminal branches. Under such conditions, it is not surprising to find such wide disparity in the three-dimensional geometry of each neuron or so large a number of anatomical synapses present in the ganglion.

These anatomical findings also complicate the question of how such organization between neurons takes place developmentally. It strongly supports the idea that proper function during development plays a role in determining the final anatomical arrangement between cells. Although contacts between cells are probably genetically determined, the neurons must have some way of knowing when the proper number has been reached. Exactly where this information is stored is an exceptionally intriguing question.

13

A Comparative Approach to the Neural Control of Locomotion

Paul S. G. Stein

Introduction

The neural mechanisms controlling locomotion have been examined in many organisms (Gray, 1968). Several authors have proposed that these mechanisms can be characterized by a set of unifying principles (e.g., Brown, 1911, 1914; Wiersma and Ikeda, 1964; Wilson, 1966a,b, 1967, 1968c, 1972; Szekeley, 1968; Lundberg, 1969; Hoyle, 1970; Evarts et al., 1971; Evoy and Cohen, 1971; Davis, 1973b; Gurfinkel and Shik, 1973; Stein, 1974, 1976; Grillner, 1975; Shik and Orlovsky, 1976; Wetzel and Stuart, 1976). Such principles are useful in that they can order vast groups of data and provide working hypotheses for the design of new experiments. This chapter will present one version of the unifying principles with emphasis on their joint application to the arthropods and the vertebrates.

The unifying principles are stated in the form of a conceptual model. The model is functional; i.e., it assigns certain logical functions to specific subcomponents of the neural network. The model has two major components: a "central" part and a "peripheral feedback" part. The components of the unifying principles can be stated as follows:

I. The "central" component

    A. Command neurons—tonic descending control

        There is a set of command neurons which serve to turn on and maintain locomotory behavior. The discharge rate of these neurons influences the repetition rate of the locomotory cycle; this latter parameter in turn influences the velocity of progression. These cells can activate a normal locomotory behavior even in the absence of sensory input.

    B. The locomotory pattern generator

        The entire nervous system is not needed to produce the rhythmic locomotory output. In fact, a restricted portion of the central nervous

Paul S. G. Stein • Department of Biology, Washington University, St. Louis, Missouri 63130.

system (CNS) is sufficient. This restricted portion of the CNS contains the locomotory pattern generator, which is activated by command neurons and can function in the absence of sensory input. The pattern generator is composed of a set of local control centers and the coordinating neurons interconnecting them.

1. The local control center—a pattern generator for one limb

There is a local control center which directs the movements of a single limb. Each limb is driven by a separate center which can organize the temporal activation of limb muscles during locomotion. Activity of the control center is driven by command neurons and can occur in the absence of input from sensory structures, other local control centers, and the remainder of the CNS. Note that while the local control center is *not dependent* on sensory or other CNS input, its activity can be *modified* by these influences.

2. The coordinating neuron—interlimb phase control

There is a set of coordinating neurons which serve to regulate the relative phase of the limbs during locomotion. These neurons transmit phase information among the local control centers. Each of these cells is active during a particular phase of the rhythm of one local control center and in turn can serve to modulate the phase of other limb control centers. These cells can function in the absence of sensory input. Note that any influence which perturbs the rhythm of a local control center will also alter the activity of coordinating neurons emanating from that center.

II. The "peripheral feedback" component

A. Amplitude modulation

There is a set of "amplitude-modulating" neurons which are driven by sensory input and serve to modify the intensity of motor neuron (MN) discharge during locomotion. Intensity of MN discharge can be altered by a change in the firing rate of a given motor unit, a change in the number of active units, or both. The amplitude-modulating neurons *do not* cause a shift in the temporal patterning of motor output.

B. Phase modulation

There is a set of "phase-modulating" neurons which are driven by sensory input and serve to alter the timing of the locomotory rhythm. This alteration in timing will cause a permanent "phase shift" in the rhythm of the local control center if the other control centers are not active. During a phase modulation, it is also possible that the amplitude of the motor discharge will be altered.

This model is derived mainly from data obtained with animals utilizing their limbs for propulsion. This model can also be applied with modification to animals which depend on axial musculature to generate the force of progression (e.g., leech: see Kristan *et al.*, 1974; Ort *et al.*, 1974). This chapter, however, will emphasize the experimental strategies characteristic of studies of limbed locomotion. For a more detailed summary of the experimental data on locomotion, the reader should consult two recent conference volumes (Stein *et al.*, 1973; Herman *et al.*, 1976) and three recent reviews (Grillner, 1975; Shik and Orlovsky, 1976; Wetzel and Stuart, 1976).

The Central Component of the Network

The Command Neuron

The term "command neuron" was defined by Wiersma and Ikeda (1964) and Kennedy (1969) as a single interneuron (IN) which when stimulated will produce a complex yet stereotyped behavior. The result of command neuron stimulation is a behavior which can be characterized by measuring a temporal series of body and appendage positions. The strategy of command neuron work has been to select a naturally occurring behavior, and then assay this behavior (videotape or cine, EMG or MN recordings). INs in the CNS are then prepared for electrical stimulation. When stimulation of a given neuron elicits a motor output which is an excellent replica of the output observed during a natural behavior, then that cell is considered a command neuron.

Command neurons which control the static position of the body in space have been termed "postural neurons" or "tonic command neurons" (Kennedy *et al.*, 1966; Bowerman and Larimer, 1974*a*, 1976*a*; Larimer, 1976; Larimer and Gordon, this volume); command neurons which produce rhythmic changes of body position that move the animal from one point in space to another have been termed "locomotory neurons" or "phasic command neurons" (Wiersma and Ikeda, 1964; Bowerman and Larimer, 1974*b*, 1976*a*; Larimer, 1976; Larimer and Gordon, this volume). In many of the situations examined among the crustaceans and the mollusks, stimulation of a single cell is sufficient to produce a complex motor pattern. In some situations, however, the excitation produced by a single cell of a cluster is not sufficient to drive a behavior; extracellular excitation of the entire cluster is needed to produce the behavior under study (Willows and Hoyle, 1969; Willows *et al.*, 1973*a,b*; Willows, 1976).

Locomotory command neurons may function either to trigger or to gate the behavior. The output of a trigger command cell may be one cycle of motor behavior, e.g., the single tail flip produced by giant fiber discharge in crayfish (Wiersma, 1947*a*; Wine and Krasne, 1972; Krasne and Wine, this volume), or several cycles of motor output, e.g., the swimming produced by an electrical pulse delivered via an extracellular electrode placed in the region of the trigger cells of *Tritonia* (Willows and Hoyle, 1969; Willows *et al.*, 1973*a,b*; Getting, 1975; Willows, 1976). Gate command neurons can drive one or many cycles of locomotory behavior, depending on the duration of the train of electrical stimuli (Wiersma and Ikeda, 1964; P. S. G. Stein, 1974). In some cases, when a higher frequency of electrical stimulation is utilized, then a higher frequency of the locomotory rhythm is produced (Wiersma and Ikeda, 1964; Davis and Kennedy, 1972*c*). In the lobster swimmeret system, the output range of any one command neuron is limited to a fraction of the entire set of movement frequencies (Davis and Kennedy, 1972*a*). The phenomenon has been called "range fractionation" and implies that different command neurons probably need to be activated in order to produce the entire range of movement frequencies.

An important property of the gate command neuron is that no specific temporal pattern of stimulation is necessary to elicit a perfectly timed locomotory output. This was initially discovered by examining the locust flight pattern produced by random electrical stimulation of the circumesophageal connectives (Wilson and Wyman, 1965). From this point of view, the command neuron serves as a general excitor to a specific group of nerve cells which we can term the "pattern generator." When the pattern generator is given a sufficient level of excitation, the normal motor output is produced. The pattern generator itself is an ensemble of local control centers and the coordinating neurons connecting them. These concepts will be discussed in subsequent sections.

It is important to determine the extent to which the command concept applies in the vertebrate systems (Grillner, 1975, 1976). There are examples of single cells in fish which when stimulated will produce a coordinated motor output, e.g., Müller and Mauthner cells (Rovainen, 1967; Diamond, 1971). I am not aware of a case where stimulation of a *single* IN in a higher vertebrate will result in a coordinated motor output. Low-intensity extracellular stimulation of a small group of neighboring cells in the sensorimotor cortex of the cat has been successful in eliciting a discrete muscle movement in the limb (Asanuma and Sakata, 1967). Low-intensity extracellular stimulation in the superior colliculus of the monkey can produce conjugate saccades of the eyes (Schiller and Stryker, 1972). It may be that in the CNS of higher vertebrates, as with the trigger cells of the *Tritonia,* the excitation produced by any one cell is not sufficient to produce a coordinated motor behavior, but stimulation of a set of related cells is needed to produce the desired motor effect. The ensemble of cells which must be activated in order to produce a voluntary movement in a vertebrate remains to be established.

It is possible to utilize part of the command neuron "strategy" in some vertebrates; i.e., the experimenter can select localized stimulation sites in the CNS which will produce an excellent replica of behavior, while temporarily ignoring the issue of how many cells need to be stimulated. This approach has led to the result that electrical stimulation of the lateral columns of the spinal cord can elicit locomotory movements in the high spinal cat (Roaf and Sherrington, 1910; Sherrington, 1910), in the intact turtle (Lennard and Stein, 1974, 1977), in the low spinal turtle (Lennard and Stein, 1977), and in the high spinal turtle (Stein, 1977). In addition, electrical stimulation of the midbrain in a mesencephalic fish (Kashin *et al.*, 1974) will induce swimming. Electrical stimulation of the "locomotor region" of the midbrain of a mesencephalic cat (Shik *et al.*, 1966) can produce walking, trotting, or galloping on a treadmill.

Stimulation of primary afferents is usually not considered "command" stimulation. Such stimulation can excite command neurons, which in turn can elicit locomotion. This is true in the arthropods, e.g., wind on the head of a locust elicits flight behavior (Wilson, 1968*a*), and in the vertebrates, e.g., dorsal root stimulation will elicit stepping motor output in a spinal curarized cat (Grillner and Zangger, 1974). Chemical stimulation of the CNS is also a useful technique for eliciting locomotion in the spinal cat (Forssberg and Grillner, 1973; Grillner and Zangger, 1974; Edgerton *et al.*, 1976; Halbertsma *et al.*, 1976). In these cases, it is thought that the chemical (DOPA or clonidine) which is injected intravenously causes excitation of noradrenergic receptors in the spinal cord (Grillner and Shik, 1973). It is an interesting hypothesis that norepinephrine may be one of the transmitters utilized for command activation of locomotion in the intact cat. There is other evidence, however, which suggests that if norepinephrine is a transmitter for activation of locomotion, then it is not the only one (Jordan and Steeves, 1976).

The experiments with higher vertebrates are very important not only because they show that electrical stimulation of a site within the CNS can elicit locomotion but also because they show that a restricted portion of the vertebrate nervous system, namely, the spinal cord, is sufficient to produce the locomotory rhythm. Such a result has also been obtained in many experimental studies with the ventral nerve cord of the arthropods. These results will be discussed in the following section on the pattern generator.

The Locomotory Pattern Generator

In multiappendage organisms, the locomotory rhythm in the several appendages can be generated by a restricted portion of the CNS. In a vertebrate, this means that the pattern generator for locomotion resides in the spinal cord (Grillner, 1975; Halbertsma *et al.*, 1976; Lennard and Stein, 1977; Stein, 1976, 1977). In an arthropod, this means that the pattern generator for locomotion resides in a chain of segmental ganglia within the ventral nerve cord (Wilson, 1961; Ikeda and Wiersma, 1964; Stein, 1971). It is desirable to subdivide the pattern generator into functional components. In both the arthropods and vertebrates, each limb is innervated by a specific portion of the nerve cord. In a tetrapod vertebrate, the lumbosacral enlargement innervates the hindlimbs and the cervical enlargement innervates the forelimbs. In an arthropod, each segmental ganglion innervates a pair of limbs. For organisms in both phyla, an isolated enlargement (Grillner and Zangger, 1974) or an isolated segmental ganglion (Ikeda and Wiersma, 1964) can produce the locomotory rhythm in the pair of limbs innervated by the local region. In most cases, it is technically difficult to bisect the nerve cord in order to show that a hemienlargement or a hemiganglion can produce the locomotory rhythm to one limb in the absence of its mirror image portion of the CNS. There is strong evidence, however, that the left and right limbs can move at different frequencies and therefore have separate control centers (Hughes and Wiersma, 1960b; Wendler, 1966; Kulagin and Shik, 1970). These data lend support to the hypothesis that the local region of the nerve cord is composed of a pair of local control centers. The properties of these local control centers will be discussed in the following section, and the neurons responsible for regulating the relative phase of the local control centers will be discussed in a subsequent section.

The Local Control Center

Each local control center has the capacity to generate the locomotory rhythm for a single limb. This rhythm can be produced in the absence of not only sensory input but also input from other local control centers and the rest of the CNS. Experiments from many organisms support this point of view (cat: Brown, 1911, 1914; Grillner and Zangger, 1974; Edgerton et al., 1976; cockroach: Pearson and Iles, 1970; Pearson, 1972; crayfish: Ikeda and Wiersma, 1964; dogfish: Grillner, 1974; Grillner and Kashin, 1976; locust: Wilson, 1961; *Tritonia*: Dorsett et al., 1969, 1973; Willows, 1976).

Further analysis of the local control center requires a more specific description of the locomotory rhythm. From the point of view of the neural output during locomotion, the discharge of a single MN to a leg muscle is rhythmic, with a burst frequency equal to the frequency of the limb movement. Each MN is coactivated with a set of other MNs. This set of MNs innervates a group of muscles which act synergically during locomotion. Each MN is a member of a synergic class.

In some nonlocomotory behaviors, e.g., the neural control of heart muscle in crustaceans (Hagiwara, 1961) and the neural control of respiration in lampreys (Rovainen, 1974), there is only one synergic class. In the control of limb movements in arthropods and vertebrates, there are always at least two synergic classes of MNs active during locomotion, e.g., flexors and extensors of the cat hindlimb (Sherrington, 1910; Engberg and Lundberg, 1969; Gambarian et al., 1971; Grillner, 1975; Grillner and Zangger, 1975), power stroke and return stroke MNs of the crustacean swimmeret (Hughes and Wiersma, 1960b; Davis, 1968a,b), and elevators and depressors of the insect wing (Wilson, 1961). During locomotion, there is rhythmic alternation between the two classes of synergic MNs. There are several situations in which a limb will have more than two synergic classes activated during locomotion (newt walking: Szekeley et al., 1969; lobster walking: MacMillan, 1975; turtle swimming: Lennard, 1975; Lennard and Stein, 1977). In these animals, the locomotory rhythm consists of the serial activation of the several synergic classes.

In order to determine what mechanisms are utilized by the local control center to generate the locomotory behavior, it is desirable to identify two areas of concern: (1) the production of synergies and (2) the production of timing. The production of synergies describes the fact that MNs to specific groups of muscles are coactivated during locomotion. The production of timing describes the fact that each synergic group is activated at a given phase of the locomotory cycle. The best hypotheses currently existing suggest that local INs are responsible for the generation of synergies and timing. In order to provide experimental proof for these hypotheses, these local INs must be identified and their properties explored.

In general, the complexity of a hypothesis concerning the IN organization of the local control center varies according to the number of synergic classes present. For a behavior with only one synergic class, only one class of INs is necessary to organize the synergy. This has been well established in the case of the crustacean cardiac ganglion (Hagiwara, 1961; Hartline, 1967; Watanabe *et al.*, 1967). It is also possible that only one class of INs is necessary to organize a behavior with two synergic classes of motor output. Some members of this IN class could excite one group of MNs while other members of this IN class could inhibit the antagonistic group of MNs. Such a situation exists in the control of the feeding musculature of the snail (Kater, 1974). In the neural control of circulation in *Aplysia,* the same IN directly excites one population of MNs and directly inhibits a second population (Koester *et al.*, 1974).

In the case of locomotory behavior, there are at least two synergic classes of motor output, and it is likely that there are at least two classes of INs. In this situation, one IN class can excite one synergic class of MNs and perhaps also inhibit the second synergic class of MNs. The second IN class can excite the second synergic class of MNs and perhaps also inhibit the first synergic class of MNs. INs within a class can inhibit the INs of the other class. This type of synaptic connectivity is sufficient to explain the MN activities observed during locomotion in a limb with two synergic classes of motor output. This type of model is essentially the half-center hypothesis of Brown (1911, 1914; see also Jankowska *et al.*, 1967a,b; Lundberg, 1969; Grillner, 1975). This hypothesis was also favored by Wilson (1968a; Wilson and Waldron, 1968) as the best explanation of the locust flight system. Experimental support for these hypotheses has been obtained in many systems with the use of microelectrode techniques, e.g., cat (Jankowska *et al.*, 1967a,b; Jankowska and Roberts, 1972; Feldman and Orlovsky, 1975; Grillner, 1975; Edgerton *et al.*, 1976), cockroach (Pearson and Fourtner, 1975; Fourtner, 1976; Pearson, this volume), locust (Burrows, 1973c, 1976, and this volume; Hoyle and Burrows, 1973b; Burrows and Horridge, 1974), and *Tritonia* (Willows *et al.*, 1973a,b; Willows, 1976).

For locomotory behavior with more than two synergic classes of motor output, it is likely that there are more than two classes of INs in the local control center. In this situation, there can be one class of INs exciting each synergic class of MNs. As before, the INs in one class may also inhibit MNs of the other synergic classes. Moreover, as before, INs within a class can excite each other and an IN in one class can inhibit INs in other classes. Such a model has been termed the "ring hypothesis" (Kling and Szekeley, 1968; Szekeley, 1968). It will be important to obtain IN recordings to provide support for the validity of this hypothesis.

Therefore, at the present time the best hypotheses for understanding the production of the limb motor synergies require networks of INs characterized by excitation within a class and inhibition between classes. Such a network can also explain the production of timing. Many workers have noted that if certain parameters of the interaction are properly adjusted, then rhythmic oscillation can be produced by model neurons displaying this connectivity pattern (Wilson, 1966a; Kling and Szekeley, 1968; Wilson and Waldron, 1968; Perkel and Mulloney, 1974). In contrast, it is known that networks of neurons can produce rhythmic oscillations in the absence of synaptic inhibition (Getting, 1974; Getting and Willows, 1974; Kater, 1974). Moreover, it is well known that single neurons can produce rhythmic oscillations in the absence of both action potentials and synaptic interactions (Alving, 1968; Strumwasser, 1968; Junge and Stephans, 1973; Barker and Gainer, 1975). There are sets of experimental manipulations which can be used to distinguish between oscillations produced by networks and oscillations produced by a membrane specialization of a single neuron (Selverston, 1974, 1976, and this volume). In the control of the pyloric rhythm of the lobster stomach musculature, it may well be that both network oscillation properties and single-cell oscillation properties are working to reinforce each other. Each mechanism might be able to produce the rhythm in the absence of the other (Maynard, 1972; Selverston, 1974, 1976; Warshaw and Hartline, 1976), but the mechanisms working in concert may in fact produce a more reliable rhythm.

It is likely that future recordings of the activity of INs in the local control center will yield further insight into the control of locomotion. One very exciting principle which is currently emerging is that certain INs in the local control center might function without action potentials. Evidence for such activity has been obtained in the neurons responsible for respiratory control of crustaceans (Mendelson, 1971) and walking of insects (Pearson et al., 1973; Pearson and Fourtner, 1975; Fourtner, 1976; Pearson, this volume). It will be important to examine other local control centers with intracellular recording techniques to determine the extent to which such cells exist in other locomotory pattern generators.

In summary, the IN composition of the local control center is understood only in the most primitive manner in both the arthropods and the vertebrates. It is clear that much productive research in the next few years can be directed toward an understanding of these control centers. It is important to note that the locomotory pattern generator consists of a set of local control centers. Since each center generates its own rhythm, it is important to examine the INs responsible for coordinating the relative phase among these centers.

The Coordinating Neuron

The term "coordinating neuron" was defined (Stein, 1971) as an IN which serves to regulate interlimb phase during locomotion. Such an IN must exist in all limbed organisms with separate control centers for each limb. This follows from the observation that each local center can generate its own timing cues. The approximate frequency of each limb center is regulated by the impulse frequency of the locomotory command neurons, but this command neuron control is not sufficient to produce a situation in which there is frequency equality and regulated phase among the local control centers (Stein, 1971, 1974, 1976). This is because gate command neurons are active at a frequency (e.g., 30 Hz) which is different from the frequency of movement (e.g., 1 Hz) and because there is no fixed timing relationship between a command neuron impulse and any particular phase of the movement.

Since interlimb phase is regulated, then the control center to one limb must be informed about the state of the control centers for other limbs. In the crayfish swimmeret system, a neural copy of the motor discharge to one limb, the coordinating neuron discharge, is sent via the interganglionic connectives to other limb control centers (Stein, 1971, 1974, 1976). This central intersegmental discharge can produce a shift in the timing of the next output cycle of the other centers. This phase modulation of one control center by information originating in other control centers can account for the regulation of phase during the metachronal beat. For further details concerning interlimb regulation, see Pearson and Iles (1973), Miller and van der Burg (1973), Stein (1974, 1976), and Halbertsma et al. (1976). It is likely that coordinating neurons are utilized by a wide variety of animals. It will be interesting to see further experimental studies in order to discern which characteristics of swimmeret coordinating neurons are shared by functionally similar cells in other species.

Summary of Part I

There is now considerable evidence that the "command neuron–local control center–coordinating neuron" formulation is a useful "model" of the central component of the neural network responsible for locomotion in some multilimbed organisms. A model is useful if predictions resulting from the formulation can be verified. It is now appropriate to probe further to determine if the details of the synaptic connections predicted by the model do in fact exist when examined in a wide variety of organisms.

The "Peripheral Feedback" Component

It is now well established that the basic locomotory rhythm can be produced without the assistance of sensory feedback. It is also clear that sensory feedback has many significant influences on the central portion of the locomotory pattern generator. In particular, any information about the organism and its relationship to the environment which is not coded in genetic information must be communicated by sensory channels to the CNS (Wilson, 1972). That information can then be utilized by the organism to produce a locomotory output which is adaptive for the current conditions. From this point of view, if an animal can utilize sensory input to modify locomotory behavior so that locomotion is appropriate under many conditions, then that organism will have a greater probability of survival under changing environmental conditions than an animal with little ability to modify its locomotory behavior. The sensory modifications of locomotion are therefore essential to any consideration of the "fitness" of an organism in response to the pressures of natural selection.

There are many different ways in which sensory input can affect locomotory behavior. The animal can use sensory input to assist in the determination of whether or not locomotion is appropriate at any given time. If the organism decides that locomotion is appropriate, then sensory information can guide the CNS in determining which modality, direction, and speed of locomotion are best suited for the current situation. There may be situations where visual guidance of the limbs is critical for adaptive behavior, e.g., if a man is stepping over rocks randomly located in a stream. This situation would require cerebral centers to provide a very strong override of the spinal centers. This chapter will not discuss these extremely important control situations, but instead will concentrate on the sensory modulations of ongoing locomotion over a comparatively uniform substrate or within a buoyant medium without major turbulence.

Under these more narrowly defined conditions, there are two major modifications of locomotory behavior which are performed by sensory-derived information, an amplitude modulation (AM) and a phase modulation (PM). An amplitude modulation of a limb consists of a change in limb position or limb force without a change in the timing of the limb's movement. A phase modulation of a limb consists of a permanent change in the timing of the limb's movement. During phase modulation, there might be a concomitant amplitude modulation, but AM is defined to exclude any PM. It is reasonable to assume that the neural circuitry underlying AM is different than that responsible for PM. In particular, direct excitation of MNs which bypasses local control center INs can, in theory, produce an AM. On the other hand, synaptic input to local control center INs is necessary for the production of a PM. The experimental evidence for the existence of both AM and PM during locomotion will be discussed in the following two sections.

Amplitude Modulation

There are reflexes which can change the amplitude and direction of a limb's movement during locomotion but which do not shift the phase of the movement within the locomotory cycle. There are many different ways to measure amplitude, e.g., position of the limb, angle of a joint, or force produced by a muscle. The neural correlates of such changes can be a change in the impulse frequencies of active MNs, a change in the number of active MNs, or both.

Amplitude modulation can be observed when an animal attempts to maintain an upright position and progress in a straight line during locomotion. Some of the most important AM systems have been described in the arthropods. In the flight system of the locust, Goodman (1965) and Wilson (1968b) demonstrated that a dorsal light reaction could produce stability in the roll plane. This stability was produced by modulating the relative lift produced by the wings on either side of the body. If the animal was rolling to one side, then the lift produced by the wing on that side must be increased to stablize the body orientation in space. Wilson (1968b) demonstrated that this was accomplished by increasing the number of MN impulses on one side. The dorsal light reaction provided the feedback cue necessary to drive the appropriate balance of motor output. Wilson noted that many animals had an inherent "bias"; i.e., in the dark they would consistently roll to one side. The possible causes of the bias might be either genetic, maldevelopmental, or caused by injury to body muscles. No matter what the cause, the AM is adaptive if it can produce a correction so that the animal flies in a straight line.

A similar AM occurs for the control in the yaw plane during locust flight (Camhi, 1970a, 1971, 1976). In this case, the detectors are wind-sensitive hairs on the head and the effectors are abdominal movements. These movements act as a rudder to correct deviations in the yaw plane (see Cahmi, 1976, for a general discussion of AM).

Another AM of importance has been demonstrated in the swimmeret system in the lobster (Davis, 1968c, 1969). In this preparation, if the lobster is rolled about its longitudinal axis the swimmerets change the vector direction of their power stroke. The force generated by the change in direction will tend to counter the imposed movement. The net result is an organism which tends to remain upright. Davis demonstrated that the statocysts were the detectors and the power stroke muscles of the swimmerets were the effectors. In particular, muscle 13, a lateral power stroke muscle, is not activated when the animal is upright, but when a roll is imposed the lateral power stroke muscle is coactivated along with the main power stroke muscles. This has the behavioral effect of producing a laterally directed power stroke with the proper vector force for producing the correction. These systems are elegant examples of AM. It is important to note that there is little known about the synaptic pathways mediating these very important reflexes.

Similarly, in the vertebrate literature, there are examples of AM of a locomotory rhythm. The best-studied case is that by Orlovsky (1972) on AM by bulbospinal pathways in the mesencephalic cat preparation. Both the lateral vestibular nucleus and the red nucleus contain cells whose axons project to the spinal cord (Brodal, 1969). Stimulation of the red nucleus in a nonlocomoting cat produces limb flexion; stimulation of the lateral vestibular nucleus in such a cat produces limb extension. If these brain stem nuclei are stimulated while the hindlimb is displaying a locomotory rhythm, only the amplitude of muscle activity is altered; the timing of the step cycle is unchanged (Orlovsky, 1972). Stimulation of the red nucleus during flexion enhances the flexor electromyogram (EMG); stimulation during extension has little effect. Similarly, stimulation of the lateral vestibular nucleus during extension produces an enhanced extensor EMG; stimulation during flexion has little effect. The full adaptive significance of this circuitry is not yet known. It is likely, however, that the AM produces adaptive changes in locomotor output.

It has been demonstrated that AM can assist in the control of body orientation during locomotion. It will be extremely important to explore more cases of AM in order to elucidate the general characteristics of this method of control.

Phase Modulation

PMs act within the CNS to alter the timing of the locomotory rhythm produced by an individual local control center. One task in which PMs can play an important role is equal distribution of load among the several appendages during overground locomotion. Such PMs become critical when the animal is moving over uneven terrain or when one or more legs of the animal are injured and unable to produce their normal share of force.

The major work on PMs by sensory input during locomotion has been performed by Pearson and his co-workers in the cockroach (Pearson and Iles, 1973; Pearson et al., 1973, 1976; Pearson and Duysens, 1976; Wong and Pearson, 1976) and in the cat (Duysens and Pearson, 1976a,b; Pearson and Duysens, 1976). These experiments examined animals which were producing walking movements. Sensory structures which are activated during natural locomotion were found and selectively stimulated. In some situations, a PM was obtained.

Pearson and co-workers examined the situations in which the impulse frequency of these sensory structures could be altered during locomotion. From these experiments, they were able to infer that some of the sensory cells can measure the load on a limb during locomotion. They reasoned that during terrestrial locomotion it is maladaptive for a limb to lift off the ground unless the load on the limb is very small. Such a minimization of load on a single limb will occur when several other limbs have touched down and can therefore support the animal when the limb with very small load on it is lifted off.

The neural circuitry which can effect this behavior is straightforward. If the load detector for a single limb senses that there is still a load on the limb, the INs in the local control center active during lift-off are inhibited. These INs are termed the "swing generator" since they drive the motor output active during the flexion (swing) phase of the step cycle. Since the INs in the swing generator are part of the timing circuit of the local control center, inhibition of those INs will cause a phase modulation in the timing of the local control center. Pearson and co-workers were able to demonstrate that the load detectors inhibit the activation of the swing generator (Pearson and Iles, 1973; Duysens and Pearson, 1976a; Pearson and Duysens, 1976).

A more complex form of PM has been demonstrated during walking in chronic spinal cats (Forssberg et al., 1975, 1976). In this situation if cutaneous stimulation is applied to the dorsum of the foot during the late extension phase of walking, then the extension is enhanced but its duration is shorter. If the stimulus is applied during flexion, then flexion is enhanced. This type of behavior has been termed a "phase-dependent reflex reversal" since the muscle which is reflexly activated will be altered according to the phase of the cycle in which the stimulus is applied. This complex form of phase and amplitude modulation demonstrates the importance of examining reflex effects during an ongoing behavior.

According to the model of locomotion presented here, whenever a PM occurs to a local control center, a concomitant PM will be observed in the "copy" of local control center activity which is carried via the coordinating neurons to other centers. From this point of view, the coordinating neurons may serve not only to produce the central pattern but also to assist in the distribution of reflex information to other centers.

Summary of Part II

It is clear that sensory-derived neural information is critical for an adaptive performance of locomotory behavior. This chapter has outlined several experimental studies which demonstrate that particular classes of modulation may be utilized in specific correction tasks. Much work needs to be done before an adequate understanding of this very important area is achieved.

Conclusions

This chapter has summarized a set of principles which can serve as working hypotheses in the study of the neural control of locomotion. In each section, the support for these hypotheses from both arthropod and vertebrate material was presented. The viewpoint is that the similarities among such diverse organisms as the crayfish, the cockroach, and the cat may be more important for the basic understanding of the biological control of locomotory behavior than are the differences among these species.

ACKNOWLEDGMENTS

The author was supported by NSF Grant BNS 75-18040 during the writing of this chapter.

Part 2

Roles of Interneurons in Behavior

14

Circumesophageal Interneurons and Behavior in Crayfish

James L. Larimer and William H. Gordon

Introduction

The intent of this chapter is to focus attention on the special role of circumesophageal interneurons (INs) in the mediation of behavior in crustaceans. In addition to summarizing our current knowledge of several classes of neural elements in these connectives, we will note the advantages and disadvantages of this segment for study. Finally, we will set forth a plan of further experimentation with the aim of gaining more direct information on the role of circumesophageal connective fibers (CECs) that underlie certain behaviors. We have selected for study not only behaviors which are reliably under environmental control but also those known to have putative underlying commands. The final step, which has not yet been completely achieved, is to obtain direct recording access to both the selected behavior and the neural activity and, by using several experimental methods, to correlate the two in an effort to define their causal relationships.

Neural Processes Comprising the Circumesophageal Connectives

Each CEC of crayfish contains approximately 3200 axons (Sutherland and Nunnemacher, 1968). Even though this is only two-thirds the number of processes composing the connectives between abdominal ganglia, the CECs lie between the two largest ganglia in the CNS, i.e., the cerebral and the subesophageal. In selecting a segment of the CNS for study, the CECs would thus appear to offer both a strategic and a numerical advantage. Other obvious advantages of the CECs include the fact that they are relatively long, readily accessible, and overlain on the ventral side by a hard, flat carapace which provides a convenient anchoring site for chronic electrode implantation. Unlike the abdominal connectives, they do not move about during activity, further stabilizing them for long-term recording or stimulation.

James L. Larimer and William H. Gordon • Department of Zoology, University of Texas, Austin, Texas 78712.

Perhaps the leading advantage of this segment of the CNS is the substantial amount of data available on the functions and locations of units within the CECs. Wiersma and his colleagues have provided extensive documentation on the primary sensory units and higher sensory INs that occur throughout the connectives of crayfish (Wiersma, 1961b; Horridge, 1968). Some 131 of these sensory elements have been characterized in the CECs alone (Wiersma, 1958; Wiersma and Mill, 1965), and about half are known to carry ascending, as opposed to descending, traffic. Such data are of great value when attempting to characterize the neural activity from chronic recordings in the CECs (see below).

Another class of neural elements, the command INs or premotor INs (Wiersma and Ikeda, 1964), are also prominent components of the circumesophageal connectives (Wiersma, 1961b; Atwood and Wiersma, 1967; Bowerman and Larimer, 1974a,b). Studies over the past decade have identified a large number of command neurons at all levels of the CNS of crustaceans. Stimulation of these neurons has resulted in the generation of an extensive catalog of behaviors ranging in complexity from simple movements to complete cyclical motor programs. As a result of such studies, the term "command fiber" has come to mean almost any premotor IN which provides a defined, reproducible motor output (Larimer, 1976). We still know little about the neural structure of command neurons or about their role in coordinating normal behaviors. Thus the term "command neuron" is currently considered to be simply a useful concept but one which will undoubtedly be defined more precisely as new information is obtained. Since our aim is, in part, to specify more directly their roles in behavior, certain of the known CEC command neurons will be described in more detail in the following section.

Finally, major behavioral modifications have long been known to result when one or both of the circumesophageal connectives are severed (Bethe, 1897a; Minkiewicz, 1907; ten Cate, 1930; Schöne, 1961), indicating their importance in coordinating the CNS centers. More recent studies have emphasized the role of CEC units in evoking swimming and escape behavior (Larimer et al., 1971; Wine and Krasne, 1972; Krasne and Wine, 1975; Schrameck, 1970) and abdominal extension behavior (Page, 1975) and in mediating various forms of locomotion, particularly those controlled by environmental light changes (Camougis, 1960, 1964; Page and Larimer, 1972, 1975b; Gordon and Larimer, 1975; Gordon et al., 1977).

We will summarize below the characteristics of some environmentally controlled behaviors and their possible neural substrates in the CECs. This background will serve to introduce our current experimental approach to the correlation of neural activity and behavior.

Behaviors Evoked by Environmental Light Regimen: Reflexive and Circadian Locomotion Requiring the CECs

We have examined two behavioral systems whose outputs occur below the brain: general locomotion and heart rate. Both of these exhibit two daily peaks of activity in individuals exposed to an environmental light cycle of 12:12 (L:D) (110 lux), one occurring at dawn (lights-on), the other at dusk (lights-off). At lights-on, both locomotion and heart rate increase with little delay of behavioral onset, and the elevated activity persists for about 1 hr. The dark phase of activity tends to increase gradually after the onset of darkness and typically persists for several hours (Page and Larimer 1972, 1975a; Pollard and Larimer, 1977).

Other experiments have shown that only the lights-off peak is circadian. Under conditions of DD, for example, the dawn peak of activity disappears, while the lights-off peak does not just persist but free-runs with a period other than 24 hr (Fig. 1). Similar data are also typical of heart rate (Pollard and Larimer, 1977). A second criterion of a circadian system (Pittendrigh, 1960) is also exhibited only by the lights-off peak, and that is the presence of transients during re-entrainment (Fig. 2). It should be noted that free-run data for both general locomotory activity and heart rate are poor and unreliable, but nevertheless are detectable in the records of some individuals. Several results suggest that the peak activity seen at lights-on is reflexive in nature and that it is driven by a retinal input. Figure 3 shows, for example, that in the presence of a light–dark regimen the lights-on peak disappears when the ommatidia are surgically removed, while the circadian peak persists.

An additional property of the rhythms in both locomotion and heart rate is entrainment by extraretinal photoreceptors (Fig. 3), presumably located within the brain (Page and Larimer, 1972, 1975b, 1976). It should be noted that we do not actually know whether retinal input participates in entrainment in intact animals, only that it is apparently not necessary. Finally, the caudal photoreceptor, the best-known CNS photoreceptor in any arthropod (Prosser, 1934; Kennedy, 1963; Larimer et al., 1966; Wilkens and Larimer, 1972, 1976), apparently does not function in entrainment in these animals (Page and Larimer, 1972) (Fig. 3).

A more important finding in the present context is that the brain and optic lobes are required for the expression of the peaks of locomotory activity and heart rate (Page and Larimer, 1975a; Pollard and Larimer, 1977). In addition, the circumesophageal connectives carry the timing information for the circadian outputs and the corresponding triggering information for the reflexive lights-on responses. Thus severing of both the CECs (Fig. 4) abolishes both the lights-on and lights-off peaks of locomotory activity and of heart rate (Page and Larimer 1975a; Pollard and Larimer, 1977). We have assumed that the loss of timing information was due to the interruption of the neural pathways since the hormonal system of the eyestalks were intact in these experiments. We do not know whether the relevant tracts in the CECs are conventional axons or whether they are neurosecretory; however, some additional data suggest that they are of the former type.

For example, the severing of the CECs alone resulted in an increased activity in the forelimb and a diminished activity in the hindlimb, even though both of the thoracic neural oscillators were presumably under hormonal control from the eyestalks (Fig. 4). In addition, removal of the eyestalks raised the levels of activity in both limbs substantially (Fig. 4, lower). This latter increase in activity was interpreted as the result of the removal of an inhibitory hormone. With or without the hormone, however, the movements apparently remained arrhythmic. We performed still another study in an effort to glean the direction of information transfer for

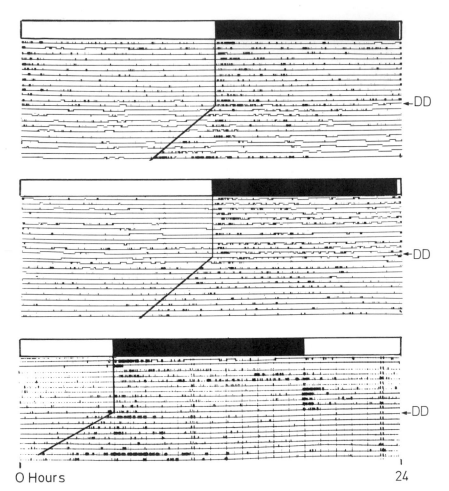

O Hours   24

Fig. 1. Three examples of the activity patterns of the crayfish *Procambarus clarkii* exposed to a light cycle of 12:12 (L:D) and to constant darkness (DD). The shaded area represents the dark portion, the unshaded are the light portion of the light cycle. There are two peaks, a short one occurring at dawn (lights-on) and a more prolonged one occurring after dark (lights-off). In DD, there is an immediate loss of the lights-on peak while the lights-off activity continues to free run. Although the free-run (lights-off) data are typically poor for this animal, its persistence and its shortened period (other than 24 hr) suggest that it is circadian. Ordinarily, this peak is undetectable after a week in total darkness. From Page and Larimer (1972).

triggering the peaks. As shown in Fig. 5, severing the connectives between the third and fourth thoracic ganglia preserved the cyclical activity toward the brain and abolished it on the caudal side of the cut. These data, too, are consistent with the hypothesis that the brain (or brain and optic lobes) contains the control center for generating the peaks of activity.

These results raise several questions regarding the number as well as the nature of the units responsible for transmitting the information along the CECs.

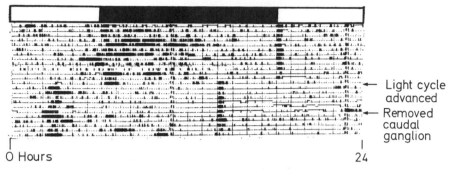

Fig. 2. An example of the continuous activity of an animal subjected to a 4 hr advance in the phase of the light cycle. The lights-on peak is advanced without transients and appears to be directly coupled to the light cycle. Removal of the photoreceptor of the sixth abdominal ganglion does not affect either peak. From Page and Larimer (1972).

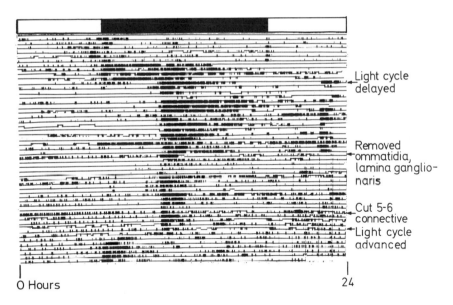

Fig. 3. An activity record of an animal undergoing two shifts in the entraining light cycle. In the first, where the animal is intact, there is some evidence of a transient in the shift of the lights-off peak, while the phase shift of the lights-on peak is not clear because of the loss of data. Removal of the retina and lamina ganglionaris immediately results in a disappearance of the dawn (lights-on) peak, while the lights-off peak persists. Again, severing of the axons of the caudal photoreceptor neurons does not appear to affect the circadian peak. Evidence for an extraretinal–extracaudal photoreceptor for entrainment is shown where the phase advance is presented to the blinded animal. Note that the shift in this case exhibits a 2-day transient before re-entrainment. From Page and Larimer (1972).

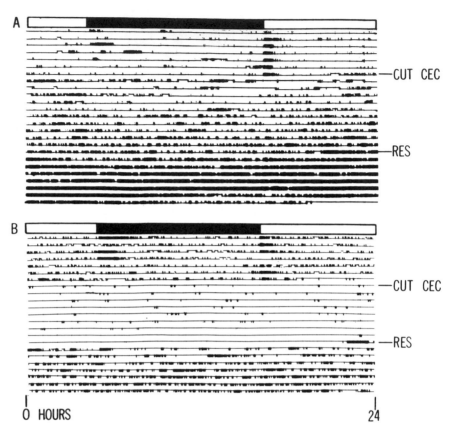

Fig. 4. Activity records taken from the right first pereiopod (A) and from the left fourth walking leg (B) while the animal was in an upside-down position. Before the circumesophageal connectives were severed (CUT CEC), both limbs showed a typical rhythm. After severing of the CEC, however, both peaks of activity were lost. In the case of the anterior appendage the total activity increased after sectioning, while the activity of the posterior appendage diminished. The increased activity in R1 may have resulted from the removal of tonic inhibition, while the decrease in L4 may represent a loss of some excitatory source. When the eyestalks are removed in addition (RES), the activity remains apparently arrhythmic; however, both limbs exhibit an increase in activity. The increased activity due to eyestalk ablation suggests the removal of a tonic inhibitory hormone. From Page and Larimer (1975a).

Premotor (Command) Fibers and Visual INs in the CECs

If we assume that the descending information that releases the lights-on/lights-off activity is neural, it is possible to suggest several types of known units that might underlie the behaviors. More immediate candidates include the locomotion-evoking units, the visually activated INs, the descending inhibitory units, and the neurosecretory elements of the cords.

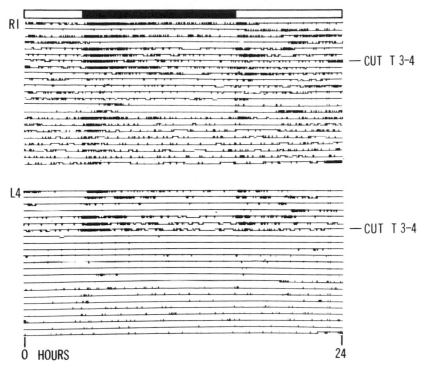

Fig. 5. Activity recorded from first and fourth pereiopods as in Fig. 4. In this case, the ventral nerve cords were severed between the two limbs (between the third and fourth thoracic ganglia). The two peaks of activity are retained only anterior to the cut. From Page and Larimer (1975a).

The INs that release locomotory behavior on stimulation of their descending axons include at least nine entities, five of which evoke forward walking and four of which evoke backward walking (Bowerman and Larimer, 1974b) (Fig. 6). This list is probably not exhaustive and does not include numerous fibers which when activated evoke noncyclical limb and body movements or other motions of various sorts (Atwood and Wiersma, 1967; Bowerman and Larimer, 1974a).

Since the effective stimulus for the reflexive lights-on response is via the retina, visual units might carry the trigger directly to the locomotory centers. There is a variable delay, however, between environmental light onset and the beginning of locomotion, which can be as long as 3–4 min. If visual units are responsible, any neural mechanism to account for this delay must be localized in the lower ganglia, since known, visually activated neurons in the CECs respond within a few seconds. These cautions aside, there are numerous visual INs present in the CECs (Wiersma and Mill, 1965; Camougis and Kasprzak, 1966).

We have considered descending inhibitory fibers as a possible triggering source because not only are such units known (Bowerman and Larimer, 1974a) but also a release from inhibition is seen in the activity of animals following sectioning

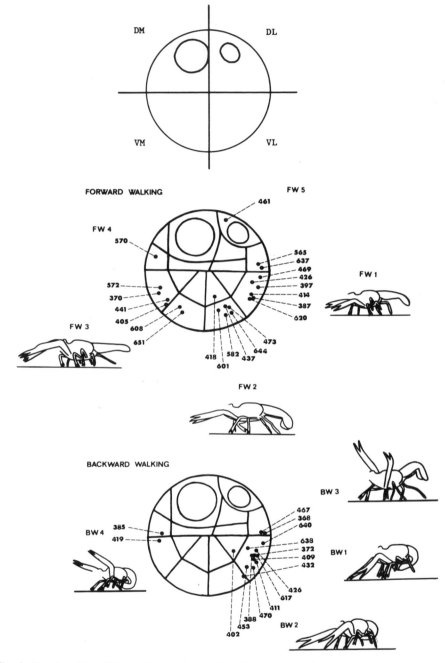

Fig. 6. Top: Locations of the surgical quadrants of the circumesophageal connectives that were assayed individually for the expression of reflexive (lights-on) and circadian (lights-off) behaviors. All quadrants with the exception of the dorsomedial (DM) were capable of mediating one, or almost always both, behaviors. Middle and bottom: Cord locations for known walk-evoking units in the circumesophageal connectives. There is a suggestive correlation between the map locations and the effective quadrants. Modified from Bowerman and Larimer (1974*b*).

of the CEC (see Fig. 4). Our knowledge of this type of unit is meager, however, and as a result map locations are not useful to guide future experiments.

Unfortunately, almost no information is available on the number of map locations or the function of neurosecretory tracts in the CECs of crayfish, although it is agreed that they do exist (Welsh, 1961; Bern and Hagedorn, 1965).

Since map locations are available, at least for the locomotion-evoking neurons and the visually activated cells, we have attempted to better localize those tracts in the connectives which carry the lights-on and circadian information with the aim of comparing their positions and distributions with those of the identified neurons.

Location of Coupling/Triggering Tracts in the CECs: Their Relationship to Command and Visual Fibers

In an effort to determine more precisely the number and location of the responsible units, we have cut one connective completely and then severed the fibers of the other connective except for one quadrant. Animals were therefore prepared with only the dorsomedial, dorsolateral, ventromedial, or ventrolateral fourths of the single connective remaining (see Fig. 6, top). Each was exposed to a light cycle of L:D (12:12) and assayed for the two locomotory behaviors. A total of 66 animals were assayed in the series, and the connective was examined histologically to verify the position of the connecting tract after each assay (Gordon and Larimer, 1975; Gordon et al., 1977). The data clearly show that coupling/triggering elements are widely distributed in the connective except for the dorsomedial quadrant. Specifically, out of 15 individuals with only a dorsomedial quadrant remaining, none exhibited either a circadian or lights-on peak; however, from 69% to 95% of the animals retaining one of the remaining quadrants exhibited one peak or, more often, both peaks. In fact, in 93% of the cases where one of the peaks appeared, the other one was also present. The data suggest that the coupling/triggering elements may actually be redundant, as well as widely distributed throughout three-fourths of the cord, since our total activity assays were indistinguishable for animals retaining different quadrants. In addition, since the two peaks of activity were seen either to appear or to disappear together, we believe that the elements responsible for mediating the two behaviors are either codistributed in the three quadrants or that they are in fact the same INs (Gordon and Larimer, 1975; Gordon et al., 1977).

A comparison of the map locations for locomotion-evoking neurons (Bowerman and Larimer, 1974b, 1976; Larimer, 1976) with the three quadrants which carry locomotory-timing and reflexive-trigger neurons revealed some positive correlations. Specifically, the dorsomedial quadrant, which fails to sustain the activity peaks, is almost devoid of known walk-evoking commands, while the effective quadrants all contain several (Fig. 6). The distribution of visual and related multimodal INs is not well correlated with the quadrants mediating the behavior since the ineffective dorsomedial quadrant, as well as the others, contains several identified visual INs.

Correlation of Descending Neural Activity with Behavior

Although the correlation between the location of walk-evoking neurons and the effective quadrants for mediating light-stimulated and circadian activity is suggestive, there is a need for more direct evidence. It would also be desirable to examine other sensory and premotor activity occurring in the freely behaving animals. We have proceeded in this direction by combining long-term neural recording techniques with methods which permit simultaneous documentation of behaviors.

Certain observations and assumptions helped to direct our experimental approach to the problem. First, of the 3200 axons comprising the individual circumesophageal connectives (Sutherland and Nunnemacher, 1968), it is estimated that approximately half, at least of the sensory classes, carry ascending activity (Wiersma and Mill, 1965). For the present purposes, however, we are more in-interested in descending units. Since the CNS neurons in crayfish do not degenerate or regenerate rapidly (Bittner *et al.*, 1974), we have the option of severing a connective and selectively recording descending activity from electrodes implanted rostral to the cut. Neural activity in such preparations is reduced as predicted, and the lower level of activity greatly simplifies the sorting and classification of recorded units.

Second, if only one of the connectives is severed, this leaves the remaining one to mediate any brain-directed behaviors to lower levels. If one further assumes that the two connectives are neurally equivalent and that one is sufficient for the transmission of at least some behaviors, this arrangement not only allows descending units to be classified but also permits a correlation of neural and behavioral activity.

Third, as described above, we have examined three behaviors which require the CECs for expression: reflexive and circadian locomotion and fluctuations of heart rate. We have, for several reasons, selected locomotion for this phase of the study. It is not only an important and easily assayable behavior, but also its known commands are fewer than those for modifying heart rate (Field and Larimer, 1975) and appear to be located in the coupling/triggering areas of the connectives. All these fluctuations are under environmental control in the sense that they can be locked to a programmed light–dark cycle. This feature also allows behavioral and neural data to be recorded continuously or sampled only during the phase of the lighting regimen in which activity is occurring.

Experimental Approach

Access to the CECs was made from the ventral side via a small opening in the labrum. One of the connectives was anchored by passing a lacquer-coated stainless steel pin through the cephalothorax. The secured connective was severed caudal to the anchoring pin and a window of cellulose acetate was fitted over the opening, allowing the connective to be viewed for electrode implantation. The chronic recording procedure utilized a bundle of three 25-μm teflon-coated wires or one or more electrolytically sharpened and lacquer-coated stainless steel electrodes.

Animals implanted in this manner were glued to a rigid rod and suspended over a low-mass, low-friction walking wheel in a water bath (Bowerman and Larimer, 1974*a,b;* Page and Larimer, 1975*a;* Field and Larimer, 1975). The axle of the walking wheel extended approximately 15 cm above the water and was fitted at the top with a continuous potentiometer which served as the upper bearing. The continuous potentiometer was incorporated into the circuit of a voltage-controlled oscillator (VCO) in such a manner that forward walking generated an increasing voltage while backward walking gave a decreasing voltage at the VCO. The oscillator thus provided an increasing frequency ramp within the audio range that indicated forward walking and a decreasing frequency to signal backward walking. With this scheme, not only could wheel movement be encoded on an audio tape recorder but also a preliminary correlation of spike data and walking could be made with an oscilloscope and audio monitor before the animal was placed on a light cycle.

The animal and walking wheel chamber were placed inside a larger light-tight box supplied with a shielded 20 W tungsten stimulating/entraining lamp. The lamp as well as various peripheral recording devices were under the control of a programmable clock.

It is possible to devise a number of experimental programs using these combined behavioral and neural recording techniques. However, we have thus far utilized only the lights-on behavior and selected descending recording leads. Here the experiments were designed to generate multiple samples of locomotory activity by optimizing the conditions for releasing reflexive (lights-on) walking. The environmental lighting regimen consisted of repeated cycles of 15 min of light (120 lux) interrupted by 105 min of darkness, with the neural and behavioral data taken in the light phase. This procedure reliably generates dozens of bouts of walking, providing an ample opportunity to correlate the neural and behavioral data (Fig. 7). Figures 7A gives an example of a continuous-event recorder output for 24 bouts of

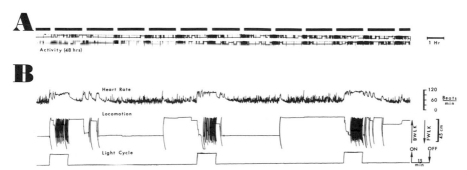

Fig. 7. A: Total activity obtained from an animal suspended over a walking wheel. The switch closures were continuously recorded on an event recorder for 48 hr. The animal was exposed to a light regimen of 15 min of light and 1 hr 45 min of darkness (see upper scale), generating 24 bouts of activity (lights-on or reflexive). B: Heart rate and locomotory data are shown for an animal exposed to the same light cycle as in A. Here the heart rate is taken from the EKG and recorded as cardiotachometer output. The locomotory activity was obtained from the voltage-controlled oscillator output from the walking wheel (see text). The oscillator output contains information about both the direction and the speed of locomotion.

walking in a 48-hr period. Figure 7B shows the effect of three illumination cycles on the heart rate and locomotion. Note that the direction, speed, and distance traveled can be obtained from the VCO output. In this case, the animal began each bout by walking in a forward direction. However, this was not always the case. Finally, there is, as expected, a very strong correlation between heart rate and locomotion regardless of whether they are being driven by the light cycle.

This procedure, combined with neural recording from the three effective quadrants, has been used as a screening procedure for activity associated with locomotion. Future experiments will utilize a lighting regimen which should reveal locomotion associated with the circadian as well as the reflexive peaks in order to help resolve whether the neurons which trigger lights-on walking are the same as or different from those timing the release of circadian locomotion and to further characterize the neuronal firing patterns.

In order to interpret the correlations, a difficult task at best, it was necessary to identify the primary sensory fibers and lower-order sensory INs in each lead. When this was accomplished, these units were eliminated from correlation analysis by windowing, and the units of interest were recorded either as amplitude histograms or as frequency graphs along with the locomotory data. We have searched for neurons whose activities preceded as well as accompanied the behaviors, since this type of correlation signature might be expected for the triggering or timing units. A procedure similar to this has been successful in revealing putative command fiber activity associated with forward walking in the lobster (Davis, 1976). Our technique has thus far utilized only recording techniques using large electrodes.

Among approximately a dozen preparations that have been studied thus far, a surprising number appeared on first examination to have units correlated with locomotion, i.e., units whose activity faithfully preceded the onset of locomotory activity and accompanied it. On careful examination, however, most correlations were believed to be spurious, or false in the sense that the accompanying neural activity arose from known sensory activity. For example, all of the following can coincide with locomotion: activity originating from tactile hairs on the cephalothorax, from contact between the dactylopodites and the walking surface, from joint receptors and head appendages as well as sensory activity ascending via the intact connective through the brain to the recording site on the severed connective. In some instances, however, neural activity appeared to fit some of the correlation criteria for a trigger source.

The records presented in Fig. 8 were selected more for the purpose of demonstrating the method of analyses currently in use than to suggest that the units represent underlying commands. The recording was taken from a chronically implanted electrode in the ventrolateral quadrant (see G, Fig. 8). Sensory mapping identified the two largest neurons (A,a) as responsive to vibration, while the remaining were responsive to both light and touch (see F, Fig. 8). Thus all were sensory INs of various complexities. Utilizing a window discriminator, three amplitudes of activity (A,B,C) were selected according to the three major peaks of an amplitude histogram of the data (E) and compared with the corresponding segment of

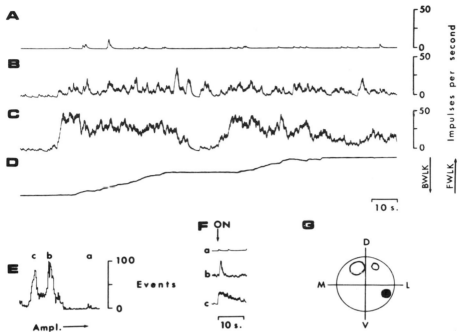

Fig. 8. Records demonstrating the methods of correlating neural and behavioral activity. A window discriminator was used to select three impulse amplitudes (A,B,C and a,b,c) for comparison with the locomotory data (D). The neural data (A,B,C) are expressed as frequencies, while the locomotory data (D) indicate wheel position from which walking direction and velocity may be obtained. The amplitude histogram (E), constructed from the same data as A,B,C, shows three major peaks (a,b,c) that were selected for correlation. The lead, however, contained activity from an estimated six neurons. The location of the recording site within the CEC is shown in diagram G. Neurons (b) and (c) responded to the onset of illumination (F). In this case, the animal, which was in the light, walked forward, paused, then continued. Activity in both neurons B and C preceded the onset of the behavior and generally accompanied it. We do not know, however, if the activity in these neurons was actually responsible for transmitting the excitation which triggered locomotion (see text).

locomotory activity. It is apparent that units B and C appear to precede locomotion as well as accompany it. We do not know, however, whether or not there is a causal relationship between the two. In fact, much more rigorous analysis as well as additional data must be obtained before a correlation can be made. In the concluding section, we have examined some of the information which must be taken into account in making a thorough analysis of neural activity that might underlie behavior.

Concluding Observations

Although the methods employed thus far reveal interesting correlations between behavior and activity in the CECs, there are numerous difficulties in interpret-

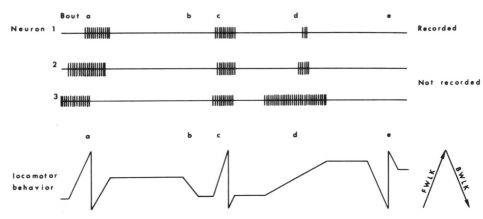

Fig. 9. A hypothetical system in which three commands might cooperate to evoke forward walking. Recording access is available for only one neuron, and its activity is to be correlated with locomotory data. It is assumed that the neuron under observation is at times recruited after the others. It is also assumed that the frequency of neural activity can be compared with the velocity of movement, that the occurrence of activity in the neuron can be correlated with direction of locomotion, and that the timing of neural firing can be compared with the onset and course of behavior. In the example given, the frequency and direction criteria are met satisfactorily; however, only in walking bout (c) is the timing proper.

ing the data. Several refinements in methodology must be introduced to overcome these difficulties, and additional precautions must be recognized in performing such experiments in general.

Considerable evidence points to the presence of several related but unique "command" neurons for eliciting each class of behavior. For example, some five excitors and three inhibitors were located which influence the swimmeret system of crayfish (Wiersma and Ikeda, 1964), perhaps 20 units cause abdominal flexion or extension (Evoy and Kennedy, 1967), at least four units evoke swimming and escape (exclusive of the giant fibers), and, as noted above, at least nine units can cause either forward or backward walking (Bowerman and Larimer, 1974b). Although some of these units can release a complete behavior, many provide only a partial behavior. In addition, a majority of commands appear to require activation at relatively high frequencies, e.g., 50–100 Hz, to produce a movement, suggesting that several related commands might normally operate in concert to provide a complete behavior. Direct evidence for the required participation of multiple commands in securing a complete behavior has in fact been obtained for the swimmeret movements of lobsters (Davis and Kennedy, 1972a). If this were the rule, one would not always expect to obtain a complete correlation between activity in a single command (premotor IN) and the behavior it is supposed to release. Consider, for example, a model based on a hypothetical array of three locomotion-evoking INs (Fig. 9). If one attempted to correlate the time of neural activity with locomotion, it would appear correct only for bout (c) since the onset is delayed in both (a) and (d), presumably because the unit under observation is recruited late in the sequence. A clear correlation can be made between frequency of firing and velocity of locomotion in the example given. However, if patterning or other coding mechanisms were used to alter the output, this too might be misleading. In addition, activity in the unit is clearly correlated with direction, but this too might not always prevail. For example, it would be confusing if in bout (d) the unit was not recruited at all, or if a forward and backward program were initiated in rapid sequence.

In a related example, we have generally assumed that neurons whose activities might underlie a behavior are duplicated, with one in each connective. If, however, the neural record is obtained from the severed left CEC (a procedure which greatly simplifies other aspects of data analysis) while the observed behavior is evoked by elements in the intact right connective, a low correlation will result if the two INs fire at different frequencies or are recruited at slightly different times.

A number of behaviors or physiological responses are always tightly coupled, and there must be assurance that neural data are correlated with the correct one. It would be easy, for example, to misinterpret neural activity that is associated with either the regulation of heart rate or ventilation for activity underlying locomotion, since all three behaviors fluctuate together. In addition, both the heart rate (Field and Larimer, 1975) and ventilation (Wilkens *et al.*, 1974) are strongly influenced by INs in the circumesophageal connectives. Such a potential error might be avoided by monitoring the EKG simultaneously with neural and locomotory behavior and then uncoupling the behaviors by evoking specific cardiac reflexes (Larimer, 1964).

Although more conjectural, there is a possibility that activity in different INs might provide for different walking gaits. It is known that crayfish constantly shift from one gait to another in normal locomotion (Parrack, 1964). The signature of "command" activity under such conditions might be inscrutable indeed.

The experimental paradigm as outlined above also excludes the opportunity to drive the putative command by electrical stimulation. Thus rigorous proof that activity in a neuron caused a behavioral output would require working in some instances with intact connectives where stimuli could be applied. This procedure, however, is not without difficulty either, since confinement of stimulus only to the units from which recordings are made is almost impossible using extracellular techniques.

In certain cases, potentially erroneous correlations between neural and behavioral data may exist when the animal undergoes several postural adjustments in preparation for locomotion. Often the antennae are waved, the abdomen is positioned, and one or more limbs are moved before a signal for walking is obtained from the VCO. If these movements evoke sensory activity, the false impression of neural activity preceding locomotion may be obtained. Some of these difficulties could be avoided by simultaneous EMG recording from selected limb muscles or by the use of cinematography to correlate behavior and neural activity.

Although we know from the voltage requirements for direct stimulation of "command" INs that they vary in size, the more important ones might in fact belong to the smallest population of neurons. Unfortunately, the techniques used in surveying a connective for premotor neurons, i.e., bundle separation and electrical stimulation, both favor the recognition of the larger axons. In addition, although the complex commands are assumed not to be directly driven by simple sensory activation, there is not as yet enough substantiating data to make this rule firm. In short, the neurons which have been assigned a command function may in fact be descending "sensory" INs.

In summary, although each of these procedures has recognized disadvantages when used alone, they have considerable merit when applied in combination as a directed approach not only for studying the activity of INs which might initiate behavior but also for examining sensory units in behaving animals.

The strategy that emerges, then, is a statistical one in the sense that comparative data on circumesophageal INs must be carefully and repeatedly assembled from the different experimental paradigms. This strategy extends previous cord mappings by adding the important capability of recording neural activity during normal behaviors. Finally, we hope to utilize this combined approach to learn more about the mechanisms of activation, coding characteristics, and hierarchical organization of the so-called command INs.

ACKNOWLEDGMENTS

Original research reported herein was supported by NIH Grant NS-05423 (J. L. L.) and by NIH Postdoctoral Fellowship NS 00942 (W. H. G.)

15

Visual Input and Motor Output of Command Interneurons of the Defense Reflex Pathway in the Crayfish

Raymon M. Glantz

Introduction

Visual systems hold a special fascination for a large number of neurophysiologists. This is due in part to the fact that the behavior of visual interneurons (INs) "more closely resembles perception than sensation" (Lettvin *et al.*, 1959) and thus conveys the illusion that we are studying something that is very close to behavior. Some excellent illustrations of this point can be found in the studies of the optic nerve of the rock lobster by Wiersma and co-workers recently reviewed by York and Wiersma (1975).

The properties of many visual INs and particularly their trigger features often invite comparison with organismic behavior. Such comparisons, however, can at best suggest that an IN is in some manner involved in a given behavior. A major obstacle for the precise determination of the role of visual information processing in behavior is that the methods generally applied to sensory system analysis are poorly suited to the requirements of elucidating the behavioral consequences of a neuron's activity. An important exception to this limitation is provided by certain sensory–motor pathways in arthropods, such as the INs associated with the visually evoked defense reflex of the crayfish *Procambarus clarkii*. The defense reflex can be elicited by simple visual stimuli such as an approaching object. This stimulus is known to be particularly effective in activating the "medium motion detectors" observed in several crustacean optic nerves (Waterman *et al.*, 1964; Wiersma and Yanagisawa, 1971) and the "jittery motion detectors" in the crayfish optic nerve (Wiersma and Yamaguchi, 1966, 1967*a*; Glantz, 1974*b*).

An additional advantage of this system is that the defense reflex can be elicited by the activation of a single IN in the circumesophageal connectives (Wiersma, 1952*a*). This finding was confirmed and extended by Atwood and Wiersma (1967) and Bowerman and Larimer (1974*a*), who have also observed other command INs in the connectives capable of eliciting the entire defense posture or components

Raymon M. Glantz • Department of Biology, Rice University, Houston, Texas 77001.

thereof. Furthermore, Wiersma and Mill (1965) observed a large motion-sensitive visual IN in the circumesophageal connectives (C99) that occupies the same cross-sectional area of the connective (75) and may be identical to a defense reflex command unit.

The subject of this chapter is a series of studies conducted to explore some of the implications of the earlier studies by Wiersma and co-workers. Evidence is examined regarding the visual trigger features and physiological response charac-
·istics of the command INs as well as tests of the adequacy of the sensory response for the promotion of the defense reflex. The functional relationship between the optic nerve afferents and the command elements are also examined and a general scheme of the excitatory pathway for the reflex is presented.

Stimulus Requirements and Habituation of the Defense Reflex and Optic Nerve INs

The three major classes of optic nerve visual INs (Wiersma and Yamaguchi, 1966) are the sustaining fibers (SF), dimming fibers (DF), and jittery motion detectors (JMD). In each case, the class name reflects the adequate stimulus or primary trigger feature of the neuronal class. Each class is thought to consist of 14 members (Wiersma and Yamaguchi, 1966), although a few motion detectors and several of the dimming units were not observed with sufficient frequency to justify their identification by the above authors. The members of a given class have identical or very similar stimulus requirements and discharge characteristics and are located in adjacent regions of the optic nerve. The only systematic difference among the numbers of a given class is their receptive fields.

Table I qualitatively indicates the relative responsiveness of the defense reflex (DR) and each of the three IN classes to a group of simple visual stimuli.

Table I. Relative Responsiveness of Sustaining Fibers (SF), Dimming Fibers (DF), Jittery Motion Detectors (JMD), and the Defense Reflex (DR) to Several Visual Stimuli[a]

Stimulus	SF	DF	JMD	DR[b]
Transient increase in illumination	++	Inhibition	−	−
Transient decrease in illumination	Inhibition	++	+	+
Stationary contrast	++	++	−	−
Jittery target motion	+	+	++	++
Approaching target	+	+	++	++
Moving edge	++	++	+	+

[a] ++, Strong effect; +, modest or weak effect; −, very weak or no effect.
[b] Defense reflex responsiveness was measured with electrodes inserted into the levator muscles at the base of the chelipeds.

Although there is good correlation of the defense reflex and motion-detector trigger features, these comparisons cannot exclude participation by the SFs and/or DFs from the reflex pathway. Habituation studies indicate that SF and DF activities are not sufficient to elicit the reflex (Glantz, 1974a,b). Figure 1A illustrates an averaged reflex habituation curve elicited with approaching target motions repeated at 4/min. Figure 1B illustrates the averaged responsiveness of the three classes of visual INs under identical stimulus conditions. The results indicate that for repetitive stimulation the SFs and DFs exhibit approximately constant or slightly facilitated outputs, while the JMDs and the defense reflex reveal parallel declines in responsiveness.

An important feature of the reflex habituation is that it is highly specific to the retinal locus of the stimulus. Shifting the axis of target motion laterally by 5° results in at least partial recovery of reflex (Fig. 1C) and JMD (Fig. 1D) responsiveness.

The simplest interpretation of this result is that motion-detector activity is a necessary although possibly not a sufficient condition for the activation of the reflex. Furthermore, these experiments place the site of habituation at or before the input stage of the sensory INs in the reflex pathway. Similar results have been obtained for the crayfish escape reflex elicited via tactile afferents (Zucker, 1972b).

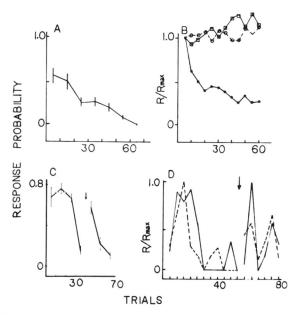

Fig. 1. A: Probability of eliciting a visually evoked defense reflex as a function of the number of successive trials ($N = 8$). B: Relative response magnitude vs. trial number, averaged for nine sustaining fibers (○), two dimming fibers (□), and 13 motion detectors (●). C: Habituation of the defense reflex and partial response recovery associated with a 5° lateral shift in the axis of stimulus motion between trials 40 and 41. D: Habituation of two motion detectors and response recovery with a 5° lateral shift of stimulus. Repetition rate was 4/min in all cases.

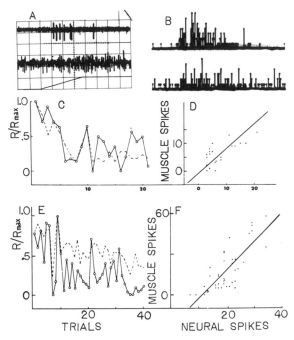

Fig. 2. A: Simultaneously monitored activity of motion unit 07 (top trace) and cheliped levator muscle (middle trace). Bottom trace indicates stimulus position vs. time. Time scale: 100 msec/div. B: Motion detector (upper) and muscle (lower) PST histograms based on 21 stimulus repetitions. Vertical calibration in first bin of each histogram: 1.0 spikes/bin. Horizontal scale: 10 msec/bin and 1.28 sec long. C,E: Habituation functions of simultaneously monitored motion detector (dashed lines) and muscle (continuous line) spike counts. D,F: Regression plots of muscle output vs. motion-detector output based on data in C and E, respectively. Correlation coefficients in D and F are 0.73 and 0.65, respectively. Continuous lines are regression functions of muscle output on nerve output. Regression slope: 0.94 in D and 2.05 in F.

Optic nerve recordings were also obtained from restrained animals which were free to move their claws in response to approaching targets. The JMD responses exhibited the expected strong correlation to cheliped levator muscle activity (Fig. 2). A similar analysis on SFs indicated that for rapidly approaching targets the SF activity consistently lagged behind the start of the reflex response, thus eliminating this class as a candidate input channel to the reflex pathway.

Examination of the defense reflex latency at various target velocities provided additional information on the input requirements of the reflex pathway (Glantz, 1974c). Figure 3A illustrates the systematic decline in the cheliped electromyogram response latencey (L) with increasing target velocities. A complete set of data for one preparation is illustrated in Fig. 3B. The continuous function represents the relationship

$$L = \frac{\Delta\theta}{d\theta/dt}$$

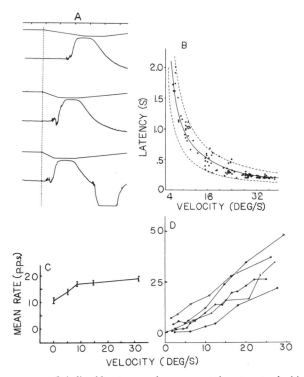

Fig. 3. A: Electromyograms of cheliped levator muscle response at three target velocities. Time calibration: 1.0-sec intervals. B: Reflex latency vs. target velocity. Continuous curve is the time required for
target visual angle to expand by 8.1°. The upper and lower dashed curves indicate times to 11° and 5°
expansion, respectively. C: Dimming fiber mean rate vs. target velocity. Each point is based on 40
observations. D: Motion-detector discharge rate vs. target velocity ($N = 5$). Each point is the mean of at
least ten observations.

where $\Delta\theta$ is a constant with the dimension of a diametric expansion and $d\theta/dt$ is the
diametric expansion velocity. $\Delta\theta$ is 8.1° in Fig. 3B.

The latency–velocity relationship indicates that the response occurs when the
target visual angle undergoes a constant increment (8.1°) or when the time integral
of the mean expansion velocity attains a certain value.

The initial conditions (target visual angle and distance) can be varied over a
wide range with nearly identical results, and comparable ones are also obtained if
the target is replaced by a cinematic projection (24 frames/sec) of a two-
dimensionally expanding black disk.

An examination of the DFs and JMDs under similar stimulus conditions resulted in the data shown in Fig. 3C and Fig. 3D, respectively. The dimming units
exhibited only very modest increases in rate with target motion, and the range of
differential responsiveness was limited to the lower 24% of the physiologically
relevant velocity range. Analysis of the DF response pattern in poststimulus time
histograms and interspike interval histograms yielded similar results. By contrast,

the motion-detector mean discharge rate varied in an approximately linear fashion over the entire velocity range (Fig. 3D) and the interspike interval histograms indicated systematic shifts of the JMD instantaneous firing rate with variations in target velocity. The poststimulus time histograms of the motion-detector discharge revealed only small latency changes with target velocity (less than 10% of the reflex range of latencies). Thus the reflex latency is not associated with a JMD threshold.

The simplest interpretation of these data is that the reflex latency is determined by the time required for a constant number of motion detector spikes to occur. A similar relationship has been noted with direct command IN stimulation (Smith, 1974a). Precedents for neural systems capable of evaluating a time integral to a constant value are legion. Some classical examples are the strength–duration curves for nerve excitation and Bloch's law for visual excitation.

Visual Input and Motor Effects of Defense Reflex Command INs

The stimulus-dependent features of the defense reflex and optic nerve JMDs establish several contraints on the sensory and motor properties of INs, such as the command neurons, that directly promote the reflex. For instance, the command INs must respond to the relevant visual stimuli with a latency that is less than the defense reflex response latency. The responses to visual stimuli that do not elicit the reflex should be much weaker, of longer latency, or both. Furthermore, direct stimulation of these neurons should evoke the defense reflex within the temporal window defined by the difference between reflex and optic nerve response latencies, i.e., 100–200 msec. In addition, since reflex habituation to repeated stimulation appears to occur in the eyestalk, the command cell's visual response should also habituate to repeated stimulation.

A study of INs in the esophageal connectives was therefore undertaken in an attempt to identify elements with the appropriate sensory trigger features and motor fields. Initially, two questions were asked of each unit isolated. Does the neuron respond to any of the reflex-eliciting visual stimuli, e.g., approaching targets or tangentially moving jittery targets, and does direct stimulation result in motor activities that in part or whole may contribute to the defense reflex?

Isolation of single neurons in the circumesophageal connectives was achieved by a modification of the method first applied by Kennedy et al. (1966). A bundle of axons isolated in the connectives and containing a large visual motion-sensitive IN was reduced to a small number of elements by successive recording and dissection. The fine bundle was isolated along the entire length of the circumesophageal connective and placed on two platinum hook electrodes 10–15 mm apart. The electrodes were modified from the design of Wilkins and Wolfe (1974) which permitted the bundle to be drawn into an oil-filled capillary. Each electrode assembly contained its own reference electrode fastened to the tip of the capillary.

Visual stimuli that normally elicit the defense reflex were presented and the sensory response was recorded in the isolated axon. A strong response elicited by an approaching target is illustrated in Fig. 4A. Figure 4B illustrates the waveform of the visually elicited spike on expanded vertical and horizontal scales. Pulses were applied to the second electrode (pulse width 0.1 msec), and the voltage was slowly increased until a spike could be discerned on the recording electrode. Figure 4B illustrates the similarity of the spike waveforms elicited by the two modes of stimulation. Precise correlation was rarely obtained because of the electrical stimulus artifact. Unambiguous identification was possible, however, since stimulation, even at very high voltages, failed to evoke another spike comparable to that elictied visually.

The isolated neuron was stimulated at rates of 1–100 Hz with a regular train, and the animal was visually inspected for indications of a motor effect. On six occasions, visual motion-sensitive fibers were isolated, and upon stimulation they elicited activity in the levator and/or the opener muscles of the cheliped. Stimulation of three of these six neurons resulted in a complete defense posture, with chelipeds raised, claws opened, and tail fully extended. The three neurons were located (1) just medial to the medial giant, (2) at the ventral margin of the connective, and (3) near the lateral margin of the connective. Position 1 corresponds to the location of a visual motion-sensitive unit (C99) identified by Wiersma and Mill (1965) and CM10, a defense reflex command unit identified by Atwood and Wiersma (1967) and Bowerman and Larimer (1974a). Positions 2 and 3 also correspond to the

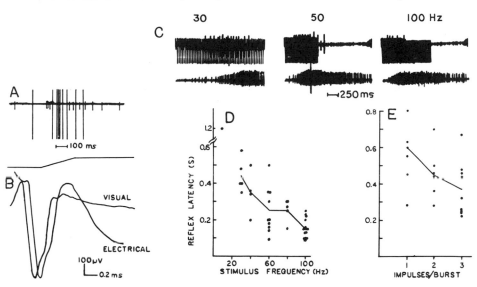

Fig. 4. A: Connective motion-detector response to an approaching black target. B: Waveforms of extracellular action potentials elicited with visual and electrical stimuli. C: Responses of cheliped levator muscle elicited with electrical stimuli to an isolated motion-sensitive connective IN. D: Cheliped levator muscle response latency as a function of stimulus frequency to connective neuron. E: Cheliped levator muscle response latency as a function of the number of impulses/burst in the stimulus train applied directly to a connective motion detector. Mean rate was held constant at 30 pps. Intraburst intervals were 10 msec. D and E are from different preparations.

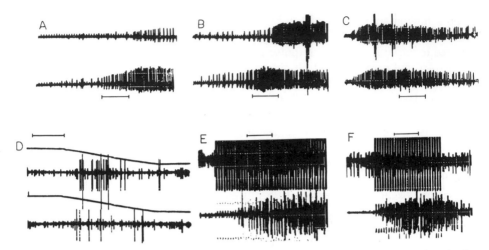

Fig. 5. A–C: Cheliped levator muscle responses exhibiting facilitation in response to successive stimulation of a defense reflex command neuron at 30 Hz (A), 50 Hz (B), and 100 Hz (C). The upper row consists of responses after a 60-sec rest. Stimuli for the lower row commenced 20 sec after the upper-row stimuli. D: Response of connective motion-sensitive neurons before (lower trace) and during an excited state. E,F: Cheliped levator muscle responses (lower traces) to 10-Hz command neuron stimulation (upper traces) before (E) and during (F) a mild excited state. Calibration marks: 400 msec in A–D and 1.0 sec in E and F.

locations of neurons eliciting the defense posture as indicated by the above authors.

Electrodes were placed in the levator or opener muscles to record the motor response. Stimulation at rates of less than 10 Hz was ineffective in most cases. Stimulation at 10 and 20 Hz resulted in response latencies of one to several seconds (Fig. 5E). Similar latencies were observed by Atwood and Wiersma (1967) for claw extensions elicited by command neuron stimulation. Figure 4C illustrates typical levator responses to command neuron stimulation at 30, 50, and 100 Hz. As noted previously (Evoy and Kennedy, 1967; Kennedy, 1968), the motor output does not follow the input train on a 1:1 basis. The data suggest that the command neuron activity is integrated over time. This feature is illustrated by the latency vs. input frequency function in Fig. 4D. Similar results have been reported for different command INs by Atwood and Wiersma (1967), Gillary and Kennedy (1969a), and Smith (1974a). The levator response generally commenced after 10–20 command neuron pulses.

The motor response latencies were considerably in excess of the previously defined temporal window established on the basis of the visually evoked reflex and optic nerve latencies. For example, the strongest visual responses evoked from these neurons exhibit eight to ten spikes at mean rates of about 30 pps after a latency of about 100 msec. The motor response latency to 30 Hz stimulation is about 450 msec. The sum of the two latencies, 550 msec, is more than twice the reflex response latency observed with the identical visual stimulus (Fig. 2A,B).

The discrepancy between the calculated and observed reflex latencies (as well as the number of command impulses preceding the response) suggests that the visually elicited activity of a single command IN is insufficient to evoke the defense reflex. Before this conclusion is accepted, it is important to examine several potentially mitigating observations.

Influence of Pulse-Train Pattern, Facilitation, and the Excited State on the Efficacy of Command Neuron Stimulation

Since the command neuron visual response typically contains one or two bursts, it is of interest to note the influence of burst pattern on the motor response. Figure 4E illustrates the decline in muscle response latency to command neuron stimulation when the electrical stimulus is adjusted to elicit 1, 2, and 3 impulses/ burst. The mean stimulus rate was held constant at 30 pps, and the intraburst intervals were 10 msec, a minimum for these units. The 30% decline in response latency associated with the three impulse/burst train (i.e., two successive interpulse intervals of 10 msec followed by an 80-msec interpulse interval) indicates that the patterning of the visually elicited activity is relevant to the functional organization of the reflex pathway. These results are in general accord with the findings of pattern generation and sensitivity in motor neurons (MNs) (Wiersma and Adams, 1950; Wilson and Davis, 1965; Gillary and Kennedy, 1969b; Smith, 1974a). Modest increases in efficacy with patterning of command neuron stimulation were also noted by Atwood and Wiersma (1967) and Gillary and Kennedy (1969a).

A second issue relevant to the efficacy of command neuron stimulation is facilitation. In a previous study of defense reflex habituation (Glantz, 1974a), it was noted that at stimulus repetition rates of 2–4/min facilitation frequently preceded habituation. Furthermore, high stimulus repetition rates (20/min) resulted in a lower rate of habituation and strong reflex facilitation in the period following high-frequency stimulation. Direct electrical stimulation of the command units resulted in substantial facilitation for stimuli spaced up to 30 sec apart (Fig. 5A–C).

An additional factor which can modify both the sensory and motor activities of an IN is the general level of excitability of the preparation. The influence of the excited state in the optic nerve is well documented (Wiersma and Yamaguchi, 1966, 1967a Aréchiga and Wiersma, 1969a; Glantz, 1974b). The excited state also enhances both the visual responsiveness of connective neurons to moving targets (Fig. 5D) and the motor responses to direct stimulation of the defense reflex command neurons (Fig. 5E,F).

These data raise serious problems for the interpretation of the quantitative results presented in Fig. 4. There is no question but that the constrained, dissected condition of the preparation required for direct IN stimulation results in a general depression of the animal's level of excitability.

The influences of discharge patterning, facilitation, and the excited state are almost certainly all expressed in the intact animal. Thus it is difficult to rigorously exclude the possibility that under appropriate conditions the sensory response of single command elements may be sufficient to elicit the defense reflex.

It can be shown, however, that the defense reflex can be elicited from intact animals in a quiescent state (Glantz, 1974a). Furthermore, the 30 pps upper limit of the command neuron visually evoked discharge also pertains to recordings from the intact, freely moving animal (Glantz and Martel, unpublished data). Thus it is unlikely but not impossible that the visually elicited activity of a single command neuron is a sufficient condition for the promotion of the reflex.

Since six different INs have been observed with the appropriate visual trigger features, overlapping receptive field and overlapping motor fields, it is likely that the behavior is normally under the control of an ensemble of parallel INs. Based on different criteria in the crayfish and other arthropods, several investigators have come to simular conclusions about several other behavior control systems (Schrameck, 1970; Wine and Krasne, 1972; Davis and Kennedy, 1972a; Burrows and Rowell, 1973; Bowerman and Larimer, 1974a; Smith, 1974a). This position is also supported by observations which indicate that the motor influences of two command elements, with overlapping motor fields, can be summed (Atwood and Wiersma, 1967; Evoy and Kennedy, 1967; Davis and Kennedy, 1972b).

Many of the visually active neurons isolated in the connective exhibited little or not responsiveness to the reflex-eliciting stimuli. These neurons responded to pulses of illumination with either phasic "on–off" discharges or low-level tonic "on" responses (Wood and Glantz, in preparation). In most instances, direct electrical stimulation of these neurons failed to elicit a motor response. On three occasions (out of 15 attempts), however, direct stimulation of the phasic on–off units resulted in motor activity of the walking legs (two occasions) or the ipsilateral antenna. In no instance has direct stimulation of an "on" sensitive unit resulted in observable activity in the chelipeds.

The receptive fields of the motion-sensitive command units were generally binocular and appeared to cover most or all of the eye surfaces. Attempts to determine the relative sensitivity of different segments of the eyes were hampered by response habituation to repetitive stimulation. The available data suggest that there are considerable differences in the activity elicited from different areas of a given eye and between the two eyes. Our tentative impression is that the three command cells examined have overlapping but different areas of maximum sensitivity.

Relationship between Optic Nerve Motion Detectors and the Defense Reflex Command INs

The sensory properties of the command INs and the optic nerve JMDs are compared in Figs. 6 and 7. The discharge of the command INs to a rapidly approaching target generally begins after a latency of 60–120 msec and consists of one or two bursts with minimum interspike intervals of about 10 msec.

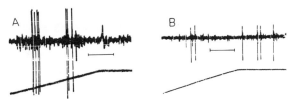

Fig. 6. Comparison of typical optic nerve (A) and connective motion-detector (B) responses to approaching targets. Time calibrations: 40 msec. The horizontal sweep was delayed for 60 msec following stimulus initiation.

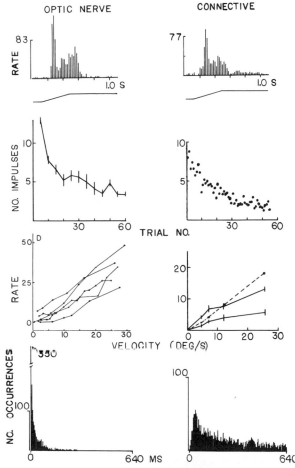

Fig. 7. Comparison of optic nerve and connective IN response features for discharges elicited with approaching targets. Top row: Poststimulus time histograms, 10 msec/bin; rate on ordinate is calibrated in pps. Second row: Habituation functions. Repetition rate is 4/min. Optic nerve data are averaged over five trials for 13 JMDs. Connective IN data are averaged for single trials for ten neurons (four command INs and six neurons with unknown motor fields). Third row: Discharge rate vs. target velocity. Bottom row: Interspike interval histograms, 5 msec/bin.

The responses of the command INs are generally weaker than optic nerve responses elicited under identical conditions. Figure 7 (top row) compares the poststimulus time histograms of the optic nerve motion detectors and command IN responses to approaching targets. The averaged time courses of the two discharges are remarkably similar, although peak rate of the connective unit is generally less than 60% of the optic nerve rate. The time courses of habituation (Fig. 7, second row) are also similar.

The clearest differences between the JMDs and command neuron responses were the output rate vs. target velocity functions (third row) and the interspike interval histograms (bottom row). The command IN firing rate tended to saturate at lower velocities. The interspike interval histograms of the command neuron visually elicited discharge generally exhibited a peak between 15 and 40 msec compared to the optic nerve motion-detector peak at 3–5 msec.

One final interesting feature of the visually sensitive command units is that only one of the three elements, C99, exhibited nonvisual input. C99 had a powerful input from the antannae and statocysts and was particularly sensitive to substrate vibration. The purely visual input to the other two cells was a surprising finding since most of the motion-sensitive units in the connective were multimodal, with input from the antennae, statocysts, legs, or combinations of these.

The strong similarity of the JMD and command neuron time course of response to approaching objects (Fig. 7) is also observed for vibrating targets (Fig. 10). Computer simulations of neural synapses (Segundo *et al.*, 1968) suggest that strong similarities in the temporal form of pre- and postsynaptic pulse trains may arise either if the synaptic efficacy is very strong or if the discharges of converging presynaptic elements are highly correlated.

We examined the correlation between pairs of JMDs recorded on the same extracellular electrode and electronically separated with a multilevel window discriminator. Figure 8 illustrates two samples of the discharge of two of the units examined. The recordings illustrate the tendency of the spikes in the first one or two bursts to occur in approximate synchrony. The scattergram of Fig. 9 is a joint peristimulus time histogram (JPST) (Gerstein and Perkel, 1972) which segregates the stimulus-synchronized activity in broad bands parallel to the ordinate and abscissa and the IN-correlated activities on a diagonal band. The strong, broad diagonal band illustrated in this JPST is associated with the first one or two post-

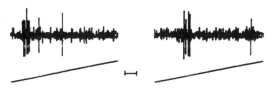

Fig. 8. Responses of two motion detectors to approaching black target. Large unit is 069 (front half of eye), smaller unit is 07 (entire eye). Time scale: 20 msec. The horizontal-sweep trigger of the oscilloscope was delayed for 60 msec after stimulus initiation.

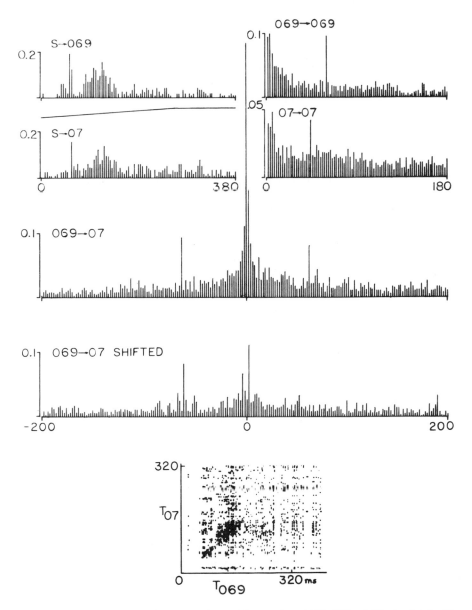

Fig. 9. Joint peristimulus time histogram and correlograms of two JMDs (069 and 07) stimulated with a rapidly approaching target. S→069 and S→07 are poststimulus time histograms; bin width is 4 msec. 069→069 and 07→07 are autocorrelograms, 2-msec bin width. 069→07 is the cross-correlogram, and 069→07 shifted is a control calculation of the cross-correlagram of frameshifted data; bin widths are 2 msec. Ordinates indicate the conditional probabilities of an event, given a reference event. N (069) = 652, N (07) = 1383.

stimulus bursts (S→069, S→07). The length and width of the band suggest that the correlation arises from a strong common input that is phasically activated by the stimulus. This interpretation is supported by the cross-correlogram 069→07) which exhibits a strong peak with a 6-msec half-width centered at the origin and secondary peaks at ±60 msec. Frameshifting one set of data with respect to the other and repeating the correlation procedure provides an estimate of the contribution of the common stimulus correlation to the neural cross-correlation (Perkel *et al.*, 1967). The histogram indicates that a portion of the broad base symmetrical around the origin as well as the secondary peaks at ± 60 msec arises from the separate correlations of each JMD to the stimulus (S→069, S→07). The central peak, however, is totally abolished by the record shift, which suggests that the synchronous activity reflects a very strong source of common excitation (Perkel *et al.*, 1967).

Results similar to those in Fig. 9 are obtained whenever the stimulus is presented into an area of overlap of the receptive fields of the two JMDs. If the target is presented across the boundary of two nonoverlapping receptive fields, relatively strong correlations are observed, but the correlations are entirely attributable to the separate correlations between the JMDs and the stimulus.

The strong correlations between converging optic nerve JMDs can provide an explanation for the marked similarity of JMD and command-unit response form as estimated from the poststimulus time histograms.

Simultaneous recordings of visual motion-sensitive INs of the connectives and optic nerve JMDs were made on a number of occasions (Glantz and Martel, unpublished data). The experimental procedures used to obtain these data did not permit direct stimulation of the connective units; thus it is not known whether the units examined were command INs for the defense reflex. The sensory properties of the connective units were studied in some detail, however, and in this regard they were indistinguishable from the previously described command elements.

Figure 10 illustrates the results of an analysis on a typical pair of units. The JPST illustrates the basic features of the two responses. A small black oscillating target typically elicited bursts with latencies of either 100 or 220 msec after stimulus onset (S→07, S→CM). Since the bursts occurred at about the same time in the two units, there is a high concentration of points at two loci along the main diagonal. The cross-correlation of the two units (07→CM) exhibits a pronounced asymmetrical peak between 3 and 7 msec that rises rapidly on the left but decays to baseline over about 10–15 msec on the right. The results of the control calculation (07→CM shifted) indicate that a segment of the underlying broad base but not the peak of the cross-correlation function may be attributed to the correlation of each of the two units to the common stimulus.

In five similar studies, the peak of the cross-correlation function was also between 2.5 and 3.5 msec. The half-width of the peak, however, varied from 1 to 12 msec, with an asymmetrical form similar to that in Fig. 10. Integrating the probabilities across the peak (+3 to +7 msec) and correcting for the stimulus correlation yields a conditional probability of 0.19 that a connective unit will discharge 3–7 msec after a given optic nerve JMD spike.

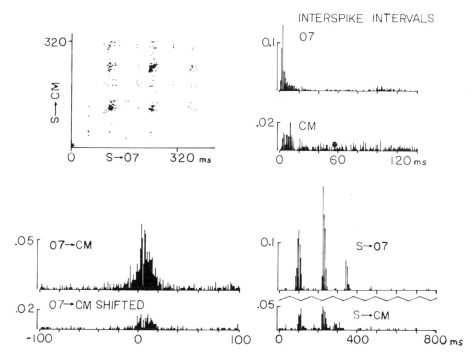

Fig. 10. JPST, correlograms, and interspike interval histograms of optic nerve (07) connective motion-sensitive INs (CM) recorded just rostral and caudal to the brain, respectively. The stimulus was a tangentially vibrating target. PST resolution: 5 msec/bin. JPST resolution: 1 msec. Interspike interval histograms, cross-correlogram, and control calculation: 1 msec/bin. Vertical scales are conditional probabilities. N (07) = 563, N (CM) = 750.

These results are consistent with the presence of a monsynaptic connection of modest strength between the visual motion-sensitive INs of the optic nerve and connective. Other interpretations are possible, however.

First, the strength of the presumed connection between JMD 07 and the connective IN may be overestimated because of the possibility that other neurons in parallel with and highly correlated to a given JMD discharge may converge on the same connective neuron and thus contribute to the 3–7 msec peak. A second possibility is that the connective IN may actually originate in the optic nerve and the 3–7 msec time lag represents the conduction delay due to the 3–5 mm spacing of the electrodes on either side of the brain. This delay would arise if the conduction velocity through the brain were about 1.0 m/sec.

Direct measurements of conduction velocity with pairs of hook electrodes spaced 10–15 mm apart indicate conduction velocities of about 3–7 m/sec for the larger visual INs in the connectives. Thus the 3-msec time lag to peak is more consistent with a range of synaptic delay of 1.0–3.0 msec (Kennedy and Mellon, 1964) than with a conduction lag.

The through-conduction argument would also imply that the optic nerve contains a population of motion-sensitive units exhibiting interspike interval distributions unlike those of the optic nerve JMDs and conduction velocities considerably smaller than those of the motion-sensitive INs of the connective. The possibility seems unlikely, but it is difficult to rigorously dismiss.

Summary and Conclusions

Based on the data presently available, it is possible to present a tentative view of the functional organization of the pathways mediating the visually evoked defense reflex. The motion detectors of the optic nerve translate target motion into a discharge in which both the mean and instantaneous firing rates are proportional to the stimulus velocity. Two features of the JMD input organization ensure that parallel members of the ensemble will fire synchronously. The first is that neurons with overlapping receptive fields derive their presynaptic input from common elements. The second property is based on the strong similarity of the response time course for different units activated by separate areas of the same stimulus. The strong ensemble correlation of the optic nerve JMDs ensures activation of the command IN on which the JMDs converge. The mapping probably consists of multiple optic nerve elements both converging and diverging to a number of command elements. High convergence ratios are indicated by the substantial increase in receptive field size of the connective units as compared to the optic nerve JMDs and the relatively modest synaptic efficacy of individual JMDs on the connective elements.

Control of the motor systems relevant to the defense reflex is vested in an ensemble of command elements for which firing pattern, level of the excited state, and recent history of activity play a role in the regulation of several segmental premotor systems. Habituation of the reflex pathway with repetitive stimuli is localized at or before the input stage of the optic nerve elements, while facilitation occurs at or more likely peripheral to the terminals of command INs.

The total number of elements in a physiologically effective command ensemble is not known. The data indicate that several neurons (at least three) which respond to the reflex-eliciting stimuli can promote the entire reflex when directly stimulated at high (probably unphysiological) rates. At least three other cells with comparable sensory properties can promote either claw opening, cheliped elevation, or meropodite extension.

ACKNOWLEDGMENTS

Several of the studies reported here were conducted by or with the assistance of Howard Wood and Michael Martel. Previously unreported experiments were supported by National Science Foundation Grant BMS 72-02010.

16

Control of Crayfish Escape Behavior

Franklin B. Krasne and Jeffrey J. Wine
in collaboration with Andrew P. Kramer

Introduction

Professor Cornelis Wiersma, whom we honor in this volume, introduced the giant fiber system of the crayfish (Johnson, 1924) into modern neurophysiology in an important series of papers published from 1936 to 1952 (Wiersma, 1938, 1947a,b, 1949, 1952b; Wiersma and Schalleck, 1947, 1948; Wiersma and Turner, 1950). Wiersma showed that the giant fibers are "command neurons" for escape, which, by a single firing, produce a fast flexion and extension of the abdomen and a variety of ancillary motor reactions involving hundreds of motor neurons (MNs) distributed along the length of the neuroaxis. A host of later workers who have built on the findings of Wiersma and his collaborators have brought crayfish escape behavior to a point where there is perhaps no equally complex behavior in the repertoire of any animal that is so well understood in neuronal terms.

As psychologists, we became interested in crayfish escape because the involvement of giant neurons made electrophysiological analysis seem promising, yet the behavior itself did not *seem* as though it were mediated by simple reflex mechanisms. Both its occurrence and its precise form seemed so capricious that it was as if, at least in the use of the tail flip, the crayfish had "a mind of its own." The purpose of this chapter is to review what is now known about why this is so.

Subsystems: Lateral Giant, Medial Giant, and Nongiant Escape Behavior

Behavior

A major step in understanding the variability of escape behavior came when it was recognized that escape is not a unitary entity (Schrameck, 1970). Crayfish can

Franklin B. Krasne • Department of Psychology, University of California, Los Angeles, California 90024.   **Jeffrey J. Wine** • Department of Psychology, Stanford University, Stanford, California 94305.

make at least three different types of escape responses that differ from one another in form and causality (Larimer, *et al.,* 1971; Wine and Krasne, 1972).

The medial and lateral giant axons (MGs and LGs) (Fig. 1A) studied by Wiersma mediate short-latency, stereotyped tail flips as responses to sudden stimuli. Latencies of giant axon firing are typically 2–10 msec, with about 10 msec more elapsing before movement begins. The MGs respond to visual stimuli or rostrally applied tactile stimuli and command a form of abdominal movement that thrusts the animal directly backward, away from the source of stimulation (Fig. 2A). The LGs fire to caudally applied tactile stimuli and produce a movement that pitches the animal upward and forward in such a way that part of a somersault is executed, again efficiently separating the animal from the source of stimulation (Wine and Krasne, 1972) (Fig. 2B).

Escape responses to stimuli of more gradual onset are *not* mediated by the giant axons. Non-giant-mediated (non-G) responses have highly variable latencies always

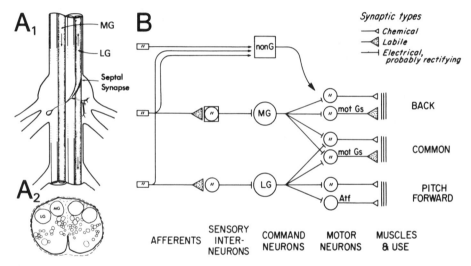

Fig. 1. A: Anatomy of giant escape command cells in abdominal nerve cord. The MGs originate in the brain and course the length of the nervous system. MG action potentials are believed to be initiated exclusively in the brain. The LGs are actually a chain of cells joined by very effective electrical (septal) synapses. Action potentials in LGs can be initiated in any one of the abdominal ganglia. Only one member of each pair of cells is shown in full. A2: Cross-section through an abdominal connective, showing the giant escape command axons and some other large axons. Traced from a plastic-embedded section cut by Joan Misch, courtesy of D. Kennedy. B: Major known features of escape behavior circuitry. Circles indicate identified neurons, ditto marks indicate a number of parallel but comparable neurons, and boxes indicate unanalyzed circuitry. IN circuitry of the MG pathway is drawn ambiguously to emphasize the possibility that it is like that of the LG pathway. Note that the populations of MNs and muscles shown are distributed over a number of segments; "mot Gs" refers to motor giants (F1 of Fig. 10); "Atf" is the large anterior telson flexor MN of the last abdominal ganglion (see Larimer and Kennedy, 1969; Larimer *et al.,* 1971). Non-G mediational circuitry is conjectured to receive input from the receptors involved in the giant fiber reaction as well as perhaps others. Some known features of this circuitry have been omitted for simplicity. Based on references cited in the text.

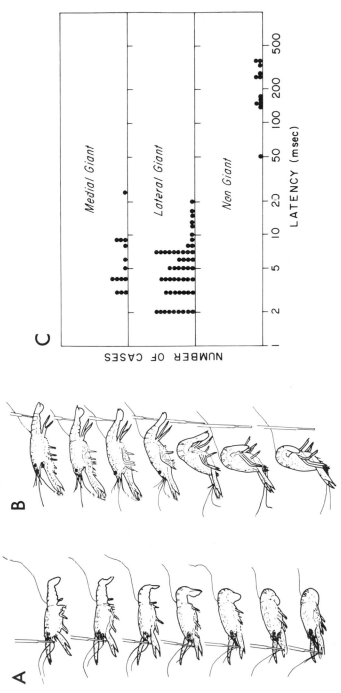

Fig. 2. Forms of escape behavior. A: A medial giant tail flip, initiated by a tap to the rostrum. Note that all abdominal segments flex and the animal darts backward along a low trajectory. B: A lateral giant tail flip, initiated by a tap to the abdomen. Note that only the anterior segments flex, so that the force of the caudal abdomen is directed downward, causing the animal to pitch forward. C: Response latencies for MG, LG, and non-G tail flips (measured to the giant axon spikes or to the start of muscle potential in the case of non-G responses; muscle potentials for giant-mediated tail flips begin about 2 msec after the spike.) Nongiant responses can take either of the forms shown, as well as a variety of other forms. From Wine and Krasne (1972).

at least an order of magnitude greater than giant-mediated ones (Fig. 2C), and they are wide ranging in form, permitting the animal to turn and rotate in all directions as it swims through the water. Non-G escape responses are produced by stimuli such as reaching for an animal or walking past its aquarium, or by noxious stimulation. Also, occasional "spontaneous" responses which occur without obvious antecedent stimulation are mediated by non-G systems. Because of their highly variable latency and form, as well as their occasional spontaneity, non-G reactions may be classified as "voluntary" to contrast them with the much more automatic giant-mediated tail flips. Crayfish escape often involves repetitive sequences of tail flips ("swimming"). The initial flip of such sequences is determined as just described, but all flips after the first are non-G mediated (Wine and Krasne, 1972).

Neural Circuitry

The major known features of the neuronal circuitry of escape behavior are shown in Fig. 1, which summarizes the findings of Johnson (1924), Wiersma (1947a), Hagiwara (1958), Furshpan and Potter (1959), Kao (1960), Kennedy and Takeda (1965b), Takeda and Kennedy (1964), Kusano and Grundfest (1965), Otsuka et al. (1967), Remler et al. (1968), Roberts (1968a,b), Krasne (1969), Schrameck (1970), Larimer et al. (1971), Zucker et al. (1971), Wine and Krasne (1972), Zucker (1972a,b,c), Selverston and Remler (1972), and Mittenthal and Wine (1973). The MNs involved in flipping the tail receive direct excitatory input from MGs, LGs, or both, as well as from as yet unidentified non-G mediational circuitry. The LGs in turn receive their most powerful excitatory input from a partially identified set of interneurons (INs) that are excited directly by tactile afferents of the abdomen. The pathway between afferents and MGs is not known, but preliminary evidence suggests that it is similarly organized, at least for the somatosensory modality (Wine et al., 1974a). Non-G mediational circuitry is almost entirely uncharted; we know only that non-G reactions can no longer be elicited after ablation of the subesophageal ganglion (Wine and Krasne, 1972; but see also Wine, 1972).

Armed with this basic information, one can generally provoke the operation of any of the three subsystems at will, at least in an alert, unrestrained crayfish. However, the ease of doing so is subject to great variation, the known sources of which we now describe.

Habituation

Each of the three mediational systems is subject to habituation; i.e., if the animal is repeatedly stimulated, the probability of a tail flip diminishes for a period of minutes to hours depending on the circumstances of testing (Krasne and Woodsmall, 1969; Wine et al., 1975) (Fig. 3).

The habituation characteristics of the subsystems differ from one another. The non-G system is particularly labile, and, within the system, habituation to one

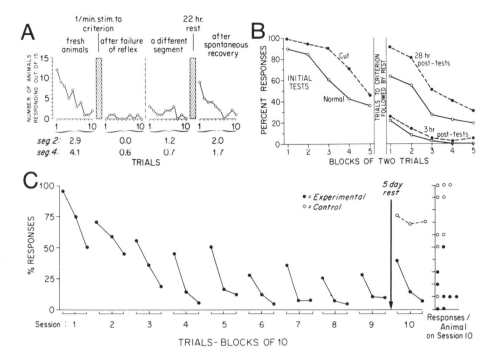

Fig. 3. Habituation of escape behavior. A: Habituation of tail-flip responses to side-to-side squeezes of the abdomen. Most responses to such stimuli are mediated by non-G systems. Trials are at one/5 min (except for overtraining to a criterion of ten successive failures indicated by the first hatched bar). Below each panel the average number of responses per animal is broken down by segment stimulated. There appears to be substantial generalization of habituation between segments; however, this interpretation must be viewed with caution because relevant receptors might not be specific to the segment squeezed. From Krasne and Woodsmall (1969). B: Habituation and recovery of LG-mediated responses to abdominal taps in normal and cord-transected crayfish. The trials plotted were at one/5 min. Trials to criterion were at one/minute in blocks of ten separated by 10-min rests until completion of a block without responses. From Wine et al. (1975). C: Long-term habituation of LG-mediated responses to abdominal taps in cord-transected crayfish. After establishment of thresholds for responses to taps, 30 trials per day were given at one/15 sec. Control animals were given only threshold tests and session 10, both at the same times as experimentals. Unpublished data; controls for the possibility of sensory damage are still in progress.

stimulus generalizes to others (Krasne and Woodsmall, 1969) (Fig. 3A). The MG system has not been formally studied, but its ability to mediate responses to visual stimuli is clearly very labile. The LG system has been the most fully investigated (Krasne and Roberts, 1967; Krasne, 1969; Wine et al., 1975; Zucker, 1972a,b). It is moderately labile, and, in contrast to the non-G system, habituation in it seems to be stimulus specific (although there are occasional indications to the contrary). A variety of experiments, most notably the elegant work of Zucker (1972a,b), strongly suggest that habituation of the LG system is due to intrinsic depression of the individual synapses between tactile afferents and INs. Moreover, there is preliminary evidence that the synaptic depression is, at least in part, specifically due to changes of the presynaptic element at these junctions (Zucker, 1972*b*; Krasne, 1976).

The intrinsic character of habituation is particularly interesting because, as will be discussed below, the LG response is modulated by a powerful inhibitory pathway that descends from the brain and other rostral ganglia and might be suspected of mediating habituation. However, removal of this influence by transection of the nerve cord between abdomen and thorax has no detectable influence on the rate of habituation of LG-mediated escape (Wine *et al.*, 1975) (Fig. 3B).

Work still in progress suggests that *repeated* exposure to the same stimulus for 10 min each day for 5–9 days causes habituation to persist for days. Again, this long-term habituation occurs in the absence of rostrally originating inhibitory influences (Fig. 3C). The physiological basis of long-term habituation has not yet been investigated in this system.

Extrinsic Modulation of Excitability

The intrinsic plasticity of the LG pathway is especially interesting because of its promise as a model system in which some of the mysteries surrounding the physiological bases of learning and memory might be unraveled. However, intrinsic plasticity is by no means the only source of variability in escape behavior.

The subsystems each produce powerful and somewhat different behaviors whose precise form is crucial for the adaptiveness of the response. Thus one would expect that activities in one subsystem should be coordinated with activities in the other systems, perhaps producing interactions that could lead to variable consequences. Moreover, escape must obviously be integrated with the remainder of the animal's behavior. Although escape is a high-priority response, there may be circumstances under which other activities take precedence, particularly in the case of non-G escape, where defending, walking away, or merely stopping or remaining motionless might be the most adaptive response.

We have documented a number of circumstances under which the basic escape circuitry is modulated. There are indications of both facilitatory and inhibitory modulation, but since the intrinsic excitability of escape seems to be high, with inhibitory effects being most conspicuous (Krasne and Wine, 1975), we shall limit this discussion to them. It is convenient to distinguish the decision process itself from adjustments which follow a decision to escape and serve to momentarily focus the nervous system's operation on the efficient execution of a particular response.

Postdecision Adjustments

It is clear that once a giant escape command neuron has fired, a host of profound adjustments in the functional circuitry of the central nervous system follow (Fig. 4, modulatory pathway I).

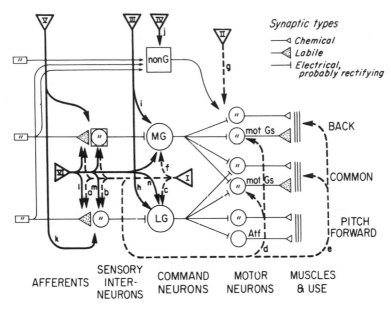

Fig. 4. Inhibitory controls. Dashed bold lines are postdecision controls; solid bold lines are pathways that influence the decision to respond. See text for explanation. (a) From Krasne and Bryan (1973) and Krasne *et al.* (1974); (b) from Krasne and Bryan (1973); (c) from Roberts (1968*a*); (d) from Hagiwara (1958), Roberts (1968*b*), and Wine (1977); (e) from Roberts (1968*b*) and Wine and Mistick, 1977; (f) from Wine (unpublished); (g) from Schrameck (1970); (h) from Krasne and Wine (1975); (i) partly conjectured; see Krasne and Wine (1975); (j) from Krasne and Wine (1975); (k) from Kramer, Lee, and Krasne (unpublished) and Block (unpublished); pathway (k) may not depend on integrity of rostral ganglia; (l) from Kennedy *et al.* (1974); (m,n) Kramer and Krasne (unpublished). Cases lacking references are conjectured from symmetry.

It should first be noted that, insofar as we can tell, exactly the same adjustments ensue whether it is an LG or an MG command neuron that fires. It might have been supposed, given the contrasting patterns of response produced by these two command neurons, that the two systems would have affected one another reciprocally—the LGs inhibiting the MGs as well as those MNs that are fired during MG but *not* LG escape, and conversely. But the system is not organized in this way (Mittenthal and Wine, 1973; Wine and Krasne, unpublished).

The inhibitory consequences that follow an escape command are remarkable for the extent of their distribution. In particular, the LG response pathway, which is the best studied, is inhibited at virtually every possible level. At first glance, this might be thought of as a particularly powerful system for ensuring that a second tail flip will not intervene until the first is over. We at first thought this and believed that inhibition at the various levels might be distributed by a single, or a few widely branching, inhibitory neurons. However, our current opinion, based on details of timing, on certain failures of distribution of the inhibitory effects, and on certain dissociations of effects, is that each inhibitory effect is probably independent and has a specific purpose.

For example, inhibition at the command neuron starts within a few milliseconds of command neuron firing (Roberts, 1968*a*), whereas inhibition at the first central synapse starts after about 10 msec, which is just prior to the onset of movement (Krasne and Bryan, 1973). Inhibition of the first synapse is therefore well suited to filtering out effects of stimuli produced by the tail-flip movements that are about to begin, whereas inhibition of the command neuron is timed appropriately for controlling the duration of the command neuron's spike train.

Even the pre- and postsynaptic inhibitions at the first synapse, although they start together, appear to have separate and special functions. One of the potential adverse effects of stimuli produced by tail-flip movements is that they would be expected to excite tactile receptors and thus lead to the kind of afferent terminal alteration (see above) that causes habituation of LG-mediated escape. However, it is plausible to expect that the presynaptic inhibitory effects produced by pathway I might spare transmitter, etc., and thereby prevent such self-produced habituation. As shown in Fig. 5, the first synapses of the LG reflex are protected from use-produced depression during the operation of the presynaptic component of the first synapse inhibition (Krasne and Bryan, 1973; Bryan and Krasne, 1977*a,b*). A special function for the postsynaptic inhibition has not been demonstrated. However, it is plausible to suppose that its purpose might be to silence afterdischarge in sensory INs that will receive no further sensory input and whose role in the behavioral sequence has terminated.

Evidence that postsynaptic inhibition of the command cell may be needed to abbreviate the duration of its spike train comes from experiments in which single, brief shocks are administered to sensory nerves in dissected preparations. Such shocks have never been observed to produce more than a single LG spike in normal preparations, yet if inhibition is reduced by bath applications of picrotoxin the same stimulus produces a long train of spikes (Krasne and Roberts, 1967; Roberts, 1968*a*).

A final piece of evidence against the notion that the entire system is simply being shut down is that the inhibitory projection to the motor system is not uniform. As far as we can tell from published literature and our own preliminary investigations, inhibition projects to MNs and muscles activated by the MGs or by the MGs and LGs in common but not to those which are solely involved in LG escape responses (Larimer and Kennedy, 1969; Krasne, unpublished observations). Moreover, inhibition projects to the "giant" MNs but apparently not to others.* We do not understand the functional significance of the differential inhibition of the motor system. However, it is interesting that the giant MN is unique among the fast flexor MNs in that its synapse with flexor muscle fibers rapidly depresses with repetitive stimulation (Kennedy and Takeda, 1965*b*; Bruner and Kennedy, 1970). Inhibition may serve to restrict the extent of depression by helping to limit the motor giants to a single spike per escape response.

---

*Although ipsp's are readily seen in the motor giant axon initial segment and soma, they have never been seen in somata, axons, or dendrites of nongiant MNs (Selverston and Remler, 1972; Zucker, 1972*c*; Wine and Krasne, unpublished; Wine, 1977).

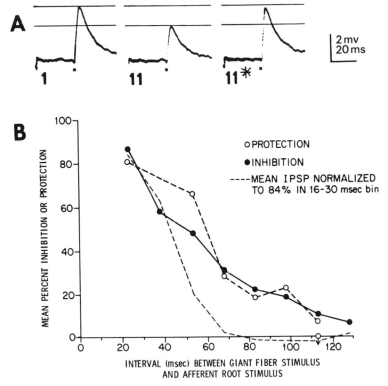

Fig. 5. Protection from habituation during presynaptic inhibition of afferent terminals. A: Epsp's in IN A evoked by electrical shocks to a root containing afferents. Traces 1 and 11 are responses to the first and eleventh stimuli of a sequence at one/4 sec; note the depression. Trace 11* is the response to the eleventh stimulus in a sequence that was identical to the previous one except that each of the first ten stimuli was preceded by activation of pathway I; note that there has been substantial protection from depression. From Bryan and Krasne (1977a). B: The time courses of protection, inhibition, and the postsynaptic component of the inhibition; note that protection outlasts the postsynaptic component of inhibition. From Bryan and Krasne (1977b).

Many of the inhibitory effects just described probably also occur during non-G flips, but the evidence is less complete because of the greater technical difficulties of investigating non-G activities. However, the non-G system can apparently exert more wide-ranging inhibitory control on the motor apparatus than the giant systems, since in the intervals between the flips in a bout of swimming the firing of the LGs has *no* visible motor consequences, whereas a similar LG firing in a similarly timed sequence of artifically produced LG firings does evoke considerable, although not full, motor output (Schrameck, 1970) (schematized as pathway II in Fig. 4).

Adjustments Affecting the Decision Process

There are also a multiplicity of factors which influence the decision to escape (Fig. 4). For example, if an intact crayfish is strapped on its back and the LG response threshold is tested repeatedly, wide swings of excitability often occur which do not seem to correlate with any particular activity of the animal. Transection of the nerve cord just above the abdomen abolishes all of the variability, and excitability rises to a level near the maximum displayed by the intact animal (Krasne and Wine, 1975) (Fig. 6A). If one does the same kind of experiment while tracking the excitability of IN A in addition to LG, one observes that the variation in the LG threshold is *not* accompanied by changes in the excitability of IN A. Hence it is clear (assuming that IN A is representative) that the inhibition operates on, rather than prior to, the LGs (Krasne and Wine, 1975) (Fig. 6B). These and other experiments lead to the postulation of modulatory pathway III descending from Higher centers (Fig. 4). When pathway III is operating strongly, it is virtually impossible to elicit LG tail flips. The potency of this pathway is very much greater than that of habituation, and for the LG system, at least, it seems to be the largest source of the variability that we originally set out to study.

A variety of ablation experiments suggest that pathway III originates in the brain and the most rostral thoracic ganglia (Krasne and Wine, 1975); however, it could be that rostral nervous tissue permits the operation of an abdominal inhibitory system rather than being the origin of the inhibitory effects.

The adaptive significance of pathway III is poorly understood. As pointed out above, it does not appear to be required for either short- or long-term habituation of the LG response. However, when a crayfish is picked up and held firmly, particularly out of water, a profound suppression of the LG response occurs (Krasne and Wine, 1975) (Fig. 7A). This form of inhibition also depends on the rostral ganglia, and it seems plausible to attribute the effect to pathway III. Similar inhibitory consequences of restraint are seen in the MG and non-G systems; this has been indicated in Fig. 4 by showing pathway III projecting to the MG as well as the LG,[*] but, for reasons that will become apparent below, a separate pathway (IV) has been indicated for inhibition of the non-G system.

It might be argued that inhibition of tail-flip escape during restraint makes adaptive sense because the energetically expensive tail flips have become useless. It is consistent with this view that *all* tail-flip behavior is not suppressed. Remaining are non-G responses to touching the uropods, which are most prevalent if the uropods are actually free to move away from the stimulus. Furthermore, a significant increase in "spontaneous" responses occurs, which become particularly likely if one's hold on an animal is relaxed so that a tail flip can free the animal (Fig. 7B). Thus, whereas the animal shuts down giant fiber and other more or less useless "reflexive" responses, its "volitional" systems may actually be sensitized for adaptive responses at opportune moments. This is one reason that pathways III and IV have been separated in Fig. 4. We would not be surprised if, as part of an optimal strategy for escape, activation of predecision circuitry for non-G escape were one means for activating pathways III and IV.

Non-G escape may also be inhibited during defensive behavior. If one tries to grasp a crayfish with forceps, it will usually escape, but some feisty animals instead

*There is no evidence on what points within the MG pathway are inhibited.

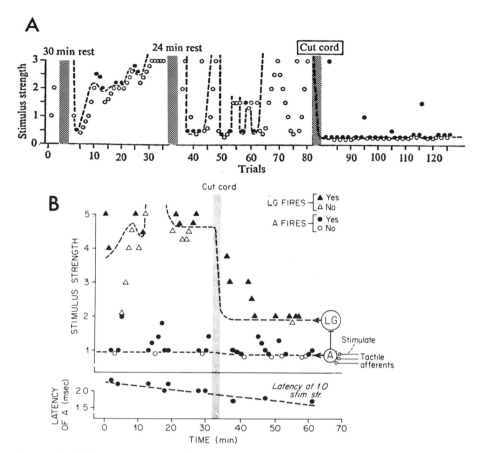

Fig. 6. Variability in the excitability of the LG response. A: The LG threshold was tracked in a restrained crayfish by administering electrical shocks of varying intensity to a peripheral nerve in the abdomen every 30 sec; dots indicate a response and circles indicate no response. The dashed line is an estimate of stimulus strength needed to evoke a response based on the data points. B: Evidence that descending inhibition operates at the command cell level. The experiment was similar to the one above, except that the threshold for IN A was also tracked. As in A, the threshold for LG excitability was high and variable in the intact, restrained animal, but low and constant following cord transection at the thoracic-abdominal level. The threshold of IN A was relatively constant throughout the experiment. (Habituation is not apparent in these experiments. We believe that habituation occurred early in the experiment and was asymptotic by the time the cord was cut, although a modest amount of habituation would have gone undetected with the compressed ordinate scale we used.) From Krasne and Wine (1975).

attack the forceps and will continue to attack in spite of stimuli that would normally evoke non-G escape. Watching animals in groups gives us the impression that non-G escape is similarly suppressed during agonistic encounters between individuals. By contrast, non-G escape becomes more excitable in crayfish that have lost their claws (Krasne and Wine, 1975). It is noteworthy that available evidence (some informal and some hard) suggests that through all such variations in non-G excitabil-

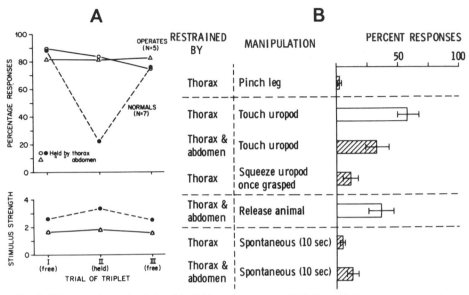

Fig. 7. Features of restraint-induced inhibition of escape. A: Inhibition of LG responses to tapping on the abdomen in normal crayfish and animals whose nerve cords have been severed between abdomen and thorax. Animals were given triplets of trials about 1 min apart; on the middle trial (II), they were held out of the water between the experimenter's fingers. B: Presumptive non-G responses under various circumstances. See text for interpretation of these results. For comparison, note that in free animals leg pinch evokes tail flips 80–90% of the time and spontaneous flips are negligible (given the observation periods used for this graph). Variability markers are standard errors of means. Based on Krasne and Wine (1975).

ity the giant responses (or at least the LG response), which are after all the ultimate fallback for a swift surprise attack, retain more or less normal excitability. We include these effects among those mediated by pathway IV (Fig. 4).

We believe it makes sense that the inhibitory effects represented by pathways III and IV should operate at the level of the command neuron rather than earlier, because the sensory input that feeds the escape circuits undoubtedly goes elsewhere, and there is no reason for sensory processing in general to be shut off simply because tail flips are at the moment inappropriate. However, there are circumstances under which transmission at the first synapse *is* inhibited. So far, such inhibition has been noted during struggling and swimmeret beating (Krasne, unpublished observations) and walking (Block, unpublished observations). These effects, the study of which is only beginning, are indicated by influence V in Fig. 4.

A final modulatory influence (pathway VI of Fig. 4) which probably has a major impact on the giant responses is the ability of tactile stimulation, even in an isolated abdominal cord, to attenuate transmission both pre- and postsynaptically at the synapse on first-order INs of the LG system (Kennedy *et al.*, 1974) and also postsynaptically on the LG itself (Kramer and Krasne, unpublished observations), starting about 5 msec after initiation of a stimulus. This effect should act as a spatial filter, allowing narrow but not sustained broad field inputs through the system (see also O'Shea and Rowell, 1976). We think it must also operate as a temporal filter, giving much greater weight to phasic stimuli of the sort to which the giant fibers preferentially respond and attenuating gradually increasing stimuli no matter how strong they eventually become. Additionally, the presynaptic component of this effect must be important in preventing a sustained source of stimulation from totally depressing the labile synapses of the tactile afferents.

Identifying INs Involved in Modulation

Summarizing the situation portrayed by Fig. 1, we see three subsystems for escape, many of whose neural elements have been identified. These systems are played upon by a superstructure of modulatory influences that serve to coordinate the operation of each subsystem with other aspects of the animal's behavior. The interactions within these networks produce behavioral properties of a kind that we ordinarily associate with "higher mental processes."

So far, the modulatory circuitry is known solely by its effects. The task of further characterizing these effects as well as of identifying the neuronal elements responsible for modulation is largely a task for the future. However, in the remainder of this chapter we describe the results of our initial attempts to find some of the modulating neurons. It should be noted that this is a new level of analysis for behavioral neurobiology. So far, most analysis has focused on neuronal circuitry that *mediates* behavior. Although this first task has only just begun, we have already learned enough to be able to start analyzing circuitry that *oversees* the direct mediational circuitry.

Some Neurons of Inhibitory Pathway I

We decided it would be efficient to start our search by identifying INs excited to discharge by the giants (Wine, 1971, and unpublished results). Neurons of pathway I would be among these, and since the distributions of pathways I and VI are so similar we hoped some elements might be common to both.

It soon became apparent that the giants drive, at short latency, a large population of "corollary discharge interneurons" (CDIs) that run up and down the cord for various distances. Because there are so many CDIs, we have focused our initial effort on two particularly large ones, CDI 2 and CDI 3, which appear to be clearly involved in mediating the presynaptic inhibition of tactile afferents that is produced by pathway I (Kramer, Krasne, and Wine, unpublished observations).

CDI 2 and CDI 3 (Fig. 8A) have their somata and dendrites in the second and third abdominal ganglia, respectively. Their axons, which are large (30–40 μm), are contralateral to their major dendrites and run without further known input back to the last (sixth) abdominal ganglion. Both neurons are driven by both MGs and LGs, and when fired by direct electrical stimulation they depolarize primary affe-

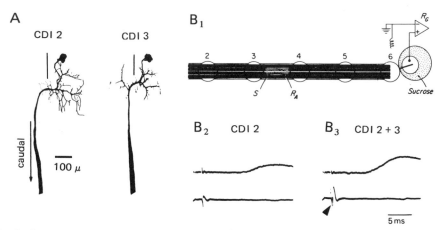

Fig. 8. Properties of CDI 2 and CDI 3. A: Dorsal views of cobalt-filled whole mounts. Midlines indicated. B: Primary afferent depolarizations (PADs) evoked by CDI 2 and CDI 3. B1: Preparation. A sucrose gap was placed at the entrance of the fourth root (almost purely sensory) to last abdominal ganglion. The MGs have been stripped from the 3–4 abdominal connective to expose CDI 2 and CDI 3. B2: Stimulus at S just suprathreshold for CDI 2, whose spike at R_A is shown on lower trace. B3: Increasing stimulus brings in CDI 3; note increased PAD. CDI 2 spike is marked.

rents of the tail fan (Fig. 8B) and inhibit transmission between these afferents and LG response INs. This inhibition occurs about 8–10 msec after initiation of a spike at the rostral ends of CDI 2 or CDI 3, which is commensurate with the time at which pathway I produces its largest effects on the first synapse. All these facts are consistent with a mediational role for CDI 2 and CDI 3 in the effects produced at the first synapse by pathway I.

Different neurons seem to mediate other pathway I effects. So far, we have been unable to detect an inhibitory influence of CDI 2 or CDI 3 on the motor giants, whereas other, smaller CDIs do produce a large ipsp in them, and although one of the large CDIs (3?) can produce postsynaptic inhibition of the LG, its contribution comes well after giant-fiber-produced inhibition of LG commences.

Motor Functions of CDI 2 and CDI 3

Given the above role for CDI 2 and CDI 3, it is difficult to understand why they have such restricted input locations (we have been unable to find homologues of them originating in other segments), and why they are so large—their spikes reach the last ganglion 2–3 msec after the giants fire, yet inhibition of the first synapse does not start for another 5–8 msec. As we have continued to study these cells, we have discovered a new set of facts that helps explain these peculiarities and expands our view of the role of these neurons (Kramer, 1976).

The rapid arrival of spikes at the last ganglion became more explicable when we discovered that CDI 3 monosynaptically excites and sometimes fires MNs of some uropod and telson phasic flexor muscles (Fig. 9C). The restricted dendritic fields of CDI 2 and CDI 3 took on meaning when we found that phasic flexor MNs that originate in the ganglion containing the dendrites of one of these CDIs and that emerge from the cord ipsilateral to its major arborization excite (although they do not necessarily fire) the neuron. These facts suggested the possibility that CDI 3, at any rate, might function as an intersegmental coordinator that would cause certain tail-fan flexor MNs to fire at a specific moment in the tail-flip motor program, namely, a few milliseconds after the third ganglion phasic flexor MNs had fired.

However, this seemed a peculiarly complex and unnecessary arrangement given that the giant axons already course the length of the cord, making direct

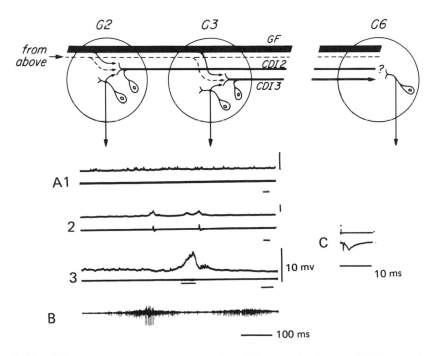

Fig. 9. The CDIs as motor coordinating neurons. Top: Diagrammatic features of CDI connections related to their hypothesized roles as intersegmental coordinating neurons. G2–G6, Abdominal ganglia 2–6; GF, giant fibers. The neurons emerging from the ganglia represent phasic flexor MNs involved in tail flips. Connections between the giants and CDI 2 and CDI 3 are drawn as monosynaptic on the basis of latency without further evidence. Connections of MNs with CDI 2 and CDI 3 are inferred from the fact that antidromic firing of MNs can summate with giant fiber input to enhance firing probability of CDI 3. Bottom. A: Upper traces, intracellular recording at the rostral end of the CDI 3 axon. A1: Brushing antenules and rostrum. Lower trace, thoracic musculature. A2: Non-G flips to squeezing legs. Lower trace, thoracic musculature. A3: Spontaneous flip. Lower trace, gross cord activity in 4–5 connective (at very low gain); the bar indicates the time of most intense activity. B: Suction electrode on exposed CDI 2 and CDI 3 in 3–4 abdominal connective. Two successive flips caused by pinching a leg are shown. In the first, CDI 2 and/or CDI 3 fired; in the second, they did not. Calibrations in A and B: 10 mV and 100 msec. C: Excitation of posterior telson flexor muscle (lower trace, extracellular recording) in response to direct stimulation of CDI 3 (spike shown in upper trace).

contacts with appropriate MNs. Where such intersegmental coordinating action would make sense is in the elaboration of non-G tail flips in which some system of relatively large neurons would presumably be needed for intersegmental coordination of MN firing. Since the exact form of non-G tail flips is highly variable and apparently under the control of higher centers, one might expect not only that large intersegmental coordinating neurons exist but also that the nature of their participation in a given response would be determined by higher centers prior to the execution of the response.

In order to examine this possible interpretation, we have prepared partially deefferented but largely intact animals for intracellular recording from CDI 2 and CDI 3 during non-G tail flips. We find that (1) stimuli which should excite the non-G subsystem produce flurries of small depolarizations in CDI 2 and CDI 3 that depend on the integrity of ganglia rostral to the abdomen even when the stimulation is applied to the abdomen; (2) about 100 msec prior to a non-G response a large depolarization builds up in these fibers and peaks near the moment of response; (3) CDI 2 and CDI 3 sometimes but not always fire at about the time that the animal flips its tail (Fig. 9A,B). These observations do seem consistent with the notion that CDI 2 and CDI 3 serve a coordinating role during non-G escape.

This hypothesis does not explain why the giants, which already directly excite appropriate MNs, should also fire these "coordinating interneurons." However, this is by no means either the only redundancy or the only undue complexity seen in the efferent projections of the giant fibers. One might similarly ask why the giants, in addition to synapsing on the motor giants of a given segment, excite at least half a dozen other phasic flexor MNs that in turn excite muscles that are already excited by the widely branching motor giants (Takeda and Kennedy, 1964; Selverston and Remler, 1972) (Fig. 10). Moreover, when one examines the exact pattern of the command cell–MN contacts, one finds that instead of simply exciting all of the MNs each MG and LG (four axons in all) excites various partially overlapping subsets of the MNs (Fig. 10B). One possible way to make some sense out of much of this complexity might be to think of the giant systems as relatively recent evolutionary products fashioned out of, or superimposed onto, a much more differentiated (but slower) complex of non-G control systems. In this view, there might have been a gradual evolution or retention of contacts between the giant axons and those portions of the non-G circuitry that would produce appropriate responses.

In summary, the characterization of CDI 2 and CDI 3 seems to be as consistent with their playing a role as intersegmental coordinators as with their hypothesized role as links in an inhibitory feedback pathway. CDI 2 and CDI 3 do produce inhibitory effects. However, since they, like the command cells, cause phasic movements, it is consistent that they also inhibit the first synapse so as to filter out reafference. Hence, instead of being in series between the command cells and other elements of pathway I, these CDI cells may simply act in parallel with the command cells to activate portions of the inhibitory pathway. Even if the latter characterization turns out to be correct, it does not necessarily follow that CDI 2 and CDI 3 are

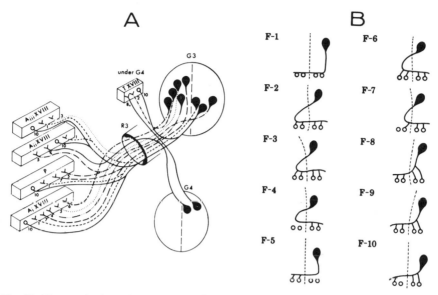

Fig. 10. Motor projections of giant axons. A: Projections of fast flexor MNs to third abdominal segment musculature (A, anterior obliques; P, posterior oblique; T, transverse muscle). Note that F1 (the motor giant) is common to all muscles except the transverse. B: Diagrammatic representation of giant axon-to-fast-flexor MN connections. F10 is an inhibitor, and is not germane to our present discussion. From Selverston and Remler (1972).

redundant elements in the inhibitory circuitry of giant-mediated escape, for they might provide essential reinforcement for both the inhibitory and the motor effects.

Conclusion

Significant advances have been made in understanding crayfish escape behavior at a neuronal level and in comprehending the reasons for its apparent fickleness. Nevertheless, we believe the job of analysis has only begun. Some of the questions for further research were sketched out above; others arise from considerations of common sense and from observations that make it clear that the picture we have presented is incomplete. For example, facilitatory modulation of escape behavior certainly occurs and must be studied; there is suggestive evidence that various hormonal factors may modulate escape behavior; feedback from postural and muscle tension receptors must surely influence the operation of escape-mediating circuitry; and so on. Indeed, we are continually impressed at what a far-reaching, subtle, and valuable model for the study of behavior Professor Wiersma provided for us by the pioneering investigations that he initiated some 40 years ago.

ACKNOWLEDGMENTS

This research was supported by USPHS Grant NS08108 (F. B. K.) and NSF Grant BNS 75-17826 (J. J. W.). We thank Sun Hee Lee and Grace Hagiwara for assistance with many of the experiments reported here, and thank Gene Block, Russel Fricke, Grace Hagiwara, and Donald Kennedy for permission to cite unpublished results.

17

The Command Neuron

William J. Davis

Introduction

Of the many important concepts that have stemmed from the prolific research of Professor C. A. G. Wiersma, perhaps the one that has had the greatest impact on comparative neurobiology is that of the "command" neuron. The term has a long history of application in the invertebrates (for recent reviews, see Bowerman and Larimer, 1976a; Davis, 1976; Kennedy and Davis, 1977) and has recently found its way into the mammalian literature (Grillner, 1975). As evidenced at this symposium, however, the concept has also stirred considerable debate. Given the importance of the topic and the incompleteness of existing data on such neurons, this debate is both inevitable and desirable. As I hope to show in this chapter, such debate can help to clarify our thinking on the subject of the command neuron and can also illuminate fruitful areas for future research.

My purposes here are fourfold: (1) to sketch briefly the history of the concept of the command neuron, (2) to summarize and interpret discussion on this topic that took place at the symposium, (3) to present new ideas on how command neurons are organized to effect behavior, based on recent data from our laboratory, and (4) to identify areas in which new studies on command neurons are especially needed. These purposes will be addressed sequentially in the four major chapter sections.

Evolution of the Concept

The literature on command neurons has been summarized and interpreted in the several recent reviews cited above. About 40 years ago, Wiersma described central neurons that elicit recognizable behaviors when stimulated electrically (Wiersma, 1938; Wiersma and Novitski, 1942). The earliest such studies were performed on crayfish giant neurons, a single one of which causes a tail-flip escape response when stimulated. In later work, Wiersma described a different central neuron in crayfish which elicits the defense posture when electrically stimulated (Wiersma, 1952a).

William J. Davis • The Thimann Laboratories, University of California, Santa Cruz, California 95064.

This neuron could be located in the same region of the circumesophageal connective of every preparation and therefore corresponds both physiologically and anatomically to the definition of an identifiable nerve cell. Wiersma thus singlehandedly extended the concept of the "identified" neuron, which originated largely from his own earlier work on crustacean motor neurons (MNs), to the central nervous system.

The term "command" was first applied to single nerve cells capable of eliciting coordinated swimmeret movements in crayfish (Wiersma and Ikeda, 1964). A variety of command neurons causing recognizable behavior or recognizable motor output patterns were subsequently analyzed, including neurons in the crayfish circumesophageal connectives causing motor output to claw and abdominal muscles (Atwood and Wiersma, 1967) and walking behavior (Bowerman and Larimer, 1974*a,b*), and neurons in the ventral cord causing flexion and extension movements of the crayfish abdomen (Kennedy *et al.*, 1966, 1967; Evoy and Kennedy, 1967) and swimmeret motor output in crayfish (Hughes and Wiersma, 1960*b*; Ikeda and Wiersma, 1964; Wiersma and Ikeda, 1964) and lobsters (Davis and Kennedy, 1972*a,b,c*). In the case of swimmeret beating, Wiersma and Ikeda (1964) showed that the rhythmic locomotor output caused by tonic command neuron stimulation occurs in deafferented preparations. Thus Wiersma and Ikeda provided one of the earliest demonstrations of a motor pattern that can be generated without the aid of sensory feedback.

The Definition Dilemma

Discussion at this symposium made clear that much of the current debate surrounding the concept of the command neuron stems from the difficulty of arriving at a generally accepted definition. Wiersma noted in discussion that he coined the term originally to account for the empirical finding that certain central neurons cause an apparently adaptive, coordinated motor act or output when stimulated. Thus the term arose as an *operational* construct. In the same discussion, Wiersma furnished the important historical insight that his thinking on the subject was strongly influenced by studies on mammals, which were beginning to suggest the existence of motor command "centers" in the brain. Given the economy of innervation in the invertebrates as demonstrated by his own earlier studies of crustacean claw and leg motor innervation, Wiersma reasoned that the same command function seen in mammals might be served in invertebrates by a smaller number of descending neurons, which he termed "command cells."

Wiersma's original observations thus suggested the reasonable and important hypothesis that invertebrates possess descending interneurons (INs) that are specialized to elicit or command specific motor output patterns that underlie behavior. Subsequent research has confirmed, extended, and refined Wiersma's original observations but has not provided an unambiguous test of this hypothesis or its corollaries. Among the most crucial unanswered questions are the following: (1) Are command neurons INs? (2) What is the hierarchical relation of command neurons to other neurons, including the motor networks they drive? (3) Are command neurons used as pathways for activating normal movements in freely behaving animals? (4) If so, are command neurons used singly or in combination with other command neurons having similar effects? (5) Are command neurons functionally distinct from other "higher" neurons that might control behavior (e.g., "trigger" neurons)? (6) What drives command neurons?

While most of these questions were discussed at the symposium, satisfactory answers were for the most part not provided. To begin, it is often difficult to determine whether or not a putative command neuron causes a "recognizable" behavioral act, since the most detailed studies have been performed by recording motor output from dissected preparations in order to monitor the effect of stimulation. However, cinematographic analysis of the movements caused by command neuron stimulation in nearly intact crayfish (e.g., Bowerman and Larimer, 1974a,b) leaves little doubt that single INs can cause recognizable behavior. Such findings do not prove that these neurons are normally used singly by the animal; on the contrary, in most cases examined carefully, the effective single INs were found to cause but a small, variable fraction, not the whole, of a behavioral act (e.g., Davis and Kennedy, 1972a). Stimulation of such command neurons in pairs results, by means of excitatory summation, in a more complete motor output pattern (Davis and Kennedy, 1972b).

As to the remaining questions posed above, answers were not forthcoming at this symposium simply because the necessary data have not been collected. For example, we do not know whether presumed command neurons are normally used to control behavior because recordings have not been made from them under behavioral conditions. It has been shown that swimmeret command INs in lobsters discharge action potentials in response to segmental sensory inputs that cause swimmeret beating in isolated abdomens (Fig. 1), but data from intact, behaving animals are not available. In the case of crayfish giant neurons, which in Wiersma's early work were shown to cause a tail flip, it was later found, in contradiction to expectation, that they are silent during the repetitive, "voluntary" tail flips that comprise swimming (Schrameck, 1970; Davis and Davis, 1973). What they actually do is mediate reflexive tail flips induced by tactile stimuli (see Kranse and Wine, this volume); indeed, they function well after transection of the cord has eliminated communication with higher ganglia (see Bittner, this volume). Do these findings disqualify these giant neurons as command elements? Opinion on this question was strong and divided in discussion at the symposium; Kennedy represented the proponents of the view that the giant neurons are properly classified as command neurons, while Hoyle comprised the opposition. If the giant neurons are classified as command neurons, then we are obligated to include in the category of command neuron all INs that participate in such simple, "automatic" reflexive acts, which seems to me to seriously distort the meaning of "command." On the

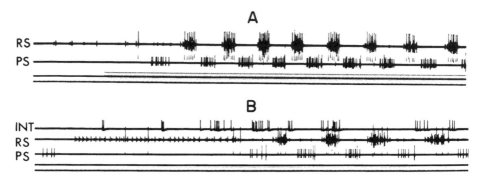

Fig. 1. Stimulating (A) and recording (B) from a swimmeret command IN in the lobster. A: Rhythmic motor output in the power stroke (PS) and return stroke (RS) nerve of a swimmeret, caused by electrical stimulation of a command neuron. The third and fourth traces are a stimulus monitor and a time base (100 marks/sec), respectively. B: Extracellular recordings from the same IN (INT) stimulated in A during tactile stimulation of the ventral surface of the abdomen. The command cell integrated inputs from all abdominal segments, suggesting that it was an IN.

other hand, if we restrict ourselves to the narrower definition of a command neuron as a cell that activates normal "voluntary" behavior, then we are faced with the extremely difficult, and in some cases hopeless, task of defining voluntary behavior and distinguishing it from simple reflexive behavior (see Kennedy and Davis, 1977).

The solution to this impasse is unclear, but there was general agreement that information on the activity of a command neuron during normal behavior is crucial to our understanding of such neurons. This information in turn requires recording from identified command elements in freely moving animals. Ayers and I attempted to obtain such recordings in walking lobsters, with the results illustrated in Fig. 2. Extracellular recordings made with glass capillary suction electrodes from the lateral circumesophageal connectives during optokinetically induced walking revealed descending neurons that discharge immediately before and during walking (Fig. 2A). These neurons were located in regions previously shown by Bowerman and Larimer (1974b) to contain walking command neurons in crayfish. Electrical stimulation through the same electrodes caused coordinated walking in only two of 31 animals, however, perhaps simply because normal proprioceptive cues were not available to the lobsters. These results suggest that neurons categorized as command elements on the basis of electrical stimulation are also active during "voluntary" execution of the same behavior. The approach of recording command neuron activity in behaving animals clearly poses formidable technical and interpretative problems, but Larimer and co-workers are nonetheless pursuing this approach with encouraging results (Larimer and Gordon, this volume).

Because command neurons have been studied mainly by stimulating them rather than by recording their activity, we know little of their hierarchical relationships with other neurons. It is possible that command neurons interact with each

A. VISUAL STIMULATION

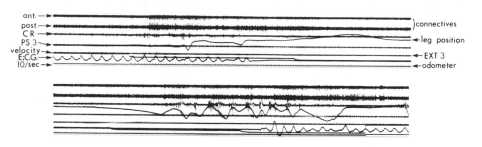

B. ELECTRICAL STIMULATION

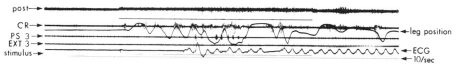

Fig. 2. Electrical activity during command fiber stimulation in lobster walking. A: Walking responses to a staircase of backward optokinetic velocities ranging from 3 to 17 cm/sec. The two records are continuous. B: Walking output driven by electrical stimulation at 70/sec through the anterior electrode on the connective. In A, the upper two traces are recordings from the anterior (ant.) and posterior (post.) suction electrodes, separated by 5 mm on the circumesophageal connectives. The velocity trace is a D.C. voltage linearly proportional to the treadmill belt velocity. A pulse occurs on the odometer trace whenever the belt moves 1 cm linearly. The leg position trace is a D.C. voltage linearly proportional to the angle of the thoracocoxal joint. Upward deflections indicate protraction movements. Extracellular myograms were recorded from the coxal retractor of the third right walking leg (CR), the power stroke muscle (PS3), and the postural extensor (EXT3) of the third abdominal segment. From J. L. Ayers and W. J. Davis (unpublished) and Davis (1976).

other and receive inputs from other central neurons, including members of the motor networks they drive (see next section). Moreover, it is entirely conceivable that some of the INs we have called command neurons are presynaptic, i.e., first order, to second-order command INs with more limited motor effects. The data of Atwood and Wiersma (1967) support this view by demonstrating that there are command neurons that control more than one motor system. Supportive evidence for this hypothesis has been provided by cinematographic analysis of command neuron effects in crayfish (Bowerman and Larimer, 1974a,b). In this case, we are probably unduly restricting our vision if we monitor only one motor system during command neuron stimulation. Moreover, if we are indeed dealing with central neurons that have a widespread motor effect, they could represent a separate class of neurons that deserve a special title. There is surely no shortage of imaginative candidate names: "trigger," "executive," "decision," "driver," and "gating" are already in the literature, and "grandmother," "godfather," "governor," and even "suggestion" neuron have all arisen in one context or another.

In this connection, it was suggested by Hoyle that command neurons should be distinguished from "trigger" neurons on the basis of their motor effects. Command neurons, it was proposed, may be ones that need to be active continuously to cause the behavior, while trigger neurons cause behavior that outlasts their own activity by many seconds or even minutes (cf. Willows and Hoyle, 1969). Studies on INs causing swimmeret beating showed that, for some, their motor effects can long outlast the stimulus (Davis and Kennedy, 1972a). It is possible that the duration of the motor effect reflects properties of the driven motor network; differentiation of higher-order INs clearly cannot be determined from properties of the different motor networks that they control. In short, functional distinctions that would require segregation of higher-order neurons controlling motor systems into different classes cannot be drawn effectively from available data, although such distinctions may well exist.

In addition to the above problems, we are faced with the disturbing possibility that some of the neurons that have been called command neurons may simply be central axons of sensory or MNs rather than descending INs. Neuroanatomical studies have not been performed on identified command neurons, and functional evidence that such cells are descending INs has been obtained in only a limited number of instances (e.g., Fig. 1).

As a final issue, the majority of studies on command elements have involved stimulating these cells while recording some index of motor output. With the exception of crayfish giant fibers (see Krasne and Wine, this volume), we know little about the organization of sensory and other synaptic inputs to command neurons simply because recordings of command neuron activity have seldom been obtained. As will be shown in the next section, characterization of inputs may be essential in assigning a normal command function to a given central neuron.

To summarize, there is widespread agreement that a command function can be operationally demonstrated in many preparations by stimulating single central neurons. This empirical observation suggests the reasonable hypothesis that there exists a special class of INs that normally operate either alone or together with other similar neurons to elicit recognizable behavioral acts. Data capable of rigorously testing this hypothesis, however, have not been previously obtained, contributing to the present ferment.

Command Neurons Controlling Feeding Behavior in a Mollusk (*Pleurobranchaea*)

Neurophysiological studies on the feeding system of *Pleurobranchaea*, performed in collaboration with Rhanor Gillette and Mark Kovac, have furnished among the first intracellular data from neurons identified by the criteria referred to at the beginning of this chapter as command neurons. In this case the command neurons control a rhythmic behavior, feeding. Although these studies involve a mollusk, the conclusions have compelled us to reassess our notions of command neurons in arthropods as well. I will first briefly summarize salient features of these studies and then discuss how they require a reevaluation of the concept of the command neuron.

The brain of *Pleurobranchaea* was previously shown by dye injection to contain the somata of many neurons that send descending axons to the buccal ganglion (Davis *et al.*, 1974). These somata comprise three discrete populations: paired metacerebral giant neurons and two clusters of somata which we have termed the paracerebral and opisthocerebral neurons (Fig. 3A).

Our investigations demonstrate that the metacerebral neurons and at least some paracerebral neurons, as well as the paired ventral white cells of the buccal ganglion (Fig. 3B), meet the operational criterion for command INs. Intracellular stimulation of one or both metacerebral neurons at physiological frequencies accelerates an

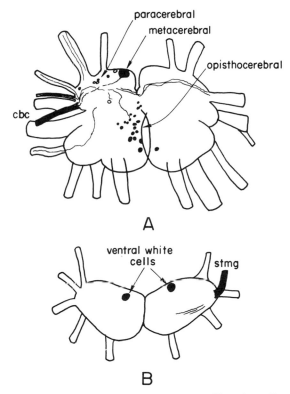

Fig. 3. Somata of feeding command neurons in the brain (A) and buccal ganglion (B) of *Pleurobran-chaea*. A: Somata of all neurons sending axons into the ipsilateral cerebrobuccal connective, identified by back-injection with cobalt chloride. B: Somata of the paired ventral white cells, identified by back-injection of the stomatogastric nerve. Functional studies show that the ventral white cell sends an axon out the contralateral stomatogastric nerve only and that the cells are electrically coupled with each other. The electrical connection is presumably responsible for the spreading of dye to the ipsilateral cell in this injection. Abbreviations: cbc, cerebrobuccal connective; stmg, stomatogastric nerve. These injections were made in collaboration with M. V. S. Siegler.

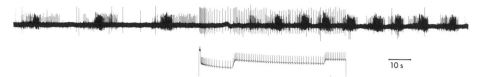

Fig. 4. Effect of tonic intracellular stimulation of one metacerebral giant neuron (MGG) on the feeding rhythm of *Pleurobranchaea* recorded extracellularly from the third buccal root (r3). The MCG contains an axonal branch in r3. This experiment was performed on an isolated nervous system. From Gillette and Davis (1977a).

ongoing feeding rhythm in an isolated nervous system (Fig. 4). Similarly, intracellular stimulation of a single paracerebral neuron causes intense feeding activity with a latency of a few seconds even in quiescent preparations (Fig. 5). Likewise, intracellular stimulation of a single ventral white cell causes intense feeding output with a short latency in quiescent preparations (Fig. 6). Both the metacerebral giant neurons and the ventral white cells send axonal branches to the periphery and may thus play a motor role in addition to their excitatory effect on the central pattern generator for feeding behavior. In contrast, we have been unable to demonstrate axonal branches of the paracerebral neurons in any buccal root or in the anterior brain nerves (large and small oral veil nerves, tentacle nerves, and mouth nerves), using either physiological (ortho/antidromic stimulation) or anatomical (dye injec-

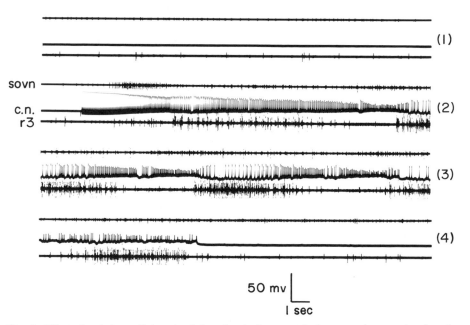

Fig. 5. Effect of tonic intracellular stimulation of a single paracerebral command neuron (c.n.) on the feeding rhythm recorded extracellularly from the small oral veil nerve of the brain (sovn) and the third root of the buccal ganglion (r3). Records (1),(2), and (3) are continuous; (3) and (4) are separated by 2.5 min of continuous current injection into the paracerebral neuron. This experiment was performed on an isolated nervous system. From Gillette et al. (1977).

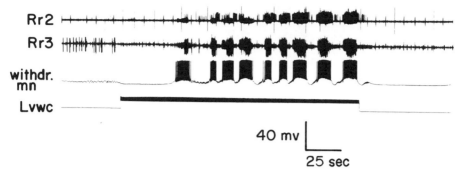

Fig. 6. Effect of tonic intracellular stimulation of a left ventral white cell of the buccal ganglion (Lvwc) on the feeding rhythm recorded intracellularly from an identified withdrawal MN (withdr. mn) and extracellularly from the right roots 2 and 3 (Rr2, Rr3) of the buccal ganglion. This experiment was performed on an isolated nervous system. From Gillette and Davis (1977*b*).

tion methods). Thus not only do the paracerebral neurons meet the functional criteria for a command neuron, they also appear to meet the structural criteria for INs, although this assertion is necessarily based on negative evidence.

The ability to impale identified feeding command neurons with microelectrodes permits intracellular recording from these cells. We have made such recordings in isolated nervous systems, during spontaneous feeding output and while feeding was driven by electrical stimulation of the stomatogastric nerve (Davis *et al.*, 1973). We have also made intracellular recordings from the command neurons under more "normal" conditions, both in semi-intact preparations and in behaving, whole-animal preparations. In all cases the findings have been similar; the command neurons are active rhythmically and are in phase with the efferent feeding activity that they drive.

This generality is documented in Figs. 7–9 for a metacerebral neuron, a paracerebral neuron, and a ventral white cell, respectively. These three classes of command neurons have been studied extensively and their synaptic relations with other neurons have been determined in considerable detail (Gillette and Davis, 1975, 1977*a–c*; Gillette *et al.*, 1977). For example, the metacerebral giant neuron makes reciprocal excitatory electrotonic connections with feeding MNs in the brain and receives inhibitory feedback from identified corollary discharge neurons in the buccal ganglion (Gillette and Davis, 1975, 1977). These demonstrated connections are adequate to explain the observed synaptic feedback to the metacerebral giant neuron and its cyclic discharge during feeding output.

The paracerebral neurons also receive synaptic inputs from identified feeding neurons, but the type of input and the neurons involved are different from the metacerebral giant neuron. In particular, the paracerebral cells make strong, reciprocal, and monosynaptic excitatory connections with several corollary discharge neurons of the buccal ganglion (Gillette *et al.*, 1977; Gillette and Davis, 1977*c*). These connections account for at least some of the synaptic feedback to the paracerebral command neurons and the cyclic discharge pattern of these command neurons during feeding output.

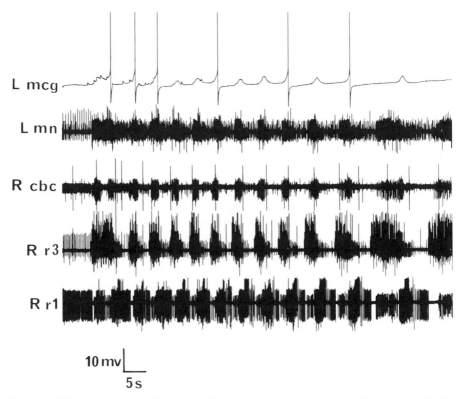

L mcg

L mn

R cbc

R r3

R r1

10 mv

5 s

Fig. 7. Activity recorded intracellularly from the left metacerebral giant neuron (Lmcg) during feeding output in an isolated nervous system. Note cyclic activity of the mcg, phase-locked with feeding. Feeding output was driven by tonic extracellular stimulation of the stomatogastric nerve. Remaining abbreviations are as follows: Lmn, left mouth nerve of the brain; Rr3, right third root of the buccal ganglion; Rrl, right first root of the buccal ganglion. From Gillette and Davis (1977a).

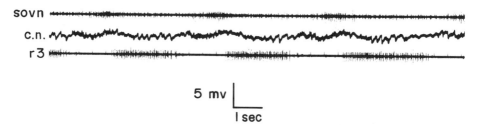

sovn

c.n.

r3

5 mv

I sec

Fig. 8. Activity recorded intracellularly from the same paracerebral command neuron stimulated in Fig. 5. Note cyclic Epsp's in the paracerebral neuron during sovn bursts, and ipsp's during the r3 burst. From Gillette et al. (1977).

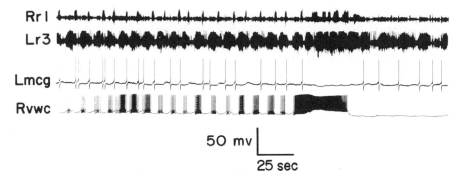

Fig. 9. Activity recorded intracellularly from a ventral white cell during cyclic feeding output driven by stomatogastric nerve stimulation in an isolated nervous system. Note cyclic activity of the vwc, phase-locked with feeding. The intense tonic burst in the vwc near the end of the record is characteristic of the activity of this neuron and shuts off the metacerebral giant neuron (mcg) by activating a corollary discharge neuron that inhibits the mcg. Feeding is monitored here by extracellular recordings from the second and third buccal roots (r2 and r3). From Gillette and Davis (1977*b*).

Finally, each ventral white cell in the buccal ganglion receives both monosynaptic excitation from several identified MNs that fire during the proboscis eversion phase of the feeding cycle and monosynaptic inhibition from single para-cerebral command cells (Gillette and Davis, 1977*b*). These synaptic interconnections with other members of the feeding network are adequate to explain the rhythmic synaptic input to the ventral white cells during feeding and their correspondingly cyclic discharge pattern.

The above findings have several implications for the control of behavior, as explored in detail elsewhere (Davis, 1976). Two of these implications are especially relevant to the topic of the command neuron. First, in the feeding system of *Pleurobranchaea* a command neuron is clearly an integral component of the net-work it excites. Because of extensive synaptic reciprocity between command neurons and other members of the feeding network, stimulation of any member of the network, including a MN, is in principle capable of secondarily activating the entire network. In this case, the accepted operational definition of a command neuron in dissected preparations becomes less useful in extrapolating to the normal role of the neuron under behavioral conditions. In particular, electrical stimulation studies alone do not furnish conclusive evidence that a neuron normally plays a command role. Certain neurons are presumably specialized to exercise the com-mand function, but such specialization may depend simply on privileged access to the central or sensory information that normally elicits the behavior. Information on the organization of central and sensory inputs to a neuron thus becomes critical in determining whether a neuron is properly considered to be a command neuron.

Second, we have identified and analyzed several command neurons for feeding behavior in *Pleurobranchaea,* and, while most of these are *sufficient* to cause feeding, without exception none is *necessary.* Any one of the command neurons studied above can be silenced by hyperpolarization, yet feeding output still occurs. It is clear that in this motor system, at least, the command role is shared among a population of neurons, an arrangement suggested also for the lobster swimmeret system (Davis and Kennedy, 1972a,b).

Present Status and Future Research on Command Neurons

Our studies on the feeding system of *Pleurobranchaea* have demonstrated that operationally defined command neurons receive potent synaptic feedback from the network they excite. The original concept of a command neuron was as a polarized, unidirectional activator of a motor network (Fig. 10A). We should add to this model feedback from the central motor network that it excites and the possibility that a command neuron can be an integral member of the network (Fig. 10B). Such command neurons would be part of a positive feedback loop that can in principle underlie network reverberation, which is of obvious significance for rhythmic behaviors. Such positive feedback may explain why some motor behaviors outlast the stimulus that causes them, as discussed above in the context of the command/trigger dichotomy. Other implications of this finding are discussed elsewhere (Davis, 1976).

The findings from the feeding system of *Pleurobranchaea* suggest that we should consider the possibility that arthropod command neurons also receive synaptic feedback from the motor networks they excite. This possibility has been overlooked previously, perhaps simply because recordings from identified arthropod command neurons have seldom been made during the occurrence of the motor behavior they drive. The few existing examples of such recordings, from the walking and swimmeret systems of the lobster (Figs. 1 and 2), furnish tantalizing but insufficient evidence of rhythmicity in command neuron discharge. It seems possible

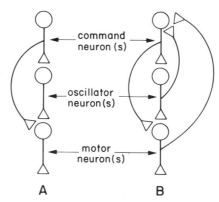

A   B

Fig. 10. Two different arrangements by which command neurons may control behavior. A: Hierarchical organization previously assumed. B: Reciprocal relationships demonstrated in the feeding system of *Pleurobranchaea*. Feedback to command neurons is illustrated here as excitatory, although inhibitory feedback has also been found.

that feedback to command neurons from the driven motor network may occur also in arthropods.

It is to be hoped that future studies on arthropod command neurons will be addressed to the issue of synaptic feedback from the driven motor network and also to the several unanswered questions posed near the beginning of this chapter. For such studies it is difficult to imagine a more ideal arthropod preparation than the one in which the command neuron was first so named, i.e., the crustacean swimmeret system. Single swimmeret command neurons can be microdissected from the abdominal nerve cord, and it should be comparatively easy to fill such neurons with cobalt chloride using the back-injection method (Kater *et al.*, 1973; Siegler *et al.*, 1974). Such morphological studies would help to assess whether arthropod command neurons are truly INs and to reveal geometric details that might aid in understanding their function. Moreover, recordings can be made from swimmeret command neurons that are dissected from the posterior nerve cord, leaving their anterior input and output connections intact and operational (e.g., Fig. 1). Therefore, it should be possible to analyze the activity of these neurons during swimmeret beating in semi-intact preparations without interrupting possible feedback loops of the kind demonstrated in the feeding system of *Pleurobranchaea*. Finally, sensory inputs that drive swimmeret beating have been characterized and include contributions from the statocysts (Davis, 1968*c*), eyes (Davis and Ayers, 1972), and abdominal exteroceptors (Davis and Kennedy, 1972*a*) (Fig. 1), all of which are amenable to quantitative experimental control. Therefore, it may be possible to analyze the organization of sensory inputs to swimmeret command neurons.

We may hope that the next decade will witness such studies on arthropod command neurons and that the results will help to clarify the many important questions that may be traced to C. A. G. Wiersma's original and pioneering studies. The results are likely to prove of general significance for motor control in all animals, including mammals, thus completing the reciprocal feedback loop between invertebrate and vertebrate neurobiologists that began with Wiersma's study of the command neuron.

ACKNOWLEDGMENTS

Original research from this laboratory is supported by NIH Research Grants NS 09050 and MH 23254. I am indebted to my colleagues, Dr. Joseph Ayers, Dr. Rhanor Gillette, and Dr. Mark Kovac, for collaboration and critical discussions of the material presented in this chapter.

18

Complex Neural Integration and Identified Interneurons in the Locust Brain

Michael O'Shea and C. Hugh Fraser Rowell

Introduction

In 1971, one of us (Rowell, 1971a) published an extensive literature review concerned with the analysis of responses recorded extracellularly from certain movement-detecting visual interneurons (INs) contained in the ventral thoracic nerve cord of grasshoppers and crickets. These units attracted attention because they are the most conspicuous ($\sim$ 3 mV) of the units which can be recorded with extracellular hook electrodes from the whole thoracic cord. They were characterized (Rowell, 1971a) and called the descending movement detectors (DMDs). They fall into two classes depending on whether they are excited by movement in the receptive field of the eye ipsilateral or contralateral to the nerve cord projection: DIMDs or DCMDs. Prior to 1971, the DMD neurons in both crickets and grasshoppers were used in studies on perception of movement and visual acuity (Burtt and Catton, 1954, 1962, 1966, 1969; Palka, 1965), color sensitivity (Suga and Katsuki, 1962), and light and dark adaptation (Burtt et al., 1963, Cosens, 1966). These studies were not directed at determining either the function in behavior or the origin, in neural terms, of the specific response characteristics. The DMDs were also studied in their own right, and by 1971 a body of work had accumulated describing their specific response characteristics (Palka, 1967a,b, 1969; Rowell and Horn, 1967, 1968; Horn and Rowell, 1968; Rowell, 1971a). The ease of extracellular recording still makes them an attractive and convenient assay for general properties of the visual system (Northrop, 1974; Palka and Pinter, 1975). Consideration of their role in behavior was introduced (Rowell, 1971a) and extended, for the DCMD, by studies in freely moving animals (Rowell, 1971b,c).

In spite of the fact that the DMDs, and especially the DCMD, of the locust were becoming among the most extensively studied arthropod neurons, they were not, strictly speaking, "identified" neurons; their anatomical identity and their input and output connections remained unknown. It was clear, however, that the DMDs were ripe for identification and that if this were done intracellular recording from

Michael O'Shea and C. Hugh Fraser Rowell • Department of Zoology, University of California, Berkeley, California 94720. Dr. O'Shea's present address is Department of Biological Sciences, University of Southern California, Los Angeles, California 90007.

their integrating regions might reveal the mechanisms underlying their already well-documented responses. It seemed to us that an understanding of the origin of their many and complex responses would provide insights into the mechanisms of high-order sensory processing because we believe that complex integrative problems have fewer neural solutions than simple ones. Severe limits must be placed by the necessity of combining many complex responses, each with its own specific demands, and therefore the likelihood of discovering general neural solutions to complex problems is high. It was in this optimistic frame of mind that we decided to attempt the identification of the locust DCMD neuron.

The DCMD is now an "identified neuron" (O'Shea *et al.*, 1974), as is the neuron which provides its primary input, the lobula giant movement detector or LGMD (O'Shea and Williams, 1974). Some of the output connections made by both the DCMD and DIMD with identified motor neurons (MNs) have been established (Burrows and Rowell, 1973). In addition, the LGMD and DCMD have been found to respond phasically to auditory stimulation (Palka and Pinter, 1975; O'Shea, 1975) and are therefore bimodal. In this chapter, we will review our recent work on the identification of these complex INs and discuss the extent to which we have been able to account for their response characteristics.

It is a great pleasure to be able to contribute this review to the volume honoring Kees Wiersma, who, as in so many areas of invertebrate neurophysiology, was the pioneer worker on the higher-order visual INs of arthropods.

Anatomy and Output Connections of the DCMD

We succeeded in determining the anatomy of the DCMD of the locust *Schistocerca nitens* by first probing in the thoracic nerve cord with procion-filled microelectrodes until we penetrated the axon (recognized from its response characteristics). The axon was marked by electrophoretic dye injection. The distribution of the DCMD's branches in the thoracic ganglia and the location of the soma were elucidated by the introduction of cobalt by axonal iontophoresis and via intracellular microelectrodes (Iles and Mulloney, 1971; Pitman *et al.*, 1972; O'Shea *et al.*, 1974).

The anatomy of the DCMD in the brain as drawn from six cobalt-filled preparations is shown in Fig. 1A, and its branching pattern in the thoracic ganglia is shown in Fig. 1B. The terminals of the DCMD in the metathoracic ganglion are extensive, and it is here that the only known output connections with MNs have been established (Burrows and Rowell, 1973). The anatomy and output connections are well correlated (Fig. 2A,B), and it appears that connections are made with MNs in the vicinity of their cell bodies. The symmetrical excitatory output connections made by each DMD neuron with both left and right fast MNs to the extensor tibiae muscle (the FETi MN of Burrows and Hoyle, 1973*a*) provide the best clue to the behavioral role of the DMDs. These MNs excite the muscles which produce rapid extension of the jumping legs and are used in only two behaviors: jumping, where they are activated symmetrically, and defensive kicking, where they are normally

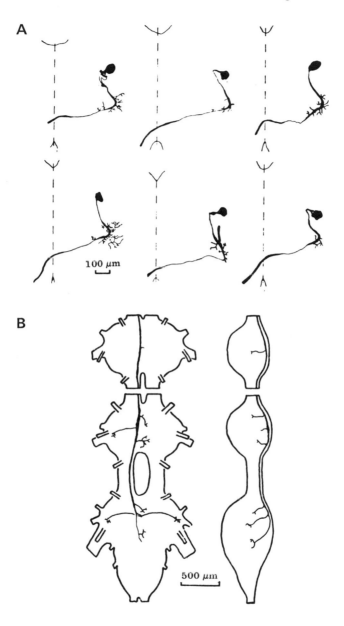

Fig. 1. A: Camera lucida drawings of the right DCMD in the brain of six different specimens. Note individual variation in position of neuron relative to the midline of the brain (dashed line), position of soma, course of neurite, curvature and form of integrating segment, and point of thickening of main axon. All these features are presumably at least partly independent of the degree of success in staining the cell. In addition, considerable variation is seen in the points of departure of the dendrites from the integrating segment, although this feature, especially, could be an artifact of staining. B: Course of the 6 ft DCMD in the three thoracic ganglia, drawn from the dorsal (left) and lateral (right) aspects.

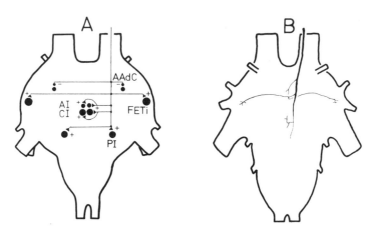

Fig. 2. Comparison of the course of the DCMD in the metathoracic ganglion as visualized by cobalt injection (B) with that deduced from electrophysiological recordings from MNs (A). The neurons may be thought of as either the right DMCD viewed ventrally or the left viewed dorsally. Burrows and Rowell (1973) constructed the connectivity diagram by drawing straight lines to the sites of known MNs. Abbreviations: AAdC, anterior coxal adductor MN; FETi, fast extensor tibiae MN; AI, anterior inhibitory flexor tibiae MN; PI, posterior inhibitory flexor tibiae MN; CI, common inhibitory MN.

active alone or alternately. The symmetrical excitatory connections of the DMDs with the FETi's are therefore highly suggestive that they are concerned with the initiation of escape jumping behavior. In addition, the well-developed novelty-detecting property (see below), high axonal conduction velocity (3m/sec), and response to loud noise are all suggestive of a role in escape behavior.

Recent work (Pearson, unpublished observations) has associated activity of the DMDs with motor activity which leads to the prejump crouch (Heitler and Burrows, 1976; Bennett-Clark, 1975). It has recently been shown (Heitler *et al.*, 1977) that the epsp of even a single DMD can elicit spikes in the FETi, provided that body temperature is in excess of 28°C. The threshold of the motor unit is markedly temperature dependent; in previous experiments (Burrows and Rowell, 1973) which failed to show spike initiation as a result of DMD activity, body temperature was too low. These data appear to provide the physiological basis for the observation that grasshoppers jump much more readily in response to visual stimuli on sunny days than on overcast ones. The jump itself appears to be released by a neuron which inhibits the flexor of MNs and thus terminates the co-contraction (when both flexor and extensor tibiae MNs are active together) period of the crouch (Heitler and Burrows, 1977). Identification of this neuron appears to be necessary before the possible role of the DMDs in this activity can be assessed.

Identification of the LGMD

It was hoped that the identification of the DCMD would provide a preparation in which the neuronal basis of some of its complex responses could be studied at a

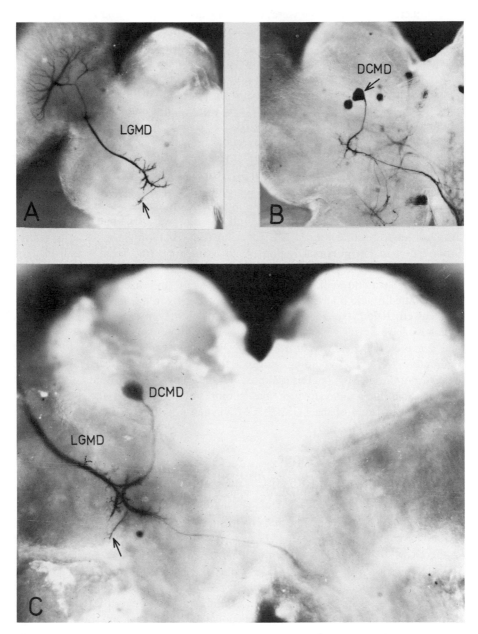

Fig. 3. A: Cobalt fill of the LGMD via an intracellular electrode inserted near the site of impulse initiation. From O'Shea and Williams (1974). B: Cobalt backfill of the DCMD (arrow) made from the contralateral neck connective. A variety of other neurons, mainly out of the plane of focus, were also filled. C: Double cobalt fill of the synaptic zone between the LGMD and DCMD. Note the apparent multiplicity of contact zones. There also remain numerous branches not accounted for. In both A and C, the branch of the LGMD which probably receives auditory synapses is marked with an arrow.

level hitherto impossible. We were, however, disappointed to find that very few of the responses of the DCMD were determined by it or by connections made with presynaptic neurons. We were able to record both epsp's and ipsp's in the DCMD's integrating segment; none of these, however, seemed to affect substantially the spiking activity of the neuron. Action potentials in the DCMD arise abruptly from the baseline and are not associated with epsp's. Extracellular recordings at the junction of the optic lobe and brain revealed spikes in a unit which preceded 1:1, with an invariant latency, those in the DCMD. This represented either a branch of the DCMD which was not revealed by cobalt injections or another neuron which relays spikes to the DCMD. In any case, it was clear that the mechanism underlying the responses of the DCMD was not to be found in its integrating segment and that the identity of the unit recorded near the optic lobe had to be established.

This was done by probing at the junction of the optic lobe and brain with a cobalt chloride-filled microelectrode until the unit was penetrated and injected. Another large cerebral neuron was revealed (Fig. 3A) which has a large fanlike arborization in the proximal region of the optic lobe (the lobula) and an axon projecting to the integrating segment of the DCMD. This cell was termed the LGMD (O'Shea and Williams, 1974). It is directly presynaptic to the DCMD as demonstrated by the injection of cobalt into both cells in the same animal (O'Shea and Rowell, 1975a) (see Fig. 3B,C). The LGMD is the only input to the DCMD for which we have a clearly established function—it initiates spikes. The various chemical synapses which are recorded in the DCMD appear superficially to have *no* integrative role! Our recordings suggest that the LGMD predicts precisely the behavior of the DCMD, but this is almost certainly a naive view. Before we consider the possible integrative role of the subthreshold inputs to the DCMD, the physiological nature of the LGMD/DCMD synapse will be described.

The LGMD/DCMD Synapse

Action potentials in the DCMD appear to arise without preceding epsp's. While this result could be obtained by recording too far from the zone of initiation to see the epsp, it was also possible that no chemical epsp existed, and that the synapse was electrotonic. If the synapse is electrotonic we would expect the spike recorded in the DCMD's integrating segment to be a compound potential composed of the LGMD spike seen through the synapse plus the DCMD's axon spike. On close examination, the potential recorded in the DCMD's integrating segment was seen to have an abrupt change of slope on its falling phase, suggesting that it was a compound potential. We were able to fractionate this potential and show that it was composed by the addition of the DCMD's axon spike with a potential derived from the LGMD (O'Shea and Rowell, 1975a) (see Fig. 4). Our evidence suggests that the potential derived from the LGMD is an electrotonic epsp, the most compelling evidence being the presence of a small potential, recorded in the LGMD terminal, which results from antidromic stimulation of DCMD. [It has, however, been stressed

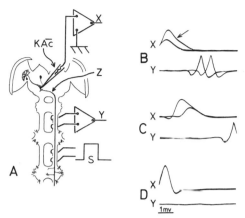

Fig. 4. Compound nature of the potential recorded postsynaptically in the DCMD integrating segment. Electrode positions are shown in A. B: The larger intracellular potential on trace X is recorded in the DCMD integrating segment during the passage of a normal, orthodromic, visually induced spike. Note shoulder (arrow) on the trailing edge of the waveform. The smaller waveform is a spontaneous "injury" spike, presumed to originate at the impulse initiation zone of the axon (Z) and to be transmitted electrotonically from that point to the integrating segment. A similar potential can be recorded by stimulating the DCMD axon antidromically from S. In C, the same two previous records are brought together by superimposing the extracellular axon spike recordings (trace Y). Note that the later part of the shoulder is convincingly fitted to the axon spike component. In D is seen the result of a visually induced orthodromic spike in the LGMD which failed to elicit an axon spike in the DCMD (note clear Y trace) because of fatigue at the IIZ caused by high-frequency antidromic stimulation from S. This represents the psp component of the compound potential. When it is summed arithmetically with the axon spike potential (the smaller potential in trace X of B), a waveform virtually identical with the compound (large waveform in trace X of B) potential is produced.

(Bennett, 1972) that electrical and chemical synapses are not readily distinguished and that only simultaneous intracellular recording both pre- and postsynaptically will suffice in itself as proof. For our complete evidence, see O'Shea and Rowell, 1975a.]

Under orthodromic stimulation, the electrical epsp is suprathreshold and transmission occurs 1:1. On rare occasions in our experiments, however, when LGMD spikes in rapid succession, the epsp can be reduced in amplitude, and DCMD may not spike in response to it. A reduction to about 80% is sufficient to prevent spike initiation in the DCMD. This shows that the safety factor at this synapse is smaller than its normal behavior suggests, and it indicates a possible function for the chemical synaptic potentials recordable in DCMD. Any permeability increase in DCMD will tend to shunt the electrical epsp and reduce the probability of spike initiation. Chemical epsp's in DCMD will tend to have an inhibitory or gating effect on the relay properties of the electrical synapse. Since both excitatory and inhibitory psp's are present, it is likely that this is not the only function of chemical synaptic potentials in the integrating segment; some may be spike initiating, for example. Our understanding of the integrative role of DCMD is clearly incomplete, but the modulation we suggest here as being theoretically possible may explain the puzzling failures in responsiveness of DCMD which are occasionally seen in animals with chronically implanted extracellular electrodes under seminatural behavioral conditions (Rowell, 1971*b,c*).

We have seen that in most experimental circumstances the DCMD acts as a relay, the response characteristics of the DMDs are not primarily a function of connections with antecedent neurons, and their origin must be sought in LGMD. Spikes in LGMD can be initiated in both the visual and auditory modalities, and since there is no subthreshold interaction and the two are essentially independent the origin of responses in each modality will be considered separately.

Visual Responsiveness of the LGMD

The LGMD responds with spikes over a wide range of adapting intensities to both negative and positive changes in illumination of a test target previously kept at the adapting intensity. It therefore behaves as an on–off unit. The response to movement is derived by summation of the relatively small responses to change in intensity of illumination over small areas of the retina; moving objects produce a succession of such local changes (see also Palka, 1967*a*). While it has been known for some time that the DMDs are excited by both on and off stimuli (Palka, 1967*a*; Horn and Rowell, 1968), there has until recently (Rowell and O'Shea, 1976*a*) been no systematic study of the response to quantitative changes in light intensity or of the effect of light and dark adaptation.

The ability of the MD system to detect movement is maximized if the system responds to very small differences in contrast between the background and the moving object. At all light intensities experienced by a diurnal insect, the DMD response saturates within 0.5 $\log_{10}$ unit of contrast, and within even less at high adapting luminances (Rowell and O'Shea, 1976*a*). Only at very low background illumination is there a greater dynamic range, a more graded response to contrast. Variations in background intensity (adapting luminance) therefore make little difference to the response elicited by a moving object as long as it differs from its background by more than a small amount in either direction. The adaptive significance is that this allows the system to respond uniformly regardless of an environment which is heterogeneous in its light intensity.

When the same area of the retina is stimulated repetitively, the response of the MD neurons decrements. Decrement is site specific; unstimulated areas of the receptive field are unaffected. This means that the process responsible for decrement must be located prior to the site of convergence of the retinotopic projection, and we can therefore reject as candidate mechanisms of decrement any which are postconvergent. A necessary condition for identifying the site of decrement is the identification of the site of convergence.

Visual stimuli of the sort which produce spike activity and decrement in the DMD neurons elicit epsp's which are at their largest in the fanlike dendrites of

LGMD and are reduced or invisible at all other sites in the neuron. The fan is therefore the zone of synaptic contact from the excitatory afferents converging on it from more peripheral or distal parts of the visual system. The ultimate site of convergence in this system is the point at which spikes are initiated on the single axon of LGMD. A change in spike threshold prior to the point of convergence is one possible mechanism of decrement (Stephens, 1973). There is, however, no evidence to suggest that decrement in the MD system involves an increase in spiking threshold (O'Shea and Rowell, 1976). The fall in the number of DCMD spikes on repeated visual stimulation is accompanied in LGMD fan dendrites by a diminution in amplitude of the compound epsp. This diminution continues beyond the point at which spikes fail to initiate in the LGMD, showing that decrement is in no way a consequence of the cell's spiking output, e.g., by recurrent inhibition. The reduction in spike number during habituation is a consequence of the decrement in epsp amplitude (Fig. 5).

The epsp seen in the fan could decrease either as a result of processes occurring at the afferent–LGMD synapse or as a result of a more distally located process. To distinguish between these and to locate the site of decrement, we had to demonstrate decrementing epsp's in the fan dendrites as a result of repetitively exciting the afferents which connect monosynaptically with them.

Fine paired stimulating electrodes were placed in the presynaptic area, and we found that single shocks produced decrementing epsp's recorded in the fan dendrites (Fig. 6). With stimulating electrodes placed in the distal part of the second chiasma, the latency of the decrementing epsp is 2.25 msec. Allowing for a conduction delay between stimulating and recording sites, we believe that this latency represents a monosynaptic connection, as the chiasma itself is devoid of synapses. The mechanism underlying decrement therefore is located either pre- or postsynaptically at the junction between the afferents of the chiasma and the dendrites of the LGMD fan. One possible postsynaptic mechanism (a change in spiking threshold) has been eliminated. Of those remaining, it can be shown that decrement is not associated with an increase in membrane conductance postsynaptically, neither is there any association between decrement and ipsp's. A telling piece of evidence against most postsynaptic mechanisms is the presence of an excitatory input which results in epsp's in the fan which are resistant to decrement at all but the highest repetition rates (O'Shea and Rowell, 1976). Currently, we favor the hypothesis that site-specific response decrement in the MD system is due to a process occurring in the excitatory terminals on LGMD fan dendrites.

Dishabituation of the MD system occurs in response to arousing stimuli and counteracts the initial decremental process (Rowell and Horn, 1968; Rowell, 1971b,c, 1974). Unlike habituation, it is not site specific, affects simultaneously the whole receptive field, and does not enhance the response to a previously unstimulated area. There is no electrophysiological event in the fan which can be recorded during dishabituation, suggesting that this is a presynaptic process. It is highly unlikely that a presynaptic process could operate in such a way as to compensate for a postsynaptic decrement without incrementing the response to nonhabituated areas

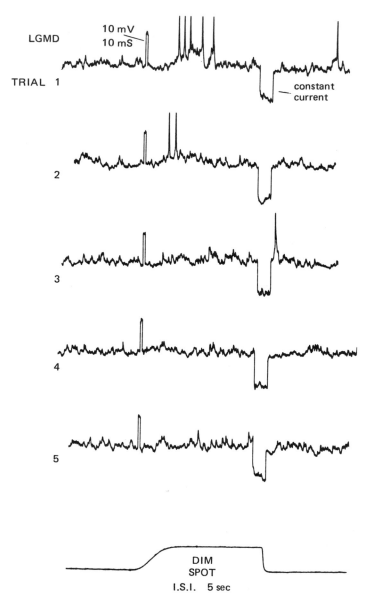

Fig. 5. Decrementing epsp's produced in LGMD by repetitive visual stimulation. A: Response recorded by an intracellular electrode in the LGMD fan during repetitive stimulation of the eye due to the dimming of a small (5°) area of the visual field. The time course of the intensity change of the test area is shown in the bottom trace, where upward indicates a decrease, and the amplitude of the change is approximately 2 $\log_{10}$ units. Interstimulus interval: 5 sec. The response consists initially of a compound epsp which generates several spikes. With repetition, the amplitude of the epsp and the number of spikes it elicited decrease rapidly; the records shown come from five consecutive stimuli. A short pulse of hyperpolarizing current injected through the recording electrode after each stimulus produces a constant voltage deflec-

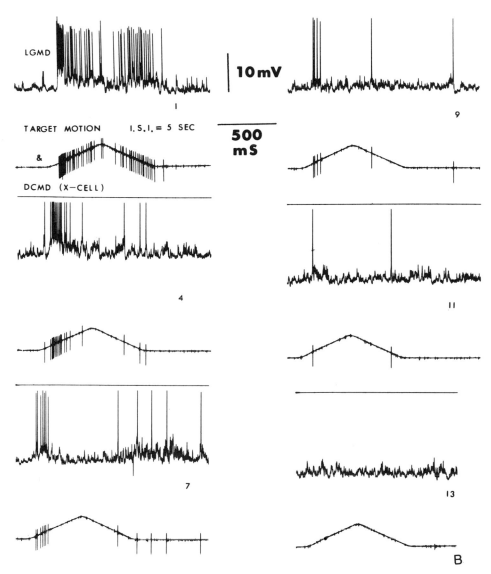

tion throughout the series; there is no indication of a marked change in membrane resistance which might account for the decreasing efficacy of the epsp. B: Upper trace as in A (intracellular record from LGMD fan) while the eye is stimulated by the to-and-fro movement of a 10° black disk against a white background. The triangular waveform corresponding to the movement of the disk is shown in the lower trace, and superimposed on it is an extracellular record of DCMD spikes in the ventral nerve cord. Interstimulus interval: 5 sec. The presentation number is indicated beside each recording. The initially large compound epsp decreases in amplitude with repetition, and the number of spikes it elicits decreases likewise.

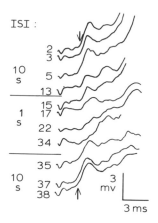

Fig. 6. Short-latency decrementing epsp produced in the LGMD fan by focal electrical stimulation in the second optic chiasma. A pair of fine bipolar electrodes were introduced into the optic lobe through a small hole in the retina and advanced into the chiasma. Their position was ascertained by measurement and subsequently verified by passing a coagulating current and examining the fixed tissue histologically. Because of the small size of the chiasma units and the large size of the LGMD fan, most attempts at stimulation in the chiasma merely excited the LGMD directly. The figure shows the shortest-latency epsp's which were recordable before this happened. The oscilloscope traces show an initial negative inflection, which is a stimulus artifact, and thereafter the start of the compound epsp which is elicted by electrical stimulation. The first inflection of this (arrows) is examined during repetitive stimulation. It shows some decrement with an interstimulus interval of 10 sec, and is rapidly eliminated by stimulating at an ISI of 1 sec; it recovers when placed once more on the slower regime. The latency of the component is about 2.25 msec. Calculation suggests that this represents a monosynaptic synapse.

(for further discussion, see Rowell, 1971b). This is yet further evidence against a postsynaptic model for site-specific decrement.

There are few examples in which the locus responsible for behaviorally significant decrement has been established. In the best known of these (crayfish escape response: Zucker *et al.,* 1971; Zucker, 1972b; the central component of the gill-withdrawal reflex in *Aplysia:* Kandel, 1974; and the giant fiber system of some insects: (Murphey, Matsumoto, and Levine, 1975; Callec *et al.,* 1971), the physiological event underlying decrement has been localized to the primary afferent synapses. There has been a tendency to generalize from these observations, and it has been suggested that the primary afferent synapse is the logical site for behaviorally significant decrement. In the MD system, however, this is not the site of decrement; it seems likely to us that this site will be determined in any particular system by at least two factors: (1) the amount of sensory processing required to abstract significant information from the receptors and (2) the number of independent behavioral systems to which the receptors contribute. Both these qualities are likely to be at their lowest in the crayfish tail-flip circuit or the *Aplysia* gill-withdrawal circuit, which are initiated by phasic receptors having little other function. In the MD system, the raw retinal cell output is processed over many synaptic layers. The same output is differentiated for many other purposes, e.g., form, movement, and direction. Retinotopic information is preserved in some and not in others. The primary afferent synapse seems an unlikely choice for decrement in a sensory system subserving and combining different functions, many of which may require decrement resistant information.

The MD neurons are on–off units (see above). The retinal receptors are on units, and all second-order visual cells so far established in insects are off units, so it seems clear that the on–off properties of the MD neurons are derived by convergence of separate on and off channels. The convergence could take place on the fan itself—i.e., the fan receives two separate on and off projections. The other alternative is that on and off channels converge prior to the lobula, and the LGMD receives a single projection of combined on–off excitatory channels. It is possible to distinguish between these alternatives on the basis of the response of the system to habituating stimuli, given that the afferent synapse to the LGMD is the site of decrement. There will be generalization of decrement between on and off channels if the projection is of a single on–off nature but not if the two classes project via separate synapses onto the LGMD. In the latter case, there will be no interaction, and habituating an area of the visual field to, say, on stimuli would not decrease the response to off stimuli. Our results (see O'Shea and Rowell, 1976) fulfill the first prediction and show that the LGMD fan is fed by on–off units via labile synapses at which decrement occurs.

The response of the MD neurons to similar stimuli in different parts of their receptive field shows that sensitivity is not homogeneous. There is a rather complex gradient of sensitivity (Palka, 1967a; Rowell, 1971a) which can be summarized by saying that responsiveness is greatest at the center of the posterior sector of the visual field, and that, in addition, sensitivity falls symmetrically dorsally and ventrally and asymmetrically in the anteroposterior axis such that anterior parts are less stimulating than equivalent posterior parts. Such variation in sensitivity could be produced by systematic variation in the properties of the small-field afferents feeding the LGMD, but it is possible to produce it in the absence of differences between presynaptic units. The shape of the LGMD fan and its relationship to the site of axonal spike initiation suggest a mechanism. Identical units synapsing with the fan will have a relative potency depending on their proximity to the zone of spike initiation and the internal geometry of the fan arborization. The retinotopic projection in the locust is twice laterally reversed in the two chiasmata, which results in the retina being mapped on to the LGMD fan in the following way. The anterior parts project to the most distal parts of the fan dendrites, the posterior retina projects onto the proximal parts of the dendrites, and the dorsoventral axis projects dorso-ventrally onto the fan. This organization suggests an asymmetrical, dorsoventral gradient (decreasing sensitivity dorsally and ventrally) and a gradient of increasing sensitivity from anterior to posterior. This is more or less fulfilled by the gradients described above. A major discrepancy does, however, exist. At the extreme posterior margin of the visual field, sensitivity falls markedly. It may be that the very thick proximal segments of the fan's dendrites, to which these posterior regions project, have a reduced input impedance, thus reducing the synaptic potency of connections there. This can account for the low sensitivity of the extreme posterior field in spite of the close proximity to the zone of spike initiation of the thickened proximal dendrites. It seems to us that the major features of the sensitivity gradient in the receptive field of the MD neurons are more likely to be determined by the LGMD than by heterogeneity among the small-field afferents. Such heterogeneity would certainly have to be specific to the MD neurons. This is because the LGMD will impose a sensitivity gradient, and to suppose that presynaptic heterogeneity compensates for this is a highly unattractive hypothesis—it implies that an array of potentially versatile units becomes the slave to a single neural system.

We have now to account for one of the most striking features of the visual responsiveness of the MD neurons—their bias in favor of small rather than large objects, and the consequent insensitivity to whole-field movements. There are many mechanisms which could account for the spatial frequency-tuning characteristics of the MD neurons, but we will see that the actual mechanism employed is to a large extent determined by the complex requirements imposed by their novelty-detecting property (O'Shea and Rowell, 1975b). Direct inhibition of the LGMD by the excited afferents could produce the preference for small- over large-area stimulation. In fact, there is such an inhibition of the LGMD; it is excited by large-area stimuli ($\geq 20°$) and can prevent the initiation of spikes in response to a concurrent small-field stimulus (Fig. 7A). The inhibitory connection is made with the branch of LGMD closest to the site of spike initiation in the visual modality (subfield C of O'Shea and Williams, 1974). Directed as it is at the site of initiation, it is postconvergent and can be recognized in extracellular recordings from DCMD because its effect is equal over the entire receptive field. This type of inhibition was first noted by Palka (1967a), who suggested that it is responsible both for suppressing the response of the DMDs to movements of the visual field caused by the animal's own locomotion and for the existence of an "optimal area" effect, which he also described.

Can postconvergent inhibition explain the preference in the MD system for small-area stimulation? We were initially attracted by this idea but were forced to reject it because we demonstrated this to be incompatible with the requirements of the novelty-detecting property of the LGMD. The ipsp is not diminished when elicited at intervals which produce rapid decrement of the excitatory small-field response. It must therefore be derived from a predecremental site and fed forward, past the site of lability, to the LGMD. Therefore, if postconvergent inhibition were responsible for the preference for small-field stimuli, prolonged whole- or large-field movements would reduce the responsiveness of the LGMD to subsequent small-field movements, and the DMDs would habituate in response to stimulation caused by the animal's own locomotion. This is clearly maladaptive and does not happen (Fig. 7B). The responsiveness of the LGMD must be suppressed prior to the site of response decrement and therefore prior to the site of convergence. Protection from habituation and suppression of response to large-field movement is achieved by lateral inhibition acting prior to the site of decrement (Fig. 7C). This lateral

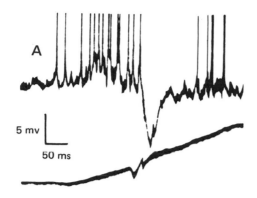

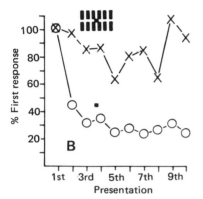

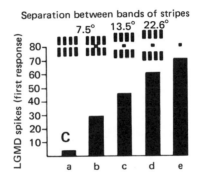

Fig. 7. A: Postconvergent inhibition in a LGMD produced by rapid displacement of the whole visual field. The upper trace is an intracellular record from a branch in the LGMD fan. The slow ramp in the lower trace is the voltage analogue of the movement across the visual field of a small (about 10°) target, which produces a barrage of epsp's and impulses. The background consists of vertical black and white stripes. About half way through the response, the background is moved abruptly for a period of 50 msec. This is indicated by inflections on the ramp. The movement of the background produces a strong hyperpolarization which suppresses the response to small-field movement. B: Response is suppressed by large-field movements at a velocity which does not produce hyperpolarization in the LGMD. The locus of the suppression is prior to the site of response decrement and therefore protects the labile synapses from depression during whole-field movements. The response to repeated movements of the small target alone shows rapid decrement from its original high level (O–O). When a large area of moving stripes is added to the stimulus in close proximity to the target, however, the response is not only depressed but also shows no significant decrement (×–×). Both curves are normalized for comparison. C: Lateral inhibition of the response to a small target. The lateral movement of two bands of vertical stripes, which extend horizontally across the visual field, at a speed corresponding to seven transitions per second at the retinal cell, produces very few spikes in the LGMD (a). This spped of movement produces no inhibition in the LGMD itself. When a small black target is added to the stripes, the response is appreciably increased (b). The size of the response is a function of the proximity of the striped pattern to the small target (b–d) and the full response to the target is not seen until the stripes are totally removed (e).

322   Michael O'Shea and C. Hugh Fraser Rowell

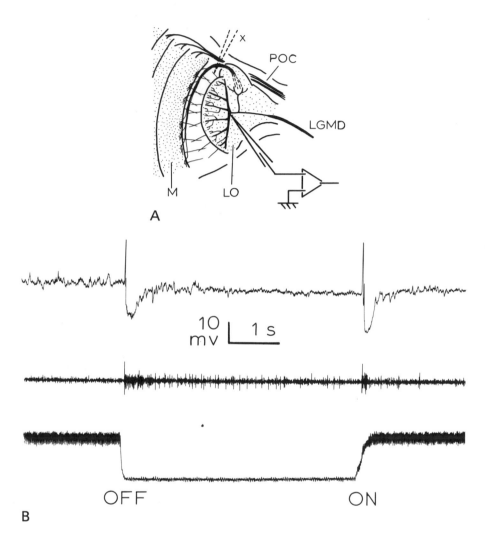

Fig. 8. Feedforward inhibition on to the LGMD. A: Frontal section of the optic lobe in the area of the second optic chiasma. M, Medulla; LO, lobula; POC, fibers running in posterior optic commissure. A recording microelectrode is placed intracellularly in the fan of the LGMD. Chiasma afferents leave the proximal face of the medulla and insert on the receiving face of the lobula. Additionally, the axons of some 200 other neurons, with 20° by 30° dendritic fields in the proximal face of the medulla, run upward across the chiasmatic projection and form an uncrossed dorsal bundle which runs slightly anterior to the posterior optic commissure and ramifies within the dorsal horn of the lobula. This area of neuropil also contains the dorsal dendritic field of the LGMD (subfield C of O'Shea and Williams, 1974). In some experiments, a lesion (X) was made in the dorsal surface of the optic lobe at the level of the chiasma, severing the dorsal uncrossed bundle and usually some fibers of the posterior optic commissure as well. B: Recordings from the LGMD fan prior to lesion. Top trace, LGMD fan, intracellularly; middle trace, ventral nerve cord, extracellularly, showing DCMD spikes; bottom trace, photocell output. The 60-Hz ripple indicates that the fluorescent room lights are on. Whole-field on and off stimuli are generated by turning the room lights on and off; the stimulus amplitude is about 0.5 $\log_{10}$ unit. Both stimuli elicit

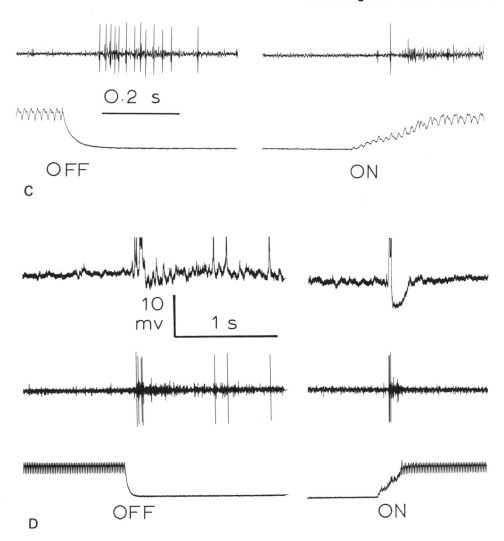

epsp's which generate one or a few spikes and subsequently large compound ipsp's which curtail spiking. C: Extracellular recording after lesion to dorsal uncrossed bundle, showing DCMD spikes. Before this record, the preparation was rested for 10 min in order to show a relatively unhabituated response. Compared with the control, the off response consists of an unprecedentedly large burst (whole-field stimuli rarely elicit more than two or three spikes at most), whereas the on response is normal. D: As in C, but this time with an intracellular record from the LGMD as well. In this case, the necessity of holding the penetration does not allow so long a rest interval since the last stimulus, and the response is therefore less than in C, although still much larger than the control. Note that the lesion has virtually abolished all the ipsp's from the off response, and instead a complex series of epsp's are revealed, comparable in duration to the spike burst seen in the unfatigued preparation in C. The on response is normal, with the ipsp intact as in the control. These experiments show that the off and on ipsp's are mediated by independent pathways, that the off ipsp is mediated by the uncrossed dorsal bundle, and that the ipsp's serve to limit the large response to whole-field stimuli which would otherwise occur.

inhibitory network is fed by phasic on–off units and is not activated at all during tonic illumination—a characteristic which distinguishes it from another, more peripheral, tonic lateral inhibitory network (Rowell and O'Shea, 1976*b*; Rowell *et al.*, 1977).

What, then, is the function of postconvergent inhibition? We found that the ipsp's which mediate it are evoked only when large areas of the visual field are stimulated simultaneously, as happens, for example, with large-field on or off stimuli, or with movement of large fields at high-contrast frequencies. At low-contrast frequencies, whole-field movements produce neither epsp's in the LGMD (attributable to phasic lateral inhibition) nor ipsp's. A simple lateral inhibition circuit cannot discriminate against transient, whole-field excitation (Rowell *et al.*, 1977); this can be achieved only by some form of feedforward inhibition. We have been able to show that the postconvergent ipsp's in LGMD derive independently from on and off units in the medulla, and so represent feedforward inhibition of this type (Rowell *et al.*, 1977). Postconvergent inhibition supplements the effectiveness of the lateral inhibition network by blanking the response to transient large-field stimuli which would otherwise occur. So, when, for example, the off inhibitory pathway is blocked by cutting of the tract of axons which mediate it, the LGMD gives a large burst of spikes in response to a whole-field on stimulus. The on inhibitory pathway is unaffected by this lesion, and whole-field on stimuli continue to elicit the ipsp which blocks spike initiation in the LGMD (Fig. 8).

Lateral inhibition supplemented by feedforward postconvergent inhibition not only produces the specific preference for small-area stimuli but also protects the labile synapses in the system from the results of self-generated afferent stimulation. Such stimulation arises from rapid movement of either the whole animal (e.g., in jumping, flight, or rapid walking) or of the head alone (e.g., during saccades, which in *Schistocerca* can produce angular velocities of up to 600°/sec: Kien and Land, unpublished). A functionally similar but very different circuit has been described in the crayfish (Krasne and Bryan, 1973; Kennedy *et al.*, 1974), where presynaptic inhibition of the afferents is derived from the animal's motor command. Lateral inhibition networks such as that described above can perform a similar function and protect against both endogenous and exogenous large-field stimuli. They may have a general role in protecting interneurons with wide receptive fields and a preference for novel and local stimulation (O'Shea and Rowell, 1975*b*).

Auditory Responsiveness of the LGMD

The response of the LGMD to sound is highly phasic; usually only one spike is initiated (Palka and Pinter, 1975; O'Shea, 1975). Spikes initiated in the auditory modality travel along the LGMD axon in the opposite direction to those initiated in the visual modality (O'Shea, 1975). The LGMD is a bimodal IN with two modality-specific sites of axonal spike initiation.

We were able to use this fact to confirm our earlier hypothesis that visual spikes are initiated at the abrupt thickening of the LGMD axon in the optic peduncle (see Fig. 3). The conduction velocity of an LGMD axon is 3 m/sec, which is effectively the same as that of DCMD (Burrows and Rowell, 1973). Auditory and visual spikes are recorded with different latencies at electrodes placed in an LGMD fan in the optic lobe, in the proximal part of an LGMD axon, and on a DCMD axon of the thoracic nerve cord (Fig. 9). This is because visual spikes are initiated distally and propagate first past the recording electrode in the LGMD axon and then down the cord to the third electrode. Auditory spikes, by contrast, are initiated at the proximal end of the LGMD axon and propagate in both directions toward optic lobe and nerve cord.

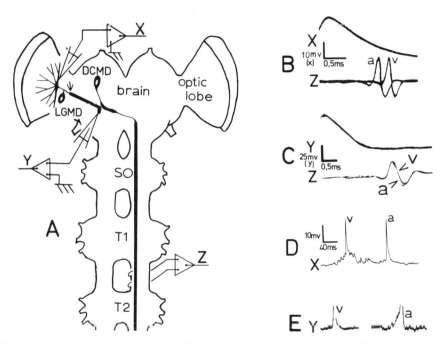

Fig. 9. A: Anatomy of the LGMD and DCMD as drawn from cobalt impregnation. The abrupt thickening of the LGMD axon is marked with an arrow. The LGMD and DCMD make electrical synaptic contact in the brain, and the DCMD extends its axon through the subesophageal (SO) ganglion and the first (T1) and second (T2) thoracic ganglia to the third thoracic ganglion. B: Upper trace is an intracellular recording from the LGMD at site X and the lower is an extracellular recording from the DCMD axon at Z. The oscilloscope was triggered from the LGMD spike and stimuli were provided in both visual and auditory modalities. Two distinct classes of latency are evident. The latency in response to auditory stimulation (a) is shorter by 0.38 msec than to visual stimulation (v). In each modality, five sweeps of the oscilloscope are superimposed. C: Upper trace is an intracellular recording from the LGMD at site Y, and the lower trace is an extracellular recording of the DCMD at Z. Here the auditory DCMD spike precedes only fractionally the visual spike, showing that site Y is very close to the initiation site for auditory spikes. D: An intracellular recording from site X in the LGMD. The first impulse is visual and arises from a compound epsp. The second (a), initiated by auditory stimulation, arises abruptly from baseline. E: At recording site Y in the LGMD, visual spikes (v) arise abruptly without preceding psp and auditory spikes (a) arise from epsp's.

Under these circumstances, the time of arrival of a spike at the optic lobe electrode and that at the cord electrode differ for visual and auditory spikes by a time equal to twice the time taken to propagate between the two zones of impulse initiation (IIZ). This time can be converted into spatial separation. The hypothesis that the abrupt axonal thickening is the IIZ for visual spikes can now be tested directly by moving the electrode from the fan and placing it in the LGMD axon the calculated distance from the thickening. At this point, there should be no difference in conduction time between auditory and visual spikes. This prediction was confirmed (Fig. 9).

We have started to identify at least one auditory IN which synapses with the LGMD. Extracellular recordings from the ipsilateral nerve cord reveal an ascending IN which makes an excitatory chemical synapse with the LGMD in the protocerebrum, close to the LGMD/DCMD synapse. Our recordings (Fig. 10) suggest that the cord unit connects monosynaptically with LGMD. In spite of this, however, spikes recorded from this neuron's axon in the nerve cord are not always followed 1:1 by epsp's in the LGMD (Fig. 10D), and recordings from the output terminals of the auditory unit, close to its connection with the LGMD, may reveal the reason for this. The capacity of the main axon of this cell to carry spikes at high frequency is not sustained by the branch which connects with LGMD. At high frequencies, the auditory spikes are truncated, presumably because they occur in the relative refractory period of the previous spike. This branch of the auditory neuron therefore appears to be far more phasic than the main axon, and the auditory response of the LGMD is even more phasic, because the diminished spikes do not release sufficient transmitter to be measured as a psp. During a dense burst of spikes in the auditory neuron, the labile synapse on the LGMD is therefore protected against synaptic depression. We are currently looking at the output connection made by this IN with metathoracic MNs, including those with which the DMD neurons also connect. Preliminary results suggest that it makes excitatory connection with the FETi.

Conclusions

There are a number of aspects of the MD system which we have not touched on in this chapter. Some have been mentioned elsewhere (e.g., Rowell, 1976). Sufficient has been said, however, to present the outline of what we believe to be the neuronal basis of the system, and to justify some generalizations.

Studies of identified INs are in their infancy. These neurons may, and almost certainly will, be found to have many functions, and it would therefore be naive of us to suppose that one IN (in our case, the LGMD) is devoted exclusively to that role which it plays in our experiments. A LGMD is integrated into the CNS and we can account for only one of its output connections. Certainly the LGMD tells us something about how or when a locust will jump, but, perhaps more importantly, it provides us with insights into more general problems of integration. One cannot, for

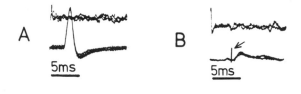

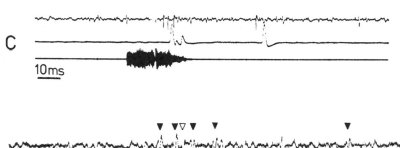

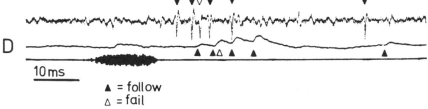

▲ = follow
△ = fail

Fig. 10. A: Upper trace is triggered from an extracellular recording of an ascending auditory unit contained in the thoracic nerve cord. The lower trace shows a simultaneous intracellular recording from the terminals of the unit in the brain, in the vicinity of the junction between the ipsilateral LGMD and the DCMD. Several sweeps of the oscilloscope are superimposed. B: The upper trace is as in A. The lower shows an epsp recorded in the LGMD close to the LGMD/DCMD synapse. The bar (arrow) marks the estimated arrival time in the brain of the spike recorded in the thorax from the presynaptic auditory unit. The latency suggests a monosynaptic connection. C: First two traces are as in A. The bottom trace is a sound monitor. Note that spikes in the brain terminals of the auditory unit (center trace) are attenuated when they follow each other in rapid succession. D: This reduced amplitude is reflected in the occasional failure of epsp's in the LGMD to follow 1:1 axon spikes of the auditory unit (upper trace). In D, the auditory unit was not penetrated prior to entering the LGMD, and it is unlikely therefore that the failure of the brain terminals of the auditory unit to follow 1:1 the axon spikes is attributable to their injury.

example, study a complex IN for long without coming up against the acute problem of deciding between what is noise and what is message in the CNS.

Consider, for example, bimodality in INs. We can ask whether action potentials in such cells are ambiguous. Bi- and multimodality are not unusual features of neurons (indeed, it is difficult to imagine the existence of truly monomodal INs). If multimodality implies a high degree of noise because individual impulses cannot be interpreted in a unique way, the CNS may indeed be largely indeterministic at the level of the single neuron. In that case, it is not sufficient to study only the single identified neuron (see John, 1972, and Bullock, 1969, for detailed treatment of this kind of argument).

The discovery of modality-coded activity in a bimodal neuron challenges this view, because the individual spike in such a cell is no longer *necessarily* ambiguous. This depends on the ability of postsynaptic units to detect the temporal differences corresponding to the two sites, and several suitable mechanisms are available (e.g., see Rall, 1964). But do multimodal cells actually work in this multiplex way? How commonly in complex INs is modality coded by its position? Are the various inputs to such a cell organized for some developmental expedient, or are the sites of spike initiation determined in the interests of integrative processes at whose nature we can only guess? Questions of this type can be approached only by the rigorous identification of more INs and the realization that current neuron doctrine is probably hopelessly naive.

In addition to allowing for informed speculation on the general role of complex INs, our "identified neuron" approach to the locust MD system has provided us with insights into many aspects of complex neural mechanisms associated with lability, stimulus filtration, and the elicitation of specific behavior in response to diverse sensory input. These aspects of behavior are clearly orders of magnitude more complex than the simple reflex response, and as such should be of interest to ethologists. Understandably, the many students of behavior have not been attracted by the neural analysis of reflex behavior that has constituted most of the research on behavior done by neurophysiologists until recently. Now that the identified neuron revolution is well under way, there is hope that a fertile interaction between neurobiologists and ethologists will develop as the more complex aspects of labile behavior progressively become accessible to electrophysiological technique.

ACKNOWLEDGMENTS

This work was supported by a NATO fellowship to M. O. and by a USPHS grant to C. H. F. R.

19

Interneurons in the Ventral Nerve Cord of Insects

Keir G. Pearson

Introduction

The majority of neurons in the nervous systems of vertebrates and invertebrates are interneurons (INs). Despite the enormous diversity in the anatomical properties of INs, in mammals at least, most can be readily classified as either *relay* INs or *local-circuit* INs (Rakic, 1975). Relay INs are those which function to transmit information from one discrete region in the nervous system to another, while local-circuit INs are those contained wholly within a localized region of the nervous system which function to integrate neural information within these regions. In addition to the anatomical and functional differences in these two classes of INs, there may be significant differences in their electrical properties since many local-circuit INs do not generate action potentials (Rakic, 1975; Pearson, 1976). Although this division of many types of INs into two classes seems reasonable, there are some obvious limitations to this classification. Some relay INs (e.g., mitral cells in the olfactory bulb) interact reciprocally with local-circuit INs and are therefore also involved in local integrative processes. Thus these INs are not strictly relay INs. Furthermore, to define an anatomically discrete region within certain parts of the central nervous system is often not possible, which means that some INs within these areas cannot be classified. To obviate these difficulties, it is probably better not to regard individual neurons as the only functional units within the nervous system (Shepherd, 1972, 1974). Spatially separated regions of certain neurons are now known to have different functions, and each region can interact locally with adjacent neurons (Nelson *et al.*, 1975; Shepherd, 1972). Thus, in some cases, it is better to regard a part of a neuron, or a part of a neuron plus parts of other neurons, as the functional unit (Shepherd, 1972).

At present, there is no generally accepted scheme for classifying INs within the nervous system of insects. The classification of INs as either relay or local-circuit applies for a number of identified neurons in insects, but the same difficulties arise with this scheme as when it is applied to mammalian systems. Indeed, in insects it

Keir G. Pearson • Department of Physiology, University of Alberta, Edmonton T6G 2E1, Alberta, Canada.

has been considered for many years that many single neurons cannot be regarded as single functional units (Hughes, 1965). Perhaps the clearest classification of INs within the insect nervous system is for those within the ventral nerve cord. Huber (1974) has made a distinction between "segmental" and "plurisegmental" INs, according to whether they respond solely to input into one ganglion or into a number of consecutive ganglia, or whether they drive motor actions organized within one or more ganglia. The most obvious problem with this classification is that it does not distinguish between those segmental INs which are contained wholly within a single ganglion and those which have axonal processes running in the connectives. For this reason, it seems more appropriate to classify the INs in the thoracic nerve cords of insects as either *intraganglionic* or *interganglionic* (according to whether they are contained wholly within one ganglion or have axonal processes running in the connectives). In the following sections of this chapter, some of the anatomical and functional properties of intra- and interganglionic INs are discussed. No attempt is made to review exhaustively all examples of these INs. For detailed information on INs, the reader is referred to articles by Miller (1974b) and Huber (1974).

Interganglionic INs

The most intensively studied interganglionic INs are the ascending giants originating in the sixth abdominal ganglion and terminating in the brain (Parnas and Dagan, 1971; Mendenhall and Murphey, 1974; Edwards and Palka, 1974) and the large descending movement-detecting neurons which originate in the brain and terminate in the metathoracic ganglion (Rowell, 1971a,b,c; O'Shea and Rowell, this volume; O'Shea *et al.*, 1974; Palka, 1969). Although the anatomy and response patterns of these groups of INs are well known, their motor functions are not clearly understood. Some of the earlier studies on the ascending giant INs indicated that they could be responsible for eliciting an escape response when cercal afferents are stimulated. This now appears unlikely since no physiological connections from the giant INs to motor neurons (MNs) initiating escape behavior have been demonstrated (Iles, 1972; Dagan and Parnas, 1970). The only motor response so far found to be elicited by the giant INs is activation of antennal MNs (Dagan and Parnas, 1970). The functional importance of this response is uncertain, but it may be related to a generalized alerting reaction in the animal. The activation of antennal MNs is unlikely to be the only function of the giant INs since processes leave their axons in each of the thoracic ganglia. This input to the thoracic ganglia may function to alter the excitability of various motor systems in preparation for an escape response. An obvious possibility which has not yet been studied is that the giant INs function to inhibit all overt behavior and thus cause a moving animal to become stationary. If this is a function of the giant ascending INs, the lack of any evoked motor responses to their activation would be understandable.

The descending movement-detecting INs have been shown to evoke mono-synaptic epsp's in the fast extensor MN in each metathoracic leg of the locust

(Burrows and Rowell, 1973). Since this MN is active mainly during jumping and kicking, it has been concluded that the movement-detecting INs are in some way involved in initiating a jump. However, observations on tethered animals have shown that visual stimuli which are known to selectively excite the movement-detecting INs very rarely evoke a jump (Rowell, 1971b) but often elicit a rapid flexion of the tibia to the fully flexed position. Full tibial flexion is a mechanical requirement for a jump to be initiated (Heitler, 1974). Thus, rather than initiating a jump, the descending movement-detecting INs may function to prepare the animal for a jump by positioning the tibia in full flexion. Muscle recordings have shown that the fast extensor tibiae MN is activated during this preparatory response, but its activation does not cause any extension movement since an unidentified fast flexor MN is activated at the same time (Pearson, unpublished observations). Since this is the only motor response so far found to be elicited by activity in descending movement-detecting INs, the function of the processes of the axons of these neurons in the pro- and mesothoracic ganglia remains a puzzle. Again, as for the ascending giant INs, these neurons may function to inhibit locomotory activity. Indeed, a very common response of walking locusts to a moving visual input is to cease walking immediately.

Another group of well-studied interganglionic INs are the ascending auditory INs of the locust (Kalmring, 1975a,b; Rheinlaender, 1975; Rehbein et al., 1974). Two different types have so far been identified physiologically and anatomically. The first are INs sending axonal processes from the metathoracic ganglion to the meso- and prothoracic ganglia but not to the head ganglia. These neurons are the first-order auditory INs directly activated by auditory afferents. The second class of auditory INs have axonal processes running from the metathoracic ganglion to the supraesophageal ganglion and are probably not excited directly by the auditory afferents. Studies on the response patterns of both types of INs to pure tones and natural sounds (Kalmring, 1975a,b; Rheinlaender, 1975) have led to hypotheses for the connectivity patterns of these INs and a detailed description of the transformational changes in auditory information as it ascends to the supraesophageal ganglion. The effect (if any) of activity in these INs on different motor systems is unknown.

Two types of interganglionic INs have been physiologically identified in the motor systems of some insects, namely, command and coordinating INs. High-frequency stimulation of what is probably a single axon in the pro-, mesothoracic connective in crickets has been shown to initiate the calling song (Bentley and Hoy, 1974). Unlike the present situation for crustaceans, where there are many examples of command INs (Larimer and Gordon, this volume), this is the only example in insects of a command IN. However, it is probable that command INs exist for initiating rhythmic leg movements during walking and wing movements during flight since stimulation of the thoracic cord, or dissected filaments of the cord, can initiate rhythmic leg movements (Elsner, 1970; Pearson, unpublished observations) and wing movements (Wilson and Wyman, 1965). Coordinating INs functioning to couple motor activity in different ganglia have been found in the cockroach walking system (Pearson and Iles, 1973) and the locust respiratory and flight systems (Burrows, 1975*a,b*; Miller, 1967). In no case has the anatomy of a command or coordinating IN been determined. Preliminary studies have indicated that the axons of these neurons are not among the largest in the cord (Bentley, personal communication), a fact which may make their anatomical identification difficult.

Intraganglionic INs

INs contained wholly within a single thoracic or abdominal ganglion were described in early anatomical studies on dragonfly larvae (Zawarzin, 1924*b*). Zawarzin described two types of intraganglionic INs, one type being axonless and the other type having a short axonlike process. He compared these with the amacrine and Golgi type II neurons which had been previously described in vertebrate nervous systems. The functional and physiological properties of these INs have not yet been determined. Quite recently, however, similar INs have been described in the metathoracic ganglion of the cockroach, and their physiological properties have been studied (Pearson and Fourtner, 1975). The total number of intraganglionic INs in insect thoracic and abdominal ganglia is unknown, but from an analysis of current data on the cockroach mesothoracic ganglion a rough estimate can be obtained. G. E. Gregory (personal communication) has estimated the number of intraganglionic INs by subtracting the number of neurons sending branches out of the lateral nerve trunks and connectives from the total number of neuron somata within the ganglion. The total number of MNs within the mesothoracic ganglion is a little over 300 (Gregory, 1974), and preliminary data on the number of neurons sending axons into the anterior or posterior connectives indicate that this number could be as high as 200 (Gregory, personal communication). Thus up to 500 somata have processes which leave the ganglion. The total number of neuron somata within the ganglion has been estimated to be approximately 1500 from soma counts in whole mounts (Gregory, 1977), which is considerably less than the figure of 3422 obtained from an analysis of serial sections (Cohen and Jacklet, 1967). This large difference probably reflects limitations in both methods for determining the total number of neuron somata. Glial tissue can be mistaken for neurons in the analysis of serial sections, while many small somata can easily be missed in whole mounts. For the present, however, it seems reasonable to conclude that the total number of somata is approximately 2000. Since up to 500 of these neurons send axonal processes from the ganglion, the surprising conclusion is reached that there are approximately 1500 intraganglionic INs in the ganglion.

Three characteristic features of all intraganglionic INs so far found in the cockroach ganglion are that they have a low resting potential (30–50 mV), they have a high level of synaptic activity, and they do not generate action potentials when depolarized (Pearson and Fourtner, 1975) (Fig. 1). Since these neurons do not have to relay information over long distances, their nonspiking behavior is understandable. However, it is not yet certain that all intraganglionic INs are nonspiking,

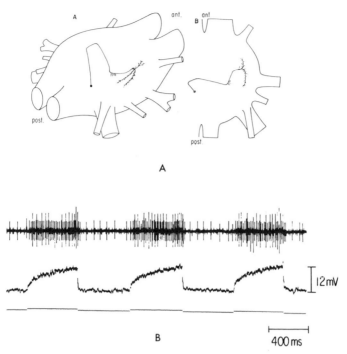

Fig. 1. IN 1 in the metathoracic ganglion of the cockroach *Periplaneta americana*. A: Structure. B: Excitation of leg flexor MNs (top trace) by application of a 10 nA depolarizing current (bottom trace) to IN 1. The intracellular record from IN 1 (middle trace) shows that the flexor MNs are excited without action potentials being generated in the INs. From Pearson and Fourtner (1975).

although preliminary data indicate that this is a good possibility. In a few cases where an unidentified spiking neuron has been intracellularly stained with cobalt, it has been found to send an axonal process out a connective or a lateral nerve trunk, while all neurons having the three characteristic features listed above have been found to be intraganglionic INs (Fourtner, personal communication).

Recent studies on the metathoracic ganglion of the locusts *Schistocerca nitens* and *Schistocerea gregoria* and the cricket *Teleogryllus oceanicus* have also revealed the existence of intraganglionic INs with electrical properties similar to those of intraganglionic INs in the cockroach; that is, the absence of spikes, a low resting potential, and a high level of spontaneous synaptic activity (Pearson, unpublished observations; Burrows, this volume) (Figs. 2, 3, and 4). Moreover, in the locust one of these INs is structurally and functionally similar to IN 1 in the cockroach (Figs. 1 and 3). This IN, when depolarized, strongly excites leg flexor MNs. A nonspiking neuron having a similar physiological effect has also been found in the cricket (Fig. 4), but its anatomy has not yet been determined. The similarity in the physiological and anatomical properties of IN 1 in the cockroach (Fig. 1) and an IN in the locust (Fig. 3) suggests there may be homologies in the organization and function of intraganglionic INs in different insect species. Many similarities of nerve tracts

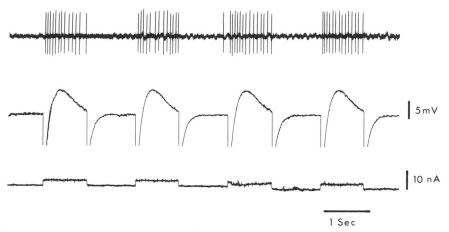

Fig. 2. Nonspiking IN exciting the slow extensor tibiae MN in the locust *Schistocerca nitens*. The activity in the MN (top trace) was recorded extracellularly from the nerve to the extensor tibiae muscle; 3 nA depolarizing current pulses (bottom trace) applied intracellularly to the IN excited the MN without action potentials being generated in the IN (middle trace). The intracellular record (middle trace) does not accurately show potential changes in the IN since the bridge circuit was not completely balanced.

within the thoracic ganglia of these animals (Gregory, personal communication) support this idea.

Conclusions

Within the past 10 years, there have been many investigations on INs within the ventral nerve cord of insects. All but one of these have been concerned with determining the anatomical and/or physiological properties of neurons with axonal processes relaying information to and from the head ganglia, or from one cord ganglion to another. As a result, most of our current knowledge about insect INs is based on the properties of these interganglionic INs. The recent discovery of nonspiking intraganglionic INs in the cockroach metathoracic ganglion (Pearson and Fourtner, 1975) and their existence in other insect species (Burrows, this volume) (Figs. 2, 3, and 4) clearly indicate that a whole new class of INs must now be considered in any future discussions of integrative mechanisms within the insect CNS. Present indications are that the majority of neurons within the thoracic and abdominal ganglia of insects are intraganglionic INs and that these INs do not generate action potentials. These conclusions parallel somewhat those in vertebrate nervous systems, where the majority of neurons within any discrete region are local-circuit INs; in many instances, these local-circuit INs do not generate action potentials (Rakic, 1975). This similarity between two diverse groups of animals immediately suggests that much integration and processing of neural information within the central nervous systems of most animals is carried out by graded interac-

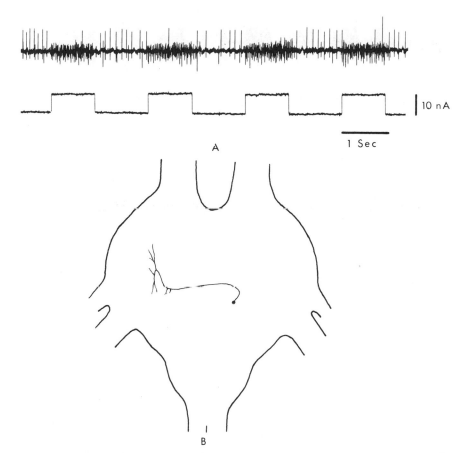

Fig. 3. A: Excitation of flexor tibiae MNs (small spikes in top trace) and inhibition of the slow extensor tibiae MN (large spike in top trace) by a 10 nA depolarizing current (bottom trace) applied to a nonspiking IN in the metathoracic ganglion of the locust *Schistocerca nitens*. MN activity was recorded with one electrode on the extensor nerve and the other in the flexor muscles. Therefore, the flexor spikes are extracellularly recorded junctional potentials from the flexor muscles and the slow extensor spike is an extracellular nerve recording. B: Structure of the IN determined by intracellular staining with cobalt. This neuron has a structure very similar to IN 1 in the cockroach (compare with Fig. 1A).

tions between small, nonspiking, axonless INs. Some of the functional advantages for this mechanism of interaction have been discussed elsewhere (Pearson, 1976).

One of the important implications of the conclusion that there exist large numbers of intraganglionic INs in the thoracic ganglia of a variety of insects is that these INs are involved in programming and patterning motor activity in most behaviors. The nonspiking intraganglionic INs described in the cockroach are considered to be involved in patterning motor activity during walking (Pearson and Fourtner, 1975), but as yet there is no direct evidence that intraganglionic INs are involved in patterning motor activity underlying other types of behavior. However,

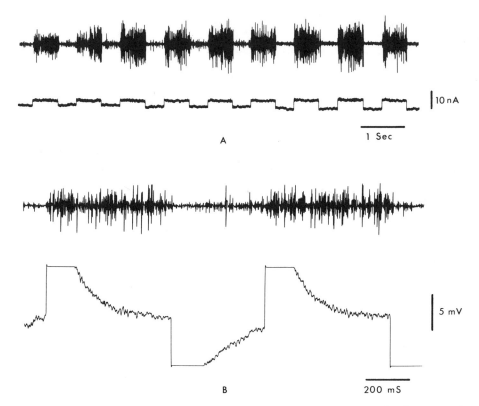

Fig. 4. A: Excitation of flexor tibiae MNs (top trace) by 5 nA depolarizing current pulses (bottom trace) applied to a nonspiking IN in the metathoracic ganglion of the cricket *Teleogryllus oceanicus*. Flexor activity was recorded by extracellular electrodes placed in the flexor muscle. Many motor units were excited by the depolarizing pulses. B: Intracellular record for the IN (bottom trace) showing the absence of spike activity in the IN during the flexor bursts (top trace). The intracellular record does not indicate D.C. changes in membrane potential since the amplifier was A.C. coupled and the bridge circuit was unbalanced. Same preparation as A.

it is clear that patterning of motor activity in locust flight (Burrows, 1973*a*), locust ventilation (Burrows, 1974), cricket stridulation (Bentley, 1969*b*), and locust jumping (Heitler and Burrows, 1976) occurs either wholly or partially at an IN level. Thus the involvement of intraganglionic INs must be considered in any future discussion on the generation of motor activity underlying these behaviors.

We are presently at a very exciting stage in our studies on the insect nervous system. The enormous increase in our knowledge of the anatomy and structure of the nervous system, combined with intracellular recording techniques, is giving us unexpected insights into the integrative events within the nervous system. We are, however, a long way from a full understanding of all these events. Just related to the problem of understanding the function of intraganglionic INs, we can ask many basic questions: (1) What is the anatomy of these INs and their distribution throughout the ganglion? (2) Can different anatomical groups be identified, and, if so, can all members of one group be classified as excitatory or inhibitory? (3) Are all intraganglionic INs nonspiking? (4) What are the synaptic mechanisms underlying graded interactions of intraganglionic INs? (5) What is the relation between the structure (gross and fine) of intraganglionic INs and their function? Many more questions readily spring to mind. Our present inability to answer these straightforward and simple questions points the way to an exciting decade of discovery ahead.

ACKNOWLEDGMENT

    I thank Drs. W. J. Heitler and C. H. F. Rowell for their valuable comments on and criticisms of the manuscript.

20

Flight Mechanisms of the Locust

Malcolm Burrows

Strategies for Neuroethology

The onus on those who choose to trace neural pathways in the central nervous system is to produce some general principles of neuronal organization. Detractors claim that this procedure produces only numerous and largely incomprehensible details relevant only to the particular piece of behavior of the particular animal under study. Just what is the task being undertaken, and will the tracing of neural pathways provide any answers? The task is to understand how a behavioral pattern is organized at the level of individual neurons. So complex are even those behavioral patterns normally considered to be "simple" that the immediate task becomes one of listing the components of the CNS and describing some of their interactions. We simply do not know what new types of neurons to expect or by what means they, or even the neurons we know already, are likely to communicate with each other.

An analysis of the components and their interactions needs to be carried out on physiologically and anatomically identified neurons during behavior. This method of analysis is not always compatible with the complexities of behavior; the unraveling of electrical activity in neurons becomes almost impossible when all pathways are active together. Two methods, behavioral and physiological, are therefore required, with continual cross-referencing between the two. Alas, there always seems to be a chasm between the two approaches which can rarely be bridged. First, there is the synthetic electrophysiological method which seeks to define connections between neurons and offers extrapolations as to how the behavior might be controlled. This method comes closest to offering explanations of behavior but usually fails because the definition of the elements of a circuit fails to predict the *emergent properties* of that circuit. Second, there is the analytical method, which seeks to make detailed observations of the behavior at an ethological level, or at the level of the action of the muscles or motor nerves. Inferences are then made about the organization of the neurons in the CNS which might have been responsible for producing the pattern. This method alone has singularly failed to give insights into neural mechanisms; given sufficient neurons, there are always many ways of inter-

Malcolm Burrows • Zoology Department, Cambridge University, Downing Street, Cambridge CB2 3EJ, England.

connecting them to produce a particular output. Over the past few years there has been a marked shift from the analytical method to the synthetic one as it was realized that the tools required are available. What is even better is a combination of both approaches in what is coming to be termed "neuroethology." Remarkable insights into mechanisms appear to be possible as a result (Elsner, 1975). I want to consider the problems and rewards that are associated with this combined approach by considering its uses in studying the flight of the locust.

Flight Machinery

During the five nymphal stages of the locust, the wing buds gradually grow but cannot be moved by the developing flight muscles. Nevertheless, first instar locusts hold their legs in a posture typical of flight when held in a wind stream, and rhythmic electrical activity can be recorded from flight muscles of fifth instars (Kutsch, 1971; Altman, 1975). On the first few days of adult life, the flight pattern is rather poor; the antagonists of one wing may alternate, but muscles of the fore- and hindwings often act together. The frequency of the wingbeats is low when elicited from newly molted locusts but increases gradually over the next 2 weeks as the locust matures, to double the original value (Kutsch, 1971). In a mature adult, flight is remarkable for the constancy of its frequency and the repeatability of its pattern. So constant is the frequency during steady flight that it can be predicted knowing the size and sex of the individual (Weis-Fogh, 1956); males have a higher wingbeat frequency than the larger females. Also remarkable is the stamina of a locust that can take on board some 15% of its body weight as fuel and they fly for some 5–8 hr covering 100 km a day, refuel by eating 1–1.5 times its body weight, and then continue flying another day. Some swarms of locusts have even been recorded to make 1600-mile flights in 60 hr across water, presumably wind assisted but nonstop and without refueling (Waloff, 1960).

The two pairs of wings of an adult are moved slightly out of phase with each other in a cycle of movement that lasts about 50 msec. Each wing is controlled, basically, by two sets of muscles that alternate, the elevators and the depressors (Fig. 1a). Such a description belies the complexity of the movement. There are about ten power-producing muscles for each wing, which are activated at a particular phase of the wingbeat cycle (Fig. 1b). The wing moves forward and downward during depression and upward and backward during elevation so that the wingtip of a tethered locust describes an ellipse (Jensen, 1956). During the downstroke the wing is also actively pronated, and during the upstroke it is supinated.

Successful flight could not be achieved by stereotyped movements of the wings. There must always be adjustments of the wings to take account of changes in the flow of air, and to allow the locust to change course. This stabilization and steering is made possible by sensors on the head and on the wings. Patches of hairs on the head give information about the direction of the wind and provide yaw, roll, and pitch stabilization (Camhi, 1970*a,b*). The antennae can control the flying speed, the amplitude of the wingstroke, and the frequency of the wingbeats (Gewecke, 1974). Campaniform sensilla on the wings monitor stress and are probably responsible for controlling the lift (Gettrup, 1966). Receptors at the articulation of the wing with the thorax exert a cycle-by-cycle influence on the flight pattern (Wendler, 1972, 1974).

All of these inputs eventually impinge upon the motor machinery that is contained within the three thoracic ganglia. When isolated from the rest of the CNS and from sensory inputs, these ganglia are capable of producing an alternating output of motor spikes to elevator and depressor muscles (Wilson, 1961). The pattern of motor spikes resembles that in normal flight except that it is of a much lower frequency. Therefore, within these ganglia is a *central pattern generator* for flight. The object of much work is to elucidate the connections between the neurons which make up this pattern generator and to see how it interacts with peripheral feedback loops and commands from the brain. This wording implies that the pattern generator is a discrete entity, separable from other neurons in the nervous system, but this may not be so.

Only about 80 motor neurons (MNs) are involved in moving the wings in flight. This small number of MNs is obviously attractive from the standpoint of analysis, but it should not be assumed that small numbers of neurons are involved at all the levels in the production of this motor pattern. Most of the MNs can be recognized as individuals either in recordings made extracellularly from the muscles (Wilson and Weis-Fogh, 1962) or in intracellular recordings from the CNS. It is this ability to work with identified neurons that makes invertebrates so useful. To use a known neuron is to allow direct comparison of experiments on different individuals and to allow the properties and connections of neuron A, as opposed to neuron B, to be determined. Such conclusions must be more useful than those that refer to only neurons of class A or class B. The separation of neurons into classes is bound to be fuzzy at the edges, for all neurons are individuals with common features as well as differences. Maps can be made of the positions within the ganglia of the somata of identified flight MNs that innervate particular muscles (Fig. 1c).

All the MNs share the following anatomical characteristics as revealed by intracellular staining with cobalt (Burrows, 1973*b*) or by backfilling with cobalt (Tyrer and Altman, 1974). The soma is devoid of dendrites and apparently receives no synapses. From the soma emerges a single neurite which plunges into the dorsal neuropil, where it dilates, giving off a profusion of side branches which themselves then branch further. It is on these fine branches that synapses with other neurons are presumed to be made, although there is no direct anatomical evidence for this in insects as yet. So profuse are the arborizations of the MNs that many problems spring to mind (Burrows, 1973*b*) which are far from being resolved. For example: In how many anatomical synapses is one physiologically defined synapse represented? What proportion of branches are inputs compared with outputs, or can a distinction be made between the two? Can different parts of a neuron act independently? And, most significant for the following discussion, what effect does a

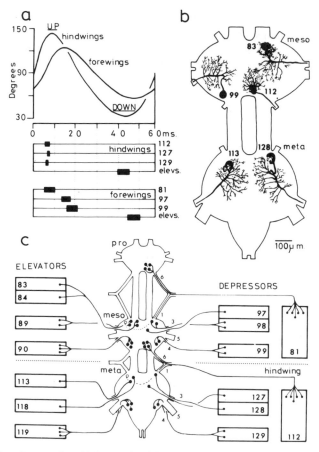

Fig. 1. MNs of the wing muscles. (a) One cycle of the wingbeat; hindwing MNs are active first so that the hindwing leads the forewing. The horizontal bars indicate the times at which the various muscles may be active. Redrawn from Wilson and Weis-Fogh (1962). (b) Structure of some flight MNs stained with cobalt. (c) Map of the positions of the somata of the MNs in the thoracic ganglia obtained by backfilling of appropriate nerve branches with cobalt chloride. The MNs and muscles are numbered after Snodgrass (1929) and are as follows: 81 and 112, dorsal longitudinal; 83, 84, and 113, tergosternal; 89 and 118, anterior tergocoxal; 90 and 119, first posterior tergocoxal; 97 and 127, first basalar; 98 and 128, second basalar; 99 and 129, subalar.

postsynaptic potential in a distant branch have on the impulse-initiating zone (IIZ) that is presumed to be at a point on the principal neurite near the edge of the neuropil?

Where to Record

The easiest place to put a microelectrode in a MN is in its soma. In locusts, these are 20–90 μm in diameter and in a rind just below the ganglionic sheath. If the soma is not itself visible, there are often visual clues to guide the electrode to the desired destination; these clues have been built up through experience because the position of an identified soma varies by only a small amount. It becomes possible to record repeatedly from the same soma in different locusts and to place several electrodes into adjacent neurons. The disadvantage is that the soma is remote both from IIZ and from the presumed synaptic sites. As recorded in the soma, the spike is a mere electronic remnant, a few millivolts in amplitude, of the potential that is propagated to the muscle. The disadvantage of recording in the soma does not become apparent until an assessment is made of what proportion of synaptic inputs impinging upon the MN will actually be recorded. Calculations on *Aplysia* neurons (Graubard, 1975), which are of larger size than those of the locust but of generally similar shape, indicate that severe voltage attenuation, particularly of transitory potentials, will occur during passage from a small to a large process. All inputs received on the fine arborizations must presumably be attenuated as they enter the principal neurite. Some indication of what a soma electrode may miss can be gained by making simultaneous recordings from two sites in the same neuron, one in the soma and the other in the principal neurite (Fig. 2). Such dual recordings have been

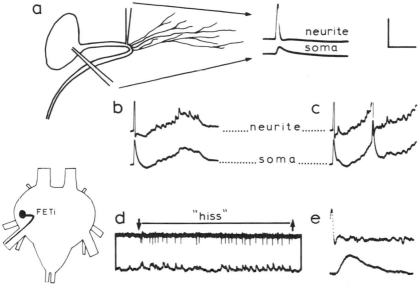

Fig. 2. Recordings from two places in the same MN. (a) Drawing of the fast extensor of the tibiae (FETi) on which have been superimposed the positions of the two recording microelectrodes, one in the soma and the second approximately 200 µm away in the neuropilar segment (the two-dimensional drawing foreshortens the principal neurite). An antidromic spike is considerably attenuated at the soma. (b,c) The tibial movement caused by an antidromic spike is restrained. The resulting strain is monitored by receptors which evoke a depolarization of the MN and sometimes an orthodromic spike. Peaks of the spikes recorded in the neuropil are omitted. (d) An ascending auditory IN recorded in a meso-, prothoracic connective evokes epsp's in the ipsilateral FETi (lower trace). (e) The average of 64 occurrences of the auditory spike more clearly reveals the epsp in the MN. Vertical calibration: (a) 35 mV, (b–d) 8 mV; horizontal calibration: (a) 16 msec, (b,c) 65 msec, (d) 100 msec, (e) 17 msec.

made from the fast MN (FETi) to the extensor tibiae muscle of the hindleg, and the results so obtained may be indicative of the general properties of other MNs. At a point approximately 200 μm from the soma, the spike in the neurite does not overshoot zero but is nevertheless some 5 times the amplitude of that recorded in the soma (Fig. 2a). It should be remembered that the surface area of a soma is greatly increased by a considerable infolding of the glia. Synaptic potentials recorded in the neurite have a faster rise time and in general appear more numerous than those in the soma. For example, a spike in the FETi causes a twitch contraction of the muscle and a rapid extension of the tibia. If this movement is restrained, receptors in the leg provide a positive feedback to FETi which depolarizes it, even to the extent of evoking further spikes (Hoyle and Burrows, 1973b) (Fig. 2b,c). As viewed in the soma, the potentials underlying the depolarization would be interpreted as unitary events. The neurite electrode, however, shows many of them to be the sum of numerous small events. Resolution of synaptic events is therefore improved, but left unanswered is the question of whether the individual potentials are caused by many different presynaptic neurons or by few neurons with terminals widely distributed on the MN. Some inputs have not been recognized in recordings from the soma. An auditory interneuron (IN) which ascends from the metathoracic ganglion to the brain evokes epsp's in the FETi (Fig. 2d). The connection appears to be monosynaptic, but even in the neurite the synaptic potential is small, so that signal averaging may be necessary to show the connection convincingly (Fig. 2e). The connection of an auditory IN with the FETi indicates the presence of a surprising loop in the CNS. In the brain, the lobula giant movement detector (LGMD) also receives inputs from ascending but unknown auditory INs (O'Shea, 1975). The LGMD in turn synapses electrically on the descending contralateral movement detector (DCMD), which synapses in the thorax on the FETi.

The neurite recordings from the MN indicate in general that care must be exercised in interpreting soma recordings. There can be a serious mismatch between synaptic activity recorded at the soma compared with the neurite. If complete circuits are to be known, soma recordings alone are probably inadequate, although the information gained by such recordings is very valuable.

Afferents

In attempting to assess the effect of afferents on central neurons, it would be advantageous to determine connections between known neurons. There are few receptor neurons in the locust that can be identified from animal to animal, although there are plenty that can be selectively activated but not distinguished from other members of their class. Fortunately, the stretch receptor of a wing can be identified anatomically and physiologically and is also a receptor whose effect on the CNS is problematical. Firmly embedded in the literature is the idea that the phasic information it provides at each wingbeat is ignored by the CNS and instead integrated into an excitatory effect with a long time constant (Wilson and Gettrup, 1963). The neuroethological approach that I advocate can be brought to bear on this problem.

Cobalt staining of the nerve innervating the forewing hinge reveals an axon with a diameter of about 6 μm which has extensive arborizations in all three thoracic ganglia (Fig. 3a). The arborizations are similar from locust to locust and allow ready anatomical identification. In the same peripheral nerve a large spike can be recorded (Fig. 3b) whose response properties upon elevation of the wing are those of the single-celled stretch receptor (Pabst and Schwartzkopff, 1962; Pabst, 1965). This axon can be traced electrophysiologically into the pro- and mesothoracic ganglia, and with the help of signal averaging into the metathoracic ganglion (Fig. 3c) from which it apparently does not emerge (Fig. 3d). The anatomical and physiological projections match so well that it is a reasonable assumption that both descriptions refer to the same neuron. The effects of this neuron can be determined by recording its readily identifiable spikes, evoked by elevating the wing, and making intracellular

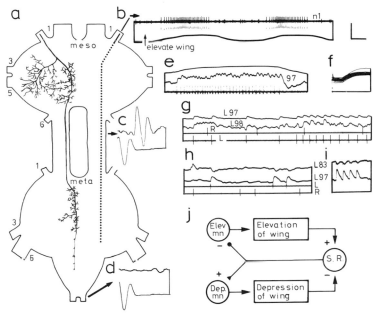

Fig. 3. Forewing stretch receptor and its effects on flight MNs. (a) Projection of a forewing stretch receptor into the meso- and metathoracic ganglia. (b) Elevation of a forewing evokes spikes of large amplitude from the stretch receptor in a branch of the wing nerve, N1d. (c,d) The spike can be traced by signal averaging into the metathoracic ganglion but no farther. (e) Each spike of the stretch receptor evokes an epsp in the first basalar, depressor MN (97) of its wing. (f) The epsp's follow with a constant latency when the axon of the stretch receptor is stimulated electrically. (g) Epsp's in other depressor MNs (second basalar, 98) are often less obvious. The contralateral stretch receptor has no effect. (h,i) Ipsp's occur in an elevator (tergosternal, 83) at the same time as the epsp's in a depressor, when stretch receptor spikes are evoked either (h) by wing movements or (i) by electrical stimulation of the stretch receptor axon. (j) Feedback loop formed by a stretch receptor. Vertical calibration: (e,f) 8 mV, (g) first trace 10 mV, second trace 5 mV, (h) first trace 5 mV, second trace 10 mV, (i) 5 mV, wing movement 80°; horizontal calibration: (b,e,g,h) 100 msec, (c,d) 2.2 msec, (f) 8 msec, (i) 200 msec.

recordings from identified flight MNs (Burrows, 1975a). The stretch receptor of the left fore wing evokes epsp's in the left first basalar MN, a depressor of the wing (Fig. 3e). Each epsp follows a stretch receptor spike with a constant latency of about 1 msec (Fig. 3f) and without failure at frequencies of about 125 Hz. The stretch receptor also evokes epsp's in other depressor MNs, although they may be difficult to discern amid the background of other synaptic potentials (Fig. 3g). In elevator MNs of the left forewing, each spike of the stretch receptor is followed after a latency of 4–5 msec by an ipsp (Fig. 3h, i). The question is raised whether or not the connection between the sensory and motor cells is monosynaptic. In practice, monosynapticity is usually undefinable physiologically. For example, I know of no experiment which could distinguish these two possible pathways between neurons A and C: (1) neuron A makes a direct connection with neuron C; (2) neuron A makes an electrical synapse on neuron B, a nonspiking neuron, which in turn makes a chemical synapse on neuron C. It is thus necessary when defining a connection to use criteria each of which is inadequate when taken separately but which in sum may be sufficient. A delay of 1 msec to the epsp in depressor MNs is generally considered plausible for a monosynaptic pathway, whereas 4–5 msec to the ipsp is not, especially as it is not compatible with the dogma that afferents make only excitatory synapses within the CNS.

The net effect of the connection of the stretch receptor is to form a negative feedback loop with the MNs of its own wing (Fig. 3j). There appears to be over-lap between ipsilateral wings of the two segments (Burrows, 1975a). In the experimental situation described above, the effects of the afferents are subthreshold so that no effect on the movement of the wing would result. If unpatterned sensory inputs from other sources are supplied or if a MN is depolarized, then a patterned input from the stretch receptor, similar to that which it would provide in flight, is now sufficient to entrain the spikes of the MN. It is reasonable to expect that in flight the stretch receptor should have some cycle-by-cycle effect on the movement of the wings. Certainly its phasic information cannot be considered to be ignored by the CNS. Just what effect the stretch receptor does have in flight might be difficult to determine because of the many feedback loops from other receptors which will be operating at the same time. Removal of the stretch receptor alone is insufficient, even it it can be done selectively, because such an experiment might reveal only the plasticity of the nervous system. Most ablation experiments are difficult to interpret because in an attempt to remove one receptor many others are unwittingly damaged, yet the results are often interpreted (Wilson and Gettrup, 1963) as if only one receptor were responsible for the observed changes in behavior. Behavioral experiments (Wendler, 1972, 1974) demonstrate the existence of fast feedback loops during tethered flight but give no indication of which receptors are responsible. The chasm between the two methods of describing pathways on one hand and of observing behavior on the other is well illustrated: the connections forming a feedback loop are demonstrated and the influence of fast loops in flight is revealed. A plausible representation of the information is that one is in part an explanation of the other. Even if this is so, the contribution that the defined loop makes to the behavior as a whole is unknown.

Such are the considerable problems involved in the interpretation of loops whose sensory neurons can be identified, but now consider those which arise when the sensory neurons are unknown. The surface of the wing is covered by a mass of trichoid hairs and campaniform sensilla, and a scolopoforous organ containing many sensory neurons exists at the wing hinge (Gettrup, 1962). What effect do these sensory neurons have on the CNS? Depression of a wing leads to a complex sequence of spikes from many axons in the sensory nerve (Fig. 4a), resulting in hyperpolarization of depressor and depolarization of elevator MNs. As yet, the sensory neurons responsible have not been identifed, and even in experiments where an extracellularly recorded spike of apparently uniform amplitude can be recognized no correlated potentials have been recorded in the soma of a flight MN. The present analysis therefore relies on the stimulation of nerve trunks containing the axons of unknown numbers of sensory neurons. Stimulation of branch 1c of any wing nerve evokes epsp's, whose amplitude is graded with the strength of the applied stimulation, in elevator MNs and ipsp's in depressor MNs (Fig. 4b). Afferents of one wing therefore influence the MNs of all four wings. The delays invoved in the transmission of these effects from hindwing nerves to forewing MNs are of the same order as the timing difference between the two wings in flight. The effects on elevator MNs are often suprathreshold, so that these receptors can also be expected to exert a phasic influence on the flight pattern. These unknown receptors form a second negative feedback loop which probably comes into play when the wing is depressed (Fig. 4c). It is only the effects of these sensory neurons that can be described, not their pathways within the CNS. For example, it is not known whether it is an individual sensory neuron that makes the widespread connections with the MNs of

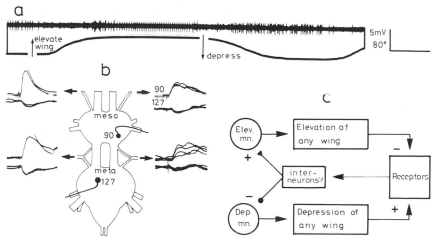

Fig. 4. Other receptors of the wing and their effects on MNs. (a) Elevation of the wing evokes the large spikes of the stretch receptor while depression activates many spikes of smaller amplitude. (b) Stimulation of the branch (N1c) of the nerve from any of the wings which contain these axons evokes epsp's in an elevator MN (first posterior tergoçoxal, 90, of the forewing) and ipsp's in a depressor MN (first basalar, 127, of the hindwing). (c) The feedback loop formed by these receptors. Horizontal calibration: (a) 400 msec, (b) 80 msec.

each wing or whether different sensory neurons do different things. The participation of INs in the distribution of these effects seems likely, especially as there is no close fit of the physiological effects with the central anatomical projections of N1c (Tyrer and Altman, 1974).

The peripheral feedback loops operating during behavior cannot be divorced from consideration of neural mechanisms. They are an integral part of the motor machinery, but their existence means that it is impossible to detect central commands unless these loops are rendered ineffective. The task is now to assess the relative contributions of feedback and central drives.

Central Loops

It should be a simple matter to remove peripheral feedback, but there are pitfalls. For example, it is not sufficiently merely to remove the region around the joint of interest (*cf.* Hoyle and Burrows, 1973*b*) because there may be unsuspected receptors elsewhere which may respond to deformation of the cuticle or stress in the tendons. With sufficient care, peripheral loops can be eliminated, but loops formed by interaction of elements within the CNS cannot; it is these very connections which are under study and which are at the heart of information processing. MNs themselves can apparently be part of these central feedback loops (Burrows, 1973*a*). An antidromic spike in either the left or right hindwing tergosternal MN (an elevator of the wing) of *Chortoicetes* is followed some 25 msec later by a wave of depolarization in both MNs (Fig. 5a–e). The waves consist of groups of epsp's which are matched in both MNs. In the contralateral MN, the waves can evoke a spike, which follows the original spike with a delay of some 40 msec. This period is equivalent to the wingbeat period in flight of this Australian locust. A single antidromic spike can set up a sequence of waves in the two MNs, and whenever an orthodromic spike is evoked the sequence is prolonged. The pathways underlying this reexcitation of the MNs are unknown but could take the general form of that outlined in Fig. 5f. The pathways could provide a mechanism whereby the left and right elevator MNs of one pair of wings spike at the same time, as they must during flight. The results suggest a reverberatory mechanism presumed to involve INs, rather than a direct cross-connection between MNs as once envisioned by Wilson (1966*a*). The contribution of this central loop to normal flight can only be surmised.

Interneurons

In all motor patterns so far examined in insects, connections between the MNs themselves appear to be rare. There are examples which may indicate electrotonic coupling between MNs innervating the same muscle (Bentley, 1969*a*) and of synaptic coupling between antagonists of the femoral joint of the locust hindleg (Hoyle and Burrows, 1973*b*). Connections between MNs sufficient to explain the genera-

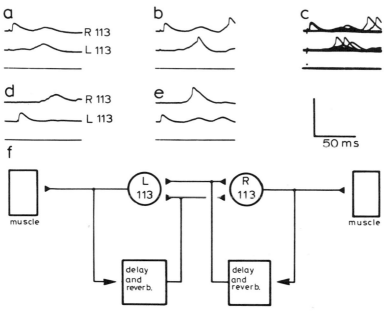

Fig. 5. Feedback loops within the CNS involving the hindwing tergosternal MNs (113) of the Australian locust *Chortoicetes terminifera*. (a,b,c) An electrical stimulus to the axon terminals within the right tergosternal muscle evokes an antidromic spike. This is followed by a wave of excitation in the left and right 113 MNs which may evoke orthodromic spikes. (d,e) Stimulation of the left muscle produces the same effect. (f) Diagram of the pathways which *might* explain the observed effects. Vertical calibration: (a,b,c) 10 mV, (d,e) first trace 10 mV, second trace 25 mV.

tion of motor patterns have not been revealed. This does not denigrate the role that MNs play in integration, nor does it indicate that they are merely the last level of a hierarchical organization of the nervous system. It simply suggests that INs and their connections to and from MNs must be involved in pattern generation. Basically, the following three methods are at present available for the study of the connections of INs in insects.

Long INs Known from Their Extracellular Spikes

The spikes of the long INs can be recorded in connectives or other tracts, and correlated synaptic potentials can be sought by intracellular recordings in other neurons. Hence pathways can be determined. This method is possible only for a few neurons which can be identified by their large extracellular spikes and unique response properties. In the absence of these means of identification, an IN can be recognized only by its output effects, and these are what are being sought. The method has allowed determination of some of the output connections of two large movement-detector neurons, the descending ipsilateral and contralateral movement detectors (DIMD and DCMD), in the locust (Burrows and Rowell, 1973). The nomenclature of these neurons implies that their sole job is to detect movement in the visual field, and is a convenient shorthand only if it does not obscure the fact they integrate information from many sources and hence probably from many sensory modalities. The DCMD, for example, also responds to sound (O'Shea, 1975; Palka and Pinter, 1975). The connections of the DCMD and DIMD are consistent with their playing some role in jumping. No direct behavioral role has been shown, either because the experimental conditions are not correct or because summation of other inputs is necessary.

INs Inferred from Common Synaptic Potentials in MNs

The existence of spiking INs can be inferred by recognizing synaptic potentials which are common to several simultaneously impaled MNs. When long sequences of such potentials are observed without failures in several MNs so that random coincidences are avoided, the inference is that they are evoked by the same presynaptic IN. This is the simplest explanation, but it may not always be the correct one. The potentials could be caused by electrically coupled populations of neurons, which in the experimental situation act as a single unit but which may become uncoupled under other conditions. The method has proved powerful in revealing the ways MNs are driven by INs (Burrows and Horridge, 1974). Some examples can illustrate this point. A forced extension of the hind tibia evokes common synaptic potentials in both the slow extensor tibiae motor neuron (SETi) and the FETi (Fig. 6a). In SETi these synaptic potentials may evoke spikes, but in FETi they remain subthreshold. Thus both slow and fast MNs may be simultaneously excited, with the lower threshold of the slow MN being due perhaps to its smaller size. Three fast MNs of the hind tibia have some common excitatory synaptic inputs (Fig. 6b). Again, these common potentials are subthreshold in the large, fast MNs but evoke spikes in the smaller, slow MNs. Remarkable for their common synaptic inputs are two MNs on either side of the metathoracic ganglion which innervate abdominal expiratory muscles (Fig. 6c). Most of their ipsp's seem to be shared and their spikes tend to occur at about the same time, although there is no indication of direct electrical coupling (Fig. 6d). The spikes occur whenever there is a pause in the bombardment of ipsp's (Fig. 6e). Release from inhibition appears to be a method of activating these MNs, and the common synaptic driving ensures that there will be a roughly symmetrical output.

One of the surprises of this method of analysis has been the extensive sphere of influence of some INs that has been revealed. Moreover, the method has shown that MNs involved in two apparently dissimilar patterns of behavior may share inputs from the same INs (Burrows, 1975b,c). There appear to be a pair of INs which synapse on 50 MNs in four ganglia and carry information about two motor patterns, ventilation and perhaps flight. They synapse on both flight and ventilatory MNs, and their present known distribution is probably no more than a rough indication of their total connections. Synaptic potentials in the left and right tergosternal (elevator) MNs of the forewings have two different periodicities; one is a slow

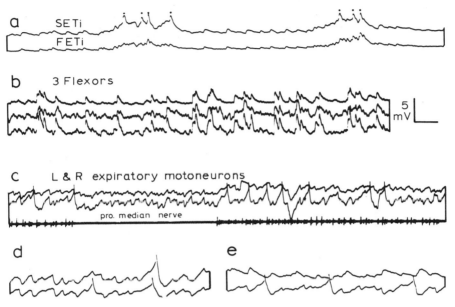

Fig. 6. Common synaptic driving of sets of MNs. (a) The slow (SETi) and fast (FETi) MNs to the extensor of a hind tibia receive common epsp's upon forced movements of the tibia. In the SETi the summed epsp's may evoke spikes (dotted). (b) Three fast flexors of the hind tibia receive spontaneously occurring epsp's. (c,d,e) Symmetrically arranged expiratory MNs on the left and right sides of the metathoracic ganglion receive common ipsp's. (d) Spikes in both neurons tend to occur at the same time. (e) The upper MN is hyperpolarized to reverse the ipsp's. Spikes are seen to arise when there is a lack of ipsp's. Horizontal calibration: (a,d,e) 100 msec, (b,c) 200 msec.

rhythm, the other is a fast one (Fig. 7a). The former is always linked to ventilation and depolarizes the flight MNs during expiration. The expiratory depolarization is broken up into a series of ripples caused by groups of epsp's (Fig. 7b) which are exactly matched in the two MNs. The ripples occur with a period of about 50 msec, which is similar to the wingbeat period of this locust, *Schistocerca*, in flight. The rhythms are present in forewing and hindwing elevator MNs (Fig. 7c) and in some forewing depressor MNs (Fig. 7d). In all, some 30 flight MNs receive these inputs. What is the purpose of depolarization of the flight MNs by these two rhythms? In the experimental situation, the rhythms are subthreshold in the MNs so that no contractions of the flight muscles occur. Therefore, they contribute no force to the ventilatory movements. The rhythms can, however, become suprathreshold when other stimulation is applied. An air stream directed onto the head is more likely to evoke spikes in the MNs during expiration and furthermore each spike is likely to occur during one of the fast ripples. The motor spikes are patterned and tend to occur at intervals that are either equal to or multiples of the wingbeat period. The circumstantial evidence might suggest that the INs play some role in the patterning of flight; they synapse on flight MNs, causing the membrane potentials to ripple at the correct frequency for flight, and are capable of evoking motor spikes during

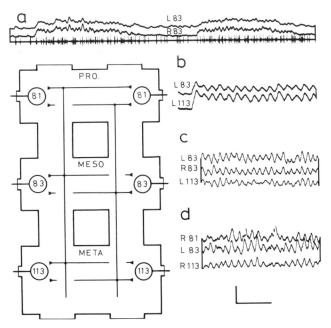

Fig. 7. Connections of INs inferred from the observation of common synaptic potentials in flight MNs. (a) Two forewing elevators are depolarized together in time with the expiratory phase of ventilation. The lower trace monitors spikes in prothoracic N6 to muscles of the neck, active during expiration. (b) The synaptic potentials in a forewing and a hindwing elevator are matched. There is a rhythmicity during the expiratory depolarization with a period similar to the wingbeat period in flight. (c) Three elevator MNs receiving common inputs. (d) Flight MNs in each of the three thoracic ganglia receiving common inputs. The inferred connections of the INs are summarized in the diagram. Vertical calibration: (a,c,d) 4 mV, (b) 5 mV; horizontal calibration: (a,c,d) 400 msec, (b) 200 msec.

expiration. However, there is no direct link between the described neural pathways and behavior. At worst, the fast rhythm may have nothing to do with the flight rhythm; at best, it may represent an output of the flight pattern generator. There are two possible ways of establishing a link. One would be to record from the MNs during flight, but there would remain the problem of deciphering complex changes in membrane potential when many pathways are active at once. Nevertheless, this is a goal toward which we must aim. The second would be to make predictions about the probable effects of these INs in flight and to test them behaviorally. One prediction is that if the INs are involved in the patterning of flight then a ventilatory modulation of flight should be discernible. This has been tested by recording extracellularly from flight muscles of a tethered locust and correlating the interval between the spikes which occur at each wingbeat with the ventilatory cycle (Burrows, 1976). The results showed that the frequency of the repetitive spikes in elevator MNs, and hence probably the wingbeat period, rises and falls by about 1 Hz in time with the ventilatory cycle. The observations of two different rhythms of synaptic input and of the modulation of flight by ventilation are compatible.

The INs also synapse on some 20 ventilatory MNs, and here their role in behavior can be established more firmly. Thoracic spiracles close during expiration and open during inspiration (Fig. 8a,b). In the closer MNs, the epsp's underlying the spikes during expiration match those in flight MNs (Fig. 8c,d). In opener MNs the ipsp's during expiration match the epsp's in the flight MNs (Fig. 8e). The INs appear to make reciprocal connections with the antagonistic MNs of a spiracle, ensuring that when one spikes the other does not. The same connections are made in each thoracic segment on the two closer MNs and the two openers (if present). Thus all closer MNs in the thorax receive the same pattern of excitory commands and all openers receive the same inhibitory commands during expiration. In the closer MNs the synaptic potentials evoked by the INs are an adequate explanation of the pattern of motor spikes. Both rhythms may be expressed in spikes; the slow rhythm determines the length of the expiratory burst, and the fast rhythm determines the patterning of the spikes within that burst (Fig. 8c). It is reasonable to conclude that the function of the INs is both to coordinate and to drive the movements of the thoracic spiracles; the described circuits are an adequate explanation of the observed behavior.

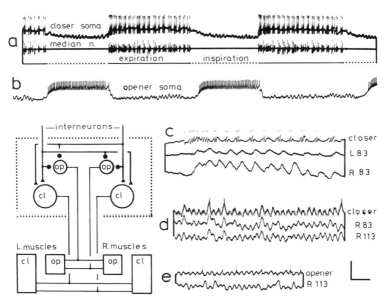

Fig. 8. Coordination of spiracular movements by INs which also synapse on flight MNs. (a) A prothoracic spiracular closer MN spikes during expiration and is inhibited during inspiration. (b) A metathoracic spiracular opener MN spikes during inspiration. (c) The spikes in a closer MN are grouped and correspond with the ripples in the flight MNs. (d) Hyperpolarizing the closer MN reveals that its epsp's match those in the flight MNs. (e) The ipsp's in the opener MN match the epsp's in a flight MN. The inferred connections of the INs on the spiracular MNs of a particular segment are shown in the diagram. ●, Inhibitory synapses; ▲, excitatory synapses. Vertical calibration: (a) 25 mV, (b) 10 mV, (c) first trace 25 mV, second and third traces 3 mV, (d) first trace 25 mV, second and third traces 5 mV, (e) first trace 10 mV, second trace 5 mV; horizontal calibration: (a,b,d,e) 200 msec, (c) 100 msec.

Local INs Known from Intracellular Recording

The method of inferring the properties of INs by observations made in the MNs must be superseded by recordings made directly from the INs themselves. In this way the inputs to the INs themselves can be determined (O'Shea and Rowell, 1975*b*). For most INs, this will be the only physiological test that will reveal their existence. This is particularly true for "local" INs, i.e., those with a restricted distribution in the CNS, perhaps an intraganglionic one. An electrode probing in the neuropil encounters two basic types of neurons which have effects on MNs: those which spike and those which do not. It seems likely that these are the two ends of a spectrum and that neurons which affect MNs by both spike and slow potential will be found, as they have been in the stomatogastric ganglion of lobsters (Maynard and Walton, 1975). The spiking neurons evoke typical epsp's (Fig. 9a,b) or ipsp's in the MNs through pathways that appear to be monosynaptic. The INs which do not produce spikes are a most interesting type, perhaps at the heart of pattern-generating

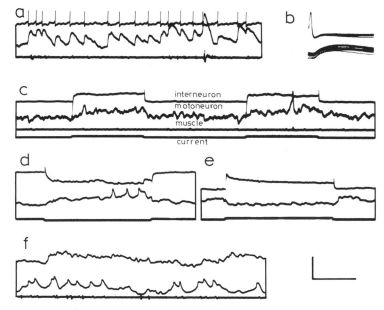

Fig. 9. Influence of INs on flexor MNs of the hind tibia. Recordings are made simultaneously from a neurite of an IN and the soma of a MN. (a,b) A spiking, presumed IN causes epsp's on the MN which may sum to evoke a motor spike (myogram of the flexor is on the bottom trace). The epsp's in the MN follow each spike of the IN with a constant latency. (c) An IN which did not produce spikes. Depolarization of it caused a slow depolarization of the MN and a spike. (d,e,f) A second IN which did not spike. (d) Hyperpolarization of it resulted in a depolarization accompanied by spikes in the MN. (e) Depolarization of this IN resulted in a hyperpolarization of the MN. (f) Forced movements of the tibia resulted in changes in the synaptic potentials in the IN. Vertical calibration: (a) first trace 20 mV, second trace 5 mV, (b) 10 mV, (c) first trace 50 mV, second trace 4 mV, (d,e) first trace 50 mV, second trace 20 mV, (f) 20 mV, current 33 nA; horizontal calibration: (a) 100 msec, (b) 13 msec, (c,d,e) 400 msec, (f) 200 msec.

mechanisms (Pearson and Fourtner, 1975). Siegler and I have been looking at the mechanism of transmission between local, nonspiking INs and flight and leg MNs (Burrows and Siegler, 1976). In these experiments, we recorded simultaneously from the soma of a MN and from a 5–8 μm diameter neuropilar process of the presynaptic IN. In this situation, the membrane potential of both pre- and postsynaptic neurons can be manipulated independently. Three different effects on MNs could be produced by changing the potential of different presynaptic INs: (1) Depolarization of the IN leads to depolarization of the MN (Fig. 9c). (2) Depolarization of the IN leads to hyperpolarization of the MN (Fig. 9e). (3) Hyperpolarization of the IN leads to depolarization of the MN (Fig. 9d). The effect on the MN is graded and depends on the strength of the presynaptic current. The effects are strong enough to control the frequency of motor spikes in a smoothly graded manner. Each IN appears to affect sets of MNs, exciting some and inhibiting others. Some MNs are influenced by several nonspiking INs, causing either excitation or inhibition. Not all MNs to a particular muscle are influenced by the same IN. For example, there are INs that cause flexion of the hindleg but do not affect the membrane potential at the soma of some flexor MNs. We believe that the INs so far studied exert their effects on the MNs by graded release of transmitter substance directly on the MNs. The INs are also modulated by resistance reflexes from joints whose muscles they affect and during evoked movements of those joints. Just what integrative role these INs play remains to be determined. Undoubtedly, they enrich but complicate an analysis of neuronal mechanisms.

Can Any Conclusions Be Drawn?

This may have seemed to be a rather pessimistic ramble through the problems of analyzing a nervous system. It is meant to be realistic and not disheartening What is more disheartening to me is the widespread tendency to suggest simple mechanisms where simplicity obviously does not exist. For example, locust flight at first glance appears to be simple stereotyped movement, but as I have indicated even the movements themselves may be complex. At the MN level, the cell numbers are small, but the task of unraveling connections among these seems unlikely to be fulfilled for some time. Moreover, the simplicity in terms of numbers may not to extend to all other levels in the neuronal organization. It seems likely that the numbers of INs will far exceed the numbers of MNs, and it is at the IN not the MN level that the organization of the flight pattern appears to take place.

It also seems likely that the majority of INs will prove to exert their effects on other neurons without producing spikes. Thus the oversimplifying tendency must be replaced soon by massively detailed descriptions of component neuronal elements. Are there general principles emerging from this ever-growing mound of details? I feel that they are emerging, although the methodology I have advocated is still in its infancy. For example, in the flight of the locust these principles are the types of feedback loops formed by receptors, the common driving of synergistic MNs and the operation of the size principle (although there are exceptions to this), the sharing of INs by MNs which participate in different motor patterns, and the control in overlapping sets of MNs by INs which do not produce spikes. These are but some of the mechanisms that I suspect will be found to be widespread.

ACKNOWLEDGMENT

This work was supported by a grant from the Nuffield Foundation.

21

Flight Motor Innervation of a Flesh Fly

Kazuo Ikeda

Introduction

A considerable number of papers have been published on the anatomy of the dipteran flight system. The early papers especially have become classical for their precise descriptions of thoracic musculature (Hammond, 1879; Luks, 1883; Ritter, 1911; Mihályi, 1935; Behrendt, 1940; Williams and Williams, 1943; Tiegs, 1955) and the central nervous system (Hertweck, 1931; Vater, 1961). In addition, histological (Mangold, 1905; Marcu, 1929; Tiegs, 1955; Auber, 1960) and electron microscopic (Shafiq, 1964) papers have appeared on the peripheral innervation of the muscles involved in flight. The neural pathway from the CNS to those muscles, however, has not been investigated well, except for some descriptions in Hertweck's work (1931). Physiological experiments performed in this area in the past have yielded incomplete or sometimes misleading results, mainly because of a lack of precise knowledge concerning the motor neurons (MNs) involved and their neural pathways. Thus an understanding of the neural organization in both the central and peripheral systems is essential in considering the flight mechanism.

The Dorsal Longitudinal Flight Muscle System

The flight system of a dipteran insect is divided into two major parts, the indirect and the direct flight systems, according to their function in contributing to wingbeat and the cytological specificities of the muscle involved. The indirect flight system is composed of the dorsal longitudinal flight muscle system and the dorso-ventral flight muscle system. The muscles in the indirect flight system are fibrillar and are attached to the thoracic cuticle. Contraction of the muscles causes deformation of the thoracic cuticle, which results indirectly in the wing movement. The muscles in the direct flight system are tubular and are attached to the base of the wing. Their contraction has a direct effect on the wing movement.

In this chapter, the neural organization of the dorsal longitudinal muscle system (DLM system) will be presented. The number of muscle fibers composing a

Kazuo Ikeda • Division of Neurosciences, City of Hope National Medical Center, Duarte, California 91010.

DLM of dipteran insects varies with the species, ranging from six to about 200 (Tiegs, 1955). We have confirmed in our laboratory that six pairs of DLM fibers are arranged similarly in the following species: *Calliphora erythrocephala, Drosophila melanogaster, Musca domestica,* and *Sarcophaga bullata.* The descriptions given here are for the flesh fly *S. bullata;* however, the general structure is common to the other species listed.

A pair of DLMs (each composed of six muscle fibers) runs longitudinally along the midline of the thorax from the scutum to the posterior phragma. The six muscle fibers composing the DLM are arranged on top of each other, so the entire medial view of the six fibers can be observed when the thorax is cut in half along the midline (Fig. 1). The entire lateral view of the six muscle fibers is obtained after removing other muscles located laterally in the thorax. These six muscle fibers are designated DLM 1 through DLM 6 from ventral to dorsal.

The DLM is innervated by the posterior dorsal mesothoracic nerve from the thoracic ganglion. This nerve runs dorsally, passing the side of the alimentary canal while giving off branches to other muscles, and reaches the ventrolateral surface of the most ventral DLM 1 (Fig. 2). At this point, it makes its first bifurcation, giving

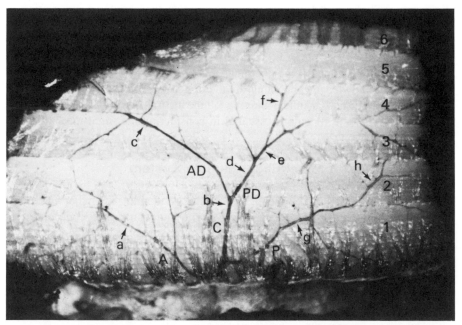

Fig. 1. Medial surface of the right dorsal longitudinal flight muscle of *Sarcophaga bullata.* The medial branch of the posterior dorsal mesothoracic nerve was stained with methylene blue. Anterior end of the thorax to the left, dorsal side of the thorax to the top. Each of six muscle fibers is recognizable by the almost horizontal line between the fibers. Muscle fibers are numbered 1 through 6 from ventral to dorsal. Structures partially covering the muscle fibers are tracheoles. A, Anterior branch; C, central branch; P, posterior branch; AD: anterior dorsal branch; PD, posterior dorsal branch.

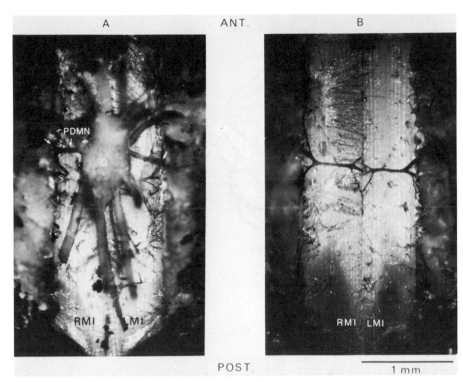

Fig. 2. Ventral view of a pair of dorsal longitudinal flight muscles. Nerves were stained with methylene blue. Anterior end of the thorax to the top. A: With thoracic ganglion (marked G, unfocused). RM1, Right-side dorsal longitudinal flight muscle No. 1; LM1, left-side dorsal longitudinal flight muscle No. 1; PDMN, right-side posterior dorsal mesothoracic nerve. Two arrows at the edge of the muscle fibers indicate the portions where the posterior dorsal mesothoracic nerve reaches dorsal longitudinal flight muscle No. 1. B: After removing the thoracic ganglion. Dark-stained horizontal bands on the muscle are the nerves. L, Lateral branch; M, medial branch.

off medial and lateral branches. The lateral branch climbs up along the lateral surface of DLM 1 and provides three further branches (anterior, central, and posterior) on the surface. These three branches lie along the lateral surface of the balance of the DLM fibers and innervate. The medial branch goes around the ventral surface of DLM 1 and then climbs up along the median surface of DLM 1, also making three further branches on its surface. These three branches (anterior, central, and posterior) lie along the medial surface of the balbance of the DLM fibers while making finer branches and innervate. Thus all six DLM fibers are innervated by lateral and medial branches of the dorsal mesothoracic nerve. This structure is illustrated in Fig. 3.

By stimulating the posterior dorsal mesothoracic nerve with fine steps of various intensities and recording the response of each muscle fiber's entire length, it was confirmed that each muscle fiber was innervated by a single excitatory neuron. As with results obtained previously with *M. domestica* (Ikeda, 1965), there was no

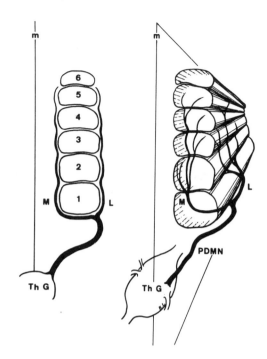

Fig. 3. Pathway of the left posterior mesothoracic nerve from the thoracic ganglion to the left dorsal longitudinal flight muscle. Left: Schematic frontal view, dorsal side up. m, Median line; ThG, thoracic ganglion; M, medial branch; L, lateral branch; numbers indicate the number of DLM fibers. Right: Schematic anterolateral view, dorsal side up. m, Median plane; PDMN, posterior dorsal mesothoracic nerve.

indication of complication from inhibitory or multiple innervation. Although a single innervation was thus confirmed, this kind of experiment is not satisfactory in discriminating the possibility that a single neuron might innervate more than one muscle fiber.

In order to overcome the above situation and identify all of the neurons involved, a separate stimulation of each neuron was necessary. For this purpose, quasinatural flight activity, so-called anesthetic flight in which these MNs were driven one by one by the higher center as they are in natural flight, was used.

Anesthetic Flight

When a fly is suspended in air and its wingbeat is initiated by a frontal air blow or by removing support for the legs, patterned activity can be recorded from each muscle fiber. A similar wingbeat can also be obtained by the application of volatile anesthetics (Ikeda, 1974). The pattern of the muscular activity and the resulting wingbeat is fixed within a certain range, independent of the kind of anesthetic or its concentration (Ikeda, 1974). In other words, if the concentration of anesthetic is within the effective range, the activity pattern is fixed, suggesting that the action of the anesthetic merely releases the preprogrammed activity. This condition provides a supreme opportunity for the use of a built-in stimulator which can drive each MN separately and sequentially. In the following section, the results obtained from anesthetic flight will be described.

Activity of the Dorsal Longitudinal Flight Muscle during Anesthetic Flight

For the experiment, a fly was mounted laterally at the opening of a piece of tubing which served as the supply duct for the air–ether mixture. The space between the fly and the tubing was sealed carefully with wax along the fly's midline. When the tubing with the mounted fly was immersed in the saline solution, one side of the fly was in contact with the saline solution and the other side with the air–ether mixture. The fly, submerged in the solution, could thus breathe with its spiracles contralateral to the side facing the solution. When the tubing was connected to a flask containing 0.7% volume-to-volume diethyl ether, it could be kept in a stable anesthetic condition for more than 24 hr. The procedure is similar to that described previously for *Drosophila* (Ikeda and Kaplan, 1974).

For the electrical recording, the lateral thorax of the fly's side facing the solution was dissected to expose the lateral surface of the DLM of that side, or the medial surface of the contralateral DLM, while maintaining the entire CNS and the posterior dorsal mesothoracic nerve intact. The initiation of anesthetic flight activity was not spontaneous but required sensory inputs. Various modalities of sensory inputs had a summative effect to elicit the activity. Under experimental conditions, the activity could also be initiated by passing an electric square pulse to the cervical connective. The duration of the activity, once started, varied from a few seconds to more than 30 min, depending on still unknown factors. The pattern was well fixed, however, giving steady experimental conditions. In this way, the activity pattern of each muscle fiber composing a DLM was investigated by the simultaneous recording of the muscle membrane potentials from various combinations of two muscle fibers at a time.

The recordings shown in Fig. 4 were obtained successively from a single fly under the application of 0.7% (v/v) ether. The activity pattern was not regular and it fluctuated within a limited range, but it certainly had a pattern specific to the species of the fly.

Each muscle fiber fired with a different average frequency, and no particular phase relationship was obtained between any combination of two muscle fibers while the frequency shift of each muscle fiber was closely correlated, except the complete synchronization in DLM 5 and DLM 6. The detailed description of the activity pattern of each muscle fiber and the relationship among them will be presented in a separate paper. As DLM 1 through DLM 4 were driven separately without discrete phase relationships and the relationship between nerve impulse and muscle activity was 1:1, it was certain that these muscle fibers were separately innervated by single neurons.

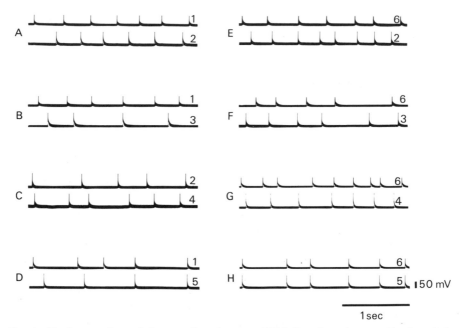

Fig. 4. Simultaneous intracellular recordings from two DLM fibers in various combinations during anesthetic flight conditions. Numbers indicate the number of DLM fibers. Any combination except that of DLM 5 and DLM 6 is asynchronously activated.

DLM 5 and DLM 6 were found to be activated synchronously at all times. There was no electrical coupling between these two muscle fibers because depolarizing or hyperpolarizing currents applied to one of them did not affect the membrane potential of the other. This indicated that DLM 5 and DLM 6 were innervated by a common single neuron. These results indicated that there must be five MNs which innervate six muscle fibers of a DLM, and each muscle fiber is innervated by a single neuron. DLM 1 through DLM 4 are innervated by four single neurons separately, while DLM 5 and DLM 6 share a single neuron. All of these DLM muscle fibers are identifiable by their anatomical localizations; therefore, the five MNs can be identified in relation to the innervating muscle fibers.

Identification of Motor Axons

In order to identify the nerve impulses of a particular axon which innervates an identified muscle fiber, nerve impulses propagating through the posterior dorsal mesothoracic nerve were monitored by an extracellular electrode while simultaneously recording from individual muscle fibers. An example is shown in Fig. 5. All recordings in this figure are from the same preparation; the nerve impulse recording was kept as stable as possible while the intracellular electrode was placed into each

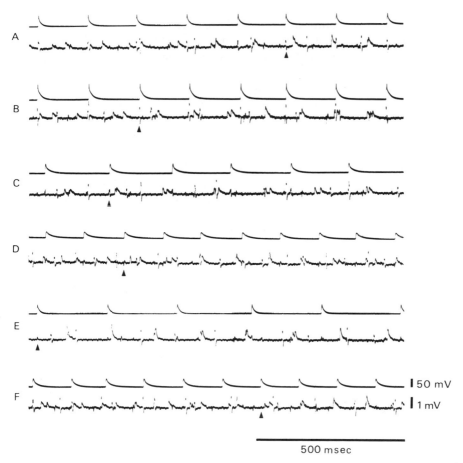

Fig. 5. Simultaneous recordings of nerve impulses from the posterior dorsal mesothoracic nerve and individual dorsal longitudinal muscle fibers during anesthetic flight conditions. Upper trace: Intracellular recording from a muscle fiber. Lower trace: Extracellular recording from the nerve. A, DLM 1; B, DLM 2; C, DLM 3; D, DLM 4; E, DLM 5; F, DLM 6. Arrows indicate discrete nerve impulses responsible for the excitation of each muscle fiber.

muscle fiber successively. The upper traces in A, B, C, D, E, and F show the responses of DLM fibers 1, 2, 3, 4, 5, and 6, respectively. The lower trace shows the nerve impulses recorded extracellularly from the posterior dorsal mesothoracic nerve. From these records, it was possible to identify the unit nerve impulse corresponding to the particular muscle fiber. The average impulse frequencies of those MNs differ, and the firing pattern is not regular; therefore, the nerve impulses sometimes showed temporal separation from each other well enough to identify each of them. At other times, superimposition of a few impulses made identification difficult. In each trace, the discrete unit impulse responsible for excitation of a particular muscle fiber is indicated by an arrow. This record shows that all five nerve impulses are identifiable and a single muscle fiber responds to the impulse from a particular axon only. There are impulses to which none of the six muscle fibers responds. They appear to be sensory impulses and are distinguished by their long duration.

In Fig. 6, a part of the recording which follows that of Fig. 5B is shown in enlargement. The lower trace is the extracellularly recorded nerve impulses passing through the posterior dorsal mesothoracic nerve. The upper trace is the intracellular recording from DLM 2. The identification of the MNs made by examining each record shown in Fig. 5 is shown by numbers under the arrows that are pointing to the identified impulses. The number corresponds to the number of the responding DLM muscle fiber except MN 5, to which both DLM 5 and DLM 6 respond. The nerve impulse recording clearly shows the activity of the identified neurons in sequence. The relationship among the firing patterns of those MNs can be discussed by making this kind of record, but it is beyond the scope of this chapter and will be reported in a separate publication.

Medial and Lateral Branches of the Posterior Dorsal Mesothoracic Nerve

The above results show that DLMs 1, 2, 3, and 4 are each innervated by a separate, single neuron; the fifth neuron innervates DLMs 5 and 6. The DLM receives terminals from both the medial and lateral surfaces through medial and lateral branches of the posterior dorsal mesothoracic nerve. Each single motor axon must bifurcate at the point proximal to the branch formation of the nerve trunk, sending bifurcated axons to both the medial and lateral branches. This structure was confirmed by histological and electron microscopic preparations. At the portion just proximal to the first bifurcation at the ventrolateral surface of DLM 1, the posterior dorsal mesothoracic nerve contains five distinctively large axons (diameter 8–10 μm) and many axons of a smaller diameter ($< 3 \mu$m). At the portion just distal to the first bifurcation, the lateral branch contains five distinctively large axons and many smaller axons, while the medial branch contains only the five large axons and no others.

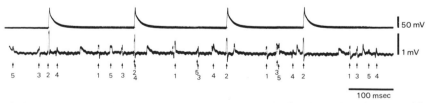

Fig. 6. Simultaneous recording of nerve impulses from the posterior dorsal mesothoracic nerve and from DLM 2. Nerve impulses identified by the records shown in Fig. 4 are marked by number. MN 1 to MN 4 innervate DLM 1 through DLM 4; MN 5 innervates both DLM 5 and DLM 6.

Ascending nerve impulses were recorded from the lateral branch in response to the mechanical stimulation of dorsal thoracic bristles but were not recorded from the medial branch; therefore, the axons of smaller diameter in the lateral branch appear to be sensory axons.

Another morphological characteristic of the posterior dorsal mesothoracic nerve presents advantages for physiological experiment. Within a certain length of nerve proximal to every branching, the large axons are always arranged on one plane parallel to the muscle fiber surface. This arrangement is common to both the medial and lateral branches. The innervation of those MNs has been studied further, using this special arrangement of axons.

Intracellular Recording of Nerve Impulses

Because of the specific structure described above, intracellular recording of the nerve impulses from individual axons was possible. Figure 7 shows examples obtained from DLM 3 and its innervating axon. In A, the upper trace shows the extracellular recording of nerve impulses at the portion proximal to the first bifurcation of the posterior dorsal mesothoracic nerve. The lower trace shows the intracel-

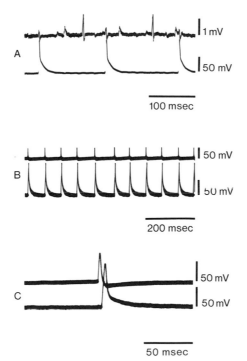

Fig. 7. Identification of neuron innervating DLM 3. A: Simultaneous recordings of nerve impulses from the posterior dorsal mesothoracic nerve (upper trace) and from DLM 3 (lower trace). B: Simultaneous intracellular recordings of MN 3 and DLM 3. C: Same as B with faster time base.

lular recording from DLM 3. The nerve impulses responsible for DLM 3 are recognizable in the same manner as in Figs. 5 and 6. In B, the intracellularly recorded nerve impulses are shown in the upper trace, while the responses of DLM 3 to them are in the lower trace. In this experiment, an intracellular electrode was inserted into an axon and then another intracellular electrode was inserted into a muscle fiber. While the electrode in the axon was held, the electrode in the muscle fiber was placed into another muscle fiber and another until it found the muscle fiber which was responding to the nerve impulses being picked up by the former. Single nerve impulses and muscle responses from the same preparation are shown with a faster time base in C. With this technique, by observing the nerve impulses passing through a particular axon, the activity of every muscle was checked for corresponding response by inserting another intracellular electrode and making a simultaneous recording with the former. For this purpose, the medial branch was preferred to the lateral because impaling of the motor axon was not disturbed by the presence of sensory axons.

Figure 8 demonstrates the simultaneous recording of axonal impulses and corresponding muscle fiber action potentials. Recording from the axon was made at the portion of the nerve located on the medial surface of DLM 1. DLM 1 was sacrificed for technical reasons; therefore, the simultaneous recording from an axon and a responding muscle fiber is shown only for DLM 2 through DLM 6. In A, B, and C, the upper trace shows intracellularly recorded nerve impulses, and the lower trace shows intracellularly recorded muscle fiber action potentials in response to the former. In A, DLM 2 responded to axon 2; in B, DLM 3 responded to axon 3; in C, DLM 4 responded to axon 4. In D, the simultaneous recordings from axon 5 (top trace), DLM 5 (middle trace), and DLM 6 (bottom trace) are shown. These record-

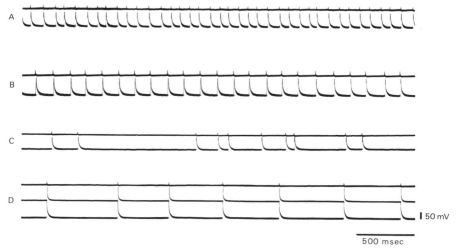

Fig. 8. Identification of neurons innervating DLM 2 through DLM 6. A: Simultaneous intracellular recordings of the activities from MN 2 (upper trace) and from DLM 2 (lower trace). B: MN 3 and DLM 3. C: MN 4 and DLM 4. D: MN 5 and DLM 5 and DLM 6.

ings give evidence that DLMs 2, 3, and 4 are innervated separately, while DLM 5 and DLM 6 share an axon.

Pathway of Motor Axons

In order to identify the axon farther along its pathway, finer branches of the medial branch of the posterior dorsal mesothoracic nerve were investigated. For this purpose, a fine branch on the medial surface was cut, the distal end of the nerve was sucked into a suction electrode for stimulation, and the response of each muscle fiber was tested by placing an intracellular electrode into each muscle fiber, one by one.

At the medial surface of the DLM, the medial branch of the posterior dorsal mesothoracic nerve divides into three major branches, anterior, central, and posterior, as shown in Fig. 1. The central branch bifurcates into anterior dorsal and posterior dorsal branches. The experiment, cutting the nerve at (a) and stimulating the distal cut end, showed that this branch contains two axons innervating DLM 1 and DLM 2, respectively; at (b), four axons innervating DLM 2 through DLM 6; at (c), two axons innervating DLM 3 and DLM 4; at (d), four axons innervating DLM 2 through DLM 6. The axons innervating DLM 3 and DLM 4 therefore are divided into the anterior dorsal branch and the posterior dorsal branch at the branch distal to (b), while the axon innervating DLM 5 and DLM 6 passes that branch without making bifurcation. At (e), three axons innervating DLM 3 through DLM 6 are confirmed; at (f), one axon innervating DLM 5 and DLM 6; at (g), two axons innervating DLM 1 and DLM 2; at (h), one axon innervating DLM 2.

As indicated by Hertweck (1931), the branching pattern of the posterior dorsal mesothoracic nerve shows some individual differences, but the larger branches such as the anterior, central, and posterior are always clearly recognizable. The axons in the proximal part of these branches do not show individual variations in number: i.e., anterior branch, two axons; central branch, five axons; and posterior branch, three axons.

Conclusion

From these results, it is concluded that DLM 1 through DLM 4 are innervated by single axons separately, while DLM 5 and DLM 6 share a single axon. All six muscle fibers and five MNs are identifiable. Thus the entire DLM system is composed of six pairs of muscle fibers and five paris of MNs. As DLM 5 and DLM 6 are innervated by a single axon, the functional units (neuromuscular or motor units) of the DLM system are five pairs. In *D. melanogaster,* Levine and Wyman (1973) reported that each of six muscle fibers in the DLM system were innervated by a single axon; thus there were six units. Levine and Hughes (1973) reported that the most dorsal DLM fiber of *D. melanogaster* (DLM 6 in this chapter) behaved differently from the other five muscle fibers and also claimed there were six MNs for the DLM system. If the most dorsal DLM fiber behaves differently from the other five muscle fibers, it would require a motor axon specifically innervating that muscle fiber.

The discrepancy between the above reports and the present results obtained from *S. bullata* might be interpreted by assuming there is a species difference in the innervation of the DLM system. Ikeda *et al.* (1975), however, reported that the DLM system of *D. melanogaster* was innervated by five motor axons. DLM 1 through DLM 4 were innervated separately by single axons, whereas DLM 5 and DLM 6 were innervated commonly by a single axon. These results from *Drosophila* are thus in agreement with the present results.

ACKNOWLEDGMENTS

This work was done in collaboration with Drs. N. Hori and T. Tsuruhara while they were in my laboratory on leave from Kyushu University and the National Institute of Health in Japan, respectively. Their excellent work on physiology and electron microscopy has made this report possible. I also extend my thanks to Misses Corinne Hartman, Vivian Sharbono, and Gail Mardock for their invaluable technical help and Ms. Lois S. Worth for preparation of the manuscript. This work was supported by USPHS NIH Grant NS 07442 and a grant from the Foundation for Research in Hereditary Diseases.

Part 3

Coding and Integration of Sensory Input

22

The Bridge between Visual Input and Central Programming in Crustaceans

Talbot H. Waterman

Prologue: Wiersma and I

By good fortune, my professional and personal friendship with Kees Wiersma began more than 35 years ago. At the time, I was a graduate student at Harvard engaged in thesis research on neuromuscular transmission in crustaceans. In the summer of 1940, I worked for 3 months in Kees's lab at Cal Tech. This marked the beginning of our close relationship (Fig. 1).

Under his tutelage, I studied the effects of ions and drugs on the claw neuromuscular system of *Procambarus*. The research itself was not earth shaking but did contribute to a paper (Waterman, 1941) comparing ionic effects in this crayfish with those in the spider crab *Maja* and spiny lobster *Panulirus*. This became part of my Ph.D. thesis (Waterman, 1943). Although Kees pursued this general topic somewhat further (Wiersma and Zawadski, 1948; Wiersma *et al.*, 1953), I never have. In retrospect, our first encounter was less notable for its scientific accomplishment than for its germinal effect on our later research in other areas.

Actually, the warm interpersonal relationship established in 1940 clearly influenced both of us in important ways. The most direct effects were three fruitful periods of close research collaboration as well as my decision to edit *The Physiology of Crustacea* (Waterman, 1960, 1961a), to which Kees contributed two important chapters (Wiersma, 1961a,b). In addition, our collaboration, mainly between 1953 and 1964, apparently had major influences on the course of Professor Wiersma's later research and on my own continual attempts to bridge the gap between visual physiology and the oriented behavior of aquatic animals.

His first publication on visual systems was an abstract; the full report was published the next year (Waterman and Wiersma, 1954). These described experiments on the *Limulus* compound eye designed to identify the spike-generating cells in this aberrant but much-studied sense organ.

Our results convinced me that the *Limulus* eye was a poor choice to model the polarization sensitivity (PS) clearly demonstrated behaviorally in insects (von

Talbot H. Waterman • Department of Biology, Yale University, New Haven, Connecticut 06520.

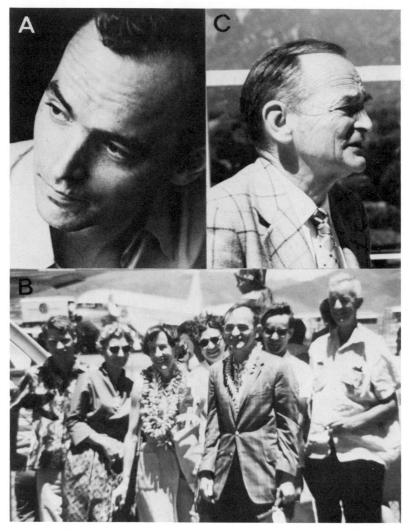

Fig. 1. C. A. G. Wiersma, then and now. A: Pasadena, July 1940, at the time of our first meeting at Cal Tech. B: Honolulu, August 1961, just after our collaborative experiments on *Podophthalmus* with Brian Bush. Left to right: Brian Bush (now Bristol), Millie vanWeel, Jane Wiersma, Mabs Campbell, Kees Wiersma, Peter Kunze (now Stuttgart), and Piet vanWeel (now emeritus, Hawaii). C: Ojai, April 1976, during the present symposium in his honor.

Frisch, 1948) and in crustaceans (Baylor and Smith, 1953). Consequently, I needed a better preparation to study the visual information processing underlying polarotaxis in crustaceans, and I hoped to apply unit-isolating techniques like those pioneered by Wiersma and van Harreveld (e.g., 1936, 1938*a*) in decapod leg nerves.

In the summer of 1955, we attempted to do this in decapod crustaceans at the Bermuda Biological Station. It was found that the eyestalk circulation had to be intact to maintain normal activity in visual interneurons (INs) at the optic peduncle level. Without developing an appropriate perfusion method, we could not use the technique of unit isolation by progressive nerve splitting that we had intended. Even so, sensory channeling in visual units was sampled extensively with needle electrodes thrust into the eyestalk. Several species were used, particularly the crabs *Grapsus* and *Goniopsis,* as well as the spiny lobster *Panulirus.*

In the lobster, sustaining units were found to be common, as were on–off elements and a third category responding to moving visual stimuli (Fig. 2). Sustaining fibers were not then studied in crabs; their optic nerves are dominated by a spectrum of movement fibers selectively sensitive to different directions and velocities of stimulus displacement. In all cases, the visual fields of such higher-order optic INs were found to be surprisingly large (Waterman and Wiersma, 1963).

After our Bermuda work, Wiersma made his own first published references to visual responses. Thus, among other INs of *Procambarus,* a few multimodal fibers

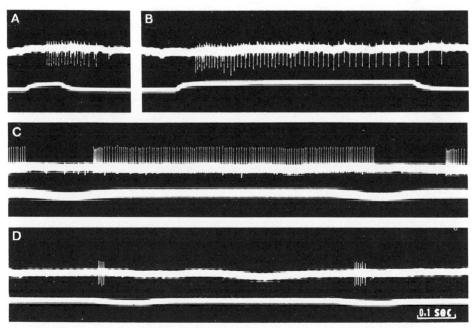

Fig. 2. Single crustacean optic nerve units recorded during the second Wiersma–Waterman collaboration which occurred in Bermuda in 1955. A and B are records of a sustaining fiber in the spiny lobster *Panulirus* responding to 0.1-sec and 0.6-sec flash stimuli, respectively. C and D compare the quite different responses of the *Panulirus* sustaining fiber and those of an off fiber in the rock crab *Grapsus,* both reacting to the shadow of a pendulum interrupting the light at intervals of 0.15 sec. We found sustaining fibers to be common in *Panulirus,* and rarer, if in fact present, in crabs. From Waterman and Wiersma (1963).

were reported to have visual input (Wiersma, 1958). Light responses were also discussed to some extent in his chapter "Reflexes and the Central Nervous System" in *The Physiology of Crustacea* (Wiersma, 1961*b*).

Again in 1961, Wiersma, Bush, and I undertook a considerable study of visual information processing in the swimming crab *Podophthalmus* (Fig. 3). This crab has extremely elongate penultimate segments in its eyestalk, which provide a long enough optic peduncle so that Wiersma-type unit isolation is possible *in vivo* provided that the afferent circulation is maintained intact.

These experiments confirmed and extended the Bermuda results (Bush *et al.*, 1964; Waterman *et al.*, 1964; Wiersma *et al.*, 1964). Among afferent fiber types found were novelty fibers as well as movement fibers maximally sensitive to specific target velocities or directions. Visual fields were estimated to include 300–

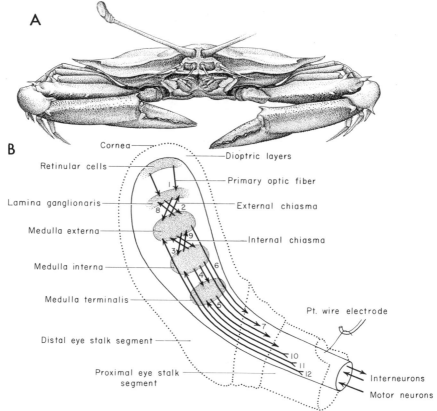

Fig. 3. The portunid swimming crab *Podophthalmus* (A) used in the experiments done in Hawaii in 1961 by Wiersma, Bush, and Waterman. The extraordinarily long eyestalk permitted single optic nerve fibers to be teased out and recorded, with the circulation and the rest of the animal intact. The eyestalk diagram (B) shows the visual information-processing system generalized from Bertil Hanström's classic studies. As discussed in the text, this basic pattern must now be altered for crayfish (and most likely for other decapods, mysids, and stomatopods) by adding a class of long visual fibers which pass directly from R_8 in the retina to the medulla externa. From Waterman *et al.* (1964).

10,000 facets, and no close point-to-point visual representation was in evidence. Movement sensitivity, in some cases at least, appeared to be the result of release from inhibition.

Study of efferent IN traffic demonstrated extensive exchange between the two eyestalks, as well as much IN information from statocysts and other mechanoreceptors of the body and legs. Thus the ipsilateral ganglia not only are informed of what the contralateral eye is sensing but also receive at least tactile and proprioceptive input from the rest of the body. Single- and multiple-modality units having moderate to large receptive fields were demonstrated. These data made it clear that decapod optic ganglia function in the integration of higher-order visual and mechanoreceptive information, both afferent and efferent.

Subsequent to these experiments on *Podophthalmus*, Wiersma's interest in visual INs proved to be self-sustaining. Since 1964, he and his other collaborators have published one or two papers a year on this topic in addition to those relating to other problems. Having suggested the relation of our interaction on the growth of Kees's research interests, let me now consider its effect on my own professional development.

Beyond my introduction to the crayfish as an important animal for comparative physiology, the most direct influence, of course, was my initiation into Wiersma's pragmatic and stimulating approach to experimental problems, including his method of isolating and analyzing single neural units. While the latter seems highly appropriate to finding the bridge between sensory input and oriented behavior, it can provide only one of many kinds of knowledge essential for this purpose. Indeed, on the IN level at which we pursued it, single-unit analysis, despite the many other things it has illuminated, did not prove to be much help in understanding PS.

I have already mentioned that our 1953 work on *Limulus* reinforced related evidence (Waterman, 1954*a,b*) that other "more typical" compound eyes like those of hymenopteran insects or decapod crustaceans would be more suitable for analyzing the mechanism of polarized light (PL) orientation. Because I had recently demonstrated that natural underwater light is partially linearly polarized by mechanisms basically similar to those acting in the clear sky (Waterman, 1954*c*), I was particularly anxious to study the relevant visual functions in aquatic animals. Hence my most direct motive in collaborating with Kees in Bermuda in 1955 was to identify the *e*-vector analyzing channels in the decapod optic nerve.

However, we were unable to find any! Despite repeated testing, no neurons unequivocally sensitive to *e*-vector direction could be located in any of the several species studied. This was true also in the later extensive experiments on *Podophthalmus* in Hawaii. Yet behavioral evidence both in the field and in the laboratory proved that the crabs *Podophthalmus* (Fig. 4), *Ocypode, Goniopsis,* and *Uca* all are quite capable of polarotactic responses. Indeed, PS appears to be a very widespread sensory accomplishment in the animal kingdom, especially among forms with rhabdom-bearing eyes (for summary table, see Waterman, 1973).

This anomaly was naturally disturbing. Its explanation seemed most likely related to failure to record from the polarization-sensitive neurons of the optic

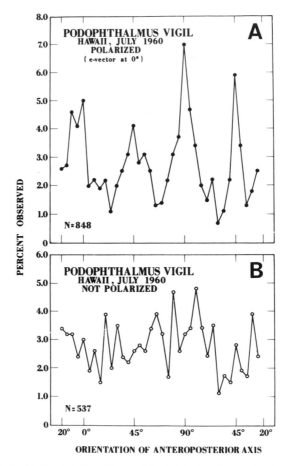

Fig. 4. Spontaneous azimuth orientation of the crab *Podophthalmus* in a vertical beam of white light (A) linearly polarized and (B) not polarized. Four preference peaks at 0°, ± 45°, and 90° to the *e*-vector are evident with the polarized beam as had been found in a number of other crustaceans and insects (Jander and Waterman, 1960). Note that despite this polarotactic behavior no clear evidence of polarization sensitivity was found in single units of the optic nerve of the same crab. From Waterman (1961*b*).

nerve, perhaps because of small diameter or similar handicap, or failure to recognize the code into which the polarization sensitivity could have been transformed. In current perspective, the actual explanation may have been our failure to give the appropriate type of light stimulus. After a considerable lapse of time, two independent workers have now reported optic nerve responses to a rotating *e*-vector in *Procambarus* (Yamaguchi, 1967), the mud crab *Scylla* (Leggett, 1976), and a stomatopod (Yamaguchi *et al.*, 1976). Ironically, Wiersma and I tested only polarized flashes with fixed *e*-vector even though we were acutely aware of the importance of movement in visual responses to unpolarized stimuli (Waterman and Wiersma, 1963; Waterman *et al.*, 1964).

However, at that time, the failure of the Wiersma–Waterman experiments in Bermuda and Hawaii to locate polarization-sensitive INs made me shift research attention to more peripheral components of the visual system. More specifically, the receptor mechanism of *e*-vector discrimination and the relation of the PS input channels to those of the other visual parameters like wavelength became major objectives of my research program.

A variety of approaches, both direct and indirect, are relevant. Thus behavioral data may provide important clues to the necessary dimensions of sensory input. Basitactic azimuth orientation to an overhead beam of linear PL* is perhaps the simplest oriented response. Since the polarization is perforce symmetrical in 180°, simple polarotaxis of that sort must yield two opposite response directions. This is borne out behaviorally, but rather than one peak in 180°, PL responses often show instead two or four peaks in the semicircle (Jander and Waterman, 1960; Geisler, 1961; Waterman, 1961*b;* Daumer *et al.*, 1963; Jander, 1963; Jander *et al.*, 1963; Rensing and Bogenschütz, 1966; Umminger, 1969; van der Glas, 1975) (Fig. 4).

In some cases at least (e.g., *Daphnia:* Jander and Waterman, 1960), the behavioral occurrence of one, two, or four peaks in 180° depends on the state of the animal or the intensity and other properties of the light pattern. However, little is known about the underlying causal relations. It is clear, however, that at least under some experimental conditions the perceived *e*-vector can give rise to multiply ambiguous orientation information. This must depend either on the peripheral *e*-vector analyzing mechanism or on the way in which the primary sensory data is processed (Macagno *et al.*, 1973).

Clearly, to use natural PL as a practical extension of a sun compass, the animal must resolve such ambiguities. Nevertheless, their occurrence under experimental conditions may well provide a means of understanding the basic mechanism. We have been analyzing such responses in fishes (e.g., Waterman and Forward, 1970; Waterman, 1972) and plan to resume similar work with aquatic arthropods shortly.

Meanwhile, a more direct physiological series of studies have been made in the retina itself. Here we were able to demonstrate PS by several techniques which illuminated its cellular, fine structural, and molecular bases.

This research has been reviewed several times recently (Waterman, 1974, 1975*a,c*), so it need not be covered again in detail here. Nevertheless, because PS seemed to have gone underground somewhere between the demonstrated mechanism in the retina and the documented polarotactic behavior, I became fascinated with the question of visual information channeling in relation to PS. The further pursuit of that topic both by us and by others is a matter of considerable current attention.

---

*Since linear PL comprises nearly all PL in nature (Waterman, 1975*a,b*), the present discussion is limited to this kind of polarization.

The Basis of Sensitivity to PL

Perceived on the rebound from the *Podophthalmus* work, Eguchi's Ph.D. thesis (Eguchi, 1964, 1965), which included a clear description of the fine structure of the crayfish rhabdom, seemed to offer a significant clue to the PS channeling problem. Specifically, it suggested that the seven regular retinular cells in each ommatidium are divided into two groups (R_1, R_4, and R_5, and R_2, R_3, R_6, and R_7, using Eguchi's, 1965, cell numbering) mediating orthogonal sensitivity to e-vector orientation. Morphologically, this two-channel organization proved to be widespread in mysids, decapods, and stomatopods (Mayrat, 1962; Rutherford and Horridge, 1965; Eguchi and Waterman, 1966; Kunze, 1967; Schiff and Gervasio, 1969; Krebs, 1972; Meyer-Rochow, 1975; Nässel, 1976).

Two such PS channels were in fact demonstrated functionally by selective adaptation of the ERG in the crab *Cardisoma* (Waterman and Horch, 1966). Maximum planes of vibration sensitivity in the central retina are vertical and horizontal given the normal eyestalk position in space. In both crabs and crayfish, these axes of maximum sensitivity lie parallel to the microvilli of their respective rhabdomeres (Eguchi and Waterman, 1967); the absorption spectrum of the intraocular dichroic element is the same as that of the rhodopsin present in the photoreceptor membrane (Waterman *et al.*, 1969).

Intracellular recording proved that both classes of wavelength-discriminating retinular cells (violet and yellow, respectively) present in the crayfish are highly sensitive to e-vector direction (Waterman and Fernandez, 1970). Surprisingly, they often yield PS ratios of 10 or more, significantly greater than the dichroic ratios obtained with microspectrophotometry of isolated rhabdoms (Hays and Goldsmith, 1969; Waterman *et al.*, 1969; Goldsmith, 1975a,b). Each ommatidium was shown by selective adaptation to contain receptor cells belonging to both PS channels *and* the two λ discriminating channels (Eguchi and Waterman, 1968; Eguchi *et al.*, 1973).

This relatively simple ommatidial input pattern in crustaceans is complicated by the widespread presence of an additional cell different from the regular retinular cells. This "accessory" or "rudimentary" unit was well known to the nineteenth-century students of compound eyes (e.g., Parker, 1891, p. 113). However, relatively few details of its structure and relations had been discovered then, and it has been given little attention until quite recently. Now we know enough about R_8 to realize that it can no longer be ignored (Fig. 5).

The key point which remained to be unequivocally proved by electron microscopy is that R_8 has a distinct rhabdomere made up of a photoreceptor membrane organized into microvilli (Mayrat, 1962; Kunze and Boschek, 1968; Eguchi and Waterman, 1973). Hence this special retinular cell must actually have some visual rather than an "accessory" or "rudimentary" function (Kunze, 1967; Eguchi and Waterman, 1973): its location, fine structure, and central connections imply a distinctive or even important role. Therefore, any effective appraisal of visual

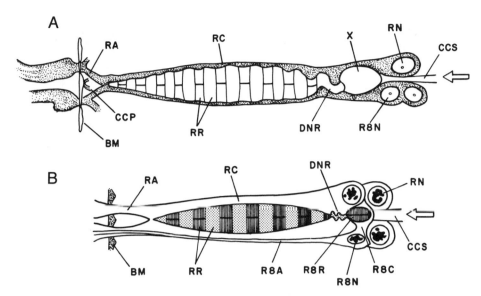

Fig. 5. Through history with the crayfish retinula. Comparison of G. H. Parker's 1895 figure for *Astacus* (A) based on light microscopy alone and Nässel's 1976 diagram for *Pacifastacus* (B) based on light and electron microscopy. Despite his extraordinary perceptivity, Parker did not realize that the egg-shaped cavity he labeled "X" contains the rhabdom of R_8 as found by Nässel (see Fig. 8). Nor did Parker identify the four-lobed cell body of this accessory retinular cell, although he suspected he saw its axon at the periphery of the retinula. BM, Basement membrane; CCP, crystalline cone process reaching BM; CCS, crystalline cone stalk through which direct illumination (indicated by the broad arrows) reaches the rhabdom; DNR, distal necklike region of the fused rhabdom; RA, retinular axon, RC, retinular cytoplasm, R8A, axon of R_8; R8C, cytoplasm of lobe A of R_8; R8N, nucleus of R_8 in lobe A; R8R, unbanded rhabdomere of R_8; RN, regular retinular cell nucleus, RR, banded fused rhabdom of R_1–R_7; X, cavity, apparently fluid filled, reported by Parker where electron microscopy shows R8R. Redrawn from the originals by Virginia Simon.

information channeling must include this unicellular pathway along with those provided by the regular retinular cells.

So far, there are no data on R_8 function in crustaceans, but the rapid growth of fine structural knowledge of these cells should soon stimulate appropriate experiments. Current studies which began some years ago on the functions of R_7 and R_8 in dipteran insect eyes (Kirschfeld, 1973*b*; Kirschfeld and Snyder, 1975) and more recently on R_9 in bees (Menzel and Snyder, 1974; Gribakin, 1975) should infuse more interest into the crustacean case, too.

To begin with, the photoreceptive cell we are interested in (R_8) lies distally in the retinula and its rhabdomere is the first to be traversed by incident light (Fig. 6). In *Grapsus*, the R_8 rhabdomere constitutes about 20% of the total rhabdom length (Eguchi and Waterman, 1973); in *Astacus*, its contribution is 12% (Krebs, 1972); in *Panulirus*, it contributes only 5% (Meyer-Rochow, 1975). It is followed in axial sequence by the well-known fused rhabdom formed conjointly by the seven rhab-

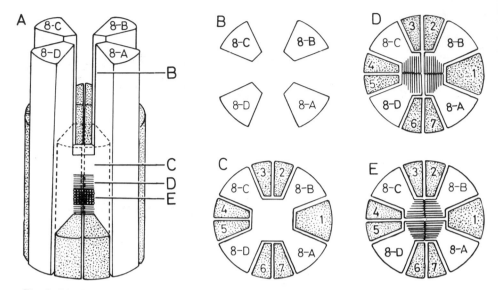

Fig. 6. Distal end of a retinula in *Grapsus* showing the apical location of the four-lobed cross-retinular cell (8-A, -B, -C, -D) as seen in a stereo view (A) and at various cross-sectional levels as indicated (B–E). Note that the R_8 rhabdomere, unlike that of the crayfish (Figs. 5B and 8), is banded and comprises two orthogonal sets of microvilli (Fig. 7). In the intermediate retinular region below the level in section E, the rhabdomeres of R_1–R_7 contribute alternately to the inner parts of the orthogonal rhabdom plates, while R_8 forms their outer parts. More proximally, only R_1–R_7 comprise the typical fused rhabdom. From Eguchi and Waterman (1973), which the reader should see for more detail.

domeres of the regular retinular cells R_1–R_7 (Waterman, 1961c; Eguchi and Waterman, 1966). Single R_8 receptor cells in this optically primary position have been reported to occur widely in mysid, decapod, and stomatopod crustaceans (Table I).

Such cells share certain characteristics with accessory retinular cells of various other crustaceans and many insects. Obviously, the optically "in series" position of R_8 in the retina establishes a tiered structure. This may be important, e.g., for wavelength and e-vector discrimination, since the first optic component can serve as a filter in front of the second (Gribakin, 1975; Menzel and Snyder, 1975; Snyder, 1975). Along with its distal position, a general feature of R_8 which would affect its optic role is the conspicuous lack of screening pigment granules in its cytoplasm.

Presumably this would leave any light filtering or blocking to its rhabdomere or to other ommatidial components. From a practical point of view, this lack of pigment granules as well as its characteristically less electron-dense cytoplasm usually allows even small sectors of R_8 to be distinguished from R_1–R_7. Even R_8 axons usually can be recognized because those of the regular retinular cells are pigmented well below the basement membrane (e.g., in *Pacifastacus:* Nässel, 1976).

Tiered, layered, or stratified rhabdoms occur in many insects eyes (e.g., the neuropteran *Chrysopa,* with two distal cells in series plus six proximal cells in parallel to one another, all with rhabdomeres: Horridge and Henderson, 1976; the

Table I. Accessory Retinular Cells (R_8) in Crustacea[a]

		Accessory cell			Regular retinular cells			
Animal	Lobes	Rhabdomere location	Microvilli direction	Microvilli band	Number	Band	Technique	Source
Mysida								
Mysis	4	distal	?	no	7	yes	LM	Eguchi and Waterman (1973)
Mysidium	4	distal	?	no	7	yes	EM	Eguchi and Waterman (1966, 1973)
Mysidopsis	4	distal	horizontal[b]	no	7	yes	EM	Nässel (1976)
Praunus	4	distal	?	no	7	yes	LM, EM	Mayrat (1956, 1962)
Astacidea								
Astacus	—	distal	?	—	7	yes	LM, EM	Parker (1895), Krebs (1972)
Pacifastacus	4	distal	horizontal	no	7	yes	LM, EM	Nässel (1976)
Procambarus	4	distal	horizontal	no	7	yes	LM, EM	Eguchi and Waterman (unpublished)
Palinura								
Panulirus	4	distal	2 orthogonal directions	yes	7	in part, yes	LM, EM	Meyer-Rochow (1975)
Brachyura								
Goniopsis	4	distal	?	—	7	yes	LM	Eguchi and Waterman (1973)
Grapsus	4	distal	vertical horizontal	yes	7	yes	LM, EM	Eguchi and Waterman (1973)
Menippe	4	distal	?	—	7	yes	EM	Eguchi and Waterman (1973)
Ocypode	4	distal	irregular	—	7	yes	LM / EM	Dembowski (1913),[c] Kunze (1967); Kunze and Boschek (1968)
Podophthalmus	4	distal	?	—	7	yes	LM	Eguchi and Waterman (1973)
Stomatopoda								
Squilla	4	distal	?	—	7	yes	EM	Eguchi and Waterman (unpublished)

[a] Accessory cells clearly or probably different from R_8 in the groups in this table have been reported in a variety of other crustaceans (e.g., Waterman, 1961c; Kunze, 1967; Elofsson and Odselius, 1975). The dashes indicate absence of relevant data.
[b] D. R. Nässel, personal communication.
[c] Clear in his Fig. 11 (Plate 40) but not mentioned in text or legend.

firefly *Photuris* and the whirligig beetle *Cyrinus,* with one distal, six medial, and one basal retinular cell, each with rhabdomeres: Horridge, 1969*b*; Wachmann and Schröer, 1975) and in crustacean groups which do not have an R_8 like that in decapods (e.g., *Artemia:* Elofsson and Odselius, 1975; *Porcellio:* Nemanic, 1975). Thus two or three sequential layers appear almost universal in compound eyes.

No doubt the most extensive tiering is to be found in banded rhabdoms where microvilli are interdigitated in such a way that light passes repeatedly from one set of rhabdomeres alternately to another. In the elongate apposition rhabdom of crabs like *Callinectes,* there may be up to 450 alternating orthogonal layers of photoreceptive microvilli (Eguchi and Waterman, 1966).

Another striking feature of the mysid, decapod, and stomatopod R_8 is that it is divided into four obliquely oriented (*vis-à-vis* vertical and horizontal) lobes, which are interconnected only by a slender bridge of cytoplasm. Hence the appropriateness of Kunze's term ''cross-retinula cell'' (Kunze and Boschek, 1968). Such R_8's are known only in these malacostracan groups. Distally, near the proximal end of the crystalline cone stalk, the lobes may be quite large (Fig. 7); they taper proximally and lie in characteristic locations sandwiched *between* cells of the following four pairs: R_1R_2, R_3R_4, R_5R_6, and R_7R_1.

One of the four lobes (the one between R_1 and R_2) contains the nucleus of R_8 and is attenuated proximally as its axon. This runs on the outer surface of R_1 through the basement membrane, as suspected for the crayfish by Parker (1895) and actually observed electron microscopically by Krebs (1972) and Nässel (1976). The proximal ends of the other three lobes terminate blindly in the distal part of the retinula. Each of the four lobes gives rise on its axial surface to about one-quarter of the microvilli of the R_8 rhabdomere (Fig. 8B). As usual in the regular retinular cells, these are normal to the optic axis.

In mysids and crayfish, all the microvilli in R_8 are closely parallel to one another, as are those of R_1–R_7 individually (Mayrat, 1962; Eguchi and Waterman, 1966).* The R_8 microvillus alignment is horizontal in *Pacifastacus* and *Procambarus* (Nässel, 1976; Eguchi and Waterman, unpublished). However, in *Grapsus* (Eguchi and Waterman, 1973) and *Panulirus* (Meyer-Rochow, 1975) the microvilli of the R_8 rhabdomere are aligned in two orthogonal directions which at least in the crab are vertical and horizontal relative to the animal's normal spatial orientation (Fig. 7). Bidirectional arrangement of R_8 microvilli thus occurs in both superposition and apposition eyes.

Finally, recent evidence demonstrates that R_8, unlike R_1–R_7, does not terminate in the most distal of the eyestalk ganglia, the lamina ganglionaris (Hafner, 1973; Nässel, 1976). The classic account (reviewed by Horridge, 1965), stemming largely from the work of Hanström, stated that all retinular cell axons in Crustacea terminate in the lamina ganglionaris. Now we know that, in the crayfish, R_8 con-

---

*Rhabdomeres and rhabdoms twisted as a consequence of retinular twisting have been well documented in insects (Grundler, 1974; Horridge and Mimura, 1975; Horridge *et al.,* 1975; Menzel, 1975*a*; Menzel and Blakers, 1975; Snyder and McIntyre, 1975) but have not been reported in crustaceans, perhaps because they have not been looked for carefully enough.

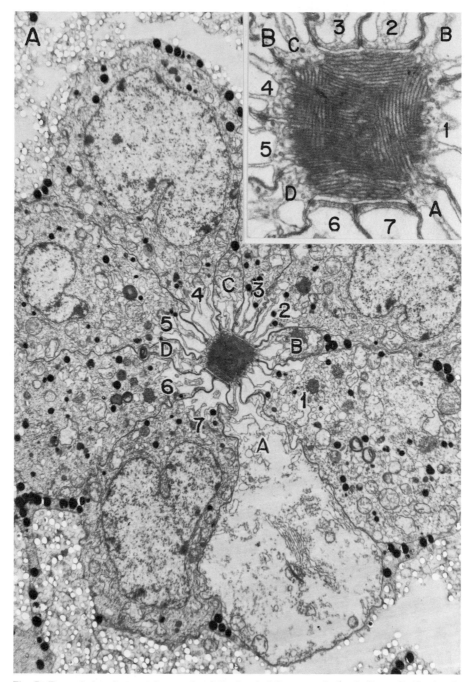

Fig. 7. Transmission electron micrographs of distal end of *Grapsus* retinula. A: Shows R_1–R_7 plus the four pigment-free intercalated lobes of R_8—A, B, C, D. × 6000. The insert B shows enlarged detail of the axial region with two orthogonal sets of microvilli originating from the cytoplasm of the lobes of R_8. × 20,000. From Eguchi and Waterman (1973).

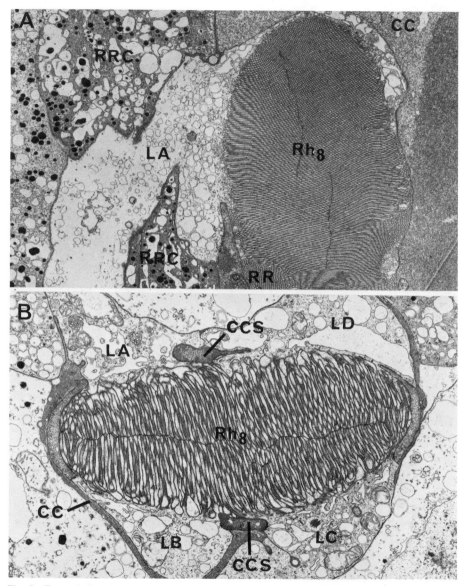

Fig. 8. Transmission electron micrographs showing details of the R_8 rhabdomere in the crayfish *Procambarus* which seems essentially the same as that of *Pacifastacus* reported by Nässel (1976). A: Axial section. × 5600. B: Transverse section. × 7400. CC, Crystalline cone stalk; CCS, crystalline cone process; LA,LB, LC, LD, four lobes of R_8; Rh_8, rhabdomere of R_8; RR, distal end of regular fused rhabdom; RRC, part of regular retinular cell. From Eguchi and Waterman (unpublished).

tinues through the distal optic chiasma to the next more central optic ganglion, the medulla externa (Fig. 3). In passing directly through the lamina ganglionaris, R_8 resembles the tiered R_7 and R_8 of Diptera and other insects as well as the basal R_9 plus two other retinular cells of the honey bee (Melamed and Trujillo-Cenóz, 1968; Horridge and Meinertzhagen, 1970; Sommer and Wehner, 1975; Strausfeld, 1976). The recent crayfish data therefore provide clear evidence for quite different information processing of the outputs of the decapod R_1–R_7 compared with R_8. There has been speculation, at least, that the decapod R_8 might be a short-wavelength receptor unit.

Furthermore, the synaptic terminals of R_1–R_7 occur at two distinct levels in the neuropil of the lamina ganglionaris in *Procambaraus* (Hafner, 1973, 1974), *Pandalus* (Nässel 1975), *Pacifastacus* (Nässel, 1976), and *Squilla* (cited by Nässel 1976). In fact, the number of cells in these two classes match those in the two orthogonal PL discriminating channels in the crayfishes (Hafner, 1973; Nässel, 1976).

There are four such neurosensory terminals in the distal plexiform layer and three in the proximal layer for each neurommatidium (cartridge) of the lamina. Their origins have not yet been traced back to specific cells among R_1–R_7, but there are two corresponding classes of secondary monopolar neurons. These synapse, respectively, with the two types of afferent receptor axons and provide one of several routes of information transfer and integration. Other neuronal types in the lamina are monopolars which in *Pandalus* receive sensory input from all seven regular retinular terminals of a neurommatidium as well as tangential fibers arising from axons which originate in the medulla externa (Nässel, 1976).

Note that, in the decapods generally, axons from neighboring ommatidia penetrate the basement membrane in four meshes (Parker, 1895; Kunze, 1967; Krebs, 1972; Meyer-Rochow, 1975; Nässel, 1976), but, at least in *Pacifastacus,* the seven retinular cell terminals of a single neurommatidium originate from three adjacent ommatidia, three from one and two each from two others (Nässel, 1976). This differs from both the dipteran and fused rhabdom patterns of distribution reported in insects (Trujillo-Cenóz, 1965; Horridge and Meinertzhagen, 1970; Ribi, 1974; Sommer and Wehner, 1975; Strausfeld, 1976)

In crustaceans, neurommatidia were thought to be well developed in crepuscular and deepwater forms (Hanström 1927; Waterman, 1961c); they are obscure or absent in the firefly *Phausis* (Ohly, 1975) and some other insects. Obviously, in such cases, a projection pattern mapping the retina onto the lamina cannot be based on repeating neurommatidial units. Strausfeld, in his elegant monograph (1976), concludes there are four types of such projections in insects: (1) neural superposition, as in Diptera, (2) optical superposition, (3) apposition with fused rhabdom, and (4) apposition with unfused rhabdomeres and open rhabdom, as in Hemiptera.

Since open rhabdoms are not known in well-studied crustaceans, only projection types (2) and (3) should occur in this group.* However, primary mapping has

*Note, however, that an open rhabdom has recently been confirmed in *Ligia* by Eguchi (figured in Waterman, 1975c, Fig. 10). This rhabdomere pattern is quite different from that reported in other isopods like *Idothea* (Peabody, 1939), *Oniscus* (Tuurala and Lehtinen, 1971), and *Porcellio* (Nemanic, 1975).

not been studied yet in Brachyura and larval Astacidea which have apposition compound eyes. Also, in the decapod superposition eyes whose lamina ganglionaris connections are known (as cited above), Nässel (1976) concludes that a sort of neural superposition (type 1 above) occurs. Whether this challenges Strausfeld's classification or merely indicates that changes or additions may be required to encompass both insects and crustaceans remains to be seen.

One obvious caveat is inherent in the banded rhabdomere pattern of mysids, decapods, and stomatopods (Eguchi and Waterman, 1966). None of the systems Strausfeld has studied has this kind of photoreceptor organelle, although it is known to occur in a few insects (Meyer-Rochow, 1971, 1974). Theories to explain the significance of such layering of microvilli from various retinular cells in the same ommatidium have usually been based on assumed optical advantages. These include yielding maximum sensitivities to I, e-vector orientation, and λ (Shaw, 1969a; Gribakin, 1975; Menzel and Blakers, 1975; Snyder, 1975), or blocking rotation of the e-vector with depth in the rhabdom and preventing conversion of linear to elliptical PL (Täuber, 1974). However, it is not known specifically whether such rhabdoms establish a special type of retina–lamina projection distinct from those categorized by Strausfeld (1976).

Among the crustaceans, all of the known banded rhabdoms occur in stalk-eyed forms, but the podophthalmic branchiopods like *Artemia* do not have banding (Eguchi and Waterman, 1966; Elofsson and Odselius, 1975). The Mysida, as cited above, have typical orthogonally alternating, toothed rhabdomeres like those of decapods and stomatopods, yet they are classified in a group of predominantly sessile-eyed forms (Peracarida) including isopods and amphipods whose eyes seem quite different in organization (Waterman, 1961c).

Explanations of these and related matters depend on new knowledge of the comparative fine structure as well as the comparative physiology of crustacean and other e-vector-discriminating visual systems. In the present lively state of interest in polarization sensitivity, continuing progress should be forthcoming.

ACKNOWLEDGMENTS

Current research is supported by National Institutes of Health Grant EY 00405; earlier projects covered by this report were variously funded by the Society of Fellows (Harvard University), ONR, NSF, AFOSR, the Guggenheim Foundation, the Japan Society for the Promotion of Science, and the National Geographic Society.

23

Modulation of Visual Input in the Crayfish

Hugo Aréchiga

Introduction

The continuous adjustment of responsiveness in sensory pathways to the changing conditions of ambient stimuli and the milieu interieur, by enabling the sensory processors to extract at any moment the most relevant information, is one of the basic operations by which the nervous system serves to optimize the coupling of the organism to the environment. It is accomplished by a wide variety of mechanisms, ranging from gross motor reactions, which modify the degree of exposure of sensory receptors to the stimuli, to the subtlest adjustments of the dynamic properties of neurons affecting specific aspects of information processing. In the crayfish, several mechanisms for modulation of visual input have been characterized, and their role in the generation of complex patterns of behavior will be discussed.

Modulation of Retinal Responsiveness to Light

For an animal such as the crayfish, commonly dwelling in shallow waters, the ample variation in intensity of environmental light far exceeds the dynamic range of the $V-\log I$ curve of the retinal photoreceptors, which extends not more than 3 log units (Glantz, 1968). So far, no differences which might suggest the type of differentiation found in insects (see Kirschfeld, 1972) are known in the sensitivity of the various retinular cells of each ommatidium in the crayfish. Nor are there light-induced variations in the shape of the crystalline elements of the ommatidium or in the position of the rhabdom with reference to the crystalline tract, as is known in some insect species (Walcott, 1971a,b). Although anatomical evidence suggests that the eighth retinular cell of each ommatidium may act as a "dim light" receptor (Nässel, 1976), the only mechanism so far known to modulate the sensitivity to light in the crayfish at the retinal level involves changes in light admittance as a function of the position of retinal shielding pigments. It was postulated by Exner (1891), as a general feature of the functional organization of the compound eye of arthropods, that the migration of both sets of shielding pigments (see Fig. 1) results in a greater

Hugo Aréchiga • Departamento de Fisiología, Centro de Investigación del IPN, Apartado Postal 14-740, Mexico 14, D. F.

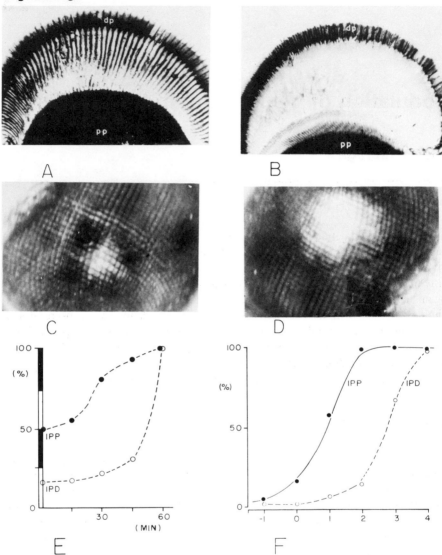

Fig. 1. Position of retinal shielding pigments in the crayfish *Procambarus* in full light adaptation (A) and when dark adapted (B). dp, Distal pigment; pp, proximal pigment. The corresponding area of glow in the cornea (clear area) is illustrated in C (light adaptation) and D (dark adaptation). The graphs at bottom represent the velocity of migration (E) and the relationship between light intensity (log units) and position (F) of proximal (●) and distal (○) pigments. Modified from Aréchiga *et al.* (1974a).

sensitivity to light and in lower visual acuity under dark adaptation, while the reverse occurs under light adaptation. This notion prevailed in the literature for several decades (see review by Parker, 1932). Crozier and Wolf (1939) showed in the crayfish *Cambarus* that the V–log I curve of flicker shifted to higher intensity values of illumination under light adaptation, or in darkness under the influence of eyestalk extracts known to promote the migration of retinal shielding pigments toward the light-adapted position. Yet De Bruin and Crisp (1957) rejected the idea that the distal pigment could contribute to the modulation of visual acuity, because the time course of its migration was too long to explain the changes in the $F-\log I$ curve they determined, and it was only the time course of migration of proximal retinal pigment which paralleled the changes in acuity. Furthermore, they challenged the role of shielding pigments in spatial resolution in the compound eye by showing that the refractive index of the crystalline tracts in the ommatidium was higher than that of the surrounding medium, thereby providing a mechanism of internal reflection that could explain the uniqueness of the information conveyed by each ommatidium. Since then, a vast amount of information has been collected on the role of the crystalline tracts as wave guides (see reviews by Horridge, 1968, 1975b). Walcott (1974), in the Australian crayfish *Cherax destructor,* found a sixfold enhancement of the acceptance angle of single retinular cells when dark adapted, without any noticeable change in the sensitivity ($V-\log I$ curve) to point sources of light. Moreover, he was unable to find any correlation between the change in light admittance and the position of both the distal and proximal pigments.

In the crayfish *Procambarus,* under dark adaptation as seen in Fig. 1, the distal pigment migrates distally, reaching the region around the cone cells near the cornea while the proximal pigment is fully rectracted below the basal membrane. In full light adaptation, the migration proceeds in the opposite way, and the rhabdoms are coated by the proximal pigment, while the distal pigment is surrounding the crystalline cone stems. The position of the distal pigment can be monitored externally by measuring the area of glow, which is proportional to the separation between the two pigment sets. Definite differences can be observed with regard to the reaction of both pigments to light and darkness. The time course of the migration is considerably faster in the proximal than in the distal pigment and, as shown in Fig. 1F, the light intensity functions are also noticeably different, the proximal pigment displaying more sensitivity, up to the point that it saturates when the distal is just beginning to respond. The time course of dark adaptation for the response to light of retinal photoreceptors (Fig. 2) shows two phases: a rapid, initial stage, which as might be expected is not paralleled by the migration of the distal pigment, and a late, slow stage, well demarcated from the first under these experimental conditions (see also Fig. 3). After 60–90 min, the time course of the response varies in parallel with the position of the distal pigment. In order to obtain further information about the role of the distal pigment, and since its migration is suppressed by ablation of the supraesophageal ganglion and by light deprivation (Aréchiga, Fuentes-Pardo, and Barrera-Mera, 1974), the time course of dark adaptation was followed both in ganglionectomized animals and in those kept under continuous darkness for several weeks. In this type of experiment, as shown in Fig. 3, a fixed amplitude of photoreceptor response is chosen, and the light intensity necessary to reach this amplitude is measured at different times during dark adaptation; it can be seen that paralysis of distal pigment results in a loss of the late stage of dark adaptation, the second phase is lost, and at the same time the adaptation is much quicker than in control animals. In all these experiments, only the sensitivity to diffuse light was tested during

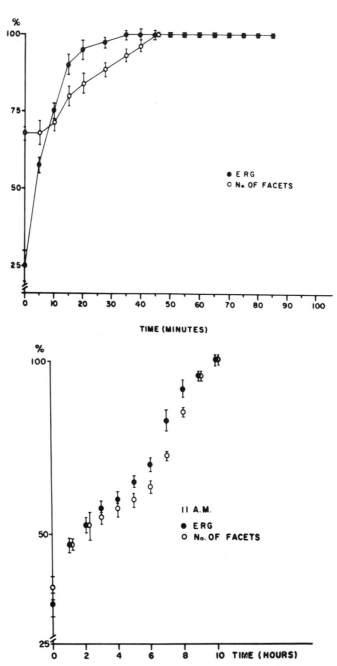

Fig. 2. Correlation between glow area (O) and amplitude of electroretinogram in *Procambarus* (●) during dark adaptation with two different time scales. In both cases, 100% is the maximum value attained at the end of the period considered in the graph. Abscissa: time of dark adaptation. From Aréchiga *et al.* (1974*a*).

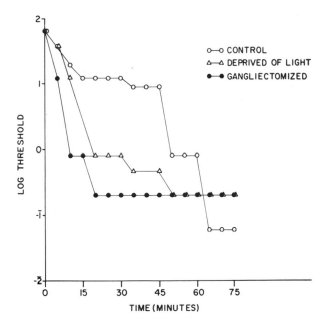

Fig. 3. Time course of dark adaptation in *Procambarus* retinal photoreceptors in control animals and its modification after paralysis of the distal pigment by ablation of the supraesophageal ganglion or by light deprivation. The threshold on the ordinate is the log of the intensity necessary to elicit a response of 200 μV amplitude. Abscissa: time of dark adaptation. From Aréchiga *et al.* (1974*a*).

recording of the mass responses of retinal photoreceptors. In order to determine if the effect is due to an enhancement of light admittance to the retina, point light sources are used, by attaching light pipes to the cornea at various distances from the recording electrodes. After full dark adaptation is attained, areas which initially were unresponsive are now excited. Under dark adaptation, the injection of eyestalk extracts, as mentioned above, promotes the migration of retinal pigment to the position of light adaptation and restores the light-adaptation type of distribution of sensitivity.

Deciding which pigment is involved in the response to eyestalk extracts has been a controversial issue. Welsh (1939) reporeted that in the crayfish *Cambarus* both pigments migrate in response to eyestalk extracts but that the distal pigment is more responsive than the proximal. In *Procambarus bouvieri,* as can be seen in Fig. 4, the only element reacting to extracts is the distal pigment. All along the range of concentrations tested, the proximal pigment remained dark adapted. On the other hand, the distal pigment light-adapting hormone has now been purified (see Kleinholz, 1966; Fernlund, 1971), and it does not promote migration of the proximal pigment in *P. bouvieri* (Villanueva, Fernández, and Aréchiga, unpublished). It seems clear then that the structure responsible for this reduction of sensitivity during light adaptation is the distal retinal pigment.

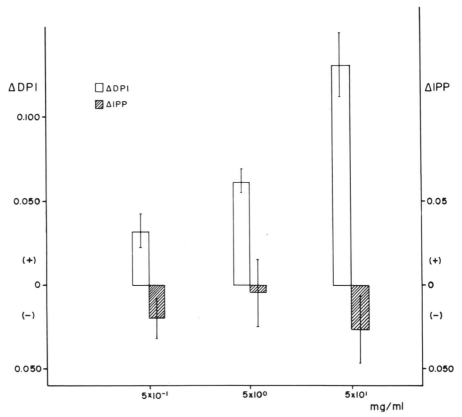

Fig. 4. Relationship between the concentration of eyestalk extract (mg wet weight/ml) and migration of proximal (ΔIPP) and distal (ΔDPI) retinal pigment. From Villanueva, Fernández, and Aréchiga (unpublished).

These differences in the behavior of the two pigments also correspond to different mechanisms of control; the proximal pigment of the crayfish is known to react to light even in the isolated eyestalk (Kleinholz, 1949), and a similar finding has been reported for other crustacean species (see review by Kleinholz, 1966). Regional differences in the migratory response of the proximal pigment among the various retinular cells contributing to the same rhabdom when stimulated with polarized light were reported more recently by Ludolph et al. (1973). Moreover, Hagins and Liebman (1962) have postulated a correlation between membrane potential and pigment migration in the squid retina. This suggests that the signal triggering the migration of proximal pigment is light impinging upon the rhabdom. The distal pigment behaves in a quite different manner; it does not respond to direct illumination, remaining motionless in the isolated retina and reacting only to local application of distal pigment hormone. On the other hand, the levels of intensity to which it reacts are considerably higher than the range encompassed by the response curve of retinular cells. This raises the question of what is the source of information about light intensity that initiates the neurohumoral reflex releasing the light-adapting hormone, given that the signal this system is reading is a level of light intensity higher than the maximum detectable under normal circumstances by the retinula. One possible explanation is that the relevant photoreceptor is not the rhabdom, as is suggested by the type of experiments illustrated in Fig. 5. The retina of a crayfish is implanted on the carapace of another animal, and the migration of

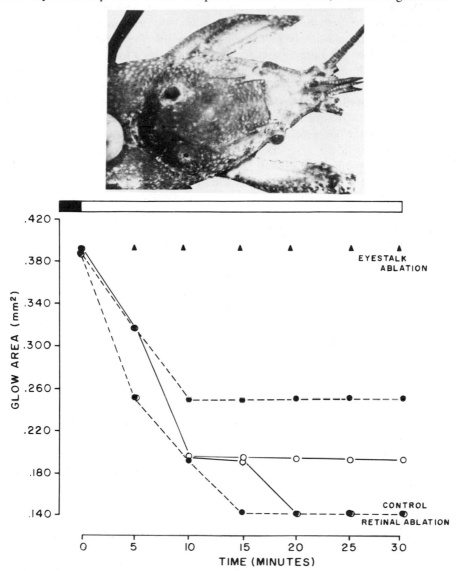

Fig. 5. Time course of migration toward the position of light adaptation in the distal retinal pigment of an implanted eye (indicated on the photograph above) in a host crayfish in control experiments (●) and after bilateral ablation of the retinae (○) and of eyestalks (▲) from the host. Ordinate: glow area; abscissa: time of illumination. From Aréchiga, Fernández and Villanueva (unpublished).

distal pigment is monitored by measuring the area of glow. The injection of light-adapting hormone following illumination promotes the migration of distal pigment both in the implanted eye and in the natural eyes of the host, with a very similar time course, and these effects persist unaltered after bilateral ablation of the host's own retinae. However, bilateral eyestalk ablation abolishes the light-induced migration, as illustrated in Fig. 5. It is a plausible assumption, therefore, that the reflex regulating the position of distal pigment is initiated at an extraretinal photoreceptor.

In conclusion, both the distal and the proximal pigment appear to participate in the modulation of sensitivity to light in the crayfish *Procambarus,* albeit with different functions. The proximal pigment operates with a low threshold and short time course, enabling the visual system to work at low levels of intensity. The distal pigment migration, in turn, shows a high threshold and a slow time course, as though its normal function is that of permitting the visual system to be desaturated at high intensitites of illumination by bringing the amount of light admitted to the rhabdom within the operation range of the retinal photoreceptors. It is interesting, in this context, that in the moths *Dilephila* and *Galleria* the sensitivity to light increases once the pigment has migrated to the light-adapted position (Höglund, 1966). It is also worth mentioning that in marine crustaceans, normally burrowing at medium or great depths (at least 30 m) and usually exposed to not more than 0.1–1 lux, the distal pigment is paralyzed in dark-adapted position. Such is the case of the Norway lobster *Nephrops norvegicus* (Aréchiga and Atkinson, 1975), and similar observations have been known for a long time for crustaceans living at great depths (Welsh and Chace, 1937).

One possible way to explain the fact that measurements of light sensitivity in single retinular cells stimulated by point lights of very small diameter fail to demonstrate any influence of the distal pigment (Walcott, 1974) is that in the crayfish, even under light adaptation, about 50% of the light impinging upon a retinular cell enters through neighbor ommatidia (Shaw, 1969b). Our own experiments with 100-μm light spots show that light can penetrate to most of the retina in the dark-adapted eye, and a similar observation was made by Kunze (1972) in *Astacus,* measuring the area of glow. Therefore, the modulatory action of distal pigment is most effective for light entering through remote ommatids. Another possible manner in which the retinal shielding pigments might exert a modulatory role on photoreceptor responsiveness in the crayfish is by acting as color filters as suggested by the observation of Woodcock and Goldsmith (1973) that when the pigments are in a light-adapted position, the peak of spectral sensitivity is shifted toward longer wavelengths.

Modulation of Receptive Field Organization of Visual INs

The consequences of changes in light admittance to the eye have been explored at higher levels of visual integration. The sustaining fibers, a group of visual interneurons (INs) whose axons run in the optic nerve, react to illumination of their receptive fields with a phasic–tonic discharge (Wiersma and Yamaguchi, 1966), the rate of which is a function of light intensity (Wiersma and Yamaguchi, 1967*a*; Glantz, 1971). Each unit has a unique field, although there is considerable overlapping among those of the various neurons. The time course of dark adaptation in these cells is parallel to that in the photoreceptors (Glantz, 1971), and there is a definite indication that the changes in light admittance described at the retinal level are also apparent in the INs. The sustaining units are organized in such a manner that light entering at any point of the retina alien to the receptive field of a given unit results in a depression of the response in that field (Wiersma and Yamaguchi, 1967*a*). This inhibition has been analyzed in *Procambarus* by Aréchiga and Yanagisawa (1973) and by Glantz (1973*a*).

When light is restricted to the receptive field of a sustaining unit, it fires a discharge lasting as long as the stimulus, and if this is strong and brief enough an afterdischarge ensues. Yet if light spreads beyond the receptive field, thus invading a neighboring, inhibitory region as shown in Fig. 6, the usual "on" response is followed by an "off" burst. When light is shined only on the inhibitory area, the off component is the only visible part of the response. In animals undergoing dark adaptation while test light pulses are applied to an area on the boundary of the

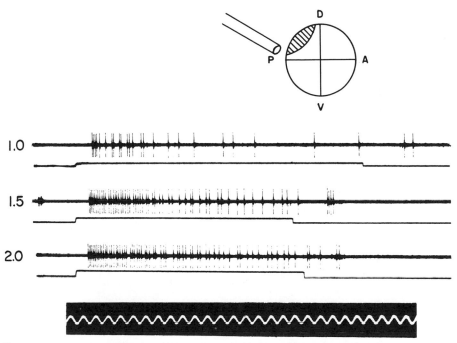

Fig. 6. Responses of a sustaining fiber (0-38) whose receptive field is the upper back rim, indicated as shaded area on the inset, which represents the whole visual field. A, Anterior; P, posterior; D, dorsal; V, ventral. The intensity of illumination is indicated at left in cd/ft². The bottom trace is of the signal from a photocell. Time signal: 20 Hz. The light pipe is covering 0.6 mm on the cornea, illuminating part of the receptive field and a small area outside of it. From Aréchiga and Yanagisawa (1973).

receptive field of a given unit, also covering part of the alien field, as dark adaptation proceeds (Fig. 7) both the on and the off components steadily increase, but after 20–30 min the off burst is greatly superseded by the on response, thus suggesting an expansion of the area encompassed by the receptive field. In another series of experiments, it was demonstrated that a point source of light which induced only inhibition on a given sustaining fiber in the light-adapted eye was capable of evoking excitation after 30 min of dark adaptation (Aréchiga and Yanagisawa, 1973). As seen in Fig. 8, the illumination of the receptive field of a sustaining fiber evokes the characteristic response, with an initial high rate which decays until reaching an asymptotic level. At that stage, another light pulse was applied on the opposite region of the eye (lower front quadrant) and the activity in the sustaining fiber was inhibited. The animal had been in darkness for only 5 min before this test was conducted. Afterward, it was left in darkness for 30 min and the procedure was repeated; however, in this case, the inhibition was preceded by a brief excitatory burst interpretable as an expansion of the receptive field. The animal was then injected with eyestalk extract (two eyestalks in 0.2 ml) and left in darkness for another 30 min. Tested again, the pattern of responsiveness had reverted to the

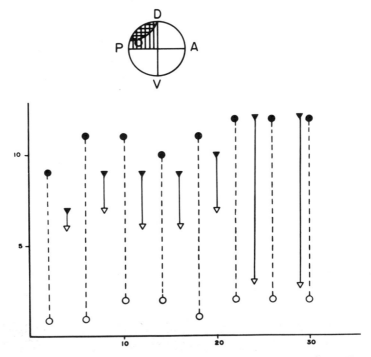

Fig. 7. Change in the organization of retinal fields during dark adaptation in *Procambarus*. The responses of two sustaining fibers were recorded at the same time: 0–38 (upper back rim field: ▼, "on"; ▽, "off") and 0–2 (upper back quadrant field: ●, "on"; ○, "off"). The inset shows the receptive fields of both units with a circle indicating the position of the light stimulus. Ordinate: number of spikes in the "on" and "off" components; abscissa: time of dark adaptation (minutes). Data from Aréchiga and Yanagisawa (1973).

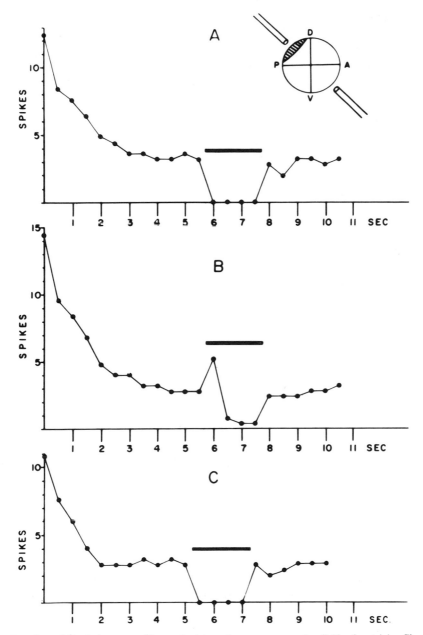

Fig. 8. Effect of distal pigment position on the interactions among receptive fields of sustaining fibers of *Procambarus*. The graphs show the effect of stimulating an area opposite to the receptive field of the IN under record (0-38, whose receptive field is represented by the shaded area in the inset). The horizontal bar indicates the time of application of the inhibitory stimulus. The excitatory light was turned on at time 0. A: Interaction when the animal had been in darkness only 5 min. B: After 30 min of dark adaptation. C: After 60 min of dark adaptation but 30 min after eyestalk extract had been injected. Ordinate: number of spikes in 0-38; abscissa: time after the initiation of the light pulse on the excitatory field. From Aréchiga *et al.* (1974*a*).

light-adapted type. Although no detailed mapping has been done of the spread of this expansion of the receptive fields of sustaining fibers under dark adaptation, it appears to be quite large, since illumination through 100-μm light pipes placed directly over the cornea can excite even sustaining fibers with receptive fields in remote parts of the eye.

It seems clear that the enhancement of receptive fields in sustaining fibers correlates with that in the light acceptance angle at the ommatidial level. No precise estimate exists for the strength of inhibition in the retina in relation to dark adaptation, but interesting in this regard is the observation by Chase (1975) that in the mollusk *Hermissenda,* commonly living on beaches, the mechanism for lateral inhibition is more developed than in *Tritonia,* which inhabits depths greater than 100 m.

Integration of Modulatory Mechanisms of Visual Input in Behavioral Patterns

Since the optic ganglia form the substrate of a highly complex set of neuronal integrations, it would not be surprising to find that the visual operations performed at this level are subjected to a wide variety of nonvisual influences. It is nevertheless striking to realize that out of the 17,000 axons composing the optic nerve of the crayfish (Nunnemacher *et al.,* 1962) fewer than 100 are known to be visual (Wiersma and Yamaguchi, 1966). The efferent nonvisual fibers so far characterized, largely by Wiersma and Yamaguchi, belong to several well-defined groups: (1) Primary mechanoreceptors from carapace hairs comprising the vast majority of the efferent population (about 12,000, from the data of Nunnemacher *et al.,* 1962; their functional significance is as yet unclear). (2) Primary mechanoreceptive axons from the statocysts, partaking in the integration of the space constancy of some visual INs. This is an operation by which those visual units selectively respond to light or movement in a given fixed position in the horizon (see Wiersma and Yamaguchi, 1967*a*). (3) Mechanoreceptive INs carrying tactile information from all areas of body surface and presumably contributing to the integration of the receptive pattern of some multimodal INs in the optic peduncle. (4) "Activity" fibers, conveying information about the level of body movements, and likely candidates to participate in the various manifestations of the "excited state," which is described below. (5) Proprioceptive INs from the joints. (6) Neurosecretory fibers arising from the supraesophageal ganglion and from more caudal ganglia (Durand, 1956). Some of these fibers have been traced up to the sinus gland, a neurohemal organ in the eyestalk, and it is conceivable from the data showed in the preceding section that these fibers transport hormones such as the one promoting the migration of distal pigment toward the light-adapted position.

Although the physiological role of most of these efferent axons is yet to be determined, there are a few instances in which a definite functional significance can be ascribed to a given set of such neurons.

Level of Arousal

In the course of experiments in partially tethered animals, Wiersma and Yamaguchi (1967*a*) noticed the occurrence of spontaneous forceful movements of the crayfish strong enough to detach the animal from the holding clamp, and they coined the term "excited state" to describe this behavioral pattern. The firing rate of the sustaining fibers under constant illumination showed a noticeable enhancement during the excited state. In freely moving animals with electrodes chronically implanted in the optic tract, Aréchiga and Wiersma (1969*a*) followed the changes in frequency of sustaining units under different levels of motor performance, from walking to struggle reactions, when confronting the preparation with another crayfish, and under various levels of illumination. As shown in Fig. 9, the facilitation of sustaining fibers is a function of the level of motor excitement. This facilitatory influence operates over a wide range of light intensities. The effect is not restricted to sustaining fibers; it is also detectable on the phasic jittery movement detectors, which respond to motion in their retinal receptive fields differently from the sustaining fibers. They give short bursts and are readily habituated (Aréchiga and Wiersma, 1969*a*), displaying a higher level of responsiveness under motor excitement. Again, this appears to be a graded function (Fig. 9).

Two efferent fibers in the optic tract of the crayfish have been considered as the most likely candidates to convey information about the excited state. Simultaneous recordings from one of them (0–71, a tonic activity fiber) and from a sustaining unit showed a close correlation between the timing and firing rates of both units, the bursting in 0–71 usually preceding by 20–40 msec the facilitation of the sustaining unit. The problem in regard to the movement detectors appears to be more complex, and no correlation has been established between the discharge in activity fibers and the facilitation of the movement detectors. In a detailed analysis of the habituation

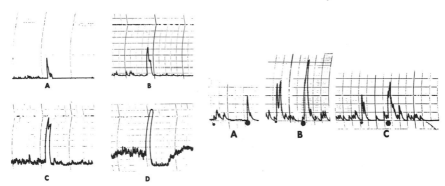

Fig. 9. Effect of motor excitement on the responsiveness of visual INs of *Procambarus*. At left, integrated responses of a sustaining fiber (0-38) to a 15-sec light pulse of 4 cd/ft² at different levels of excitement: A, from a "sleep" attitude; B, walking; C and D, strong motor excitation during struggle reactions. At right, a similar phenomenon in a multimodal IN in the periesophageal commissure (C-120) responding to mechanical (•) and visual (●) stimuli. At A, response in a quiet animal, which is "awakened" at B, and then tested when the motor excitement is subsiding. From Aréchiga and Wiersma (1969*a*).

of these units in *Procambarus,* Glantz (1974*b*) observed that the performance of spontaneous body movements was capable of "dishabituating" the motion detectors and that picrotoxin mimicked this effect; the responses under those circumstances could be even higher than in the controls.

The source of input for those INs and the locus of their output have not yet been determined. When the time course of the movements during excitement is correlated with the discharge in the activity fiber, the movement comes first, and then, after a "buildup" period, the activity unit attains its maximum frequency; on the other hand, passive movements of body parts are not capable of triggering any response, ruling out joint proprioceptors as the source of input to the activity fibers. The most likely possibilities are muscle proprioceptors or collaterals of motor neurons (MNs) feeding directly or indirectly into these INs. Since this facilitatory influence does not reach the receptors, its site of action may be at the visual INs. It may be of a permissive nature, since it is incapable of triggering the units by itself and only potentiates the activity evoked by specific visual inputs, or it may be spontaneously generated, as is the case in the sustaining fibers after several hours of dark adaptation.

If we assume that the excited state in its various degrees is reflecting the general level of arousal in the crayfish, it can be predicted that its influence would not be restricted to the visual pathway and that is indeed the case. Body movements are known to dishabituate tactile INs of the crayfish (Aréchiga *et al.*, 1975). Yet the coupling between the level of arousal and the responsiveness of sensory elements varies widely from one system to another. While the firing rate of sustaining units is closely related to that in the activity fibers, the motion detectors do not show a consistent relationship with the level of bodily activity (Glantz, 1974*c*), and in the rock lobster there is a depression of responsiveness in visual INs during strong excitement (Wiersma and York, 1972). It is to be expected that different mechanisms play a role in the neural modulation of visual elements under various levels of arousal and that the sign of the modulatory influence prevailing at a given moment should depend, as pointed out by Wiersma (1974), on the output task of the modulated neuron.

From a comparative viewpoint, the correlation between the level of arousal and the impulse traffic in sensory pathways appears to be conservative. Facilitatory activity fibers have been described in every crustacean species in which the neuronal components of the optic nerve have been functionally analyzed (Wiersma, 1969, 1970). Rowell (1971*b*) described a similar phenomenon in an insect *Schistocerca)*, and a mutual facilitation among sensory modalities mediated by sympathetic fibers innervating receptor cells is known to take place in the frog (Chernetski, 1964).

The Escape Reflex

The changes in visual input during the tail flick characteristic of the escape reflex still await a detailed analysis, but it is interesting to note in this regard that Yamaguchi (1967) observed a concurrent supression of the responses in the jittery movement fibers during the tail flick and that this effect persisted after the eyecups had been immobilized. The pathway for this influence and its mechanism of action remain unexplored. The more recent developments on the modulation of mechanoreceptive input to the lateral giant fibers of *Procambarus* (Zucker, 1972*a*; Krasne and Bryan, 1973; Wine *et al.*, 1975), however, do suggest a well-defined pattern of neural organization controlling sensory input during the execution of the escape behavior.

Other Behavioral Integrations

Much less information is available about the role of vision in other complex behavioral patterns. The type of interaction suggested by Maynard and Dingle (1963) between visual and chemosensitive input in feeding behavior of the lobster *Panulirus* poses an interesting problem concerning the role of modulatory mechanisms in the crayfish, as does the visual involvement in learning described long ago by Gilhousen (1927).

Circadian Rhythmicity

The mechanisms of modulation of visual input that have been considered above are also interacting along the 24-hr cycle, their level of activity being driven by the nyctahemeral environmental oscillations and the endogenous activity of a circadian pacemaker. In *Procambarus,* Aréchiga and Wiersma (1969*b*) described a circadian rhythm of responsiveness in the sustaining fibers. From the same study, it turned out that both the photoreceptors and the activity fibers were contributing to the rhythmicity. At the three levels of integration, the activity was higher during the subjective night than during the day phase. The spontaneous activity of the sustaining fibers in darkness displays a similar rhythmicity. Figure 10 shows a continous record during the night–day transition of a circadian cycle in a sustaining unit. Both the response to light and the spontaneous activity during darkness are changing in parallel. The notion was then advanced that a common synchronizing influence was acting at the different levels involved, modulating the responsiveness of the photoreceptors and the spontaneous activity of visual INs, as well as that of nonvisual units, as is the case of the "activity fibers." The demonstration that eyestalk extracts were capable of depressing the activity of elements in various parts of the nervous system (Aréchiga *et al.*, 1973; Aréchiga, 1974) was suggestive of neurohumoral cyclic influence. On the other hand, it has been known for a long time that the proximal (Bennitt, 1932) and distal (Welsh, 1939) retinal pigments undergo a circadian rhythmicity, as does the locomotory activity (Kalmus, 1938). Therefore, the interaction of the three rhythms could be responsible for the rhythmicity in the visual system.

The ablation of the supraesophageal ganglion suppresses the circadian rhythms of distal pigment migration and of response to light in the retinal photoreceptors

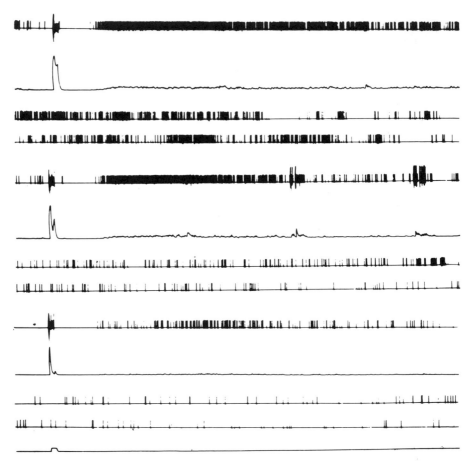

Fig. 10. Transition from night phase to day phase in a sustaining fiber (0-38) of *Procambarus*. Each trace is a 10-min record, and from top to bottom the records are continuous. Light pulses of 4 cd/ft² and 15 sec duration were applied once every 30 min (see the integrated responses). The rest of the time the animal was in darkness.

(Aréchiga *et al.*, 1973). Similar results have been reported by Page and Larimer (1975*b*), who have also postulated an analogous influence on the rhythm of loco-motion (Page and Larimer, 1975*a*). These results seem to rule out any role of the proximal pigment in the integration of rhythmicity in the retinal photoreceptors, but Barrera-Mera (personal communication) has recently found that by keeping the animals at low levels of illumination after the excision of the supraesophageal ganglion it is possible to detect circadian rhythmicity at the photoreceptor level. This finding is not surprising, given the intensity response curves for the two retinal shielding pigments shown in Fig. 1F.

It seems, therefore, that at least two concurrent circadian systems, quite dif-ferent in their functional organization, determine the rhythmicity of visual input.

The rhythm of distal pigment migration depends on the cyclic release of a neurohormone (Aréchiga and Mena, 1975), while the rhythm of neuronal activity is under the control of another neurosecretion, also released in a circadian manner (Aréchiga *et al.*, 1974*b*; Aréchiga, 1974). In this case, especially considering the rhythm of locomotion, an axonal link between the circadian pacemaker and the neural "effectors" has also been postulated (Page and Larimer, 1975*a,b*), and the possibility of endogenous rhythmicity, at least in some neurons, cannot be ruled out.

24

Crustacean Optomotor Memory

Richard Hirsh

Introduction

In order to know where the process of information storage can be observed, almost all attempts to determine the physiological basis of memory have begun by trying to localize a storage site. At the same time, there is no widely agreed-on operational definition of memory storage which controls for all of the other processes that various schools of psychology have thought to be attendant upon the performance of learned behavior. As a result, none of the candidates for storage sites that have been advanced so far has gained widespread acceptance. However, an alternative approach is available. It begins by determining what information is remembered. Then, by applying a knowledge of the information-processing abilities of the nervous system in question, it attempts to localize storage sites. This rather tall order is more likely to be achieved in invertebrates because of the smaller number of neurons present and the relative ease with which functionally identifiable neurons may be located. In any case, however, determining the content of a memory will not be wasted effort. The ultimate step in demonstrating that a particular medium stores acquired information is showing that a given piece of information is encoded by it. Such a demonstration requires a knowledge of what has been remembered.

Instances of learning are not ideally suited for determining the information content of memory. In order to show that the emergence of a new behavior is the result of experience rather than innate factors, learning experiments utilize arbitrary stimulus–response relationships. For instance, the ringing of a bell, after Pavlovian conditioning, elicits salivation. Many other stimuli can be used; the nature of the stimulus is not particularly relevant. Such arbitrary relationships place few constraints on learning theories. Thus the nature of the information that is acquired by a given species in a given learning situation is likely to be a topic of lively debate, as are the processes underlying performance of the learned behavior.

There are, however, many cases in which behavior directly reflects remembered information, thus allowing analysis of the content of memory. Usually they occur in situations where the evolution of the species has resulted in a general solution to the problem confronting the animal, and all that is required of the individual specimen is remembering the particular values of the relevant parameters

Richard Hirsh • Department of Psychology, McGill University, 1205 McGregor, Montreal H3A 1B1, Quebec, Canada.

of the situation. An example is the dance of the scout bees on their return to the hive. The orientation of the dance reflects the direction of the pollen source, while its distance from the hive can be discerned from the rate at which the abdomen is wagged. No learning, in the sense of problem solving, occurs in this case, but information is definitely remembered.

Memory-Evoked Optomotor Responses

C. A. G. Wiersma and I worked on a simpler case in which behavior directly reflects remembered information: optomotor memory in crustaceans, which was first studied by Horridge (1966a). It has been observed in two species of crabs (Horridge, 1966a; Wiersma and Hirsh, 1974), rock lobsters and crayfish (Wiersma and Hirsh, 1974), and also an insect, the locust (Horridge, 1966b). It can easily be demonstrated by placing a crab within a stationary striped drum. The animal is allowed to view the background for some time before the onset of darkness, at which time the drum is moved. Upon reillumination, the new stationary position is revealed and the animal moves its eyes in the direction of apparent background movement. It can be inferred that the new position is in some manner compared with the old one, which, since it is no longer present, must in some way be remembered. The alternative possibility, that a fixation on some innately determined background feature is maintained, is unlikely, as the eyes in question are not foveal. Other evidence against this hypothesis is presented below.

Unlike Horridge, we recorded the action potentials of the fibers innervating the muscles responsible for moving the eye in the horizontal plane. There are two sets of such fibers, one causing clockwise movements and another mediating counterclockwise movements. When one set of fibers is excited, the other is inhibited.

During the dark period, the firing rate of the motor fibers frequently declined no matter in which direction the drum turned, although excited states were not uncommon. There was no systematic change in activity reflecting the direction of rotation, as there would be if the drum had been visibly revolved. When the drum had been turned in the direction in which the fiber being observed caused the eye to move, the frequency upon reillumination was greater than the background, as is shown in Fig. 1A1. Such turns will be termed "positive." The firing rate was inhibited after revelation of drum turns in the opposite direction (as shown in Fig. 1A2), which will be labeled "negative." Spike activity was recorded for processing by a histogram-compiling computer, using 1-sec bin width. Responses were discernible for an average of 30 sec after reillumination, although the bulk of the changes disappeared within 5 sec (Fig. 1B).

Measuring the Properties of Memory

The sign of the response proved to be useful in gauging various properties of memory. For instance, the duration of memory was measured by increasing the

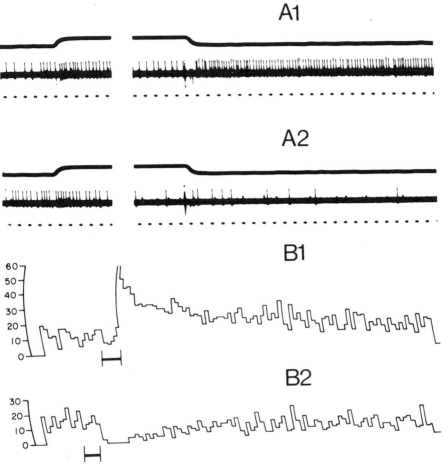

Fig. 1. A: Activity of a crab optomotor neuron during positive (A1) and negative (A2) trials. The neuron is responsible for moving the eye counterclockwise. Lower traces: time (10/sec); upper traces: light level. A raised trace indicates darkness. Four seconds of record has been removed from the dark interval. A1: Before and after a counterclockwise displacement of 3°. A2: Before and after a clockwise displacement of equal size. B: Histograms for complete positive (B1) and negative (B2) trials for a crab optomotor neuron responsible for clockwise movement. Bin width: 1 sec; displacement: 3° in both cases. The bars indicate the dark periods.

length of the dark period. If memory persists, the response after a positive turn should be excitatory while that after a negative drum turn should be inhibitory. However, as the length of the dark period increases, the firing rate prior to it becomes less relevant to the firing rate after reillumination. This problem was overcome by subtracting the number of action potentials occurring in the first 5 sec after a negative turn from the same value for a positive one. A truly excitatory response should consist of more action potentials than truly inhibited activity.

The strength of memory declined exponentially with a time constant of approximately 200 sec, with some being present even after 8 min of darkness. Both the excitatory and inhibitory responses were diminished. These results agree with those of Horridge (1966a). The exponential decline in memory is similar to that for various other forms of short-term memory. The decline in memory is evidence against the possibility that the response represents maintenance of a fixation on an innately determined feature of the background.

The establishment of memory was measured by varying the amount of time a background position was exposed before it was displaced during a dark period of 5 sec. Responses after short exposures were small and difficult to distinguish from background activity. Thus it again proved useful to take the difference between the number of spikes following revelation of a positive turn and that elicited by a negative background displacement. The strength of memory increased exponentially as a function of exposure time, with a time constant of approximately 5 sec. Some memory is detectable even after an exposure of 0.5 sec, with the strength of memory being at asymptotic levels after 30 sec exposure. These results are in good agreement with previously published data (Shepheard, 1966). Note that memory is forming even while the eye is moving in response to the previous displacement.

In the preceding experiment, the background was exposed for more than a minute, displaced during darkness, and then exposed for a varying amount of time. After this test exposure, it was moved exactly back to its original position. The response to reillumination of the original position was measured. Responses following complete turnback are solely due to the new memory, because no displacement from the original position is apparent. However, if the background is turned only halfway back (Fig. 2A) the response will be an expression of both the old and new memories. If the new memory is stronger the sign of the response will reflect the direction of the turnback, but if old memory is stronger the sign will reflect the direction of the initial displacement. Thus when old memory is stronger than new memory, the result of subtracting unit activity following a negative turnback from that following a positive turnback (Fig. 2B) will be a negative number. It can be seen that an old memory declines right from the beginning of exposure of a new position. After 3–5 sec it is weaker than the memory for the new position, and after 30 sec it has disappeared altogether. This disappearance is much faster than that which occurs during darkness, indicating that the old memory is being actively erased under the influence of the new background position.

One of the most significant experiments we did was to determine the size of the memory response as a function of background displacement. Initially, we were interested in the smallest angular change that could be detected, regarding it as a loosely defined index of visual acuity. Because responses following small displacements were small, the number of spikes following negative turns was subtracted from that following positive ones, as was done in measuring the duration and establishment of memory. Using the same gauge for the sensitivity of memory to angular change and the strength of memory as a function of time is, to a large extent, an equation of the two. This is logically justifiable in only a somewhat limited class of theories as to the nature of memory.

The results for the crab *Pachygrapsus* are presented in Fig. 3. These crabs could reliably detect displacement as small as 0.1°, a value in accord with previous

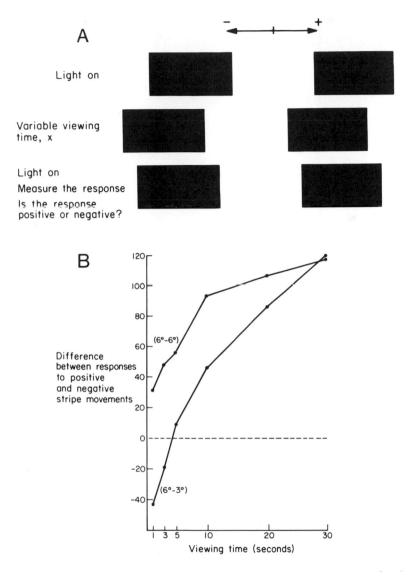

Fig. 2. A: Paradigm for measuring the relative strengths of an old and a new memory as a function of exposure time for a new stripe position. The stripes are exposed in the initial position for at least 1 min. They are then moved 6° in the negative direction during 5 sec of darkness. The new position is exposed for a variable time before the stripes are moved 3° in the positive direction during 5 sec of darkness. If new memory is stronger, the sign of the response following the turnback will be positive. If old memory is stronger, the response will be inhibitory. Complementary trials in which the first turn was negative and the turn halfway back was positive were also run. B: Competition between memories for old and new stripe positions plotted as a function of the viewing time for the new position. The upper curve represents the uncontested strength of the new memory. The lower curve represents the conflict between old and new memory. Both curves represent data for the same animals. Thus the difference between them represents the strength of old memory. Unit activity was measured in terms of the number of action potentials occurring in the first 5 sec after reillumination. From Wiersma and Hirsh (1974).

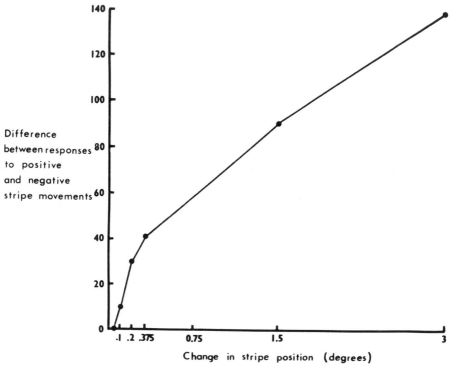

Fig. 3. Response strength as a function of displacement. The ordinate is as in Fig. 2B. The intercept with the abscissa represents the threshold for detection of displacement.

findings (Horridge, 1966c). This threshold is only a small fraction of the acceptance angle of a single ommatidium, indicating that responses from many ommatidia are integrated during memory formation.

The Nature of the Remembered Information

Most significant from the point of view of determining the content of memory is that the relationship between the size of the memory response and displacement is a linear, continuous one. Since displacement is in part determined by remembered information, namely, the position of the background prior to being moved, the relationship between the remembered information and the size of the response is also linear. Thus by systematically varying stimulus parameters and observing concomitant variation in response size it is possible to determine what information has been remembered.

One of the simplest experiments of this type was to vary the number of stripes present in the visual field of an eye. A single stripe was placed to one side of the visual field and displaced. A second stripe was then added, with the response to displacement being measured. This process was repeated until the visual field was filled with stripes, each placed to subtend 12° from its nearest neighbor. The results are presented in Fig. 4A. Generally, the size of the memory response is directly proportional to the number of stripes present, with saturation occurring due to filling of the visual field. The relationship between the responses to displacement of one and two stripes is due to alternations of the space surrounding the stripes. This effect of spacing is described in more detail below.

Since each additional stripe results in an equal increment in response strength, it can be inferred that each stripe is remembered individually and that memory forms in all parts of the visual field equally well. The latter inference was confirmed in separate experiments with single stripes (Wiersma and Hirsh, 1975a).

That stripes are individually remembered was confirmed by the discovery of an illusion. After a viewing period, a block of four black and three intervening white stripes, all of which subtended 12° angles, was displaced 27° in the positive direction, or 21° in the normally negative direction. After positive displacement of 27°, one of the black stripes is quite far from any former stripe position in the positive direction, but the other three are only 3° in the positive direction away from former stripe positions (Fig. 5). After 21° negative turns, one stripe is far away from any former stripe position in the negative direction, but each of the other three is 3° away from a former stripe in the positive direction, as is the case after the positive displacement of 27°.

If the memory response results from maintenance of a fixation of some feature of the background or if it is based on the distance between such a feature and a fixed external reference point, the signs of the responses in the two situations should be opposite. A piecemeal analysis, in which the stripes are remembered individually in terms of their initial position on the retina, predicts excitatory responses in both cases. Although to a human observer the direction of displacement is obvious, the responses in the two cases were excitatory, as shown in Fig. 5. Furthermore, the responses following the positive 27° displacements and the negative 21° ones were not consistently different in size. This indicates that those stripes far from former stripe positions were without effect and thus that the influence of memory is essentially local. This was confirmed by increasing the size of the positive and negative turns so that only two stripes were close to former stripe positions. Although now smaller, the responses in the two cases were again equal in size.

A stripe may be resolved into two borders, as has already been done in the case of optokinetic responses (Kien, 1974). In order to be able to move one stripe border while the one on the other side remains stationary, a rotating drum containing slats and windows within a stationary drum was developed. Displacements of 3° in the positive direction were used. The border on the positive side of the stripe will be termed "leading" and that on the negative side "trailing."

Displacement of only leading or trailing borders results in memory response, with those to the leading border being approximately twice as large (Wiersma and Hirsh, 1975b). Within the apparatus, stripe movement could also be simulated. Differences between the responses to stripe movement and the sum of the responses

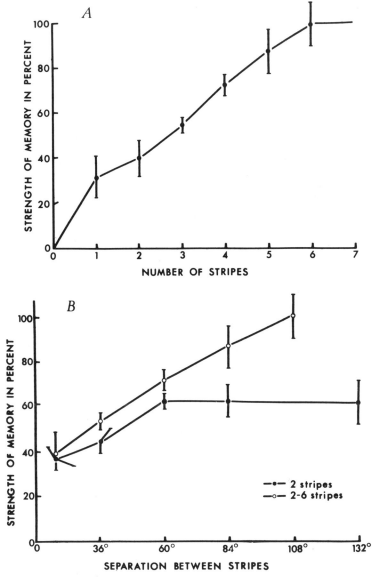

Fig. 4. A: Relative response strength plotted as a function of the number of stripes present in the visual field. Response strength was defined as in previous figures. The value for a given number of stripes was divided by that for seven black stripes, the standard pattern, and converted to a percent. Thus by definition the value for seven stripes is 100. Displacement was 3° occurring during 5 sec of darkness. B: Relative response strength plotted as a function of the angle between two stripes (lower curve). The upper curve is the data of Fig. 4A, representing the effect of the number of equidistant stripes present, replotted as a function of the angle between the inner borders of the outermost stripes. For explanation, see text. Note that for angles of up to approximately 60° the effect of stripe separation offsets that of the number of stripes present. From Wiersma and Hirsh (1975a).

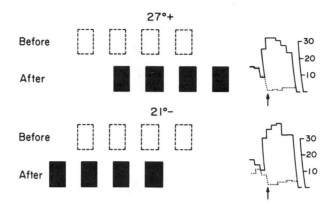

Fig. 5. Demonstration that the position of the background is remembered in terms of the positions of the individual stripes on the retina. The relative positions of the stripes prior to and following a positive displacement of 27° and a negative one of 21° are presented on the left. The phantom stripes (dotted) represent the stripe positions prior to displacement. The black stripes were 12° wide, and separation between stripes was 12°. The dark period was 10 sec. Histograms of unit activity are presented on the right. Bin width: 1 sec. Note that in both cases three of the four black stripes are 3° away from former stripe positions in the positive direction. From Wiersma and Hirsh (1974).

to leading and trailing border movements were slight and inconsistent (Wiersma and Hirsh, 1975*b*). Thus it appears that the memory for stripes is composed of independent memories for border position.

A Zone Theory of Optomotor Memory

These facts led to the development of a zone theory of memory, depicted in Fig. 6. Within the optic system, zones are held to form on either side of a border between lighter and darker areas. The zone on the white side of a border becomes sensitive to blackness, while that on the black side becomes sensitive to white. Changes in the zone to the clockwise side of a border excite fibers moving the eye in that direction and inhibit their antagonists. Changes in zones on the counterclockwise side of the border have the opposite effect. Simultaneous zone activation is summed. Black-sensitive zones are considered to be twice as effective as white-sensitive ones, since the response to leading border displacement which activates black-sensitive zones is twice as large as that for trailing border displacement which activates white-sensitive zones. Because maximal responses occur after displacement of approximately 3°, that is considered to be the width of the zone. The sensitivity of the zones is held to decline as distance from the engendering border increases, since responses to small displacements are proportionally greater than those to larger ones.

The simplest test of this theory involved displacing a single border. The presence of only one border was achieved by making one-half of the visual field black

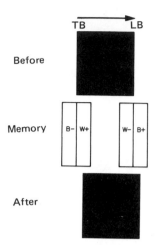

Fig. 6. Location and sample activation of change-sensitive memory zones. The arrow indicates the positive direction as in the following figures. Before: Stripe position prior to displacement. LB and TB denote the leading and the trailing border for positive displacements, respectively. Memory: Position of the black- and white-sensitive agonistic and antagonistic zones on the retina relative to that of the stripe borders. After: Position of the stripe with respect to the memory zones following displacement. The B+ and W+ zones are partly activated, giving rise to an excitatory response.

and the other white, while the heterolateral eye was covered. According to zone theory, the size of the response should increase to a maximum which is then maintained because as the positive displacement is increased the zone is increasingly, and then completely, changed (Fig. 7A). The responses were computed as a percent of standard, which was the mean of responses to displacements of 3° presented just prior to and after the test trial. This procedure was employed to overcome rather large variations in excitability both within and between preparations. The results, which are presented in Fig. 7B for black-sensitive zones, confirm zone theory. The responses for white-sensitive zones were too small and variable to permit interpretation.

The existence of antagonistic zones was confirmed in the apparatus for displacing leading or trailing borders alone. Here, borders face in opposite directions. Thus antagonistic as well as agonistic zones are present according to the theory. Moreover, displacement of leading borders will activate only black-sensitive zones, while trailing border movement will affect only white-sensitive ones. The predictions of zone theory are illustrated in Fig. 7C. Again, the response should rise to a maximum which is then maintained as the agonistic zones are increasingly and then completely activated as displacement is increased. However, after sufficiently large displacements—those exceeding the width of the white stripes minus 3°, or in this case 9°—antagonistic zones will be activated, and the size of the response should decline. Further, the rising and declining phases of the curve representing the relationship should be symmetrical, since first the proximal and then the distal portions of the agonistic zone with respect to the engendering border are activated as displacement is increased, while the opposite is true for the antagonistic zone. As can be seen in Fig. 7D, these predictions are in the main correct for both black- and white-sensitive zones. The peaking of the curves at 6° may indicate that the zones are somewhat wider than 3°.

According to zone theory, the response to stripe movement is simply the sum of the responses to border displacement. Thus the shape of the curve representing response size as a function of displacement of a regular pattern of equally wide black and white stripes should be similar to that for border displacements alone when stripes are initially of the same width. This is the case (Wiersma and Hirsh, 1975*b*).

In the most sophisticated test of zone theory, single black or white stripes of various widths were moved various distances in the positive direction. The predictions of zone theory are presented in Fig. 8A. As before, the response size should rise to a maximum which is maintained for some time as the displacement is increased. However, when displacement exceeds the width of the stripe minus 3°, the antagonistic zone on the negative side of the leading border is activated. In the case of a black stripe, this antagonistic zone is white sensitive. After displacements of one stripe width, it is completely activated, totally offsetting the effect of the white-sensitive agonist. Since the response is now, in effect, solely due to activation of the black-sensitive agonistic zone, it should be two-thirds as large as the maximum response. When a white stripe is turned through its own width, the black-sensitive antagonistic zone is completely activated, and thus the response should be reduced by two-thirds from the maximum level.

The unopposed agonistic zone, the one to the positive side of the leading border, is less than fully changed when stripe displacement exceeds the width of the stripe. Thus the response should decline in size, disappearing altogether for displacements in excess of the width of the stripe plus 3°.

Results of such experiments are presented in Fig. 8B,C. The shapes of the curves are as predicted. In five of the six cases examined, the rather exacting quantitative predictions for the size of responses to displacements of one stripe width were confirmed.

When a regular pattern of stripes, in which the white ones are wider than the black ones, is displaced, the resulting curve, according to zone theory, should be similar to that for single black stripes except that when positive displacement exceeds the width of the white stripe minus 3°, the response should change from being neutral to being inhibitory, as the antagonistic zones at the former positions of the trailing borders of the neighboring stripes are activated. These predictions were confirmed (Wiersma and Hirsh, 1975*b*).

The primary assumption of zone theory is that the response results from changes from white to black, or *vice versa*, within zones. It is not necessary that the border that caused the zone to form be displaced. This assumption was tested by placing thin black strips, subtending 1.5°, within the distal halves of the agonistic

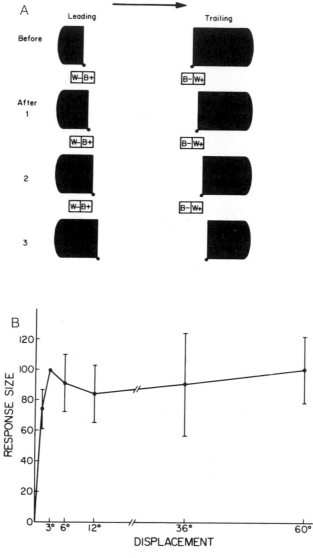

Fig. 7. A: Zone activation after increasingly larger displacements of a single leading or trailing border. Before: Border position prior to displacement. The curve represents the border of the visual fields. The small boxes represent the position of the memory zones. Displacement of the dot represents drum movement. After: The position of the border upon reillumination. The above format is employed in succeeding figures. (1) Agonistic zones are partially changed. (2) The zones are completely altered. (3) No further alternation occurs. B: Size of the memory response as a function of positive displacement of a single leading border. As in following figures, the response is defined as the number of action potentials occurring in the first 5 sec after reillumination minus that occurring in the 5 sec just prior to the dark period. This value was then expressed as a percentage of that resulting from 3° displacement. The dark period was 10 sec. From Wiersma and Hirsh (1975*b*). C: Zone activation resulting from increasingly

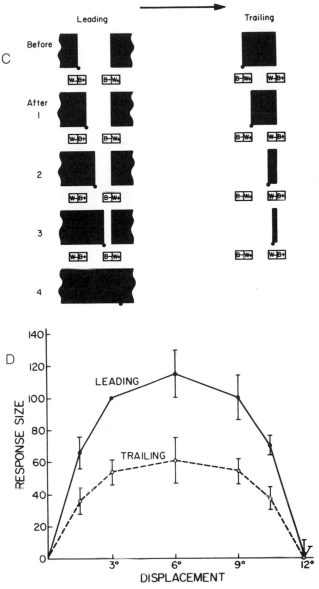

larger positive displacements of leading or trailing borders when stationary ones of the opposite type are present. The position of one displaced border relative to its stationary neighbor is represented in each column. (1,2) The agonistic black- or white-sensitive zone is partially and completely activated. (3,4) As a result of still larger displacements, an antagonistic black- or white-sensitive zone is also partially and completely activated. Note that the agonistic and antagonistic zones in each of the situations have similar sensitivities. D: Size of the memory responses as a function of positive displacement of many leading or trailing borders. Responses are presented as a percent of that to the standard displacement (3°) of the leading border. The dark period was 5 sec. Note the similarity in the shape of the curves. From Wiersma and Hirsh (1975b).

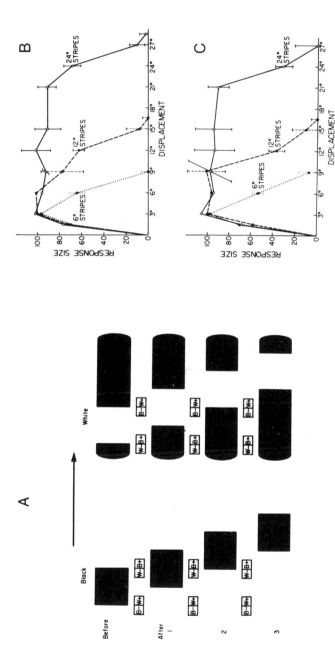

Fig. 8. A: Zone activation resulting from increasingly larger positive displacements of single black or white stripes. (1) Displacement has resulted in complete activation of both the black- and white-positive agonistic zones. (2) A larger movement also activates the white-sensitive antagonistic zone, in the case of the black stripe, and the black-sensitive antagonistic zone, in the case of the white stripe. (3) A still larger displacement leaves the agonistic zone in front of the leading border unaltered. B: Size of the memory response as a function of displacement of single black stripes of 6°, 12°, or 24°. Response strength is presented as a percent of that for 3° displacement. Note that response strength begins to decline after displacements larger than the width of the stripe minus 3°. C: Size of the memory response as a function of displacement of single white stripes of 6°, 12°, or 24°. Unlike in B the declines are at first rapid and then slow, reflecting the increasing activation of the antagonistic black-sensitive zone and the decreasing change in the agonistic white-sensitive one. From Wiersma and Hirsh (1975b).

or antagonistic zones adjoining borders during periods of darkness (Fig. 9). This was done in an apparatus which simulated displacement without involving rotation.

If changes within zones are sufficient to elicit memory responses, then placement in agonistic zones should result in excitatory responses while that in antagonistic ones should cause inhibitory responses. Since the responses were small, the number of spikes following modification of the antagonistic zone was subtracted from that for agonistic zone modification.

As a control for the white space separating the strip from the stripe not being resolved, which would result in the appearance of border movement, white strips were placed in the distal portion of either the agonistic or antagonistic white-sensitive zones. Thus the white spaces separating strips from stripes in the experiments involving black- and white-sensitive zones were equally wide. However, in the latter case failure to resolve the separation would not result in the appearance of border movement. In the control condition, too, unit activity following agonistic zone activation was greater than that after antagonistic activation.

Discussion

The zone theory of memory has stood up well to the tests to which it has been subjected, so that it is worthwhile drawing inferences from the theory about the processes responsible for generating memory and also their location. The foremost among these is that the generation of sensitivity to change, which in effect constitutes the memory, is analogous to the lateral inhibition occurring within the eye of *Limulus*. Both processes are initiated by the presence of a border. Sensitivity to black–white reversal decreases exponentially with increasing distance from the border.

Involvement of a process analogous to lateral inhibition eliminates the photopigment as a candidate for the site of memory. If a pigmental afterimage were

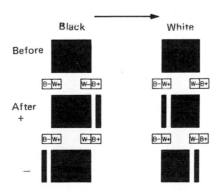

Fig. 9. Paradigm for demonstrating that zones can be activated without border displacement. Before: Stripe position prior to the dark period. After: The situation upon reillumination. In order to test black sensitivity, a thin black strip has been added to the agonistic (+) or antagonistic (−) zones. Similarly, to test for sensitivity to white, a white strip has been added to the agonistic or antagonistic zones.

involved, the strength of memory should be proportional to the intensity of the image. Thus the memory should be stronger as distance from the border increases, but this prediction is contradicted by the facts. At the same time, it is likely that the site of memory is not more central than the lamina. The position of a border is remembered in terms of its position on the retina, and topographic representation of the receptor surface is maintained only in the outer layers of the eye.

It also may be surmised that the output of memory sites is to fibers traveling horizontally across the eye. This inference arises from a consideration of the problem of directionality. A black-sensitive zone, for instance, may be generated anywhere in the visual field. It may be established by a border which faces left or one which faces right, with equal probability. In one case, agonistic fibers are to be excited and antagonistic ones inhibited. In the other, the opposite should be true. Having two distinct sets of black-sensitive memory elements is a rather uneconomical solution, but how, otherwise, could variation in the communication between memory sites and the motor fibers be achieved?

The answer lies in the fact that sensitivity to change decreases as distance from the border increases. The simplest way to capitalize on such a gradient is by means of fibers running across the retina. The memory elements can then contact these fibers in a manner which preserves their topographical order. The horizontal fibers activating movement to the right would respond only when the input was ordered from left to right, perhaps in terms of intensity or latency. The opposite would be true for fibers activating movement to the left. Such arrangements are analogous to those thought to be responsible for direction-sensitive movement detectors. Since rectification occurs postsynaptically, all of the memory elements could be in contact with fibers of both types.

The preceding discussion of inferences about the process responsible for memory formation is at best incomplete and tentative since it is based solely on zone theory. To our knowledge, there is at least one other process involved which is beyond the scope of zone theory. This is evident from the effect of the separation between stripes. As can be seen in Fig. 4B, the size of the memory response is proportional to the width of the separation between two black stripes. This process tends to offset the effect of the number of stripes present. As described earlier, equal displacement of different numbers of stripes results in unequal responses. However, as the number of stripes present in the visual field increases, the space between them tends to decrease.

It is now clear that close spacing when present only prior to or following displacement will result in memory responses of reduced size (Hirsh and Wiersma, 1977). The effect of close spacing during read-in is, of course, mediated by some form of memory, and the amount of the reduction in response is proportional to the length of the dark period. So far, it has proven difficult to determine decisively whether or not the basic sensitivity of the memory zones is modified by the effect of spacing during read-in.

The absolute size of the reduction in response strength resulting from close spacing present during readout alone is not affected by the length of the dark period

(Hirsh and Wiersma, 1977). This effect has been shown to be a function of the white space separating an activated zone from the nearest neighboring border rather than the distance between them (Hirsh and Wiersma, 1977). How the effect of readout spacing is integrated with zone processes is still unresolved.

There is also some possibility that memory may be affected by reafference. If so, additional and even contradictory inferences might be made. As already mentioned, memory zones form while the eye is in motion. In our most recent experiments, the double drum was visibly revolved in the positive direction. In one phase only the leading borders of the stripes seen by the animal moved, while in the other only the trailing borders moved. During both phases, an optokinetic response occurred.

When the slats of the inner drum are black, agonistic zones have time to form at leading borders of the stripes during the phase of trailing border movement, while antagonistic zones can form at trailing borders during the phase of leading border movement. This results in an excitatory supplement being added to the optomotor response during the transition from trailing to leading movement phase and an inhibitory decrement during the reverse transition. Close scrutiny of the times when these modifications occur might reveal whether correction for the effects of the eye being in motion are occurring. Such a correction would have to be central in origin because the oculomotor muscles in crustaceans lack proprioceptors (Horridge and Sandeman, 1964; Wiersma and Oberjat, 1968). Reafference would thus provide a strong clue in pinpointing the location of memory as well as being highly interesting in its own right.

25

Mechanistic Teleology and Explanation in Neuroethology: Understanding the Origins of Behavior

G. Adrian Horridge

Introduction

Neuroethology is the explanation of behavior in terms of neurons. These words deserve examination.

Explanation, the most difficult word to expand upon, has long fascinated man, and types of explanation are in short supply. First, we can *explain* in terms of antecedent material causes modeled on the blow of a stone that breaks another stone. Second, we can explain by invented unseen abstractions, like the spirit of heat that explains what passes from man to wood in the making of fire. The history of modern science has been the story of material antecedent causes replacing invented abstractions as causes, but when material causes are examined more closely they too are found to be full of invented abstractions. Third, we can explain in terms of future needs. A system is made in a particular way in order to perform a function. Purpose or design of animal parts is perfectly respectable since Darwin's elucidation of natural selection as the basis of purposive design. During evolution, animals grow components in combinations that will subsequently interact in ways that ensure survival of the whole population. Thereby a circle of material causes is completed and a happening at any time in the cycle can be explained by causes that act at any other time in the cycle, earlier or later.

Behavior includes all that happens when motor and secretory neurons are active, so that salivation, gut movements, and change of color are as much parts of behavior as patterned song, discrimination, or learning. *Neurons* are the only components of nervous systems so far known to be really significant in generating behavior. Where the components of a system can be discerned or inferred, the mechanisms of that system are understood, in the usual sense of that word, only when they are worked out as the consequences of the interactions of the components. This mechanistic explanation of what goes on is a prerequisite for any other form of explanation that may be added. The arrangement of the connections be-

---

G. Adrian Horridge • Department of Behavioural Biology, Research School of Biological Sciences, The Australian National University, P.O. Box 475, Canberra, A.C.T. 2601, Australia.

tween the neurons is just as relevant to mechanistic explanation as synaptic potentials, spikes, slow waves, synthesis or release of secretions, and so forth. If components other than neurons, such as glial cells, are shown to be active in behavior, they will have to be treated in the same way as the neurons. The problem is to get beyond this reductionist approach.

Some Current Forms of Explanation

Let us now take a look at some of the explanations that we actually use or seek in neuroethology.

Reductionist or Mechanistic Analysis

At the present time, we understand that the discovery of progressively more detailed material causes is the road of progress. First, we list the components and forces of chemistry and physics that are acting in the particular system we study. We analyze every little twist and detail to uncover what acts on what. Later, the interactions are described quantitatively, and we obtain mathematical expressions which not only fit the observed interactions but also embody in the theory a breakdown into the interactions and components that act together in producing the observed result. Theories without this characteristic are suspect. Invertebrate nervous systems are particularly approachable by this kind of analysis; with their identifiable neurons and simple circuits, they reveal principles of interaction that are seminal in the understanding of more complex systems like the human brain, which cannot be analyzed so cleanly.

Drawbacks of Reductionism

Mechanistic analysis with a description of all detail is not, however, of itself sufficient, for several reasons. The question is, how can the function or relevance of neuron activities be introduced into the mechanistic analysis? An undisclosed set of rules guides researchers and journal editors about what is useful or what is significant science. On what principles should these guidelines be based? I take the view that details of neuron activity that are not related to behavior in a rather direct way are not acted on by natural selection, and therefore they cannot be treated as if they are a meaningful part of the system. Most of the vast amount of unquoted results on behavior, especially of man, and of neuron activity and anatomical detail, especially of vertebrates, in the literature of the past 50 years are dead because no functional relevance can be found for them.

In a mechanistic analysis of neuron activity, the detail becomes tedious because the interactions and complexity are potentially infinite and no one beyond the original investigator will ever be interested. Analyzing the interactions of all neurons could occupy the human race for all time, if only because the more they knew the more ways of analysis they would know, and the more of their own neuronal activity they would have to describe. Even for one species of insect, the whole activity of all neurons is more than we seek. We seek *principles of action,* mainly, and detail becomes significant only when it elucidates principles. We still have the question with us, however, as to what principles of action we accept as fulfillment of the investigator's task, and in what way can the complexity of nervous systems be explained.

Methodological Objection to Reductionism

In the study of a small part of a nervous system, it is a temptation to think that the output is understood when all interactions and nonlinearities of neuron activity are known. The operative word is "all," and turning the sentence around soon reveals that the "all" is no more than a hope. "When the output is understood, all interactions and nonlinearities are known." That is to say that we go on looking for interactions in the system while there remains something to be explained in the output. This is an excellent formula for bread-and-butter elucidation of components and their activity. The catch is that the outputs and behavior of the nervous system are always far simpler than the inputs and central processes. Therefore, the behavioral or motor neuron (MN) outputs can be fully explained without necessarily making use of all the activity within, and all the possible interactions of inputs. One can never know *all* interactions inside, or when the complete list of nonlinearities has been found. The system is an open-ended one that we progressively reveal, not a circumscribed one in which the components and processes have already been listed. So much for pure mechanistic analysis: I believe that even as a self-contained exercise on a small subsystem it cannot be complete, and, besides, it is unsatisfactory because relevance and optimization are omitted.

Reductionism Is Description, Not Explanation

When every detail of what goes on in a small part of a nervous system is described, what do we have? We see how the sensory inputs are processed by components on the input side of the watershed of the central nervous system. Interneurons (INs) act on each other to generate behavior patterns that are carried out by MNs. The initial *belief* that the components work the one upon the other, in the way that components of an engine or radio act upon each other, is to a large extent vindicated. Descriptions of interaction, however, fall short of an understanding of why the structure and function of the system are as they are. The engineer putting together components has in mind the *function* of the machine that he makes; he does a good or a bad job insofar as the machine is effective in its intended function. In the living nervous system, natural selection acting over many generations has ensured that components work together: the system fulfills a function. Behavior, from the beat of a jellyfish to the thought processing of man, fits the real world. A deeper understanding of the structure and function appears when the mechanistic analysis has proceeded far enough for us to propose that all parts of the system are as they are because they are optimized to a particular function or display a compromise between optimizations for more than one function. When that is possible, we really begin to understand what we are studying.

A Clue from the Biophysics of Small Components

When we turn to the small components of nervous systems, we find that much more is known about the way they act. Moreover, many details of their physics and biochemistry can be related in considerable detail to their function. Often the mechanisms can be taken right down to components at the molecular level. *Form and function then cease to be separable ways of thinking about the same system.* At the next level of complexity, the cellular level, the acceptable current view is that the action and the anatomy lie within rigid limits that are set by the laws of physics acting in relation to the supposed *functions* of the organs or cellular organelles. Anatomical examples are the fine details of receptors, particularly auditory and visual receptors, in terms of the properties of sound or light; the spacing and adhesions of membranes; dimensions of nodes, axons, and dendrites in terms of space constants; the forms of synapses in terms of the diffusion laws; and the architecture, on large and small scale, of the effector organs such as cilia or muscle filaments. The two arguments for biophysical explanations of this type are as follows: First, this approach is heuristically successful as shown by the agreement between the efficient performance of the organelle and the laws of physics by which it is supposed to work. We readily accept the conclusion that form and function are together optimized. Second, the same structures occur throughout the animal kingdom. Sensory cells, details of neurons, synapses, cilia, and muscle fibers, including details of their operation, are surprisingly constant throughout the animal kingdom from coelenterates through vertebrates. We accept that they are perpetuated by the historical process of evolution and at the same time determined by the laws of physics in the form that we find them. The issue is whether we use the physical analysis in conjunction with the important assumption that each subsystem, and the whole working together, has been optimized by natural selection for a particular functional compromise, and that components are not merely a legacy, appropriate or otherwise, inherited from previous models. For small components that are well understood, the physical explanation as to why they are as they are is always conceived in terms of the function to be performed. My thesis is that to make nervous systems comprehensible the neurons and their fields must be treated in the same way.

Why Nervous Systems Are as They Are

A major difficulty is to explain many of the easily discoverable facts of neuronal organization: for example, why one neuron should run to two muscles in the crayfish claw, or why the common inhibitor neuron of the thoracic ganglia of some insects sends a branching axon to many muscles; why the cricket has ears on its elbows; why many insects with binocular vision have eyes that are close together. A new question this year is why should there be nonspiking INs in insect ganglia? The quest appears to be for an explanation as to how that particular arrangement comes about and why it persists. We really want to know why that particular arrangement is the best or an optimum. In standard tests we often find two quite different types of explanation offered, neither of which depends on previous completion of the reductionist analysis of what goes on.

The Legacy of Evolution

The animal has a history. History is a powerful determiner of process. Only certain ways of evolving are possible on account of the constraints against other lines of change for the inherent properties of the system. It may be that nerve ganglia appeared early in evolution of the phyla because only in the ganglia can the nonspiking INs interact closely with each other. More advanced forms may have progressively improved the interaction between nonspiking local INs without being able to get away from the basic mechanism itself. Increased interaction between nonspiking neurons is provided by the fusion of ganglia in the process of cephalization that has happened many times in evolution. The ganglia of mollusks and the ladderlike nerve cords of arthropods, the details of eyes, ears, and in fact all parts of all animals present us with many structures that are explicable in terms of *history*. One can't escape this: animals are not designed from scratch according to principles of optimization. They are optimized in different ways from a historically given ancestor. This, however, is not an explanation of how they work, or how the working mechanisms are optimized.

Design around the Properties of Components

The second type of explanation of why a particular arrangement comes about is made in terms of a mechanical effectiveness of necessity that derives from the properties of the materials of construction, from the geometry of the situation, or from limitations on what can be grown in development. The nervous system is in fact composed of most unpromising materials. Usually our inability to produce this kind of explanation, and therefore our tendency to continue the search, springs from lack of sufficient detail about the way the system works, and therefore the complete mechanistic analysis is a prerequisite. Essentially, this type of explanation is the demonstration that what is found is a good way of using the available materials, and that it makes sense in terms of function. In the same way, we cast a knowledgeable eye over any highly developed human construction, such as a sailing boat, a bicycle, or a cup and saucer, and see that it is so built because the nature of the materials has allowed and encouraged optimization along particular avenues but not along others. A further twist in this explanation is that in development the proteins can fit together only in certain ways.

The Classical Analysis of Neuron Function

In the classical and much current analysis of nervous systems, first the MNs and INs were isolated as components, and their inputs in some cases and their outputs in others were described. The main contribution was functional anatomy based on the neurons as excitation pathways. In many invertebrates, it is possible to name each neuron uniquely and return to it over and over again in different animals, so that its properties can be progressively worked out as ideas progress. In vertebrates, only classes of neurons can be identified, so that neuron properties are always representative or statistical, and one can rarely return to the same neuron. With difficulty, one can find pairs of neurons, one of which acts directly on the other, but in general in vertebrates the chain of causation is based on probabilities. This itself sets a severe limit on how much the chain of causation can be worked out between components. The invertebrate named neurons provide the seminal ideas.

In this type of analysis, the *input field* of the neuron, together with the output field, is the property to be described, and actions of neurons may be quantified as transfer functions. The field is not yet seen as a joint consequence of the laws of physics and natural selection acting on that part of the neuron activity which eventually appears in behavior. This kind of mechanistic analysis, however, must continue until the components and their basic properties are listed.

The next stage is the description of the interactions between identified neurons. This becomes the study of the flow of excitation to higher-order cells, with three main themes:

1. Fields of sensory neurons, and progressive pattern abstraction as these become fields of higher-order neurons.
2. Patterns of behavior that are generated from the arrangement of the connections between neurons.
3. Analysis of behavior to include feedback loops from the animal's surroundings.

One deficiency of this method is that it omits all the slow, hormonal, secretory aspects of the nervous system, and these are probably as important as the impulses seen on oscilloscopes. Another defect is that the results of recording fields at different levels, even in the best-studied systems, simply do not provide enough data for us to see in detail which neuron acts on which others. Present indications are that this method is not adequate to yield a reductionist description in an isolated and simplified subsystem. The situation is impossible to analyze where there are a number of parallel pathways and where any stimulus is likely to excite an unknown number of neurons, *however indirectly*. The imponderable is the activity in neurons other than those observed by the recording electrode. In these circumstances, an input–output relation, or an interaction of one neuron and another, recorded even in identified neurons, is *not* an isolated interaction, but is one part of a complex system with other activity going on at the same time. We rarely test for univariance, give proof of which anatomical synapses are responsible for our interaction, or exclude parallel activity. *Analysis depends on having the system extremely restricted.* Where there are pathways in parallel, some leading toward behavioral outputs, it is an essential but almost impossible part of the analysis to discover how the excitation is partitioned between them, and how the partitioning changes under different circumstances. Therefore, except in systems of few fibers, the method of recording at different levels in a nervous system simply fails to give a complete picture. The result is that worker after worker records from a restricted subsystem and then, having gone as far as possible, builds a model with inferences extended beyond the observations, before turning to a new system to analyze.

Explanation with and without Consideration of Design

On the basis of the above discussion, I therefore distinguish between descriptive reductionism and a higher form of mechanistic analysis as follows: A mechanistic or reductionistic explanation in terms of components sets out to describe the causes of the activity of the nervous system, i.e., the origin of behavior in terms of what component acts on what, how it does it, and when. Mechanistic analysis at its best reveals what acts on what and employs all the relevant laws of physics, but, first, it can never be complete, and, second, its ultimate aim is in the wrong direction.

Quite different is the explanation of why the system, or its individual components, or its behavioral output, is as it is, because they are optimized to fit in with each other and with the environment. Both forms of explanation are valid in that they are sought by scientists and accepted when demonstrated. Explaining why things are as they are requires all the relevant laws of physics, but in addition considers the function of the system and the function of each component. With the help of comparative data, where compromises between different demands can be seen to be met in different ways in different animals, we can show that each variant of the system and its components are beautifully adapted to the diversity of the needs that are met. They are optimized within the limitations also set by history, by the properties of materials, but primarily by the laws of physics. Revealing exactly how these compromises, limitations, and optimizations apply is a valid form of explanation that I call "mechanistic teleology" because it is the physical explanation of the stringent design criteria that are needed for selective advantage. Numerous elegant examples are available showing how primary sensory cells, and sense organs such as the eye or ear, for example, are superbly adapted to make best use of the physical principles which govern light or sound. There are also brilliant accounts of the appropriateness of neuron fields in that they select exactly the combination of inputs that are of greatest selective advantage. The MIT foursome (Lettvin *et al.*, 1959) illustrate this very well. However, that pioneering work did not have the influence it deserved. The mainstream of neurophysiological analysis continues to publish *our* reading of neuron activity, not the nervous system's reading of it. The study of central neuron fields has not been combined with the appropriate physical principles and analysis of optimum compromises that have been applied so successfully to the sense organs. The optimization, however, must apply right through into the behavior, because it is the whole flow of excitation to the behavioral output that is acted on by selection.

Function Finding with Identified Neurons

In the mechanistic analysis, we record from identified neurons and hope to show what acts on what. If a deeper explanation of neuron fields is to be made, the function of each identifiable neuron must be found. Moreover, we have to make the bold assumption that because neurons are identifiable components of the nervous system each will in fact have an identifiable function which in some sense stays with that neuron. As indicated by work in maturation of vertebrate nervous systems, in which neuron properties depend on previous experience, this fundamental assumption is going to break down at some level of analysis, at least in more complex systems, but it holds so far for invertebrates.

Functions of Single Neurons

Throughout the animal kingdom, there are numerous examples where the expression of a behavior pattern is linked in a direct causal sequence with the excitation of an identifiable neuron or of a group of neurons that are permanently connected together in a relatively isolatable system. There are numerous examples where a behavior pattern is brought about by a single MN. In these cases, *without a good reason,* one might as well study the behavior as the neuron. One reason is that intracellular records from the MN soma may reveal synaptic potentials which show part of the input to it. Through-conducting nerve nets and epithelial conducting pathways in coelenterates and giant fiber systems of annelids and of some arthropods are the classical examples of the effective evocation of a behavior pattern by a single neuron. In a few examples, a single sensory neuron sets off a complete behavior pattern, in which case the sensitivity of a single receptor acts as the abstraction mechanism that determines when a particular behavior should be triggered. Much more commonly, a class consisting of many hundreds of receptor neurons, with at least some field properties in common, sets off a stereotyped behavior.

A striking example is the ability of the bee to navigate by the plane of polarization if the light is ultraviolet. Work by von Helversen and Edrich (1974) and unpublished work by Menzel have shown that the spectral sensitivity curve of discrimination of the e-vector is close to the spectral sensitivity curve of the ninth retinal cell in the ommatidia of the bee eye. The optics of the bee ommatidium are such that this spectral sensitivity is close to the absorption spectrum of the protein rhodopsin, with peak sensitivity near 360 nm. Therefore, we have an aspect of the behavior that is dominated by a clearly defined property of a protein molecule. But again the *explanation* can go deeper. To show why the short wavelengths are most effective and why the polarization of the sky is useful for navigation, I can trace the story back to Tyndall's lecture of 1869, published in *The Forum* in 1888. Tyndall's first experiment was to show "that by the scattering action of minute particles, the blue of the sky can be produced." He did this by forming fine solid particles by chemical reaction between two gases while illuminating from the side. Tyndall then demonstrated that the plane of polarization of the scattered light is at right angles to the illuminating beam. He examined the polarization of the blue of the sky and correctly identified the plane of polarization as perpendicular to the direction of the sun. Tyndall, like the natural selection acting on the bee, found that the shorter the wavelength the greater the scattering and therefore the greater the polarization, because it is the scattered light which is polarized.

Müller's Law

The examples where the input–output relation of a single neuron is closely related to some aspect of behavior have led to the simplification known as Müller's law (Müller, 1835), which is, in brief, in modern terms, that each neuron, as a unit of the nervous system, generates its own definable effect. Normally, each neuron has one axon which carries one message. Change in impulse frequency of the axon, or depolarization of some part of the neuron, represents only the intensity of the signal, and by implication, therefore, the labeling of the activity is by axon identity.

Two major practical problems are set by this axiom. One is that where two neurons a and b act on a third c, the effect of a on c is contingent on the activity of b, which is not necessarily known by the observer to be present when only a and c are observed. As nonlinearities such as facilitation and inhibition soon emerge from the simplest interactions, the components and their circuits are impossible to define by inference. The presence of b is inferred from the lack of fixed relation between a and c. A modern interpretation of Müller's law allows for this lack of a fixed relation between input and output as part of the properties that can usually be given to an identifiable neuron. The proviso is that the contingent changes which modify the input–output relations are definable by experiment. From being a hypothesis about residual unexplained effects, the contingent changes become another dimension of the field properties of the identified neuron.

The other problem is that neuron fields are never fully mapped. For all neurons except a few specialized receptors, function finding is an open-ended search for further properties of the field. In this context, Müller's law says that contingent changes are restricted, that fields of neurons do not extend indefinitely as the experimenter dreams up new stimuli, that there is a definable function for each neuron, and that the function can be tied down to the anatomical identification. Analysis of invertebrate identified neurons has provided some of the background for these working hypotheses. Apart from their heuristic success, the only basis I know for accepting these principles is that neuron properties appear to be optimized for particular functions, a state of affairs for which there is only one explanation, namely, that the definable functions of these identifiable neurons are in fact acted on by natural selection, which maintains the optimization. In short, neurons have definable functions on which natural selection acts. If so, mechanistic teleology is a valid approach in the study of neuron fields.

Analyzing Neuron Activity

More often than not, it is impossible to read the message in the axon, to relate IN properties directly to a behavioral output or to the physics of the sense organ. More important, we do not know the whole situation but only a very small fraction of it. This is not surprising, because, in a complex system with many neurons in parallel, the effects of each neuron are contingent on the activity of others. The question is how to allocate functions to the components when faced with this situation.

By sampling at different points in the system with a defined stimulus, one records activity that originates from what we infer to be a causal chain, including final behavior. One way of analyzing such a situation is to work downstream from the properties of the receptor fields to the properties of low- and then high-order IN fields, and so trace the perturbations and combinations of the stimuli into the output. Although there is still a place for random recording from unidentified neurons and for describing the effects of every possible stimulus, that approach leads straight into the morass of recording every damn thing that presents itself, and frustrated efforts to work out what acts on what. I believe that understanding is generated during the progress of this very necessary descriptive work by assuming that Müller's law (each component is designed for a function) holds, and then by mapping the function of that part of the neuron activity which is clearly participating in behavior and therefore optimized by natural selection. I am aware that this is an extraordinarily tedious process, and especially that it requires repeated insights into the workings of the particular animal studied. What the animal abstracts from its own neuronal activity is very slowly discovered, but without it the recording equipment will churn out vast amounts of neuron activity without the discriminating filter of the higher-order neurons.

At each stage of abstraction, even by the sensory neurons at the front end of the nervous system, there is an enormous amount of detail in the neuron activity (especially if we take cross-correlations between different neurons) compared with the puny information content of the ensuing behavior. The best indication of whether or not a stimulus is appropriate is therefore the activity of the next higher IN along the line, and ultimately the behavioral response, but certainly not the recording gear itself. These objections expressed by Horridge (1968, 1969a) are largely avoided by working back from the behavioral output to the MNs and thence via central driving neurons into the sensory processing mechanisms as proposed by Hoyle (1964, 1975a), because when working upstream in this direction the outputs that are relevant are already partially identified, but the problem is then that the appropriate combinations of stimuli can never be found. Further discussion will be found in Barlow (1961).

Introducing Optimization, Compromise, and Adaptive Design

The rejection of neuron activity that is not picked up by other neurons and is never represented by any wrinkle in the behavior pattern has one consequence of enormous significance for the study of nervous systems. The aspects that appear in the behavior are those that can be acted on by natural selection and therefore we can expect in them a high degree of *optimization,* which is one of the powerful methods of the exact sciences, particularly in the mathematical treatment of physics. If we deal with quantitative aspects of nervous activity that appear in behavior, we can use methods derived from mathematical optimization in order to understand why things are as they are. I called this approach "mechanistic teleology" because the mechanisms are restricted to interactions that are measurable in terms of efficiency in subsequent behavior and can be called "design." The optimization usually refers to a compromise that can be seen as a result of natural selection pushing in two or more incompatible directions.

Over the past few years I have been studying the structure, optics, physiology, and stimulus-gathering and stimulus-splitting properties of the compound eye of insects and crustaceans. The primary photoreceptors are neurons in that they have axons. They divide up the visual world into a large number of information-carrying channels. In the compound eye, the channels are not confounded; i.e., they each carry a message about one parameter at a time. Because of the limited amount of energy available in the stimulus, there is an unavoidable compromise between the number of receptors and the sensitivity (or rather signal-to-noise ratio) of each. There is a related compromise between the resolution of each receptor and its sensitivity because small fields allow high resolution but reduce sensitivity. There is another compromise in that increase in the number of facets on the compound eye gives a greater number of sampling stations but reduces the sensitivity and resolution of each. A further compromise relates to the fraction of a compound eye that can be devoted to a fovea, where the visual axes are crowded together and in this type of eye are therefore farther apart elsewhere. Other compromises also have their basis in simple physical principles. For example, if all light is caught by a receptor, it is black, and so special provisions must be made for color vision; if receptors with different spectral peaks make color vision possible, then sensitivity and perhaps resolution suffer. New life styles are made possible by being able to make use of very dim light. There is also a compromise between seeing a wide range of object sizes and improving performance by concentrating on one size. It may be true that a generalized eye requires as much resolution and sensitivity as possible, and that photon noise and intensity discriminations must be considered, but an object of a particular size subtended at the eye is best seen when the receptor field subtends the same angle as the object, and there may be specialized eyes with some of the field sizes matched to the expected sizes of objects that are looked for. The lesson is that *matching input fields to function* is an effective way of improving performance and reducing numbers of neurons. The principle applies to all neurons.

Most neuron fields, however, are not so clear-cut as those of the eye. It is common to find a class of neurons all of which respond, but in different proportions and with overlapping fields in many dimensions, to a group of related stimuli. At present, the insights to read the message by our instruments are lacking: only the next neurons down the line can do that. The same kinds of compromises apply; in particular, there is an optimum field overlap in each dimension depending on the number of neuron responses that are seen simultaneously by the next neurons down the line, and the number of discriminations that have to be made.

For the primary photoreceptor neurons of the compound eye, we found that field properties of a photoreceptor could not be explained except in terms of the ultimate needs of the animal, which is another way of describing the selection pressures acting throughout life. In other examples, however, the principle is pretty obvious. A color receptor will have its spectral sensitivity curve in the right place in the spectrum, which implies a match with the wavelengths it is adapted to see. Chemoreceptors are usually designed to respond to a molecule of significance in behavior, mechanoreceptors to a particular loading, auditory organs to threshold levels of a particular carrier frequency, and so on. The teleological nature of this matching of input field with expected stimulus pattern has not previously been stressed. The exponents and the critics of reductionist analysis appear to have missed the point that knowing the function is part of the analysis. My own conviction is that the design of the nervous system, in the sense that engineers use the word "design," will not be comprehensible until we match the properties of the input field with the functions of the output for each neuron. This adds another major obstacle to those which already complicate the study of function finding for neurons.

There are some who will realize that I am trying to go further than the enormous past and current efforts to map sensory fields, or find the optimum stimulus for any named neuron which may be sensory, inter-, or motor. That is merely describing what is there, and such work fills the literature. Most of those recordable properties of neurons are not seen at a later stage down the line, are not of interest to the animal, and have not been honed down by natural selection. The work is therefore much simplified when we concentrate on those aspects of the fields that show through into a behavior pattern. The need is for biologically trained neurobiologists to replace the incentive to *describe* by an incentive to *explain* the design. One way to do this is to adopt the attitudes of the few imaginative engineers or informal physicists (e.g., Glegg, 1969; Feynman *et al.*, 1971), and to move from the anecdotal toward the principles of optimization.

Return to Compromises in Design

Consideration of the physical factors affecting field sizes and their overlap, and hence the number of receptors in the compound eye, showed us, in our research, exactly how the compromises relate to function. It is easy to define adaptation for one function, but given numerous functions it is very difficult, even knowing the final structure, to separate the different priorities and kinds of weighting that have been acted on by natural selection. It is well-nigh impossible if the functions and the structure have not all been specified with complete clarity. That is why explaining why things are as they are is a test of the completeness of the descriptive analysis. A curious fact about the consideration of adaptation is that approximate measurements are often adequate for the explanation but they must be the right measurements. The problem is that the functions have to be discerned before the proper descriptive measurements are made. One can only go so far without individual naming of neurons. Often one gets more insights by introducing a wide range of comparative data into the mechanistic analysis, as in the study of the fields of the compound eye. Furthermore, design considerations always apply to variants on a definite model, which is equivalent to a drawingboard specification, or a working model, and never to a statistical statement about populations of neurons or of animals. This is one reason why studies on vertebrates lag behind those on invertebrates, and identified neurons place the seminal ideas before us.

Laws of Physics vs. History

It is often said that at the molecular level the laws of physics and chemistry are the only ones that play a role. At the next level, as natural selection acts on the complex products of protein molecules, the fact of adaptation becomes the acceptable way of explaining purposive design. At the higher levels, the physicochemical laws can no longer explain most of the biological phenomena, which are too far removed from physics. They still invite explanation.

"Explain biological phenomena" here means "explaining the details in terms of function" and can sometimes be sharpened down to something like "explain why these particular features are the optimum (selected) ones in terms of what the structure does in the life of the animal." This latter kind of explanation is what the physicist seeks when he looks at components in living animals, but it can be presented only when the component's function is known. Similarly, the physics and chemistry of a particular sense organ can be understood to be as they are only when it is known when the next neuron down the line, and ultimately the animal, responds to that sensory neuron. The same holds even for the receptor molecules which react with the stimulus, because they have *been selected for their effects*. Similarly, the field of every neuron is selected because having that field the neuron works in the system as a whole. Therefore, for every sensory cell and neuron we must take those effects into account. With Edelman (1974), "My purpose is not epistemological, nor shall I attempt an analysis of the reductionist or holist *position*, for I believe that in their most extreme forms there is a fruitless opposition implied by these terms." My purpose is not to attack current neurobiology but to make teleology respectable and try to make descriptions of neuron actions more relevant to understanding why neurons are as they are.

Relevance and Purpose: A Red Herring

A cybernetic revolution swept through biology in the postwar period as a result of analogies with control systems, and discoveries of real control systems as components of animals. As the output of a feedback loop returns to be added to the input, the input–output of any component can be related to the behavior of the whole animal only when the loop circuit has been worked out. There can be an impression of purpose when a control mechanism compensates for perturbations that are artificially introduced into the system. Feedback loops, however, are a red herring in this context: first, within the loop each neuron has its own input–output–relevance; second, *the loop as a whole can be regarded as a single component* with a single input–output–relevance.

Bringing Optimization Theory into Neurobiology

An explanation of the size and properties of neuronal fields in terms of the part played by their *outputs* in normal behavior is not just an academic exercise to satisfy man's demand for elegant or relevant explanations. This particular issue becomes prominent where a physical argument is based on a process of optimization. For two decades there has been a question as to whether information theory, which refers to the amount of information carried by a transmission system, applies to the nervous system. Practicing neurobiologists ignore information theory because it is about optimized systems and its main conclusions appear inapplicable. In particular, there appear to be far more channels in nervous systems than an engineer would need for controlling the same behavior, and the rate of information transfer in single neurons appears to be far below optimum at most times. This difficulty is in part overcome when we use optimization theory only for those forms and activities of receptors and neurons which show through in the behavior, and when we try to work out the compromises in the adaptations for particular purposes, given only limited components. There are three aspects of the relevance: (1) Why the input–output function of that neuron has certain properties will be understood only when the chain of behavior, of which it forms one link, is also known. (2) The output of that neuron will mostly be thrown away at the next stage of analysis; only a small part of the information carried by that neuron is carried to the next neurons down the line. (3) Lines must be kept free for rarely encountered options. In brief, information theory can be applied to the real system if we consider only that part of the information *at the input which can be used in the output.* In the past, information theory has been rejected by electrophysiologists because they have related it to all that they can record. However, in dealing with optimum systems we consider only the information in the input which can be used. For this, it is necessary to know which fraction is used.

Every neuron has a *field,* which is represented quantitatively as the pattern of contours of sensitivity, sometimes in many dimensions of the stimulus. Only a part of this field is useful for behavior, therefore subjected to natural selection for optimization, and therefore amenable to information theory, or interesting for explaining nervous system functioning. In recording from neurons, let us adopt an attitude of mind which concentrates on field properties that appear in the output of later neurons and in behavior.

What Is the "Problem of Reduction" in the Nervous System?

The attempt to reduce the phenomena of life to physical interpretation has been progressively more fruitful over the past centuries. There is no attempt here to reverse this trend. I define "mechanistic teleology" as the philosophical approach by which the experimentalist must look at the later events subsequently caused by a living process (in this case, activity of a neuron) as well as the direct mechanical causes of the events themselves. In other terminology the input–output function needs to be extended to the input–output–relevance function. No reasonably well-informed neurobiologist can have any doubts that most of our subject, as presented to the world, falls desperately short of the interest it would contain if the relevance were completely known.

Types of Explanation Available—Summary

Three characteristic forms of explanation are in use in neuroethology.

The first type of explanation, *mechanistic reductionism,* explains behavior as the product of interactions between components of the nervous system. This is the philosophy required to motivate the actual work of analysis. Mechanistic reductionism really only describes what goes on. Except for small localized and restricted regions where numerous small neurons and hormonal or similar effects are excluded, descriptions obtained by mechanistic reductionism are unsatisfactory in that they are always incomplete, and also they do not explain why components and interactions are as they are.

The second type of explanation brings in the *legacy of evolution.* By this approach the components and interactions are as they are because selection has acted on what the ancestors have provided. Experimental analysis takes this for granted.

Although at worst a cloak for ignorance, at best the evolutionary approach reveals the compromises of the past, and the shortfall from perfect performance because evolution is not complete.

The third type of explanation, *mechanistic teleology,* in setting out to explain why components and interactions are as they are, interprets the knowledge of how the system works in terms of the efficiency in performing a function. Mechanistic teleology relates mechanisms to ends on the assumption that adaptive evolution acting over long periods of time has evolved structures and physiological properties to be efficient for particular functions. With this assumption, the principles of physics and chemistry can help to explain why things are as they are, because they meet the quantitative requirements for an optimized physical system. Mechanistic teleology therefore requires a more exact and deeper understanding than any other approach. Explanations of varying degrees of rigor, relating structure to function, have been common in biology for many years, but analysis of the nervous system has hardly yet reached the level of analysis where quantitative mechanistic teleology is possible. We are now reaching a stage, however, where the fields of receptor neurons can be treated in this way, and a start can be made on central neurons.

When sufficient detail is known of both input field and the output as seen by the next stage down the line, it is profitable and enjoyable to apply principles of optimization and the laws of physics to the design of the system. Through the laws of physics, mechanistic teleology relates the functionally significant part of the input to the functionally relevant part of the output. No other type of explanation provides a comparable understanding of why the system is as it is. This type of explanation is not a figment of the human mind because the optimization as the quantitative expression of the evolutionary process, fits the properties of each neuron to the demands set on behavior by the outside world.

26

Nonimpulsive Afferent Coding and Stretch Reflexes in Crabs

Brian M. H. Bush

Introduction

Like most other branches of crustacean neurobiology, that of the physiological responses of individual proprioceptor neurons was pioneered by C. A. G. Wiersma and co-workers. Impulses in the single afferent fibers of the crayfish abdominal muscle receptor organs (MROs) were first recorded by Wiersma *et al.* (1953). Later, Wiersma was the first to record single-unit responses from the chordotonal organs of crustacean legs, distinguishing movement-sensitive and position-sensitive afferent fibers for either direction of the joint (Wiersma and Boettiger, 1959). Proprioceptive information in crustacean limbs, therefore, as in other jointed-limb animals including vertebrates, undergoes "parallel processing" (*cf.* Wiersma, 1962, 1974) via multiple afferent channels, and is encoded and conducted centrally in the most prevalent manner, namely, a frequency-modulated pulsatile code. This applies to all the joints in the thoracic limbs of decapod crustaceans except the most basal, thoracicocoxal joint.

The Thoracicocoxal Receptors

A single "muscular receptor" occurs at the base of each leg, lying largely or entirely within the thorax, and in parallel with the leg promotor muscle (Alexandrowicz and Whitear, 1957; Alexandrowicz, 1958, 1967). The essentials of its gross morphology and fine structure in crabs (Brachyura) are illustrated in Figs. 1d and 2 (see also Bush, 1976; Krauhs and Mirolli, 1975; Whitear, 1965).

Early Recordings from the Coxal Muscle Receptor

The first electrophysiological study of these thoracicocoxal receptors was carried out by one of Wiersma's former students, S. H. Ripley (*cf.* Ripley and Wiersma, 1953) while on leave in G. Hoyle's laboratory in Glasgow in 1960.

Brian M. H. Bush • Department of Physiology, University of Bristol, Park Row, Bristol BS1 5LS, England.

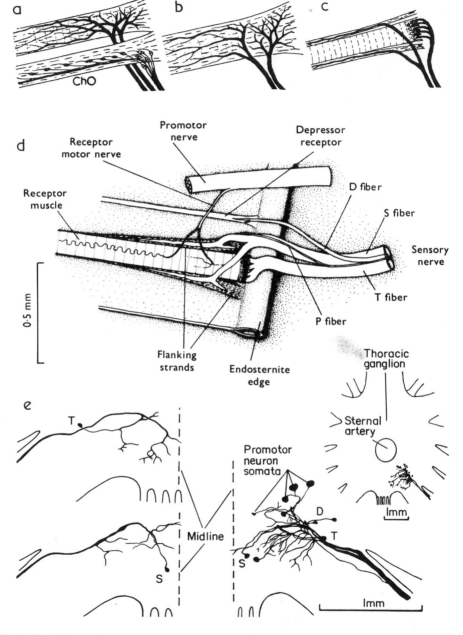

Fig. 1. Morphology of proximal region of thoracicocoxal receptors in (a) Astacura, (b) Palinura, and (c,d) Brachyura. (e) Cobalt-stained sensory and promotor neurons in the posterior thoracic ganglion of *Carcinus*. D, P, S, T, Sensory fibers or cell bodies; Cho, chordotonal organ. From (a–c) Alexandrowicz (1967), (d) Bush and Roberts (1971), and (e) Bush (1976).

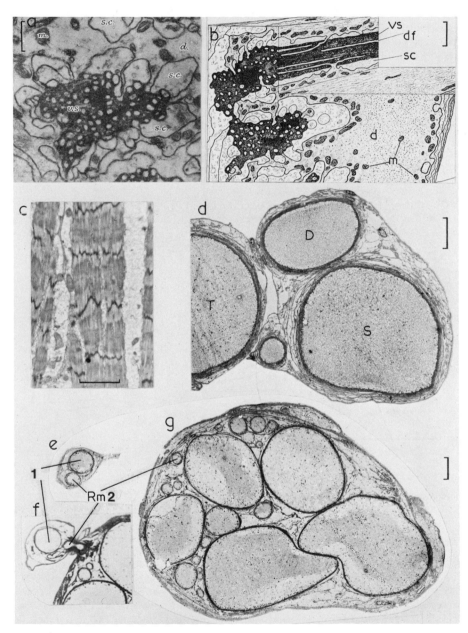

Fig. 2. Ultrastructure of muscle receptor components. (a,b) Sensory terminals, (c) receptor muscle, (d) afferent nerve, and (e) receptor motor nerve distal to (f) its branching off (g) the promotor nerve. d, Dendrite; df, dendrite finger; m, mitochondrion; sc, string cell; vs, vacuolated string. D, P, S, T: sensory fibers; 1, 2, receptor motor axons. Scales: (a,b) 1 μm; (c) 5 μm; (d–g) 10 μm. From (a,b) Whitear (1965), (d) Bush (1976), (c) Bush (unpublished), and (e–g) Cannone (1974).

Recording extracellularly, or in a few preparations intracellularly, Ripley could not detect any impulses in the sensory nerve from the muscle receptor in *Carcinus* (personal communication). Instead, he obtained only slow depolarizing potentials, graded with intensity of the mechanical stimulus and decrementing with distance toward the thoracic ganglion (Fig. 3a). These observations were corroborated on South African river crabs (*Potamon* spp.) and rock lobsters (*Panulirus* sp.) in 1967 (Bush and Ripley, unpublished).

Subsequently, with an intracellular microelectrode in one sensory fiber together with an extracellular suction electrode on the whole receptor nerve, we established unequivocally the "nonimpulsive" nature of the afferent response (Fig. 3b), evoked either by remotion of the joint or by direct stretching of the receptor

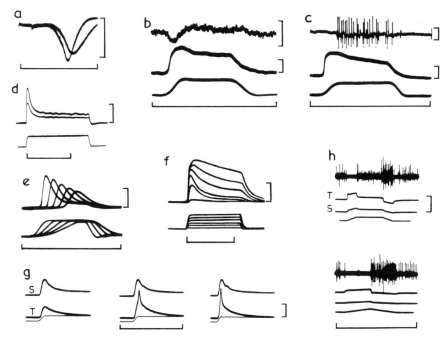

Fig. 3. Evidence for nonimpulsive afferent responses to receptor muscle stretch. (a) Extracellular recordings from two points 7 mm apart on the receptor nerve of a large crab, in response to a brief stretch. (b) Extracellular response of whole receptor nerve (top trace) and intracellular response of S fiber to stretching the receptor muscle *in situ*. (c) Reflex discharge of promotor nerve (top trace) and concurrent T fiber response to receptor stretch. (d) Intracellular responses from two electrodes 2 mm apart in a T fiber. (e) Graded velocity and (f) graded amplitude stretches eliciting graded responses in a T fiber and D fiber, respectively. (g) Graded active membrane responses in a T fiber with three stretch velocities. (h) Chordotonal organ nerve (top traces) and T and S fiber responses to stretching the two receptors simultaneously, at two velocities. a–f, *Carcinus*; g, *Potamon*; h, *Homarus*. Bottom traces are receptor length monitors, stretch upward; other traces are as indicated. Calibrations: 1 mv (a) and 100 μV (b,c) extracellular; 20 mV intracellular; 10 msec (a), 100 msec, 1 sec (h). From (a) Ripley (unpublished), (b) Ripley *et al.* (1968), (c) Bush and Roberts (1968), (d–f) Bush and Roberts (1971), and (g,h) Bush (1976).

muscle (Ripley *et al.*, 1968). Proof that these afferent responses were physiologically "normal" came in the discovery of a strong reflex discharge of impulses in several motor axons to the "extrafusal" promotor muscle, concurrently with the slow potentials in the sensory nerve (Bush and Roberts, 1968) (Fig. 3c). Furthermore, depolarizing current injected into an afferent fiber also elicited reflex discharge in these promotor neurons, without any sign of impulse generation in the afferent fibers. Clearly, the graded (Fig. 3e,f), decrementally conducted (a,d), depolarizing potentials recorded in the afferent fibers in response to receptor muscle stretch were true receptor potentials. The structural and electrical properties underlying this unusual neuronal behavior will be considered later.

Other Coxal Receptors

Essentially similar afferent responses have been recorded from the homologous muscle receptor in a variety of other decapod crustaceans, including Astacura (Figs. 1a,3h), and even in large crabs (*Cancer* and *Maia*) with sensory nerves almost 2 cm long (Bush, 1976). Similarly, two nonmuscular "innervated elastic strands," the *depressor* and *levator* receptors, associated with these muscles of the coxobasipodite joint (Alexandrowicz, 1958, 1967) also lack impulses in their smaller-diameter afferent fibers (Fig. 3f). In contrast to the foregoing nonimpulsive sensory neurons with their central somata, the astacuran thoracicocoxal chordotonal organ (Alexandrowicz and Whitear, 1957) (Fig. 1a) does exhibit afferent impulses (Bush, 1976; Bush and Cannone, unpublished observations). However, unlike the coxobasal receptor organ (Bush, 1965a), its peripherally situated bipolar sensory neurons all respond to shortening of the receptor strand, and none responds to lengthening of the strand (Fig. 3h). This receptor organ thus appears to complement the neighboring muscle receptor in its response to joint movement (*cf.* Alexandrowicz's 1958 hypothesis).

Other Nonspiking Neurons

Several more examples of nonspiking neurons have recently come to light, apart from vertebrate visual receptors and certain other sensory cells not usually regarded as neurons. These include four mechanoreceptive cells of a stretch receptor organ at the base of the uropod in the sand crab *Emerita,* also having giant afferent processes and somata in the central nervous system (Paul, 1972), and the decrementally conducting axons, up to 11 mm long, of the peripherally located visual receptor cells of the lateral eye in the barnacle (Shaw, 1972). Nonspiking interneurons (INs), which influence the firing frequency of identified motor neurons (MNs), have also been encountered, both in crustaceans (Mendelson, 1971) and in insects (Pearson and Fourtner, 1975; Burrows and Siegler, 1976; see also Burrows, this volume; Pearson, this volume). It may well turn out, therefore, that signal transmission by neurons which do not support propagated, all-or-none impulses is much more widespread than hitherto suspected, even perhaps in vertebrate central nervous systems.

Analysis of the Afferent Response

Transducer Mechanism of the Receptor Neurons

The fine structure of the sensory terminals of the S and T fibers suggests that the small-diameter "dendrite fingers" (Fig. 2a,b) might be the site of mechanoelectric transduction (Whitear, 1965). This hypothesis is supported by Krauhs and Mirolli (1975), who demonstrated a 25% reduction in cross-sectional diameter of the dendrite fingers from maximally stretched receptors compared to those from receptors fixed at minimum length *in situ*.

As in other mechanoreceptors (e.g., Terzuolo and Knox, 1971), the primary transduction process probably constitutes an increase in receptor membrane permeability. Thus constant-current pulses injected into the S or T fiber result in decreasing potential changes with increasing stretch (Fig. 9c), and receptor currents are recorded even under voltage clamp conditions (Bush, 1976; Bush *et al.*, 1975b). Ion substitution (Fig. 4a) and voltage clamp experiments indicate that the receptor currents are carried predominantly by sodium ions (Roberts and Bush, 1971; Godden and Bush, unpublished observations), although other ions, including calcium and potassium, are probably also involved.

Properties of the Afferent Nerve Fibers

The S and T fibers in medium-sized shore crabs are 4–6 mm long and 40–70 μm in diameter. Each fiber is ensheathed in several layers of Schwann cells (Fig. 2d), thus exhibiting a thicker membrane than motor axons of comparable diameter (Fig. 2g). The fibers are enclosed in a common sheath with the D fiber of the depressor receptor and the small P fiber, which terminates in the ventral flanking strand near the S fiber terminals.

The voltage/current relations of the S and T fibers are usually almost linear over a wide range (Roberts and Bush, 1971) (Fig. 4d). Their input resistance varies from about 0.4 to 1.2 MΩ. Apparent length constants range from about 3 to 16 mm in *Carcinus,* giving electrotonic lengths from 1.0 to 0.3 mm. The higher values of λ are probably more reliable since any damage to the fibers would tend to depress the membrane input resistance. Membrane time constants vary from 3 to 11 msec (Roberts and Bush, 1971).

The membrane potential of the S and T fibers of unstretched muscle receptors in *Carcinus* is -50 to -70 mV. Although it is potassium dependent, other factors are implicated by the maximum slope of only 30 mV per tenfold change in external potassium concentration (Roberts and Bush, 1971). Recent observations indicate that an electrogenic sodium pump contributes a significant fraction to the resting potential of both S and T fibers in *Cancer* (Mirolli, 1974; and personal communication) (Fig. 4e) and *Carcinus* (Bush and D. A. Lowe, unpublished). Mirolli also reports a high resting permeability of the sensory terminals to sodium ions and

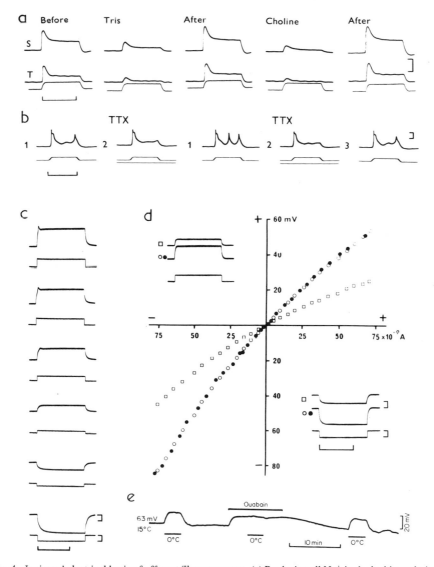

Fig. 4. Ionic and electrical basis of afferent fiber responses. (a) Replacing all Na^+ in the bathing solution by tris or choline results in large, reversible reduction in stretch-evoked receptor potentials of S and T fibers. (b) Tetrodotoxin (TTX, 0.3×10^{-6} M) reduces the initial spiky transient and abolishes any (graded) active membrane responses superimposed on oscillations in the receptor potentials of a T fiber (sample records of two sequences shown). (c) Membrane potential changes (upper traces) in response to graded current pulses (lower traces, depolarizing upward), with two electrodes about $50\,\mu m$ apart in an S fiber showing slight depolarizing electrogenesis. (d) Voltage–current curves and sample records from another S fiber, impaled by two voltage-recording electrodes approximately $100\,\mu m$ (circles) and 2.5 mm (squares) from the current-injection electrode (open and closed symbols represent currents varying in opposite directions). (e) Resting membrane potential changes in response to cooling before, during, and after bathing in 10^{-3} M ouabain in the saline, in an S fiber of a relaxed muscle receptor in *Cancer*. Calibrations: 20 mV; 20 nA (lower traces in c,d); 100 msec, or 10 min (e). From (a–c) Roberts and Bush (1971), (d) Roberts and Bush (unpublished), and (e) Mirolli (personal communication, published in Bush, 1976).

suggests that this will reduce the time constant of the fiber, thereby facilitating transmission of fast transients along its length. This apparent short-circuit condition at the input end can exist by virtue of the sodium pump in the main body of the fiber, which in turn will help to boost the afferent signal by increasing the driving potential for the depolarizing response to stretch. The overall effect of these two spatially separated current sources, Mirolli suggests, is to enable the cell "to use the precision of analog signalling over substantially longer distances without losing the information embodied in the time-course of the stimulus."

Some S and T fibers show a small, graded, active membrane response at the onset of strong depolarizing currents (Fig. 4c). Similar small, spiky transients are sometimes superimposed on the receptor potentials in response to stretch (Fig. 3g). These local, nonpropagated responses are due to a small degree of depolarization-sensitive sodium activation in the afferent fiber membrane, since they are abolished by tetrodotoxin (Roberts and Bush, 1971) (Fig. 4b). Possibly they may serve to speed up afferent conduction, although they evidently do not constitute an important afferent component of the stretch reflex (see below). It is perhaps noteworthy that such active membrane responses were commonly encountered in the swimming crab *Portunus,* which swims mainly by rapid "cycling" movements of its posterior legs (Hoyle and Burrows, 1973c).

Characteristics of Afferent Responses to Stretch

The receptor potentials recorded intracellularly in each of the S and T fibers show distinct dynamic and static components, with a close temporal relationship to the corresponding phases of a ramp-function stimulus (Bush and Roberts, 1971) (Fig. 5a). In shape and time course, the S fiber response usually resembles a simple sum of the length change and the rate of change of length, with both a positive and a negative velocity component, and a more variable initial spike-like transient.

The dynamic component of the T fiber is larger and more complex in form. With slow pulls (Fig. 5c), it can sometimes be resolved into an initial brief spike (α), probably representing an active membrane response of the afferent fiber, followed by a true initial response (β) of the transducing element of the receptor, and then the main velocity component itself, which at the higher stretch velocities often shows a progressive decline. The dynamic component amplitude increases systematically (nearly logarithmically in the T fiber) with velocity of stretch. Over the physiological range, the T fiber's dynamic response increases with stretch velocity more steeply than the S fiber, indicating a greater velocity sensitivity. This difference is also reflected in the much larger potential excursions of the T fiber with sinusoidal oscillations in receptor length, as well as in its more marked phase advance and skewed form (Fig. 5b).

On cessation of stretching, the membrane potential of both S and T fibers rapidly falls toward a new level, related to the amplitude of stretch. On subsequent

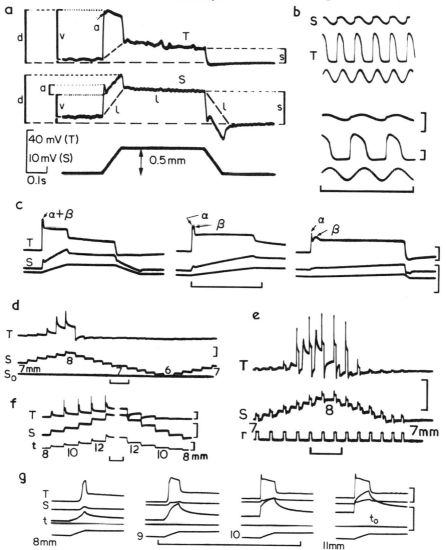

Fig. 5. Characteristic waveforms, and velocity and length dependency, of T and S fiber receptor potentials and (f,g) passive tension, in response to imposed receptor length changes of different forms: (a,c,e,g) ramp function, (b) sinusoidal, and (d–f) stepwise in equal increments (receptor lengths indicated in millimeters but not monitored on CRO records). Symbols: S, T (in this and other figures), afferent fiber membrane potential traces (depolarization upward); d (in a), "dynamic" component peak amplitude; s, "static" component amplitude; l, length; v, velocity response; a, ?"acceleration" response; α & β components (shown in c), see text; S_0 (in d), maximum membrane potential level of S fiber (with fully relaxed receptor); r (in e), ramp-function stretch monitor trace; t (in f,g), tension recorded at distal end of receptor muscle; t_0 (in g), zero tension level (with slack receptor). Receptor length ranges *in situ*: (d,e) *Potamon*, approximately 7–10 mm; (f,g) *Carcinus*, approximately 8–12 mm. Calibratoins: (a) as indicated; (b–g) 20 mV (S and T fibers); 20 mg (t); 1 sec (b,c,g) or 10 sec (d–f). From (a) Bush and Roberts (1971), (c,g) Bush (1976), and (b,d–f) Bush (unpublished).

shortening, the T fiber hyperpolarizes to a varying extent before slowly returning toward its resting potential, reflecting the electrogenic sodium pump component in the fiber membrane potential. The negative dynamic component of the S fiber, on the other hand, mirroring as it does the positive dynamic component, appears to be a function of the mechanical linkages of the receptor endings, and therefore may have significant sensory information content.

The membrane potential of the S fiber varies almost linearly with receptor length (Fig. 5d–f), whereas that of the T fiber shows a much less consistent relation to length, often with a pronounced hysteresis in its responses at successively increasing and decreasing lengths (see Bush, 1976, Fig. 3.11).

At short initial lengths, the interstretch interval can have a marked influence on the dynamic responses to a constant stretch. For example, when the muscle receptor is relatively slack, the T fiber's dynamic component duration increases progressively with increasing interval (Fig. 6e). Possibly this reflects rupture of interfilament cross-bridges by successive stretches, and their spontaneous re-formation in the absence of stretch (*cf.* Hill, 1968). This variability in the T fiber response to a constant stimulus directly affects the resulting reflex output (see below).

Tension Changes in Response to Stretch

In view of the complex viscoelastic properties of the receptor muscle and mechanical linkages between this and the sensory endings, the afferent responses to imposed stretch might be expected to reflect the resulting tension changes more closely than the actual length changes (*cf.* Brown and Stein, 1966). This proves to be the case, as can be shown with a small tension transducer mounted in series with the receptor muscle (Bush and Godden, 1974). The passive tensions recorded in this way are, of course, a function of both the receptor muscle itself, and its enveloping sheath and flanking strands. Accordingly, the "tension waveform" and its variation with stretch velocity and receptor length are intermediate between those of the S and T receptor potentials (Fig. 5f,g, 6a). If tension rather than length is made to vary with constant velocity (Bush *et al.,* 1975a), the receptor potentials in this "tension clamp" mode resemble a ramp function much more closely (Bush, unpublished observation).

Effects of Receptor Motor Stimulation

Isometric Contraction of the Receptor Muscle

Repetitive stimulation of the motor nerve results in smooth, tetanic tension development at a rate dependent on the frequency of stimulation, being very slow at low frequencies. This leads to depolarization of the T fiber, almost linearly related to isometric tension, but usually has little or no effect on the S fiber membrane

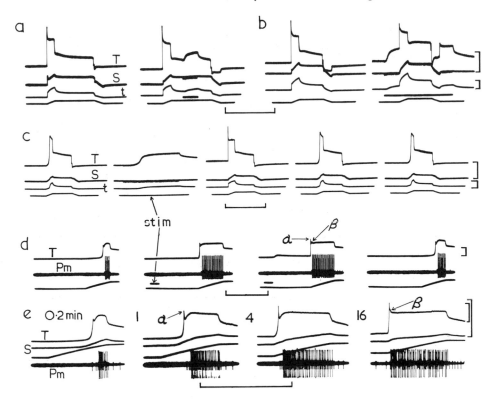

Fig. 6. Influences on the stretch-evoked T and S receptor potentials and (a–c) tension and (d,e) reflex promotor neuron (Pm) discharge, of (a–d) 100 Hz stimulation of the receptor motor nerve (bars and artifacts) or (e) varying interstretch interval. Resting receptor length (approximate range *in situ* 8–12 mm): (a) 10 mm, (b) 11 mm, (c–e) 8 mm; intervals between successive stretches: (a–c) 10 sec, (d) 5 sec, (e) as indicated (in minutes). Note independent development of α and β components in (d,e). Calibrations: 20 mV (S and T); 20 mg *(t)*; 1 sec. From (a–c) Bush and Godden (1974) and (d,e) Cannone (1974), and Bush (1976).

potential (Fig. 7a). In some preparations, high-frequency stimulation of the receptor motor nerve does result also in a small depolarization of the S fiber (Fig. 7a,c). This could be due to stronger contraction of the receptor muscle distally so as to stretch the S fiber terminals in parallel with its proximal end.

Intracellular recording from the receptor muscle at any point along its length during repetitive motor stimulation shows typical depolarizing, excitatory junctional potentials (ejp's) (Fig. 7b,d). They mostly have a slow time course compared with promotor muscle fibers, so generally show considerable summation, and sometimes also marked facilitation. Active membrane responses are lacking. These properties,

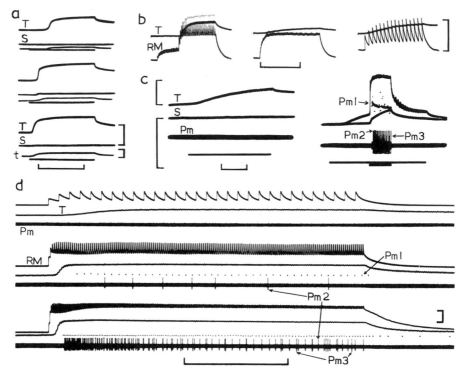

Fig. 7. T and S fiber and (c,d) reflex promotor neuron (Pm) responses to neurally evoked, isometric contraction of the receptor muscle, recorded together with (a) receptor tension *(t)* at three different lengths, or (b,d) intracellular ejp's of two different receptor muscle fibers at several stimulation frequencies. (b) Evidence of dual excitatory motor innervation and its effects on the T fiber: left, smoothly increasing stimulation intensity recruits first one receptor motor axon, giving small ejp's, and then another, giving large, compound ejp's and T fiber depolarization; middle record, high-frequency stimulation of the "small" axon only (low intensity) is necessary to depolarize the T fiber, whereas (right) quite low frequencies of the higher-threshold axon are effective. (c) 100-Hz motor stimulation (thick bar) superimposed upon a 10-Hz train (thin bar) elicits a large T fiber and small S fiber depolarization and strong promotor reflex, (instantaneous frequency points for fiber Pm1), whereas the 10-Hz train alone causes only a slow, small T fiber response. (d) Increasing motor stimulation frequencies (downward) causes increasing ejp summation and T fiber depolarization, and progressive promotor neuron recruitment, with central adaptation of the reflex with sustained T depolarization. Calibrations: 20 mV (T, S, RM); 20 mg *(t);* 1 sec. After (a) Bush and Godden (1974) and (b–d) Cannone (1974) and Bush (1976).

together with its fine structure (Fig. 2c), recall typical slow crustacean muscle, thus accounting for the tonic contractile response to tetanic stimulation.

Careful gradation of the intensity of receptor efferent stimulation sometimes reveals dual motor innervation (Bush and Cannone, 1974). This is most readily manifested as two amplitudes of ejp's (Fig. 7b), while two corresponding increments of tension and T fiber depolarization are generally evident only at high stimulation frequencies. No evidence of any inhibitory innervation to the receptor muscle has been found.

Contractile Effects on Stretch-Evoked Responses

The tension changes and concomitant T fiber potentials, resulting from active contraction and superimposed stretch, summate (Fig. 6a). In addition, receptor contraction causes a marked enhancement of the negative dynamic component of the T fiber (Fig. 6b). Even more striking is the enhancement, by preceding motor stimulation at relatively short receptor lengths, of the positive dynamic component (Fig. 6c,d). Many seconds or even minutes after a brief train of receptor motor impulses, the duration of the T fiber dynamic component, and the underlying tension response to a constant velocity stretch, is markedly prolonged, compared to its duration in the unstimulated, slack receptor. Subsequent stretches at the same short initial length, but without conditioning motor stimuli, lead to a rapid reversion to the original, brief, dynamic component (Fig. 6c).

Reflex Activation of Promotor Neurons

As described previously, the thoracicocoxal receptor muscle in crabs lies within the coxal promotor muscle, in parallel with these "extrafusal" muscle fibers. It is therefore stretched by re-motion of the limb and shortens with pro-motion. Passive remotion of the limb reflexly excites several promotor MNs (Bush and Roberts, 1968) in a typical resistance reflex analogous to those of the more distal limb joints (Bush, 1962b, 1965b). This reflex is mediated by the muscle receptor, the only stretch receptor in crabs responsive solely to movements of this basal limb joint: it is abolished by cutting the receptor's sensory nerve.

The Stretch Reflex

Stretching the deefferented muscle receptor directly by its isolated distal end excites one or more promotor MNs, while receptor shortening inhibits them (Bush and Cannone, 1973; Cannone, 1974; Bush, 1976) (Figs. 3c and 8a). These MNs have been designated Pm1 (promotor neuron 1), Pm2, Pm3, etc., in order of their thresholds for recruitment in this reflex. The lowest threshold unit, Pm1, is often tonically active, and its discharge frequency increases sharply with receptor stretch. Pm2 and Pm3 commonly respond only during the dynamic phase of stretch, dropping sharply to a lower frequency or stopping altogether as soon as the new, longer length is reached. Because of their very similar thresholds and impulse amplitudes, these two units are often difficult to discriminate, although Pm3 tends to have slightly smaller impulses and a somewhat more phasic discharge. Two further units, Pm4 and Pm5, are often also recruited at relatively high velocities of stretch. Still higher-threshold, phasic units, giving up to nine or ten in all (Cannone, 1974), become evident only in "lively" preparations, with high stretch velocities and initial lengths resulting in very large dynamic depolarizations of the afferent fibers (see Fig. 10b,d).

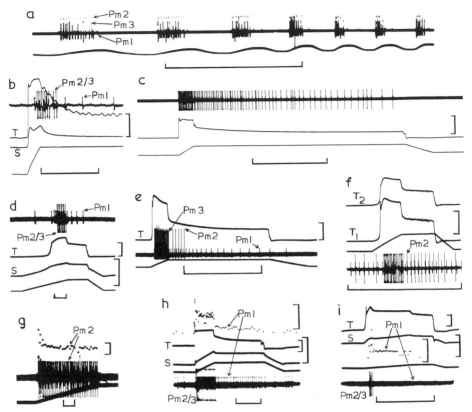

Fig. 8. Promotor neuron (Pm1,2,3) reflex and associated T and S fiber responses to receptor stretch at various velocities. (a) Oscillating receptor length elicits reflex discharge only during stretching. (b,c,e) "Adaptation" in the reflex discharge frequency follows that in the concomitant T fiber receptor potentials. (d) Successive recruitment of Pm1,2,3, with slowly depolarizing T fiber, in a slack receptor. (f) Despite considerable decrement in this T fiber response, recorded simultaneously at two points approximately 2 mm apart, the promotor reflex is still strong. (g–i) Instantaneous frequency displays for Pm2 (g) and Pm1 (h,i) show close reflex "following" of T fiber receptor potentials. Pm1, with the smallest spikes, is sometimes tonically active (f,h); Pm2 and Pm3, owing to their similar spike amplitudes (and thresholds), are not readily discriminated, but in those records where they are distinct (e.g., a,e) Pm2 generally has slightly larger spikes than Pm3. Pm4–10 are not recruited in these records (but see Fig. 10b,d). Calibrations: 20 mV (T, S); 100 Hz (instantaneous frequency plots); 1 sec (100 msec in b,d,g). From (h) Bush and Cannone (1973), (c,g,i) Cannone (1974), (d,e) Bush (1976) and (a,b,f) Cannone and bush (unpublished observations).

Correlation between Afferent and Efferent Responses

Simultaneous intracellular monitoring of the afferent fiber responses to receptor muscle stretch, and the resulting reflex promotor neurons' discharges, shows a close correspondence between them (Fig. 8b–i). The latency of the reflex response, measured from the onset of stretch, can be quite variable, being particularly dependent on the initial length and stiffness of the receptor muscle and on the velocity of stretch (*cf.* Fig. 8b–d). When compared directly with the accompanying receptor potentials, however, especially that of the T fiber, the input–output relationship becomes much clearer (e.g., Fig. 8d,f). Yet the afferent–efferent latencies are difficult to measure, particularly with the more slowly developing afferent depolarizations occurring in slack receptors. Nevertheless, minimum latencies, obtained from fast stretches of taut receptors, and with afferent and efferent conduction distances of around 4 and 8 mm, respectively, are in the range 6–12 msec (about 10 msec in Fig. 8b).

In view of these rather long latencies, the correspondence between sensory and reflex response becomes more evident with relatively slow ramp-function stretches (Fig. 8c–f). Thus the highest reflex discharge frequencies occur during the dynamic components of the receptor potentials, when depolarization is maximal. At the top of the ramp, the T fiber depolarization and the reflex frequency both fall abruptly, with a latency comparable to or somewhat longer than that following the rising phase. Any remaining promotor neuron discharge usually continues to decline slowly, roughly mirroring the gradual repolarization or "adaptation" of the T fiber during a sustained stretch (Fig. 8c,e).

Recordings of the instantaneous frequencies for each responding promotor neuron further clarify the relationship of the individual efferent and afferent responses (Fig. 8g–i). The general shapes of the frequency envelopes for each promotor unit, especially Pm1–3, reflect the waveform of the corresponding phases of the receptor potentials in the T fiber remarkably closely, and accordingly differ substantially from those of the S fiber. This striking resemblance between the reflex and T afferent responses holds true for any velocity or amplitude of stretch, and whatever the initial length or degree of efferent activation of the receptor muscle. Even the true initial response (β component) of the T fiber's dynamic component, at least with slow stretches, is represented by an initial high-frequency burst (Fig. 8h,i); there is no clear evidence, however, that the α component of the afferent response has any reflex effect. Furthermore, the tonic discharge frequency of Pm1 depends directly on the existing level of depolarization of the T fiber.

Receptor Efferent Influences on the Promotor Reflex

Repetitive stimulation of the receptor motor axons results in reflex driving of the same promotor neurons as are activated by stretch of the receptor (Bush and Cannone, 1973; Cannone, 1974). The extent of this driving varies directly with the degree of depolarization of the T fiber, and hence also with frequency of efferent stimulation (Fig. 7d). Brief, high-frequency stimulation during a longer, low-frequency train can be made to evoke T fiber depolarizations and corresponding reflex discharge patterns resembling those elicited by ramp-function stretches (Fig. 7c). Moreover, if the stimulus intensity is gradually increased so as to recruit first one and then the second receptor efferent, the reflex discharge increases suddenly at each threshold by an amount proportional to the increase in T fiber depolarization.

The reflex promotor neuron responses to receptor efferent stimulation, like the T fiber's receptor potentials, summate with the responses to receptor stretch. A fast stretch superimposed on strong isometric contraction of the receptor muscle, for example, can elicit very high reflex discharge frequencies, with recruitment of anything up to ten promotor neurons, including the large-amplitude, high-threshold, phasic units which are seldom encountered at other times. Conversely, a brief receptor motor tetanus enhances the reflex response to subsequent stretch. As already seen with the T receptor potentials, this effect is most pronounced when the receptor muscle is at short resting lengths (Fig. 6c,d). The dramatic influence on the dynamic reflex in this condition highlights a major potential role for the efferent control of this receptor, namely, its capacity to maintain the high responsiveness or "gain" of the receptor to imposed length changes.

Effects of Cutting the S or T Fibers

The foregoing observations on the stretch- or contraction-evoked reflexes strongly suggest that the T fiber provides the dominant afferent input to the promotor neurons. This hypothesis is supported by the reflex effects of either cutting or passing depolarizing or hyperpolarizing current into the individual S and T fibers. Transsecting the whole receptor nerve (see Fig. 2d) strongly excites a number of promotor MNs, including two or three large-spike, phasic fibers. Thereafter, no further reflex can be obtained on stretching the receptor muscle. Cutting either the S or T fiber individually produces a similar reflex discharge, that from the T fiber being the stronger. Now, however, the stretch reflex can still be elicited if only the S fiber has been cut, but not if the T fiber alone is severed.

Current Injection into the Efferent Fibers

Depolarizing current injected into the S or T fiber results in reflex discharge of promotor MNs (Bush and Roberts, 1968; Bush and Cannone, 1973; Cannone, 1974) (Fig. 9a–f). However, whereas a few millivolts' depolarization of the T fiber is usually sufficient to excite from one to three promotor neurons (Pm1–3), at least 10–20 mV depolarization of the S fiber is generally needed (Fig. 9e,f). The higher-threshold promotor units are also more readily excited by the T fiber, apart from one small unit which is driven only by the S fiber. In general, the curves relating reflex promotor neuron frequency to afferent fiber depolarization (Fig. 9d) are much steeper for the T than for the S fiber, and are roughly linear over much of their frequency range. The activation threshold and slopes of the curves for Pm2 and Pm3 are often quite similar to each other—the thresholds sometimes being reversed for S fiber activation—but are generally greater than those for Pm1. Afferent depolarization resulting from current injection sums with that from receptor stretch or contraction in eliciting reflex promotor neuron discharge (Figs. 9c,h and 10d). A variable degree of adaptation is usually evident in the reflex response to a long, constant-current pulse (Fig. 9c, cf. Fig. 9e,f). This will, of course, supplement the often rather larger component of adaptation of the stretch reflex attributed to the progressive decline in the level of depolarization during the static component of the T fiber's response to prolonged stretch (see Fig. 8c,e).

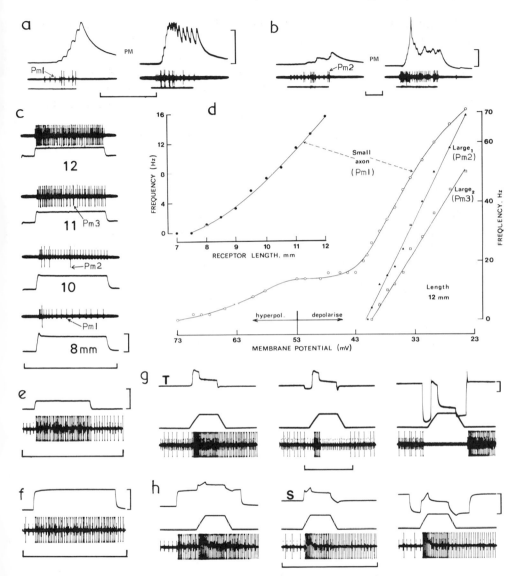

Fig. 9. Reflex promotor neuron responses to constant-current pulses injected into (a–c,g) the T fiber and (f,h) the S fiber, with simultaneous intracellular recordings from (a,b) two different promotor muscle fibers, (c,e,g) the T fiber, and (f,h) the S fiber. (a,b) Facilitation and summation of intracellular ejp's evoked by Pm1 (a) and Pm2 (b), the latter leading to an active membrane spike at high frequency. (c) Equal-current depolarizing pulses at increasing receptor muscle lengths (indicated in millimeters) result in decreasing potential changes, but increasing depolarization levels and therefore reflex frequencies. (d) Relationship between reflex promotor neuron frequency and receptor length, or current-controlled T fiber membrane potential. (e,f) Depolarizing current into either T (e) or S fiber (f) excites Pm1–3, much more effectively with T than S; current and stretch-induced depolarization sum (h; not shown for T). Hyperpolarization of the T fiber (g) but not the S fiber (h) inhibits the stretch reflex. Calibrations: 20 mV (PM, T, S); 1 sec. From (a–c) Cannone (1974), (e–h) Bush and Cannone (1973), Bush (1976), and (d) Cannone and Bush (unpublished observations).

Hyperpolarizing current injected into the T fiber reduces or, if strong enough, abolishes any ongoing tonic activity in promotor neurons (Fig. 9d,g). Furthermore, the reflex response to stretching the receptor muscle is also inhibited by T fiber hyperpolarization, to an increasing extent with increasing current intensity (Bush and Cannone, 1973; Cannone, 1974) (Fig. 9g). Hyperpolarization of the S fiber, however, has no apparent effect on the stretch reflex (h), even with high current in preparations in which strong depolarization of the S fiber produces substantial reflex driving (f). This therefore constitutes further evidence for the dominant role of the T fiber in mediating the promotor stretch reflex.

Synaptic Transmission in the Promotor Reflex

The close reflex "following" of the stretch-evoked receptor potentials in the T fiber, noted above, and the low threshold and high sensitivity of the three promotor neurons, Pm1–3, to depolarizing current in the T fiber, suggest that they may be monosynaptically excited by this fiber. Direct evidence for this hypothesis is as yet lacking. Reflex latency measurements, etc., with peripheral recording sites and the relatively slowly rising, graded, afferent inputs are not very helpful. Consistent with a monosynaptic connection, however, is the extensive overlap in neuropilar arborization fields of the promotor and sensory neurons, particularly the T fiber (Fig. 1e), with an evidently close apposition of branches in some preparations (Luff, Godden, and Bush, in preparation). Further speculation, however, is pointless without additional evidence, preferably involving simultaneous intracellular monitoring of pre- and postsynaptic events (in progress).

The sensory nerve of the muscle receptor in *Carcinus* contains relatively high concentrations of choline acetyltransferase, the enzyme which synthesizes acetylocholine (Emson *et al.*, 1976). This strongly suggests cholinergic transmission at these synapses, as in other crustacean sensory systems (Florey, 1973). If the reflex is indeed monosynaptic, the rather long afferent–efferent delay encountered (see above) would also be more compatible with chemical than with electrical transmission (*cf.* Burrows and Siegler, 1976). Of course, part of this delay comprises peripheral conduction time, although possibly only 1–2 msec, assuming an afferent "conduction velocity"—insofar as it can be measured, with decremental conduction, from records such as Fig. 3a—of, say, 5–10 m/sec. The reflex effect of T fiber hyperpolarization could probably be accounted for by a decrease in a continuous, spontaneous release of transmitter from the afferent terminals, possibly even in a fully relaxed receptor. Nevertheless, the possibility that electrical coupling may be involved in the reflex cannot be excluded.

Reflex Excitation of Receptor MNs

With a fine-tipped suction electrode on the receptor motor nerve distal to its separation from the promotor nerve, impulses can often be recorded when the receptor muscle is stretched (Bush and Cannone, 1974; Cannone, 1974) (Fig. 10a).

Normally, spikes of only one amplitude are seen, but with high stretch velocities one or two smaller impulses may occur in a second fiber. As in the promotor stretch reflex, the response frequency of the larger receptor efferent increases with stretch velocity, and hence with the dynamic amplitude of the T fiber receptor potential. However, it never reaches the high frequencies seen in the lower-threshold promotor neurons, and, except in occasional, highly active preparations (e.g., Fig. 10b), it usually responds only during the dynamic phase of stretch.

Like the promotor MNs, the receptor efferents also respond to direct depolarization of the T fiber by injected current (Fig. 10c). Depolarization of the S fiber, however, even with large currents, does not excite the receptor MNs. As before, direct depolarization of the T fiber sums with the stretch- or contraction-evoked depolarization to enhance the reflex discharge of the receptor efferents, often recruiting the higher-threshold, small axon during the dynamic phase of stretch (d). Again, hyperpolarization of the T fiber blocks the reflex response of both receptor MNs to receptor stretch (e), whereas S fiber hyperpolarization has no effect (f,g).

A Dual-Axon Positive Feedback Reflex?

As described above, both receptor motor axons give ejp's which, with sufficient facilitation and summation on repetition, lead to slow, tetanic contraction and consequent depolarization of the T fiber. Evidently, therefore, the reflex excitation of both these receptor efferents is a positive feedback reflex. Two questions arise before the functional significance of this self-excitatory reflex can be considered. First, does either of these two receptor MNs also innervate the "extrafusal" (promotor) muscle; and, second, how does the system behave in the closed-loop condition?

Increasing intensity stimulation of the whole promotor nerve, proximally, recruits first one and, at a higher intensity, the second, receptor efferent axon (Fig. 7b). However, when the promotor nerve is stimulated distal to the point where the receptor motor nerve leaves it, only the smaller ejp's are recorded and accordingly only one level of isometric contraction of the receptor muscle is obtained, as reflected in T fiber depolarization. Serial 1-μm sections through this region of the motor nerve clearly showed that the smaller but not the larger of the two axons to the receptor muscle branches off a promotor axon (Cannone, 1974) (Fig. 2e,f). That is, the smaller axon is shared with the promotor muscle, the other being specific to the receptor muscle—a situation analogous to β and γ innervation, respectively, of vertebrate muscle spindles. The observation that the unit with the smaller impulses—presumably the smaller-diameter, shared axon—has the higher threshold for reflex excitation (Fig. 10d) no doubt has functional significance.

Closed-Loop Behavior

The behavior of this proprioceptive system in closed-loop conditions is a more difficult question and as yet has not been directly investigated, but some preliminary observations bear on the matter. A number of "lively" preparations showed occa-

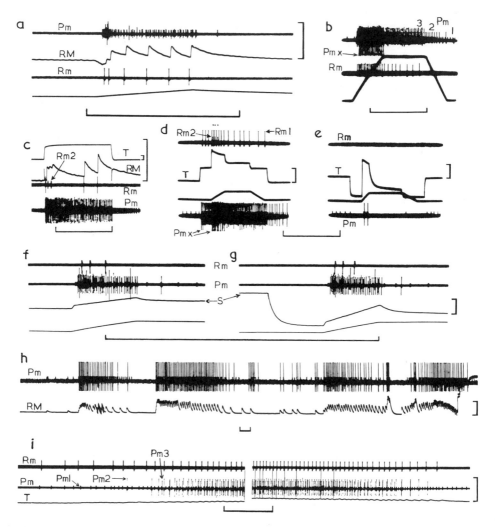

Fig. 10. Receptor motor (Rm) and concurrent promotor (Pm) reflex responses to (a,b,d–g) receptor stretch and (c–e,g) current injected into an afferent fiber, together with (a,c) intracellular records from a receptor muscle fiber (RM). Strong T fiber depolarization, (c) by current alone or (d) together with stretch, may excite both receptor MNs (Rm1 and Rm2) and sometimes also extra, high-threshold promotor neurons (Pmx); these latter are occasionally recruited by stretch alone (b). Hyperpolarization of the T fiber (e), but not the S fiber (g, compare with f), blocks the receptor motor stretch reflex. (h,i) "Spontaneous" receptor motor activity commonly starts roughly simultaneously with similar promotor discharge, suggesting "coactivation"; the resulting isometric contraction of the receptor muscle causes slow T fiber depolarization. Calibrations: 20 mV (RM, T, S); 1 sec. From (a,d) Bush and Cannone (1974), (b,e–g) Cannone (1974), and (h,i) Bush (1976).

sional spontaneous bouts of activity, evidently centrally initiated and lasting from a few seconds to a minute or more (Cannone, 1974). These involved increasing discharge frequencies of several promotor neurons, accompanied by slow depolarization of the T fiber, followed by decreasing promotor activity and T fiber repolarization. In a few preparations in which simultaneous recordings were obtained from the receptor muscle or its intact motor nerve, the larger of the two MNs discharged together with the promotor bursts, but at a lower frequency than the most active promotor neurons. Significantly, although it occasionally started to discharge a second or more before or after the first promotor axon, the receptor efferent more commonly began firing at about the same time as the promotor discharge (Fig. 10h,i).

In these experiments, the gradual depolarization of the T fiber was clearly a consequence of slow, isometric contraction of the receptor muscle. In the intact animal, such receptor motor activity would tend to prevent the receptor muscle from slackening when the promotor shortened during nonisometric contraction. That is, the function of such receptor efferent coactivation could be seen as one of maintaining the gain of the receptor, in particular of the T fiber, in conditions of unloading during centrally commanded promotor contraction.

A similar role might be attributed to the positive feedback stretch reflex of the two receptor MNs, since this occurs concurrently with promotor activation through its stretch reflex. The problem of oscillation, inherent in control systems with positive feedback, is probably obviated in this case by the slow rate of contraction of the receptor muscle.

Behavioral Role of the Thoracicocoxal Receptors

Being the only known stretch receptor at this basal limb joint (except in Astacura, with their additional chordotonal organ), the crustacean thoracicocoxal receptor must undoubtedly play an important role in the regulation of the joint and hence of the whole limb. The strong promotor stretch reflex, following so closely the afferent input via the T fiber, clearly implicates this receptor in some sort of servocontrol capacity comparable to that of other muscle receptors. As yet, there is no direct evidence on its normal behavior *in situ*. What information there is from dissected preparations suggests that coactivation of receptor and promotor units may be common. Possibly, therefore, this invertebrate muscle receptor functions as a load-canceling device to provide "servoassistance" for promotor contractions and hence for posture and movement of the basal limb joints.

Such a role would be consistent with prevailing views on the role of mammalian muscle spindles (see Matthews, 1972; R. B. Stein, 1974) and the crayfish abdominal muscle receptor (Fields, 1976). Nevertheless, the thoracicocoxal muscle receptor *could* also function in the "follow-up length servo" mode (*cf.* Fig. 7d), as originally postulated by Merton in 1953 for the mammalian spindle, and later discussed for the crayfish abdominal MRO (Fields *et al.*, 1967; Page and Sokolove, 1972). Perhaps in addition it "sets" a postural base level, by central nervous control of the efferent bias, as suggested *inter alia* for the myochordotonal organ (Evoy and Cohen, 1971). In any event, there can be little doubt that the dual excitatory motor supply to the receptor muscle plays an important role in maintaining the gain of the receptor, and particularly its dynamic sensitivity to both stretching and shortening under conditions of unloading when it would otherwise be relatively ineffective (Bush, Godden & Cannone, 1975).

Other reflexes mediated by, or otherwise involving, the thoracicocoxal muscle receptor organ probably also contribute to intra- and intersegmental coordination within the limb, and possibly between adjacent or contralateral limbs as well. A likely candidate would be a "resistance reflex" to the antagonistic remotor muscle, on relaxation of the thoracicocoxal receptor. Preliminary experiments, however, have revealed no more than a weak reflex discharge in response to receptor relaxation in one or two small remotor axons, despite strong promotor neuron discharges during stretching. Moreover, the observation of strong resistance reflexes in the remotor motor nerve during passive promotion of the joint prior to further dissection to expose the receptor muscle suggests that other, as yet unidentified, proprioceptors may mediate this reflex—possibly cuticular stress detectors (Clarac, 1976) or tendon receptors (MacMillan, 1976).

One intersegmental reflex arises from the carpopropodite joint, presumably mediated by the CP chordotonal organs (Moody, 1970). "Bending" (pro-duction) at this joint excites, and "stretching" (re-duction) inhibits, a motor fiber (one of two?) to the thoracicocoxal muscle receptor in the crayfish. Moody also reported that the same receptor MN was excited by relaxation of the thoracicocoxal receptor itself, in contrast to our finding of a self-excitatory stretch reflex (Bush and Cannone, 1974; Cannone, 1974). Whether this discrepancy represents a true species difference remains to be ascertained.

In any event, the fact that the thoracicocoxal receptor muscle—and also the promotor muscle (Moody, 1970)—is reflexly influenced by movements of the carpopropodite joint, i.e., the only other joint of the walking legs moving in the same, anteroposterior direction as the thoracicocoxal joint, might well prove to be significant. This situation is reminiscent of the strong intersegmental reflexes (Bush and Clarac, 1975) from the coxobasal chordotonal organ to the excitatory MN supplying the myochordotonal organ in the meropodite, which senses movement of the merocarpopodite joint (Cohen, 1963). These two joints also operate in the same plane, namely dorsoventral. Accordingly, it may also be significant that the thoracicocoxal receptor was *not* found to reflexly influence the myochordotonal organ MNs (Bush and Clarac, unpublished observations), since these two joints move in planes at right angles to each other.

ACKNOWLEDGMENTS

Thanks are due Drs. Al Cannone, David Godden, Maurizio Mirolli, and Sherman Ripley for permission to refer to unpublished data, including those from Cannone's Ph.D. thesis, and the M.R.C. and S.R.C. (U.K.) for research grants.

27

Development of Insect Nervous Systems

David Bentley

Introduction

As this is the first of a series of articles presented on the development of the nervous system in hemimetabolous insects, I would like to sketch the general sequence of events in this process as it is now understood and to indicate some major current approaches and problems. Most of the work in this area has involved orthopteran insects, primarily locusts, crickets, and cockroaches. These are large insects with a surprisingly sophisticated behavioral repertoire. Interest has focused on the simpler, highly stereotyped behavior patterns such as rhythmic or episodic behavior. The basic coordination underlying such patterns has been shown to be generated within the central nervous system by circuits of motor neurons (MNs) and interneurons (INs), whose output is then modulated to varying degrees by sensory input. The behavior is thus encoded in the physiological and structural properties of the central neural elements, all of which may be unique cells (Bullock, 1974; Goodman, 1976). We are interested in discovering how these neural programming circuits and their composite neurons are uniquely differentiated during development. The analysis currently involves three primary questions: (1) What are the sources of information which specify the properties of these networks? (2) How, in a descriptive sense, is a circuit constructed; that is, what are the directly observed changes in physiological and structural features during construction? (3) What are the underlying mechanisms guiding construction? How is the information translated from original sources into differentiation?

Information Sources

Ultimately, there are only two possible sources of information for guiding differentiation, those internal to the animal and those external. Internal information is, of course, transmitted genetically. Externally derived information is more variable. In its purest form, external information could be a pattern provided by an external model which is then adopted by the developing system. In this fashion, for example, white-crowned sparrow parental song guides the development of song

David Bentley • Department of Zoology, University of California, Berkeley, California 94720.

pattern in juveniles (Marler and Tamura, 1964), and the orientation of lines seen during development influences the properties of line-detecting neurons in kitten visual cortex (Blakemore and Cooper, 1970). In a more subtle form, the external world and its properties could be a link in a feedback loop in which sensory input is used to modulate motor output. Such a system operates through visual input during locust flight (Wilson, 1968a), and must be common in learning of motor acts through practice in vertebrates. From this level, external influences grade into ever more derived and less direct states. Ultimately, of course, it is not possible or even meaningful to completely separate external and internal sources of information for development. Nevertheless, there are clearly great differences possible in the balance of external and genetic information in the development of different nervous systems.

In our laboratory, we have been interested in the development of neural circuits underlying the behavior of crickets *(Teleogryllus oceanicus* and *T. commodus),* particularly in jumping, flight, and singing. Singing behavior offers an unusual opportunity to evaluate the relative contributions of genetic and external information in specifying a pattern because the song pattern is remarkably emancipated from the effects of current sensory input. In fact, it is possible to record from an isolated central nervous system a calling song pattern which is indistinguishable from the pattern of normal song (Bentley, 1969b). Consequently, the pattern is relatively unaffected by the "noise" of the current sensory situation, and is a correspondingly accurate monitor of the properties of the neural circuit which were established during development. Therefore, the contributions of genetic and environmental factors can be assessed by changing them independently and observing the effect on song pattern.

For guiding a species-specific song, the most obvious external information cue would be acoustical. To test the effect of songs heard during development, crickets were raised under three different circumstances: (1) they were deafened and heard no songs; (2) they heard only their own efforts at singing; and (3) they heard only the "wrong" songs of other species during development. In none of these cases was there a detectable effect on song pattern. Tree crickets and cicadas are also capable of producing normal songs when prevented from hearing the species-specific song as juveniles (Shaw, 1968). Therefore, acoustical input does not seem to be an important influence on the development of the song-pattern-generating neural circuit.

The role of use or practice in development of motor patterns can be evaluated by comparing patterns of naive and experienced animals. To test song patterns, we exploited a technique discovered by Huber (1960b). He found that lesions of the mushroom bodies, a restricted part of the cricket brain, sometimes released continuous singing. Last instar nymphal crickets with such lesions also attempt to sing (Bentley and Hoy, 1970). They have had no previous singing practice and still lack wings, so no sound is actually produced. However, the song muscles are innervated by only a small number of MNs, usually one to three "fast" neurons, and by implanting electrodes in the muscles the output of identified MNs can be observed.

The output can then be compared to the pattern of the same neurons during singing of an experienced adult. In Fig. 1, a juvenile pattern of this sort is illustrated, along with the sound pulse pattern of adult calling song. Judging by the durations of the longer and shorter intervals, the numbers of intervals, the switch between interval types, and the alternation of antagonistic units, the naive nymph could immediately generate a normal, adult pattern. Weber (1972) has reported similar results for the European field cricket, *Gryllus campestris*. Using a different approach, Altman (1975) studied the development of flight pattern of the Australian plague locust, *Chortoicetes terminifera*. Newly molted adults were divided into two experimental groups: one was allowed flight experience, while the other had fixed wings to prevent normal flight sensory feedback. After varying periods, the flight patterns of naive and experienced individuals were compared by recording the output of identified motor units. No experience-related differences could be found between the two groups, although certain maturation-related changes in flight pattern do occur during the first weeks of adult life (Kutsch, 1971; Altman and Tyrer, 1974). In crickets, Weber (1972) has graphically analyzed changes in flight pattern during the first few flight attempts of nymphs and compared them to adult patterns. Although the rhythm is present in naive nymphs, there appears to be a definite improvement in the stability of the wing-stroke interval with experience. Although there may well be adjustments in such motor patterns as a consequence of use, it seems clear that these factors do not play a major role in establishing the fundamental output properties of the circuits involved.

Obviously, only a few of the many possible kinds of external influences on the development of these circuits have been tested. However, considering the number and precision of orthopteran motor patterns and the noticeable lack of effect of those external inputs which have been tested, it seems safe to conclude that such factors play a relatively small role in the development of these circuits.

The alternative source of information is genetic. One method of assessing the contribution of genetic information to a motor pattern is to alter the genome while holding the environment as invariant as possible and then to compare the output of

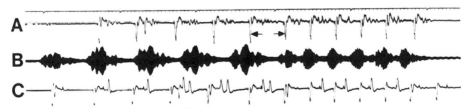

Fig. 1. Comparison of motor output of a nymph with the actual song of an adult. A,C: Muscle action potentials recorded from a last instar nymph. B: Sound pulses recorded from an adult (see text). A is a recording from the second basalar muscle (wing opener); note how closely the number and spacing of nymphal muscle potentials correspond to the adult pattern. C is a push–pull recording from subalar muscle (downward spikes, wing opener), and remotor muscle (upward spikes, wing closer); this demonstrates reciprocal firing of antagonists (closing movement produces sound pulse). Arrows indicate the switch (long intervals to left, short intervals to right), in both adult and nymphal patterns, from long to short intervals between pulses. Time calibration: 5 msec per small division.

individuals with different genetic backgrounds. Continuing with cricket song, we manipulated the genome by hybridizing *T. oceanicus* with a sibling species, *T. commodus,* which has a quite different calling song, and by backcrossing the F_1 to the wild types (Bentley, 1971; Bentley and Hoy, 1972). Sound pulse patterns during calling song were examined, as was the output of identified MNs. Figure 2 displays the output during the initial part of calling song of two MNs, innervating a wing opening and a wing closing muscle, when the neurons are built according to five different sets of genetic specifications. In contrast to experiential influences, genetic alteration produced a very powerful and predictable effect on output pattern. All features of the pattern, such as the interval between the chirp phase and the onset of the trill phase or the number of pulses in the trill phase, faithfully reflect the proportions of wild-type genes. A statistical analysis of 18 song-pattern parameters indicated that none of the parameters was controlled by single genes and, moreover, that genes influencing some parameters appeared to be on the X chromosome, while others were on autosomes. As might be expected, the genetic complement influencing this neural circuit seems to be complex, involving multiple genes and chromosomes.

Direct recording from the motor units allows a more precise analysis of the output pattern. Such analysis reveals that at remarkably fine levels there are consistent differences in discharge patterns of the different genotypes. For example, in the

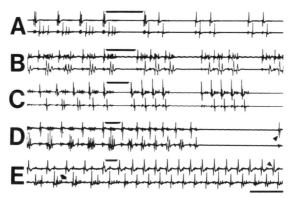

Fig. 2. Motor unit firing patterns responsible for the calling sone of *Teleogryllus* wild types and hybrids. Records are as follows: A, wild type, *T. oceanicus;* B, backcross, *T. oceanicus* ♀ × F_1 ♂ (shown in C); C, F_1, *T. oceanicus* ♀ × *T. commodus* ♂; D, backcross, *T. commodus* ♀ × F_1 ♂ (shown in C); E, wild type, *T. commodus.* Traces show muscle action potentials recorded from single, identified fast units and elicited by single MN impulses (triangles, D and E). The upper trace shows a wing opener unit (unit 1, subalar muscle), and the lower trace shows a wing closer unit (unit 2, promotor muscle); wing closing produces the sound pulse. The portion of the phrase shown is the transition (bars) from the chirp (left of bars) to the sequence of trills (right of bars). Motor unit activity corresponds to, and determines, the sound pulse patterns. Details of differences in firing patterns of homologous single MNs from different genotypes are seen. The transition interval (bar) decreases steadily from *T. oceanicus* (A) to *T. commodus* (E). Motor unit bursts per trill increase from 2 (A) to 14 (E). Genetic information is precise enough to specify a difference of one burst between the trills of *T. oceanicus* (A) and the backcross (B). For many units, this difference is only a single impulse. In some traces, the smaller promotor unit (arrow) partially obscures the recording. The bar at the bottom shows 100 msec.

trill portion of the song, *T. oceanicus* opener units normally fire twice, whereas homologous units of the backcross discharge three times (Fig. 2B), a consistent difference of only a single nerve impulse. Considering the length of the chain of events between the genes and the song and the actual amount of time involved in producing a mature animal from an egg, the accuracy with which the song pattern monitors genotype is very impressive. It demonstrates that, in this system, genetic information is an extremely powerful influence in determining the properties of the neural circuit.

The effects of hybridization on production of song pattern have also been studied in field crickets (Leroy, 1966; Bigelow, 1960), ground crickets (Fulton, 1933), grasshoppers (Perdeck, 1958; von Helversen and von Helversen, 1975), and *Drosophila* (Ewing, 1969), and in all cases a strong effect of genotype was reported. In other insects, particularly *Drosophila,* single gene alterations have also been demonstrated to have profound effects on motor patterns (Ikeda and Kaplan, 1970; Suzuki *et al.,* 1971; Konopka and Benzer, 1971). While the number of insect motor patterns which have been investigated genetically is still small, it already seems clear that genetically stored information is overwhelmingly dominant over external, experiential input in determining the basic features of coordination.

Developmental Events

Having, at least to a first approximation, identified the sources of information which specify the properties of insect neural circuits, it is appropriate to consider the developmental sequence. An initial step is to produce a basic description of the main events in this process. When do the neurons arise and what is their lineage? When are axonal and dendritic arborizations grown? When do various physiological features of the cells appear? When are elements of a circuit connected into a functional unit? Do all elements of a neuron or a circuit mature at the same time, or is there temporal displacement of maturation depending on differential behavior deployment?

In crickets, eggs are laid individually and development does not begin until after oviposition. At 30°C, embryonic development requires about 13 days. Hatching is followed by a substantial postembryonic period of gradual development. This involves eight to ten larval instars and consumes about 45 days or at least three-fourths of the total developmental period. Most adult features are acquired gradually, but certain elements such as the wings and ovipositor appear in a functional form only with the final molt.

As a beginning of this analysis, we have examined the functional assembly and maturation of neural circuits underlying exclusively adult behavior patterns. Our strategy has been to select an easily initiated behavior pattern which can be characterized precisely by the output of a selected set of MNs. These neurons are then recorded at each stage of development while the stimulus for the behavior pattern is presented. The response capability of the neurons is recorded and the stage of maturation of the circuit is surmised by comparison with the adult pattern.

For these experiments, flight was the behavior selected, rather than singing, because it is easily and reliably elicited by suspension of nymphs in a wind tunnel and does not require brain lesions. Flight in *Teleogryllus* involves many of the same muscles and neurons as singing. Both sets of wings are utilized, with the hindwings leading the forewings by about a third of a wingbeat cycle. For the purpose of monitoring neural output, an elevator and a depressor of each set of wings were selected. The normal coordination of these four units in flight is illustrated in Fig. 3: elevators and depressors alternate, and the hindwing neurons fire in advance of their forewing counterparts. These four monitor units were recorded from during each nymphal stage that showed elements of the flight pattern. The first features of flight pattern began to appear about halfway through postembryonic development, or at least four instars preceding adulthood. At this stage, a few rhythmical cycles of discharge approximating the flight frequency could be elicited from hindwing depressor neurons. In subsequent instars, features of the adult flight pattern were

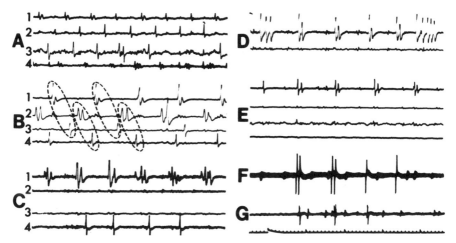

Fig. 3. Progressive development of adult flight pattern in nymphal crickets. The recordings are muscle action potentials that reflect the discharge of single MNs. In each record (A–G), the top trace is the hindwing subalar muscle (wing depressor); the second trace (if any) is the hindwing remotor muscle (wing elevator); the third trace (if any) is the forewing subalar muscle (wing depressor); the fourth trace (if any) is the forewing remotor muscle (wing elevator). Recordings were made from all four muscles in each animal, but some traces were deleted if the muscles were inactive in flight (one could confirm accurate electrode placement because the muscles are bifunctional and used in walking). In the adult pattern, the wing depressors and elevators alternate in each segment, and the hindwings lead the forewings; broken lines (B) indicate this phase lag. A: Adult. B: Last instar. C: Second to last instar. D: Second to last instar. F: Third to last instar. G: Fourth to last instar. E: This nymph, while also a second to last instar, will become an adult one molt earlier than the other animals of the figure, i.e., after the ninth molt rather than the tenth (see text). The figures illustrates the gradual emergence of the adult motor pattern during nymphal development; key features are appearance of short bursts in the hindwing depressors, generation of sustained bursts, recruitment of antagonists and of the forewing motor units, development of the adult burst frequency (further discussion in text). In the second to last instar, it appears that some small units of the hindwing elevators are active, e.g., D, second trace. Time calibration: 5 msec per small division.

steadily acquired. These included (1) increased numbers of cycles of rhythmic discharge, (2) increased numbers of impulses per unit within a cycle, (3) recruitment of additional units which participate in the adult pattern, and (4) achievement of correct relative timing. When new units were recruited, they always fired with the correct rhythm, but might show improper coordination. Thus coordination was secondarily acquired. By the last instar, the neural circuit underlying flight, like that for singing (Fig. 1), was assembled and could generate a fully coordinated pattern. However, the frequency of the pattern remains much slower in nymphs than in adults. Unlike singing, input from wing-movement-sensitive receptors is essential for maintenance of normal flight frequency in crickets (Möss, 1971) and other orthopterans, (Wilson, 1968b), and it seems likely that the low frequency of the nymphal pattern reflects the absence of this input. These data support the hypothesis that the neural circuit underlying flight is progressively assembled during the latter half of postembryonic development, that the changes seen reflect the construction of effective synapses between elements of the circuit, that rhythmic driving, which may reflect connections between serially arranged elements in the circuit, is achieved before correct relative timing, which may require synapses between elements of the same level, and that this process is essentially completed before the animal reaches adulthood. There is no evidence that neurons themselves are being constructed; connection could be either established or greatly strengthened between previously elaborated arborizations.

The development of flight pattern has also been studied in the desert locust, *Schistocerca gregaria,* and the migratory locust, *Locusta migratoria* (Kutsch, 1971, 1974), and in the Australian plague locust, *C. terminifera* (Altman and Tyrer, 1974; Altman, 1975). In locusts, the main sequence of events appears similar to that seen in crickets, but the timing is somewhat shifted with respect to the life cycle so that the pattern is not fully coordinated until just after the final molt. An interesting aspect of this arrangement is that the shift from uncoordinated to coordinated firing of antagonists appears capable of appearing in a remarkably short time, perhaps even less than 24 hr (Altman, 1975). Continued observation of adults reveals that the flight frequency continues to increase for several weeks after the final molt (Kutsch, 1974; Altman, 1975). Although this is still a small sample of behavior patterns and species, it does indicate that functional assembly of neural networks used by adults, but not by nymphs, is postponed until the last part of postembryonic development.

What is the status of the component neurons of these and other circuits earlier in development? In the brains of house crickets (Panov, 1966), katydids (*Tettigonia viridissima:* Panov, 1960), cockroaches (*Periplaneta americana:* Neder, 1959), and milkweed bugs (*Oncopeltus:* Johansson, 1957), neural proliferation continues during postembryonic development. However, in the thoracic and abdominal ganglia, where motor patterning circuits for flight and singing are located, dividing neuroblasts are not found after hatching in house crickets (Gymer and Edwards, 1967; Panov, 1966) and locusts (Sbrenna, 1971), and neuron counts remain stable throughout the postembryonic period. Therefore, it is unlikely that additional neurons are produced after embryogenesis. However, several significant phenomena do occur. First, there is an enormous absolute growth of the nervous system. Gymer and Edwards (1967), for example, measured a fortyfold increase in the volume of the terminal ganglion of the house cricket. Second, there is substantial relative growth of the neuropil, containing the neuron arborizations, with respect to the cortex, containing the cell bodies. In *Schistocerca,* this increase in neuropil volume is about double that of the cortex (Sbrenna, 1971). If the cortical growth is taken as an index of expansion commensurate with the increase in body size, the additional growth of neuropil suggests true differentiation in this area. Finally, there is a great proliferation of glial cells, e.g., from 1000 to 17,000 in the terminal ganglion of the house cricket (Gymer and Edwards, 1967). This may indicate insulating or "hardening" of recently established connections. Therefore, although all the nerve cell bodies are present hatching, it seems possible that there is continuing differentiation of processes during the early postembryonic period.

To test some of these possibilities directly, we have begun examining the structure of identified neurons at different stages of development. The first neuron selected is the contralateral, dorsal longitudinal MN of the metathoracic ganglion. This neuron seems a good candidate for delayed development because the muscle it innervates, the dorsal longitudinal muscle, is used primarily in flight, an exclusively adult behavior. Unlike other flight muscles, the dorsal longitudinal is not bifunctional for walking and undergoes a massive hypertrophy during the last instar in preparation for flight activity. The neuron soma is unusual in that it is located contralaterally to the innervated muscle (Fig. 4). Arising from it is a long neurite which gives off only a few simple ipsilateral branches, but which, after crossing the midline, forms an extensive contralateral arborization and then sends an axon through the first nerve. The arborization is characterized by a long posterior branch, a medium-length anterior–ventral branch, and very numerous side branches. With the cobalt chloride diffusion technique, the structure of this neuron has been observed in the adult and in instars down to the fifth. Even at this stage, the major branches of the arborization can be identified (Fig. 4B), although fewer secondary branches can be seen. Thus, at least by halfway through postembryonic development, the main structure of the neuron has been elaborated. This is consistent with data from ganglion measurements and cell counts suggesting that if postembryonic structural differentiation does occur, the most dramatic part is completed by the halfway point, and is also compatible with the notion that functional maturation seen in the last part of the postembryonic period reflects development of functional connections between neurons which are already present.

Developmental Mechanisms

The work reviewed above is primarily descriptive. It indicates what happens during the course of development, but not why. Experiments are also being conducted which are designed to expose the lines of information flow or causal

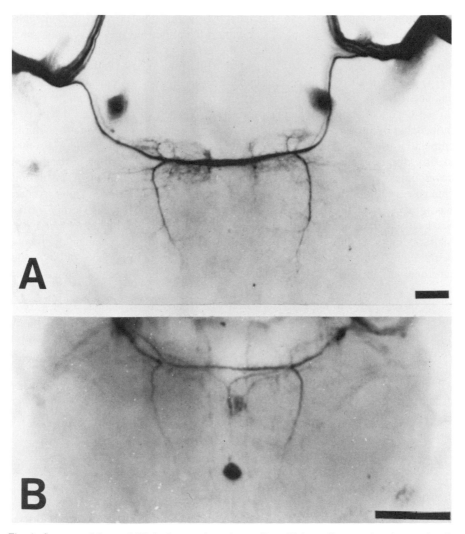

Fig. 4. Structure of the two MNs in the metathoracic ganglion of *Teleogryllus oceanicus* innervating the metathoracic dorsal longitudinal muscle. Cells were filled with cobalt chloride by axonal diffusion. A: Somata, arborizations, and axons of the two neurons in an adult cricket. After exiting the ganglion through the first nerve, the axons join with four other axons from the mesothoracic ganglion. B: The same two neurons filled in a sixth instar nymph. The major processes are already present (the dorsal unpaired median neuron has also filled). Calibration: 100 μm.

mechanisms operating in these developmental sequences. The strategy of these investigations involves alteration of selected developmental influences early in the postembryonic period, and then examination of the physiological or anatomical consequences in the adult nervous system. Several kinds of early manipulations have been made. Sensory nerves can be severed, resulting in rapid degeneration of the central axon terminals, so that the postsynaptic INs develop without either structural connection or electrical stimulation from their normal presynaptic innervation. In the house cricket, *Acheta,* the effect of this operation on the adult structure (Murphey *et al.,* 1975*b*) and also the physiology (Palka and Edwards, 1974) of identified INs has been examined. Both the morphological and functional characteristics of the cells are altered by this early deprivation, although the neurons do not degenerate and do continue to operate. These experiments are discussed in more detail by Edwards (this volume). Another possibility is to provide supranormal stimulation to INs whose stimulus selectivity is known. Murphey and Matsumoto (1976; Murphey, this volume) have employed this technique during postembryonic development of house cricket INs and again have found that there are definite changes in the physiological response properties of the neurons in adults. Another possibility is to employ genetic manipulations as a tool for investigation of interactions early in development. In this case, the strategy is to find mutants which have a malfunction that interrupts the flow of information during development of a known neural pathway. By examining the pathway in adults, the importance of the deleted information can be evaluated. In our laboratory, we have been pursuing this approach.

Crickets prove to be reasonably well suited for genetic studies. They have an acceptably short generation time of about 6 weeks when raised at 35°C, and have a high fecundity of 1000–2000 nymphs per female. Since their development is gradual, many adult behavior patterns such as jumping, walking, and foraging are also employed by nymphs immediately after hatching. The convenience of being able to search for behavioral mutants after only the 10-day embryonic period makes it possible to screen large numbers of individuals. Adult males and females were exposed to 0.025 M ethylmethane sulfonate, a powerful chemical mutagen, in drinking water. After mating, eggs were collected for several days, and the resulting nymphs were screened for behavioral abnormalities 1 day after hatching. Putative mutants were raised to adulthood and were mated in a series of Mendelian test crosses to establish the genetic nature of their malfunction. Confirmed mutants were then bred in isolated lines so their nervous systems could be examined under various experimental regimes (Bentley, 1975).

Our search was concentrated on mutations affecting jumping because this behavior is immediately displayed by hatchling nymphs and because it can be initiated by an intensively studied neural pathway (for recent review, see Edwards and Palka, 1974). The main components of the pathway are (1) cercal sensilla, (2) sensory neurons whose axons enter the terminal ganglion, (3) identified INs which are excited by the sensory neurons and send axons to the thoracic ganglia, and (4) MNs and INs of the thoracic ganglia which mediate the jump motor program. To screen for mutants, nymphs were scanned with an air-puff machine followed by a suction tube leading to a disposal flask. Individuals showing the normal response were thus vacuumed up, leaving only the nonjumpers. In processing about 40,000 nymphs, several nonjumpers were detected.

The most interesting nonjumper proved to be a single-gene sex-linked recessive. Examination of the nymphs revealed that at hatching they are lacking all of the sensilla which form the first element of the jump pathway (Fig. 5). These sensilla are long, articulated hairs called "filiform hairs." There are normally 52 on each cercus of a first instar, with the number increasing to about 650 in an adult. Two classes are found, transversely vibrating and longitudinally vibrating (Palka and Schubiger, 1975), and both are sensitive to sound pulses or other air displacements (Edwards and Palka, 1974). In the mutants, these sensilla remained absent throughout the developmental period.

Two additional types of hair sensilla are found on the cerci. Clavate hairs are gravity receptors (Bischof, 1975) and increase from one in first instars to about 100 in adults. Appressed hairs are multiply innervated, probable chemoreceptors (Schmidt and Gnatzy, 1972) which increase from 14 to about 3000. These sensilla types are present in the mutant in normal numbers at hatching, and increase in normal fashion during the postembryonic period. However, after the molt to adulthood, first all the clavate hairs and then all the appressed hairs are lost over the course of a few weeks. This selective loss provides an opportunity to examine independently the role of each class of sensilla. For analysis of the jump pathway, however, young adults which had been deprived only of filiform hair input were used.

What is the consequence of this deprivation on neurons of the jump pathway? Sensory cells were examined by sectioning the cerci through the empty hair sockets of mutants at different stages of development. Examination of the sections in the light microscope revealed that a receptor was present under every socket, and that the cells had a normal-appearing soma, a short, truncated dendrite terminating under the socket, and a normal-appearing axon which entered the cercal nerve (Fig. 6). Transmission electron microscopic sections of the first instar cercal nerve showed that the correct number of axons, within normal variation, were present, that the axons had normal ultrastructure, and that the size distribution of the axons did not show any missing classes. In young adults, electrical stimulation of the cercal nerve does drive the INs which are normally stimulated by the filiform hair receptors, indicating that at least some axons make functional synapses (this test is not conclusive since it is not known whether other sensory cells also drive these INs). Since the filiform sensory neurons are present, have normal somatic and axonal structure, and send axons into the terminal ganglion, it seems likely that they do make potentially functional synapses with the INs. Therefore, at the current level of analysis, the loss of the sensilla has no effects on the sensory neurons except for the unavoidable abnormality of dendrite structure (loss of appressed hairs from adult cerci is accompanied by degeneration of about 90% of the axons in the cercal nerve; since this number corresponds to the number of appressed hair neurons, and since these neurons have dendrites extending to the tip of the hair shaft, it appears that this class of cell is dependent on integrity of the sensilla) (Fig. 7).

Although the structure of the filiform sensory neurons is essentially unchanged by the mutation, impulse traffic should, of course, be greatly affected. The cells should be totally unresponsive to their normal stimuli, and the number of action potentials per unit time arriving at central terminals should be correspondingly reduced. What is the effect of this deprivation on the interneurons?

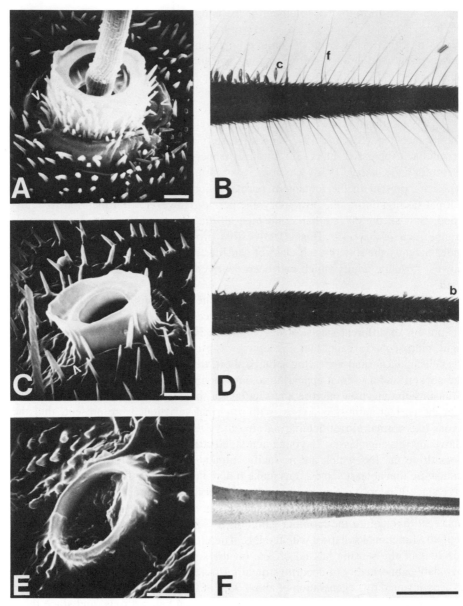

Fig. 5. Effects of *fl* mutation on sensilla. A: Wild-type filiform hair and socket, first instar cercus (arrows indicate campaniform sensilla). B: Wild-type adult cercus (*f*, filiform hair; *c*, clavate hair). C: Empty filiform socket of *fl* mutant, first instar (arrows indicate campaniform sensilla). D: Young *fl* mutant adult cercus (*a*, appressed hairs). Filiform and clavate hairs (save one) are missing (the long hairs at the base of the cercus are a special subclass of appressed hairs). E: Empty appressed hair socket of mature adult *fl* mutant. F: Mature adult *fl* mutant cercus. All hairs are missing. Calibrations: A,C,E, 5 μm; B,D,F, 1 mm.

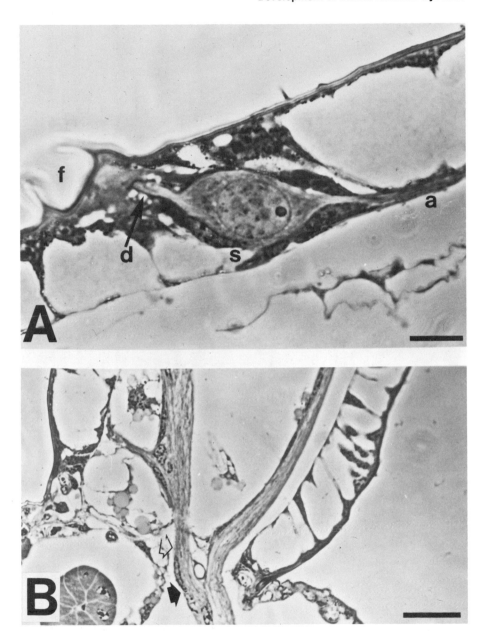

Fig. 6. Sensory neurons in the filiform mutant. A: Sensory cell underlying an empty hair socket (*f*) in a first instar nymph. The truncated dendrite (*d*), soma (*s*), and axon (*a*) joining the cercal nerve can be seen. B: Cross-section of the cercus showing a cercal nerve of normal size and configuration (arrow; electron microscopic sections at this point confirm normal number of axons). Calibration: A, 10μm; B, 25μm.

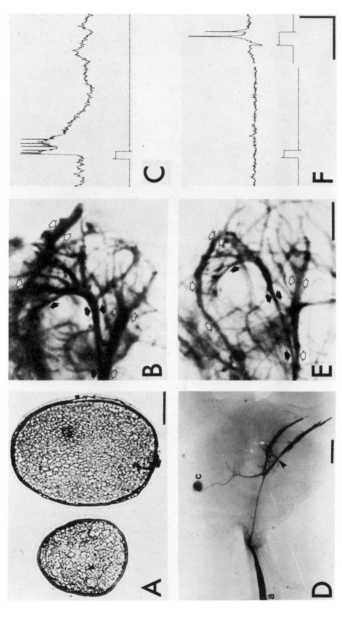

Fig. 7. Effects of *fl* mutation on neurons. A: Cross-sections of *fl* mutant (left) and wild-type (right) mature adult cercal nerves. Most axons in the mutant are degenerating, but some clusters (arrow) remain healthy. B: Major dendrites of the MGI (open arrows indicate two branches) and LGI (solid arrows) filled with cobalt dye, showing normal size in the wild type (ventrolateral aspect). C: Intracellular recording in dendrites of the MGI showing response to a standardized air puff in the wild type. D: Adult *fl* mutant MGI filled with cobalt through the recording electrode (dorsal aspect; *c*, cell body; *a*, axon; arrow, third-order dendrite where measurements were taken: see text). E: Major dendrites of the MGI (open arrows) and LGI (solid arrows) in *fl* mutant showing reduced diameter; the age, magnification, and aspect are the same as in B. F: Intracellular recording in dendrites of the MGI in an *fl* mutant, showing the absence of response to a standardized air-puff stimulus (lower trace indicates delivery of stimulus). The inset (right) shows an action potential in the MGI elicited by current injection (lower trace) through a microelectrode. Calibrations: A,B,E, 50 μm; D, 100 μm; C,F, 100 msec; 20 mV, 2×10^{-9} A.

The two most carefully studied interneurons are the medial giant interneuron (MGI) and the lateral giant interneuron (LGI) (Murphey, 1973; Edwards and Palka, 1974). Both are driven by transversely vibrating filiform hairs (Palka and Schubiger, 1975). We have concentrated on MGI, whose configuration is shown in Fig. 7D. From the soma, a thin neurite runs to a small ipsilateral arborization. This, in turn, is connected across the midline to a massive and exceedingly complex contralateral arborization which receives the input from filiform hairs of the contralateral cercus. From this primary arborization, the large axon arises and enters the contralateral connective. In wild-type and mutant adults, these neurons were filled selectively with cobalt chloride either through microelectrodes or by axonal diffusion. Details of the primary arborizations of MGI and LGI in mutant and wild-type individuals are illustrated in Fig. 7. Compared to the wild types, INs in the mutants appear to have a withered or atrophied arborization. Direct measurements of homologous processes confirm that the mutant fibers have substantially smaller diameters than their wild-type counterparts (Bentley, 1975). However, all of the characteristic branches are present, at least down to the third order. Fewer fourth-order branches are seen, but if they were smaller they could be below the level of resolution of the light microscope. There may be another difference which is more difficult to quantify: in normal INs, the branches seem more robust, differentiated, and clearly separated from each other than in the mutants. In any case, there does appear to be a definite effect of the absence of the sensilla on the growth of these INs. Although the consequences of complete cercal removal (Murphey *et al.*, 1975*b*) could be attributed either to the lack of physical connection of the IN to the presynaptic cell or to the absence of impulse traffic, in the case of the mutants it seems likely that the sensory neurons do form synapses on the INs. Therefore, the missing factor may be associated with the loss of electrical activity and its consequences. It is interesting that in other systems where deprivation effects are being studied, such as mammalian visual cortical neurons (Blakemore, 1974), electrical activity rather than connectivity also seems to be the key factor. Whatever the factor involved, these experiments do indicate that one of the mechanisms active in achieving normal neuron morphology during development is serial information flow through pathways.

Is normal physiology similarly dependent on information flow? This is rather difficult to test in practice because in the mutants, of course, there is no response to driving by normal stimuli. This problem can be circumvented by arranging a quasi-competitive situation. Normally, MGI is very effectively driven by input to the primary arborization contralateral to the soma and driven weakly, if at all, through the secondary, ipsilateral arborization (Edwards and Palka, 1974). If the primary arborization were innervated by "silent" synapses from mutant sensory neurons and the secondary arborization were excited by active synapses from wild-type neurons, would the input–output physiology of the IN be altered so that the pathway through the secondary arborization became more effective? This situation was arranged by transplanting cerci in the early postembryonic period (Edwards and Sahota, 1968). Within 1 day of hatching, the cerci were removed from wild-type and mutant nymphs; during the first instar, cercal regeneration began so that a small cercal bud appeared after the first molt. On the day after this molt, cercal buds were exchanged between wild-type and mutant nymphs so that each nymph would have one wild-type and one mutant cercus (Fig. 8). Transplanation of regenerating buds rather than whole cerci greatly increased the percentage of successful operations. The transplants continued to grow during the remainder of postembryonic development, and reached approximately normal size before adulthood. During this period, sensory neurons arise *de novo* from cercal epidermal mother cells and send axons into the CNS. Since the sensory neurons do not normally cross the midline (Palka and Edwards, 1974), arborizations on one side of the host ganglion would receive input from mutant tissue, while the other side was innervated by normal tissue. Therefore, of the pair of MGIs in the host, the IN with its soma ipsilateral to the mutant cercus would have "silent" synapses on its secondary, ineffective arborization and active synapses on its primary arborization. The contralateral homologue, however, would have active synapses on its secondary arborization but "silent" synapses on its primary arborization. The physiological consequences of this situation were examined in young adults.

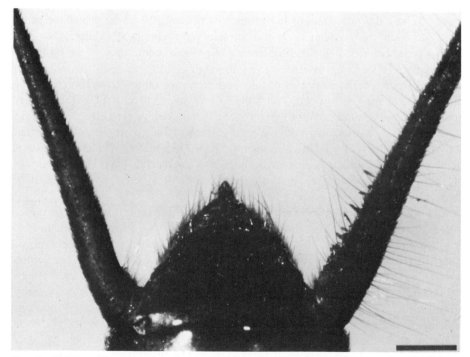

Fig. 8. Abdomen of an adult mutant cricket *(Teleogryllus oceanicus)* with a transplanted wild-type cercus on the (animal's) left side. The cercus was transplanted immediately after the first molt and has grown to normal size. Note the lack of filiform hairs on the mutant cercus. Calibration: 1 mm.

An essential control in evaluating the physiological results was a demonstration that, in the mutants, synapses really are silent with respect to normal stimulation. This was tested by recording intracellularly from the primary dendritic arborization of MGI in mutant and wild-type individuals while delivering a standardized air-puff stimulus to the cercus (neurons were subsequently identified by cobalt injection). In wild types, the stimulus was rapidly followed by a 20–30 mV excitatory synaptic potential which initiated a burst of several impulses in the axons. In INs of mutants, however, the stimulus produced no depolarization and no impulses (Fig. 7), confirming that the pathway from stimulus to CNS is effectively lesioned. The IN itself remains physiologically viable and can generate normal impulses in response to current injected through the microelectrode.

When the transplant animals reached adulthood, we recorded extracellularly, simultaneously from both MGI axons while applying air-puff stimuli to the cerci or stimulating the cercal nerve directly with electrical pulses (Fig. 9). Stimulation of the wild-type cercus resulted in a burst of impulses in the MGI axon ipsilateral to the cercus, confirming that the cell is driven in its normal fashion through its primary arborization. At the same time, one or two impulses regularly appeared in the contralateral MGI axon, suggesting that it is driven through its secondary arborization. When the same stimulus was delivered to the mutant cercus, there was no

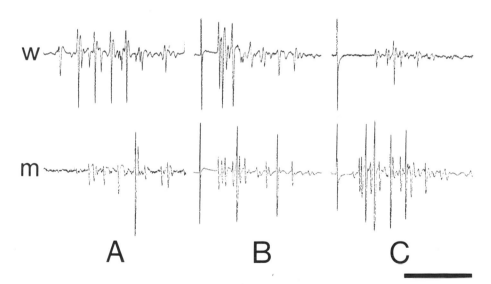

Fig. 9. Simultaneous extracellular recordings of MGI/LGI impulses in the connectives of a cricket with one mutant and one wild-type cercus. Upper traces (w) are recorded from the connective ipsilateral to the wild-type cercus; lower traces (m) are from the connective ipsilateral to the mutant cercus. A: An air-puff stimulation of the wild-type cercus elicits a burst of impulses ipsilateral to the cercus but also drives the contralateral axons. B: After removal of the cerci, electrical stimulation of the wild-type cercal nerve again drives axons in both connectives. C: Electrical stimulation of the mutant cercal nerve drives the ipsilateral giant axons, showing that cercal/IN synapses are functional, and fails to drive the contralateral axons. Calibration: 10 msec.

response in either MGI axon, as would be expected if the pathway is effectively interrupted. To control for spread of the stimulus, the cerci were then removed and the wild-type cercal nerve was stimulated electrically. Again, a burst of impulses was generated in the ipsilateral MGI axon and anomalous impulses were produced in the contralateral MGI axon. The latter response indicates that the MGI, with its primary arborization on the mutant side, is being effectively driven through wild-type sensory neurons synapsing on the secondary arborization. Stimulation of the mutant cercal nerve initiated a normal burst of impulses in the ipsilateral MGI, but only occasional impulses in the contralateral axon. Thus there seems to be a clear difference in the response properties of the two MGIs to stimulation of their primary or secondary arborizations, depending on whether or not they have received normal input during postembryonic development.

Palka and Edwards (1974) have also studied the physiological consequences of asymmetrical input during development in the house cricket. In their experiment, crickets were raised during the postembryonic period with one cercus removed. This resulted in a very marked enhancement of the response of the contralateral MGI. The physiological abnormality was much less pronounced when both cerci were removed and therefore appeared to result from the imbalance rather than from the deprivation. Under these circumstances, whether the signal for imbalance is due to connectivity or to electrical activity cannot be determined. With the mutants, it again appears likely that electrical activity is the key factor. In either case, attainment of normal physiological as well as morphological characteristics seems dependent on the flow of information along neural pathways.

The genetic experiments (Bentley, 1975), the degeneration experiments (Palka and Edwards, 1974; Murphey et al., 1975b), and the supranormal stimulation experiments (Murphey and Matsumoto, 1976) all indicate that one of the mechanisms involved in guiding physiological and structural differenciation of insect neurons is the establishment of expected neural connections, whatever the monitors of this situation may be. Although this mechanism has a definite role to play, it is equally clear that it is not the only or even the dominant factor in differentiation of the system. In fact, the degree of indifference of the neuron to this sort of manipulation is quite impressive. In marked contrast to the effects on mammalian neurons of similar interference, the insect cells do not degenerate, lose branches, slough off connections, or greatly distort their physiological properties. It is not really helpful to conclude that these experiments demonstrate once again how "genetically programmed" insect neurons are. A genetic program, no matter how dominant, must still be read out through developmental mechanisms. What these experiments do demonstrate is that we have not yet altered many of the really key mechanisms guiding differentiation of these systems.

Perhaps this is because many or even most of the critical developmental signals and interactions are occurring during the embryonic period. The embryonic development of orthopteran nervous systems has been the subject of numerous descriptions (Roonwall, 1937; Kanellis, 1952; Malzacher, 1968; Scholl, 1969; for a recent review, see Anderson, 1972). The thoracic and abdominal ganglion chain arises from a contiguous belt of three to five enlarged epidermal cells (neuroblasts) lying on either side of the ventral midline. The neuroblasts are highly organized into a two-dimensional array of rows and columns which forms the ground plan of each ganglion (Carlson, 1961). In *L. migratoria*, Bate (1976*a*) has shown that this plan consists of seven rows of four to ten cells plus a single midline cell which comprise a fixed number of neuroblasts for each ganglion. At least some of these neuroblasts are individually identifiable. The neuroblasts undergo a series of divisions which generate a stack of neurons above them. The clusters of neurons separate only secondarily to form ganglia (Fig. 10A). Viewed in this context, the problems of recognition encountered by growing neurons may be somewhat different from those usually contemplated. Traditionally, the emphasis has been on pathfinding to distant targets, whereas most central neurons in segmental ganglia may be within growth cone "touching" distance early in development. Where long distances must be traversed, as in the establishment of connections between peripheral sensory neurons and central neurons, different mechanisms may be employed. In various insect appendages, Bate (1976*b*), Sanes and Hildebrand (1975), and Edwards (this volume) have identified "pioneer" neurons which appear to fulfill this role. In the naive microcosm of the developing embryo, conditions may be radically different from those found later, so that, for example, regeneration may be a less faithful model of mechanisms involved in embryogenesis than has been supposed.

In *T. oceanicus,* we have begun looking at the establishment of connections between central ganglia during embryogenesis. Figure 10B is a transmission electron micrograph illustrating the connectives between the terminal and ninth abdominal ganglia in a 90% developed embryo. Several interesting conclusions can be drawn: there are 1381 axon profiles in the right connective and 1362 in the left. These axons are primarily interneuronal, since most of the sensory neurons have yet to develop, and may represent a substantial percentage of the total IN complement. Figure-eight or "hourglass" profiles suggestive of growing axon tips are seen, so that at this stage the connective may be in the process of active differentiation. The axons of at least three and probably four individually identified INs are recognizable, as well as another identified cluster of four profiles (Mendenhall and Murphey, 1974). These neurons can be identified by their size and location, and it is noteworthy that even at this early stage the axons assume a specific position in the connective profile which they will maintain throughout the developmental period despite the enormous growth that occurs. In regard to these INs at least, the whole embryonic connective is an exquisite miniature which could fit easily inside an adult MGI axon, or in any of several other large axons. A similar situation is found in crayfish connectives at the hatching stage (Kennedy, 1974). These observations confirm the notion that connections between many neurons are established, however tentatively, very early in development. Much of the later growth, especially for interganglionic interactions, must reflect the strengthening or elaboration of these connections rather than the establishment of new ones. Therefore, it seems unavoidable that to penetrate the mechanisms guiding differentiation of these systems it will be necessary to deal with this initial recognition between "naive" neurons.

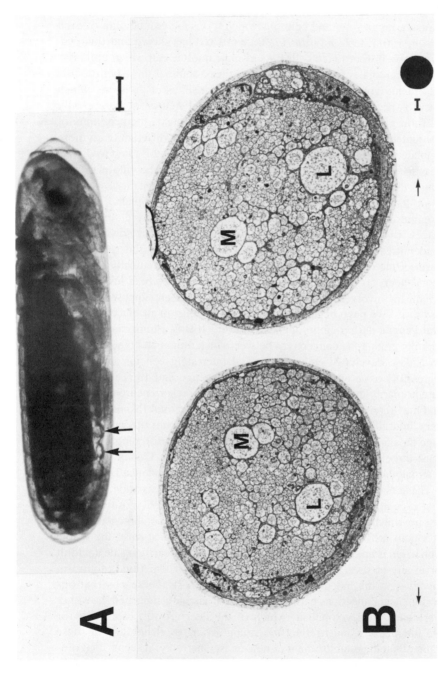

Fig. 10. A: Photograph of a living, 90% developed cricket embryo (*Teleogryllus oceanicus*) after the egg has been cleared with sodium hyposulfite. Arrows indicate abdominal ganglia in early stages of separation. B: Electron micrograph of the connective of a 90% developed cricket embryo just anterior to the terminal abdominal ganglion. 1381 axon profiles are found in the right connective and 1362 in the left. MGI (M) and LGI (L) and other identified INs can be distinguished. Arrows indicate the diameter of MGI in an adult. If the micrographs are taken to represent an adult connective, the black dot shows the relative size of the embryonic connective. Calibration: A, 200 μm; B, 1 μm.

Summary

What can be said, finally, about the development of these systems? First, our information is very sketchy; we still have only a few glimpses of how a few neurons in a few pathways are developing. From these glimpses, a highly hypothetical schema of the development of neural pathways and circuits can be erected. The nervous system arises from a strictly specified ground plan of neuroblasts; in the ventral ganglia, all of the neuron somata arise during the embryonic period. During this period, many specific connections between cells are made which are later elaborated. The conditions under which connections are made in the embryo are very different from those during regeneration in older animals, and the mechanisms for establishing primary connectivity may be correspondingly different from those in reestablishment. In the early postembryonic period, rapid growth of the nervous system continues, especially in neuropil. This may reflect continuing construction of intraganglionic arborizations. By half way through the postembryonic period, the main arborization framework even of neurons used primarily in adult life is present. During the second part of postembryonic development, neural circuits underlying adult behavior patterns are functionally assembled. This assembly is graded and progressively involves more neurons and a more complete representation of the adult pattern. It is completed during the last larval instar or just after the adult molt. This period may reflect the construction of effective synaptic junctions between arborizations. External sources of information appear to play only a minor role in specification of the properties of pattern-generating neural circuits; genetically transmitted information is the critical factor. Mechanisms involved in the readout of genetic information remain largely obscure. Several kinds of experiments show that one element of this process is serial interaction between neurons within a pathway. Such interactions are only a part of the story, however, and many additional factors remain undiscovered.

How can these factors be exposed? Ideally, one tries to restrict the possibilities to a limited number of hypotheses, and then to devise experiments which will distinguish decisively between them. Success in erecting such hypotheses depends on a firm body of background information. It is worth pointing out how little of this basic information is available, yet how much of it appears within the capabilities of current technology. For example, we do not know how many neurons, exactly, are involved, how much variation occurs in the number of neurons, when the various parts of the neurons differentiate, when and in what order connections are made in the circuits, when physiological features mature, and, especially, what the spatial and temporal boundary conditions are like. When this information does become available, sound hypotheses about mechanisms and how to test them should be abundant.

ACKNOWLEDGMENTS

I thank the Alexander von Humboldt Foundation for a U.S. Senior Scientist award. Additional support was provided by DFG Ku 506/74, NIH NS 9074-07, and NSF BMS75-03450. The electron micrographs were done by Ms. A. Raymond.

28

Pathfinding by Arthropod Sensory Nerves

John S. Edwards

Introduction

In the cellular sociology of Metazoa, no cells discriminate in their associations more than neurons. It is true that positional individuality may be highly developed in other epithelia such as insect epidermis or in embryonic primordia, but neurons are unique in expressing specificity in contacts often much removed from near neighbors. Just how specific and how flexible neuronal relations must be and how they are achieved have long been focal questions in neurobiology. And yet, despite contributions of well-known experimental studies exploring development and regeneration in the lower vertebrate visual system by Sperry, Gaze, Jacobson, and others (Hunt and Jacobson, 1974), there is much contention about the significance of such things as chemical specificity, the nature of gradients in space and time, and trial and error and functional validation as causal mechanisms. One reason why so many elegant experiments should lead to such an impasse is the level of resolution that can be achieved in measuring specificity. Most studies are concerned with populations rather than individual neurons. Other approaches to neural development include experimental modification of the developmental milieu of such well-known cell types as are found in the cerebellum (Sidman, 1974). But with the exception of the Mauthner neuron (Hibbard, 1965), single-cell interactions have been beyond the resolution of vertebrate studies.

The promise of arthropods as material for developmental neurobiology is that they offer a variety of uniquely identifiable cells in fixed positions. The great value of such cells for electrophysiological and integrative studies, as shown by Wiersma's pioneering studies and his demonstration that parts of the crustacean central nervous system could be physically and electrophysiologically dissected (Wiersma, 1958), was an important factor conducive to a climate which encouraged attack on the development of the nervous system at a cell-by-cell level.

Developmental neurobiology of arthropods is in its infancy. There is a long history of descriptive study, but, with a few isolated exceptions, experimental studies did not get under way until the past decade. The most telling experiments are yet to be done, but available techniques and background information bring us to the brink of two-cell developmental neurobiology.

John S. Edwards • Department of Zoology, University of Washington, Seattle, Washington 98105.

The objective of this chapter is to discuss some recent studies on developmental neurobiology of arthropods, most of which depend on the use of identifiable giant interneurons (INs) in the house cricket *Acheta domesticus*. Some other relevant studies of neuronal pathfinding involving arthropods will also be discussed.

Of the two approaches to the mechanisms involved in the development of neuronal connections—embryology and regeneration—the latter has held center stage for some years. The formal advantage of sensory regeneration is that the central target is a completed system, assumed to be reasonably fixed and to manifest the essential structure built during embryogenesis. Regenerating sensory axons arise in the integument and find their way to, and set up functional synapses with, central neurons. But it must be remembered that the relevance of regeneration to embryogenesis in the nervous system is not clear, for it cannot be assumed that the mechanisms of selective connection are the same in the two processes, and both must be studied in their own right, with the objective of distinguishing common elements. Another caution is in order here: The Taoist classic of Lao Tzu begins with the assertion, "The path [Tao] that can be told is not the true Tao." Without enveloping neuroembryology in mysticism, the statement can be applied in a literal sense: there are surely a number of factors and mechanisms involved in determining the path a neuron takes to establish functional contact, and any experimental intervention intended to isolate or analyze one of these will affect others also. Reduction of possibilities to two contrasting mechanisms, e.g., flexible gradients vs. rigid chemical specificity, may help to focus argument, even to sharpen experiments, but it probably does not adequately acknowledge the real situation.

Establishing Central Connections

Leaving speculation aside for now, the questions raised above will be narrowed to our own recent studies. How does a sensory axon of an insect, the product of an erstwhile epidermal cell, establish contact with the appropriate central cells? We have explored the cerci of the house cricket *A. domesticus*, which regenerate vigorously and have a relatively simple population of sensilla that project to a small number of giant INs (Edwards and Palka, 1974; Palka and Edwards, 1974). The problem of reestablishing central connections when cerci regenerate during postembryonic development may be divided into two phases: (1) the path to the ganglion, and (2) the formation of specific connections within the ganglion.

The Path to the Center

Functional cerci are regenerated by cricket larvae even when they have been repeatedly deprived of regenerates through successive instars of the nine that lead to the adult insect. The proximal parts of the cercal sensory axons degenerate rapidly after the cercus is amputated, carrying with it the peripheral cell bodies. When the cercus is removed at hatching, and subsequent attempts to form a regenerate are thwarted for several instars, the initially minute stump of cercal sensory nerve sheath regresses and is lost, so that the deprived ganglion no longer bears any mark of the entry site of the cercal sensory nerve. Afferent fibers from cercal sensory neurons which arise *de novo* from integumental cells are nonetheless able to cross the intervening space from cercus to ganglion, enter it, and make functional connections with the giant INs (Palka and Edwards, 1974). The prolonged delay between amputation and regrowth effectively eliminates the possibility that some "homing signal" emanates from the deprived ganglion to guide the growing axon through the forest of muscle strands, tracheal trunks, gonad, and fat body that lies between the base of the cercus and ganglion. It must be borne in mind that the basic architectures of the arthropod and vertebrate are very different. Whereas the regenerating vertebrate nerve traverses clefts and passages between closely investing tissue (Hughes, 1968), the arthropod nerve must traverse an open hemocoel space from integument to central structure. It may be that the lack of normal cercal sensory fibers elicits some sort of signal from the deficient neuropil, but it seems unlikely that this could be a simple chemical gradient, with the ganglion a source of material that is released to the hemolymph that bathes the tissues, because the ganglion is immersed in hemolymph, which in this region flows away from the ventral region of the body to the dorsal pericardial sinus, and a simple diffusion gradient between the ganglion and the site of the cercal regeneration could scarcely be set up under these conditions.

One experimental approach to the question of pathfinding or beacon homing by regenerating axons is to substitute an implanted ganglion for the native ganglion. This proves to be impracticable, for the terminal abdominal ganglion is involved in regulatory functions, e.g., the neurosecretory control of water balance, and the cricket does not survive for long without it. Severing the connectives immediately anterior to the ganglion also disrupts regulatory functions of the terminal ganglion and is lethal within too short a time scale to make significant regeneration experiments. An alternative approach is to implant a supernumerary ganglion adjacent to the base of the cercus so that incoming fibers might be faced with a choice between the implant and the native ganglion (McLean and Edwards, 1976). Implanted ganglia are promptly supplied with tracheae and they establish neural connections with neighboring tissue. They grow in volume, and despite their isolation from the remainder of the CNS the neurons and glia appear viable. The operation deprives the giant INs of most of their axoplasm, and their arborizations are, of course, deprived of their peripheral input. The final connections made by regenerate cercal neurons in such cases are always with the native ganglion (Fig. 1), even when a cercus has been absent up to the time when regeneration is permitted. We cannot say whether or not some fibers entered implanted ganglia and failed to persist, for we examined only the final neuroanatomy in the adult. We can, however, assert that the final pathway ignored a more closely placed implanted ganglion in favor of the native ganglion. Regenerating sensory nerves recognize the intact nervous system in preference to "correct" termination sites in an implant.

A small number of sensory fibers terminated in the implant ganglion only when the cercal motor nerve was severed at the time of implantation (Fig. 2a). This nerve serves the extrinsic musculature at the base of the cercus, and is separate throughout

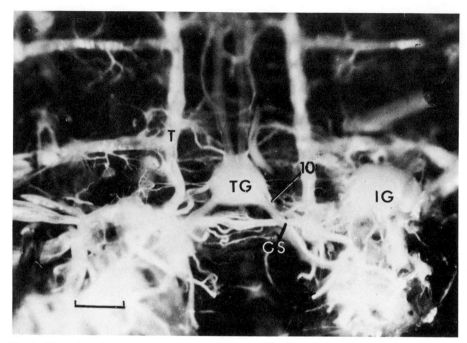

Fig. 1. Dissection of adult *Acheta domesticus* abdomen showing native terminal ganglion (TG) receiving a regenerate cercal sensory nerve (CS) entering the ganglion at lower right and bypassing an implanted terminal ganglion (IG) which has become tracheated and established diffuse neural connections with the host. T, Ventral longitudinal tracheal trunk; 10, cercal motor nerve. From McLean and Edwards (1976).

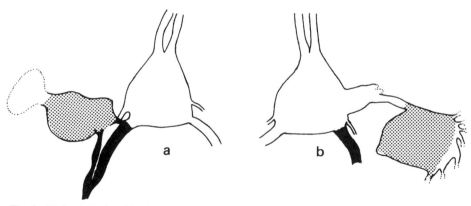

Fig. 2. Native (white) and implanted (shaded) ganglia showing paths of regenerate cercal sensory nerves (black). Dotted margins indicate diffuse tissue connections between implant ganglion and host tissue. (a) Cercal motor nerve cut at time of cercal amputation and ganglion implantation. Most cercal sensory fibers enter the mature ganglion. Of those that enter the implanted ganglion, most pass through to enter the native ganglion, but some terminate in the implant in the region of giant fiber arborizations. (b) Native terminal ganglion wounded at time of implantation. Neural connections are established between implant and native ganglion, but all regenerate cercal sensory fibers bypass the implant.

its entire length from the sensory nerve. It may be that regenerate sensory neurons depend on a source of information carried by the cercal motor nerve, although it cannot be a simple case of contact guidance because the resultant adult cercal sensory nerve is invariably separate from the motor nerve. Recent studies of the fine neuroanatomy of the terminal segments (Hustert and Edwards, unpublished) have revealed fine branches of noncercal nerves in the region of the cercus base, and they also could be involved in a guidance mechanism, but, again, the final regenerate nerve may vary from animal to animal, and in some cases is double or multiple instead of single, suggesting that successful "pioneers" on more than one route have been followed by subsequent axons.

Extensive wounding of the native ganglion on one side gives rise to complex interconnections with an implanted terminal ganglion, but in this case, also, the path of the regenerating cercal sensory nerve leads directly to the native ganglion, bypassing the implant (Fig. 2b). Further, when a terminal ganglion is implanted in a thoracic segment close to the base of a leg, and a cercal regenerate is transplanted to the leg stump, the regenerating cercal sensory nerve bypasses the implanted ganglion, to make connections with the thoracic ganglion of that segment.

We believe that the experiments with implanted ganglia rule out the possibility that a wound or deprivation signal is a major factor in the pathfinding by regenerate neurons. If that had been the case, more nerves should have shown evidence that their initial path led to, through, or nearby the implant.

In a very instructive series of experiments, also following the classical paradigm of developmental neurobiology—surgical intervention in orientation and spatial relationships—Palka and Schubiger (1975) have altered the periphery. Rotating and exchanging grafted cerci, they explored the implication of theories concerning gradients and positional information as it relates to specific connectivity in the CNS. A decisive factor in the success of these experiments is the presence of two sets of markers on the elongate, conical cerci. One of these is a patch of club-shaped sensilla unique to the mesial base of the cercus; the other is the orientation of filiform mechanoreceptor sensilla which oscillate in response to air movement. Transversely oscillating (T) hairs are situated middorsally and midventrally. Longitudinally oscillating (L) hairs clothe the lateral walls. T hairs provide the major input to two of the largest of the giant fibers, the median and lateral giant INs. Thus there are superficial markers on the cercus, and specific responses of identifiable cells centrally. Palka and Schubiger (1975) manipulated the orientation of the L and T hairs by amputating and skilfully grafting cerci at their bases, either on their original base or after exchanging left for right. They showed clearly that axial rotation of the T hairs on the cercus, or transfer from left to right, does not alter the pattern of their central connections; i.e., the "personality" of the cells is not altered by changing their position in the bodily coordinates. They preserve their central addresses and laterality; they do not distinguish left and right. These results, together with transplant experiments to other segments of the abdomen (Schubiger and Palka, unpublished) or the thorax (Edwards and Sahota, 1967), clearly indicate that the ingrowing sensory fibers are able to locate appropriate central connections in the neuropil when faced with a journey through strange territory.

Pathfinding within the Neuropil

The central termination of the afferent fibers brings us to a second aspect of pathfinding: determining the mechanisms for locating precise sites for synaptic contact. What are the rules by which the sensory fibers, having found entry to the neuropil, find their synaptic sites? For arthropods, the crucial events are to be sought in the late embryonic development when the first functional fibers enter the neuropil. At this time, in the cricket, just a day or so before completing embryonic development, about 100 fibers enter the open-textured neuropil and make their synaptic contacts in the arborizations of the giant fibers. During the nine subsequent instars, the population of cercal sensilla increases from about 100 to about 10,000 in successive waves, associated with the differentiation of new sensilla, in each instar. We have followed the methodology of the now-classic studies on vertebrates in examining postembryonic regeneration of sensory connections. These results have been reviewed elsewhere (Edwards and Palka, 1976), and it will suffice here to mention some of the basic findings (Palka and Edwards, 1974).

1. Sensory fibers can reestablish connections, as precisely as can be measured, after prolonged postembryonic deprivation of cerci.
2. Laterality is strictly observed in the normal animal, but errors are introduced by asymmetrical development, when some normally ipsilateral fibers cross the midline to make contact with the contralateral counterpart of their normal termination site.
3. Disoriented sensilla produced by rotating or exchanging cerci left for right project nonetheless to their proper INs.
4. Minor inputs to the giant INs are enhanced in their effectiveness when cercal input is removed.

As in the ganglion implantation studies discussed above, these observations are based on the final disposition of sensory neurons; they tell us nothing of the behavior of the cells during their passage through the neuropil. We have not yet examined such fibers; it is no easy task, for there are few neurons from the early regenerates. Later, more numerous neurons enter the ganglion as the regenerate grows, but these can follow the pioneers. If the behavior of the developing visual system of *Daphnia* (LoPresti *et al.*, 1973) is a guide to events in the regenerating cercus, we might expect only the pioneer fibers to have a growth cone. LoPresti *et al.* (1973) found that lead axons from retinal ganglion cells that grow into the developing lamina have growth cones, but associated axons that follow them do not. The growth cone is presumably involved in recognizing and contacting appropriate cells.

Pathfinding in the Embryo

Postembryonic regeneration of the cerci of crickets reveals many instructive facets of the behavior of neurons, but it has an inherent limitation as an approach to mechanisms involved in establishing selective connections in the nervous system, for it serves to renew connections originally made in the embryo. The original contacts may, perhaps, leave a lasting label on cells; the embryonic processes of selective contact may give rise to labels or signposts for subsequent neurons. We must turn to the embryo for insight into the process of cell recognition and specificity in generating functional circuits. Recent observations on embryonic development and metamorphosis, which can be thought of as a belated manifestation of embryonic development, give new insights into the process of pathfinding by neurons.

In order to appreciate the chronology of sensory development in the cricket, it will be necessary to review some milestones in their embryogenesis. As in all Orthoptera, in the course of development the cricket embryo undergoes two elaborate migrations within the egg. At an early stage, the embryo travels around the posterior pole of the egg and dives deep into the yolk. Anlagen of cerci appear at the posterior tip of the embryo at this stage. A return movement ensues, in which the embryo makes its way quite rapidly back to a peripheral position in the egg, and the original spatial relations are restored. During this process, the head turns through 180°, and the body follows, the embryonic cerci eventually coming to occupy a posterior position in the egg (Fig. 3a). They finally tuck under the body, and the tips grow forward between the legs and antennae (Fig. 3b). Throughout this period, the embryonic epidermis is ensheathed by a delicate, chitin-free, expansible membrane, and no sensory structures are present other than anlagen of the developing com-

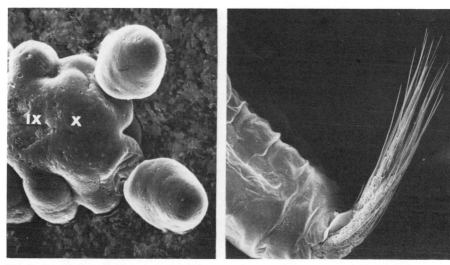

Fig. 3. Scanning micrographs of embryonic cerci of *Acheta domesticus*. (a) Late katatrepsis at the time of differentiation of pioneer fibers. The lower cercus is displaced slightly to reveal a lumen providing access to terminal ganglion situated below the epidermis of terminal segments 9 and 10 (IX, X). (b) Shortly before hatching. The embryonic cuticle has been peeled away to the base of the cerci to reveal first instar cuticle with sensillar hairs that will come to lie perpendicular to the cercal cuticle when it is expanded following the molt.

pound eye. As soon as the embryo has reached its final external form following dorsal closure, an embryonic chitinous cuticle is secreted. This is the cuticle of the so-called embryonic instar, a cuticle that will be sloughed off after hatching. Unlike all subsequent integuments, this cuticle lacks sensilla and subsequently serves as a protective sheath (Fig. 3b) during hatching and burrowing of the so-called vermiform larva to the surface; then it is promptly sloughed off to reveal the first instar cuticle. Sections of the embryonic cercus, at a stage when it is no more than 100μm in length, reveal a small group of profiles that are unmistakably axons in terms of profile and cytoplasmic appearance (Fig. 4). They differ distinctly from the more densely staining, lobate, extensions of epidermal cells. This small population of axons runs the length of the cercus and arises from cells at the tip. The axons have not yet been traced centrally, but it seems most probable that they project to the embryonic ganglion and that they do so before any of the giant INs are visibly differentiated. As the cercus elongates, these fibers are drawn out, a process recognized by Harrison (1935), who coined the term "passive stretching."

At a late stage in development, the embryo molts within the egg and forms a further cuticle, that of the first instar. This cuticle differs from the previous one in having the sensilla of the first instar. In the final days of embryogenesis, the axons from these sensilla make their way to the terminal ganglion by following the path laid down earlier by the pioneer axons of the embryonic instar, to complete the first instar complement of about 100 axons. The pioneer connections between cerci and the terminal ganglion are established by cells which produce axons but which are not associated with functional sensilla. The axons of the subsequent instar, the first by standard reckoning. follow pioneers laid down when the distance to the center is no more than 100μm. These fibers enter a rudimentary neuropil.

The events described above closely resemble events in the embryonic antennae and legs of *Locusta* described by Bate (1976b), who presents provocative evidence for projections from the periphery being the first contacts made by neurons, and suggests that the centripetal, presensory fibers rather than (MNs) lay down the foundation of contact between center and periphery and provide the paths for subsequent fibers.

The pattern of events in the embryo is strikingly comparable to that in the formation of the lepidopteran antenna. The adult antenna develops from a small nest of cells, the antennal imaginal disk, which lies at the base of the minute larval antenna but is not a functional part of it. Sanes and Hildebrand (1975) have described the development of sensilla in the adult antenna. They found a group of axons in the pupal antenna which they traced to a nest of cells at the apex of the antenna. As in the embryonic cricket described above, the pupal instar lacks sensilla on the appendages, and this small population of pupal neurons is not associated with functional sensilla. They elongate as the antenna extends rapidly during metamorphosis, and so form a pathway through the elongate appendage along which the axons of the developing adult sensilla can find their way to the antennal center. In effect, a bridge was set up between periphery and center when they were situated in close proximity. Thus both embryos and imaginal disks, which are in effect delayed

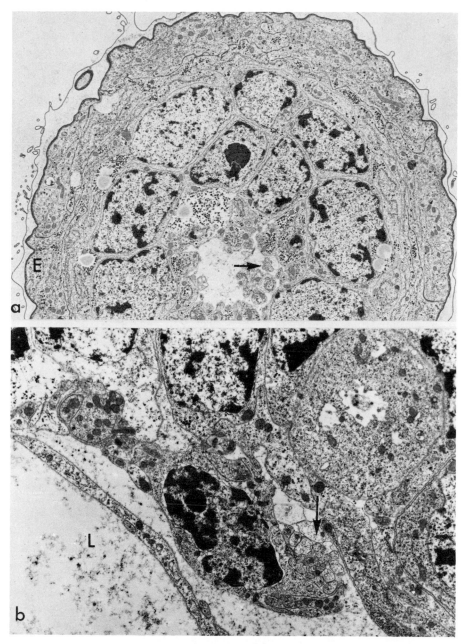

Fig. 4. Electron micrographs of embryonic cerci of *Acheta domesticus*. (a) Transverse section of embryonic cercus near tip. Epidermal cells (E) are secreting the cuticle of the embryonic instar, which has no sensilla, shortly after dorsal closure. Within the lumen, a bundle of axonlike profiles (arrow) arising from apical cells are putative pioneer fibers. (b) Detail of embryonic axon bundle (arrow) in lumen (L) of embryonic cercus at a slightly later stage than (a).

embryonic structures, have neural connections that seem to be guides to morphogenesis rather than sensory in function. But at least in some dipteran imaginal disks there are sensilla: Poodry and Schneiderman (1970) found dendrite-like ciliary structures in a leg imaginal disk of *Drosophila,* and van Ruiten and Sprey (1974) describe four apical scolopophore mechanoreceptor cells as well as a seemingly precocious chordotonal organ in leg imaginal disks of third instar *Calliphora erythrocephala* larvae.

We may further pursue the matter of pathfinding by antennal fibers because they are instructive, even though they cannot be said to project to uniquely identifiable central INs but rather project to the compact neuropil of the olfactory center in the deutocerebrum of the brain. The cricket can be induced to regenerate a heteromorphic antenna when the compound eye is ablated (Edwards, 1967), and the supernumerary antenna so formed sends fibers to the deutocerebrum. Their precise terminations within the brain segment that contains the antennal centers were not ascertained, but a parallel is suggested with the finding of Maynard and Cohen (1965) on the projection of the fibers from heteromorphic antennae of *Panulirus.* More recently, Sandeman and Luff (1974), working with the Australian freshwater crayfish *Cherax destructor,* have shown that supernumerary heteromorphic antennules regenerating from severed eyestalks can mediate antennular reflexes. Antennules implanted in an eyestalk also established central connections. In both cases, at least some of the afferent fibers must have located functionally appropriate synaptic sites after traversing an abnormal path for such axons.

A new approach to the question of pathfinding has been taken in an examination of the terminations of sensory axons from an Antennapedia mutant in *Drosophila* in which the normal antenna is replaced by a leg (Stocker *et al.,* 1976). In *Drosophila,* as in *Manduca* discussed above, the adult antenna develops from an imaginal disk, a nest of embryonic cells carried through larval life that differentiate to form the adult structure during metamorphosis. In the Antennapedia mutant, the antennal disk gives rise not to an antenna but to a leg. The observation mentioned above, that cercal sensory nerves can find their correct central terminations on the giant INs even when transplanted far from their normal site, suggests that axons from leg sensilla might find their way to the thoracic centers where they normally terminate. That would be a much longer journey through the brain: down the connectives to the thoracic ganglion, and from there to the rather well-defined areas where leg sensilla normally terminate. But we know that neurons can make long foreign excursions from the recent report of Constantine-Paton and Capranica (1975), who found that when eye anlagen of the embryonic leopard frog were moved to an evacuated ear position the optic fibers entered the hind brain, turned caudally, and continued for some millimeters down the spinal cord. Leg axons of the mutant *Drosophila* appendage should have been able to reach the thorax, and that would have been consistent with a level of specificity found in many transplant experiments. However, they did not. Instead, they behaved very much as if they were antennal fibers. Their terminations, as revealed by degeneration and cobalt-filling methods, were in the olfactory glomeruli. No degenerating fibers were found in an ultrastructural examination of thoracic ganglia in which the homeotic appendage was severed and the material fixed, when any degenerating axons should have been apparent. Perhaps here again prefunctional pioneer fibers from the early antennal anlagen laid down a path to the antennal glomeruli and subsequent fibers followed their path, to make their terminations in the first available region with unoccupied postsynaptic sites.

Metamerism and Specificity

Metameric segmentation of higher Metazoa may be a fundamental factor in specifying development of pathways in the nervous system. Experimental modification of segmental relationships has been a basic method in the study of vertebrate neuroembryology. In these cases, the behavior of neurons is not resolved at the single-cell level, but in arthropods this is possible, and may prove to be their major contribution to ideas about neural specificity. For example, comparison of maps of motor cell bodies in the meso- and metathroacic ganglia of the cockroach *Periplaneta americana* by Young (1969) show that the externally visible segmental homologies extend to the cells of the CNS, and by transplanting limbs from one segment to another Young (1972) has elegantly demonstrated that motor neurons of one segment recognize homologous limb muscles of another with great precision. Perhaps the metameric body plan, with variations on a module, simplifies choice in setting up connections. The sensory neurons of the homeotic mutant appendage in *Drosophila* discussed above send their sensory axons to a brain segment that is appropriate to the appendage, possibly because they follow pioneer fibers that have recognized a segmental specificity *per se*. In the cercal afferent system of the cricket, discussed above, there may be some things to be learned about specificity and segmental homologies. The cercus is an appendage of the eleventh abdominal segment. It projects to a compound ganglion composed of elements from segments 7 through 11, in which it has been suggested (Mendenhall and Murphey, 1974) that the giant INs may be serial homologues. The projection pattern of cercal fibers in the terminal ganglion shows sites throughout the ganglion. In this, they conform to a common pattern shown also by noncercal sensory fibers that enter the terminal ganglion through segmental nerves, some of them terminating in the vicinity of their entry point, others projecting to more anterior segments. The massive input from the large cerci has perhaps "captured" more anterior giant INs in the terminal ganglion, and a detailed examination of the exploration of embryonic neuropil by cercal pioneer fibers may reveal early contacts with a segmental series of central targets in a simpler geometry than the final disposition. That is for the future.

ACKNOWLEDGMENTS

I thank Dr. Margrit Schubiger for her critique of a final draft. Work described in this chapter was supported by NIH Grant NB 07778.

29

Does Experience Play a Role in the Development of Insect Neuronal Circuitry?

Rodney K. Murphey, S. G. Matsumoto, and R. B. Levine

Introduction

Historically, the invertebrate nervous system has been thought of as a machine (Fabre, see Teale, 1949), a machine whose invariant design and function are determined by genetic factors alone and are therefore relatively inflexible. Modern-day invertebrate neurobiologists refer to this aspect of their specimens' nervous systems as "hard-wired" or lacking in plasticity. A major thrust of invertebrate neurobiology has been the elucidation of the "wiring diagrams" of a wide range of nervous systems as a first step toward determining how nervous systems control behavior. As other chapters in this volume demonstrate, this approach to the invertebrate, particularly the arthropod, nervous system has led to insights into the organization of locomotory behaviors in all animals. In general, it has been assumed that the uncontrolled experience of an individual does not affect the wiring diagram of the nervous system in any significant way. This view, that the invertebrate nervous system is relatively inflexible, has received support from experiments which show that "experience" plays no role in the development of motor functioning. For example, rearing crickets in isolation does not affect the development of the songs they sing as adults (Bentley and Hoy, 1974). Similarly, rearing lobsters without swimmerets does not alter the motor program controlling swimmeret beating (Davis, 1973a).

There are, however, numerous behavioral studies which demonstrate that the experience of an individual invertebrate can produce modifications in its behavioral repertoire. Crabs "remember" the position of stripes in the visual field, locust thoracic ganglia "learn" to maintain certain leg positions, digger wasps "recall" the location of their nests, snails home to resting places or food sources, and *Aplysia* remain habituated to tactile stimuli for extended periods. The duration of these effects ranges from seconds to months. This suggests that the patterns of connectivity, or at least the efficacy of certain pathways, can be altered by experience.

We became interested in the question of what role, if any, experience plays in the development of the neuronal connections observed in adult invertebrate nervous

Rodney K. Murphey, S. G. Matsumoto, and R. B. Levine • Department of Biological Sciences, State University of New York, Albany, New York 12222.

systems. In order to study this question, we have begun to examine the effect of use and disuse on the development of invertebrate neural pathways. Disuse has been shown to have a very powerful effect on the organization of the vertebrate visual system (e.g., Wiesel and Hubel, 1963; Hirsch and Spinelli, 1970). These experiments suggest that the nature of synaptic input to visual cortical neurons can be modified by experience. We wondered whether analogous phenomena occurred in invertebrate nervous tissue. In particular, we wanted to know whether a change in patterns of synaptic input could be induced in uniquely identified interneurons (INs) by use or disuse of the afferent pathways which impinge upon them.

The organism we decided to study is the common cricket *Acheta domesticus*. We have examined two large INs in the abdominal nervous system of this organism. These two large INs, known as the medial and lateral giant interneurons (MGI and LGI), receive powerful synaptic influence from mechanoreceptors located on the animal's cerci (Edwards and Palka, 1974) (Fig. 1).

A number of reports suggested that we look for experience-related modification in the nervous system of the cricket. First, Palka and Edwards (1974) reported alterations of the response properties of the MGI and LGI following deafferentation. The observed change suggested that synaptic pathways not directly affected by the deafferentation procedure had been altered. Second, we proceeded to show that the lengths of the dendrites of the INs were altered by the same deafferentation paradigm (Murphey, Mendenhall, Palka, and Edwards, 1975). Third, Bentley (1975) discovered mutant crickets which lack normal sensory input to the INs because the hairs which serve as the mechanical part of the transduction mechanism are absent. The afferent neurons are intact but forever silent. These mutants display alterations in the morphology of MGI which are presumed to be causally related to the diminished afferent input to this IN. The work we present here, combined with the other just cited, suggests that the response properties of cricket giant INs are susceptible to modification during development. Thus there appears to be a fair degree of "plasticity" in this system of neurons, and experience may alter its function. We have examined this aspect of the cricket nervous system (1) by determining the patterns of connections between afferents and INs, (2) by using these pathways intensively and examining the effects of excessive use on the response properties of the INs, and (3) by depriving the INs of normal afferent activity and thereby examining the effect of disuse on the response properties of MGI and LGI.

The Wiring Diagram

The MGI and LGI are activated by low-frequency sounds, and it is this response which will be examined in this chapter. The receptors, which serve as transducers of the auditory stimulus, consist of delicately hinged, filiform hairs located on the cerci (Fig. 1). Each filiform hair is innervated by a single sensory neuron (Edwards and Palka, 1974). The filiform hairs on each cercus can be classified into two major groups: those whose morphology allows them to vibrate

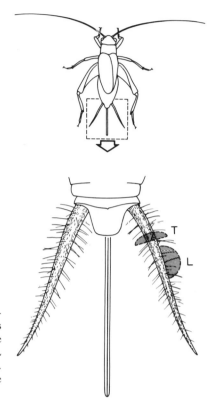

Fig. 1. Gross anatomy of the cercus and associated receptors. The drawing indicates the positions and planes
of movement (shaded) of the filiform hairs on a single
cercus. T hairs are located dorsally and ventrally; L
hairs are found medially and laterally on the cercus.
Note that T hairs on one cercus will vibrate in a plane
nearly parallel to L hairs on the opposite cercus.

freely in a plane transverse to the cercal axis (T hairs), and those constrained to
vibrate in a plane parallel to the longitudinal axis of the cercus (L hairs). Intracellular recordings from sensory cell axons demonstrate that the receptor neuron is
activated when sound causes the hair to vibrate in this preferred plane. Thus each IN
can potentially receive four classes of sensory input from filiform hairs on the left
and right cerci: from right and left T hairs and from right and left L hairs (Fig. 2).

Three different methods have been used to demonstrate the patterns of connectivity between the afferents and the MGI/LGI. First, extracellular recordings from

Fig. 2. Summary diagram of known connections between
afferents and INs in the normal animal. Excitatory connections are indicated by +; inhibitory connections by −. No
suggestions concerning the number of synapses in a pathway
are intended.

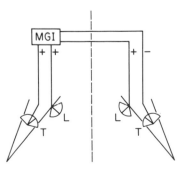

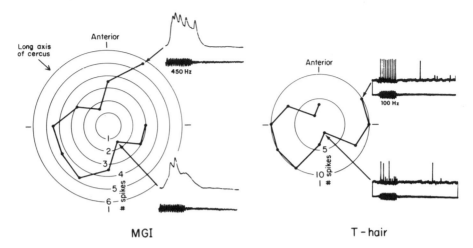

MGI   T – hair

Fig. 3. Directional sensitivity of MGI and of a single T hair. A: The directional sensitivity of MGI as determined intracellularly. Points on the graph are means of four trials. B: The directional sensitivity of a single T hair ipsilateral to MGI as recorded from the afferents' axon. Note the similarity between angles of peak sensitivity of the two elements. The number of spikes elicited by a standard tone is plotted along the radii. The angular position of the speaker is indicated by angle of the appropriate radius. The angular position of the long axis of the cercus is indicated at the left. The insets are sample recordings from MGI and from a single T hair, respectively.

the axons of MGI and LGI have been taken before and after immoblization (covering the hairs with petroleum jelly) of different classes of hairs. The extent of the changes in IN response properties resulting from these procedures is taken as an indication of the strength and nature of the pathway being tested (Palka and Olberg, in preparation). Second, intracellular recording has been employed to determine whether a specific class of hair is capable of exciting or inhibiting MGI. This is accomplished by immobilizing all but one class of hairs and then recording the response of the MGI to standard stimuli. Third, all but a single hair was immobilized and intracellular recordings from MGI revealed psp's correlated with the standard tone pulses (Matsumoto and Murphey, in preparation). A diagrammatic summary of a survey using these methods is provided in Fig. 2. All four possible afferent-to-IN connections are found to exist, and it is the strength and sign of these synaptic inputs which determine the response properties of the MGI and LGI.

The strength and the sign of the afferent inputs to MGI and LGI result in in a directionally sensitive response of these cells to sounds. For example, a polar plot of the tone-evoked responses of MGI shows that it is maximally sensitive to speaker positions which maximally excite ipsilateral* T hairs (Fig. 3). In addition, the intracellular methods referred to above showed directly that stimulating ipsilateral T hairs with tones is the most powerful way to excite MGI and LGI (e.g., Fig. 4A).

*The position of MGI or LGI is always with reference to its axon (i.e., ipsilateral to MGI means ipsilateral to MGI's axon).

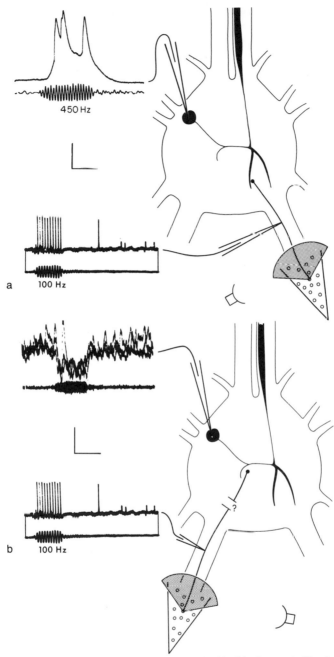

Fig. 4. Diagrammatic summary of the two pathways examined in this chapter. A: The dominant excitatory drive on MGI (and LGI) comes from ipsilateral T hairs. Note that this response in MGI was obtained when only the ipsilateral T hairs were free to move. The figure shows schematically the site of the recordings. The sample records were obtained for the speaker position indicated. Calibration: vertical, 10 mV upper; horizontal, 20 msec upper, 100 msec lower. B: The crossed inhibitory pathway. A speaker in the position indicated activates the T hairs contralateral to the MGI, and an inhibitory potential is recorded from MGI. Calibration: vertical, 1 mV horizontal, 100 msec.

This synaptic pathway determines the overall directional sensitivity of MGI, while other pathways merely modulate the response.

T hairs contralateral to MGI and LGI inhibit these INs. This can be demonstrated directly by recording intracellularly from MGI. Specifically, if a speaker is positioned to stimulate contralateral T hairs, and all ipsilateral hairs are immobilized, a clear inhibitory potential is obtained (Fig. 4B). It is not known whether this pathway is mono- or polysynaptic. The crossed inhibitory pathway accentuates the directional sensitivity of MGI and LGI.

We have obtained apparent alterations in the two T hair pathways and will concentrate on them for the remainder of the chapter. Both pathways can be examined using extracellular recording method; the remainder of the results presented here have been obtained using these methods (see Murphey and Matsumoto, 1976, for details of interpreting the extracellular records).

Effects of Altered Input

Excess Use

The first successful method of environmental modification we tried was powerful long-term excitation of the receptors. We knew that MGI and LGI responded well to low-frequency tones, and therefore we chose to stimulate specimens with short (250 msec), low-frequency (500 Hz) tone pulses repeated twice per second throughout the period of postembryonic development. This procedure had no detectable effect on the response of MGI and LGI to single tone pulses. However, when the dynamic properties of the excitatory pathways were examined, a difference was detected. The LGI and MGI of treated specimens were more resistant to a habituating stimulus than control specimens (Fig. 5). In other words, the treated specimens habituated more slowly than controls (Murphey and Matsumoto, 1976). While the differences were small, the results were encouraging. We are therefore examining the response decrement itself in an attempt to determine the mechanism by which this change comes about.

Disuse

We decided for a number of reasons to examine the effects disuse had on the response properties of MGI and LGI. First, we thought we might obtain results complementary to those just described. Second, it is easier to produce disuse unilaterally, and such a procedure would provide within-animal controls. Third, disuse has been very successfully employed in other nervous systems. We chose to use two different methods for restricting sensory input: (1) we employed short periods of unilateral deafferentation produced by amputating one cercus early in postembryonic life; (2) sensory *deprivation* was produced by blocking the movement of mechanoreceptive hairs. Somewhat to our surprise, these two very different

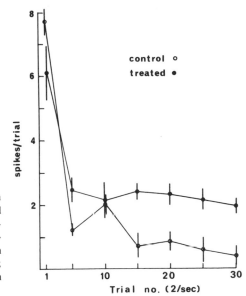

Fig. 5. Response decrement of MGI and LGI in treated and control specimens. The treated specimens were exposed to 250-msec tones repeated twice per second for the entire postembryonic period of development. Each point on the control curve is the mean of 15 specimens; bars indicate standard error of the mean. From Murphey and Matsumoto (1976).

paradigms gave similar results. In both experiments, the major excitatory pathway (ipsilateral T hair to MGI/LGI) was much weaker to treated neurons than to controls, and the crossed inhibitory pathway (contralateral T hair to MGI/LGI) exerted a stronger effect on treated neurons than upon control ones.

Deafferentation

Unilateral cercectomy during the first two to four instars followed by regeneration of the cercus leads to depressed MGI/LGI responses in the INs ipsilateral to the regenerate cercus. We have assessed the pattern and quality of synaptic connections with MGI and LGI by determining their directional sensitivity characteristics. Polar plots of the directional sensitivities of right and left INs of control specimens are always very symmetrical (Fig. 6A) (see also Edwards and Palka, 1974). By contrast, deafferentation early in life (first three instars) followed by regeneration of the cercus leads to quite different results (Fig. 7A): the reinnervated neurons are less responsive at all target positions than are homologous neurons of the control side.

This depression of the excitatory input to MGI and LGI could be due to any number of mechanisms. Some of the more obvious are (1) incomplete regeneration of the periphery, (2) an increase in the efficacy of the crossed inhibitory pathway from the control cercus, or (3) incomplete reinnervation of MGI and LGI by the regenerating sensory neurons. To differentiate among these possibilities, we examined the regenerate cercus itself and found its external morphology to be closely similar to that of the control cercus: the lengths of the two cerci as well as the

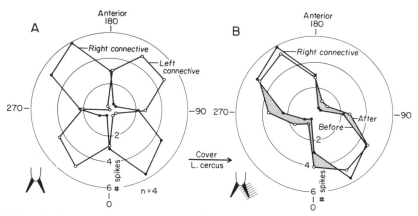

Fig. 6. Directional sensitivity of control INs. A: Polar plot of the sensitivity of the right and left giant INs as a function of the position of the sound source. B: Directional sensitivity of the right INs before and after inactivation of the left cercal afferents by covering them with petroleum jelly. The polar plot becomes more symmetrical due to a decrease in crossed inhibition (stippled area) and a decrease in crossed excitation in the region of maximum sensitivity. From Murphey *et al.* (1976).

number of filiform hairs on them were identical (Murphey *et al.*, 1976). Thus the periphery appears to have regenerated completely.

We then examined the crossed inhibitory pathway from the contralateral cercus to the treated MGI and LGI and found that it was more effective than normal (Murphey *et al.*, 1976). This was demonstrated by determining directional sensitivities of the reinnervated MGI and LGI and then covering the control cercus with petroleum jelly and redetermining directional sensitivity. In control specimens, this operation causes an expansion of the directional sensitivity curves in the region of low sensitivity (Fig. 6B). In other words, the MGI and LGI are released from an inhibitory influence (there is also a depression of response at the peak sensitivity, but this will not be discussed here). In treated specimens, the MGI and LGI ipsilateral to the regenerate cercus exhibited a much stronger release from inhibition than did the control specimens which were tested similarly. As few as 14 days (first and second instars) after deafferentation, begun at hatching, this effect was observable. Enhancement of the inhibitory pathway did not occur when a similar period of deafferentation was initiated 7 days after hatching (i.e., in the second instar). These results suggest that the balance between excitatory and inhibitory inputs to MGI and LGI can be altered irrevocably by short periods of deprivation early in life. It also suggests that there is a critical period for this effect early in life (the first 14 days of postembryonic development).

In summary, the crossed inhibitory pathway is strengthened by the deafferentation–reinnervation paradigm we have employed. One possibility is that a balance normally exists between the excitatory and the inhibitory pathways and that deafferentation by removal of ipsilateral afferents shifts this balance in favor of the inhibitory pathway. Whatever mechanism is postulated to explain this effect must

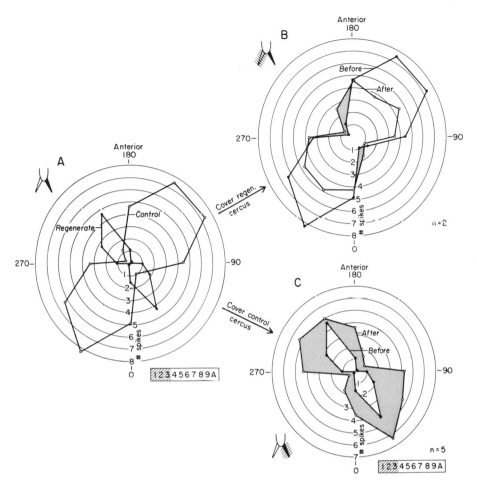

Fig. 7. Effects of deafferentation on response properties of giant INs. A: Directional sensitivity of normally innervated neurons (control) and INs reinnervated after three instars (19 days) of deprivation (regenerate). B: Directional sensitivity of the control neurons before and after inactivating the afferents on the regenerate cercus by covering them with petroleum jelly. C: Directional sensitivity of the reinnervated neurons before and after inactivation of the afferents on the control cercus by covering them with petroleum jelly. Note the enhanced cross inhibition (stippled area) on the reinnervated INs (C). From Murphey *et al.* (1976).

account for the existence of the sensitive period observed and for the permanence of the increased efficacy of the inhibitory pathway (once the balance is altered, ingrowth of new afferents as the specimen grows does not lead to normalization of the response).

Furthermore, the excitatory pathway appears to be weakened because removal of the inhibitory pathway does not lead to normal levels of sensitivity. This change in the excitatory pathway could be due to (1) incomplete reinnervation of the giant

INs by regenerating cercal afferents, (2) a change in the synaptic efficacy of the reinnervating afferents, or (3) strengthening of unknown inhibitory pathways from afferent to giant INs.

Immobilization of Filiform Hairs

Decreased afferent activity can be produced by blocking the movement of filiform hairs during postembryonic development. The filiform hairs on one cercus are immobilized by placing a thin layer of petroleum jelly or cleansing cream (Clinque) on one cercus immediately after hatching and again after each molt through the seventh instar. The immobilization lasts the duration of the instar and the hairs become free to move again only after shedding of the old hairs and cuticle during a molt. Thus the immobilization can be reversed at any point in the life cycle by merely allowing a molt to occur and leaving the hairs free to move. Since additional receptors are added to the cercus at each instar, the treatment may be affecting the original and the more recently acquired receptors differentially.

There is no evidence for sensory cell degeneration following this treatment. Examination of the cercal nerve electron microscopically after brief and prolonged periods of deprivation showed no evidence of degeneration. The cercal nerve of the treated side appeared normal in all respects.

Polar plots of the directional sensitivity of control and treated MGI and LGI were very similar to those obtained for the deafferentation paradigm. The responsiveness of the LGI and MGI of the treated side was again reduced (Fig. 8).

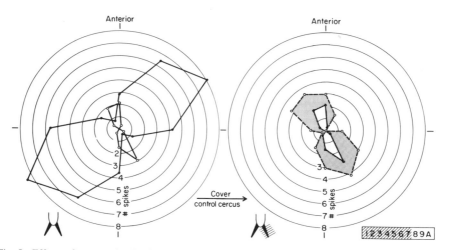

Fig. 8. Effects of sensory deprivation on the response properties of giant INs. A: Directional sensitivity of control neurons (●) and deprived neurons (○). Deprivation was produced by immobilizing the cercal hairs for the first seven instars (inset). B: Response of the deprived neurons before and after covering of the control cercus with petroleum jelly. The stippled area indicates the release from inhibition. One specimen represented.

However, in this case there can be no artifacts due to surgery, deafferentation, or the regeneration process. We can conclude that the excitatory pathway has been altered by disuse (Matsumoto and Murphey, 1977).

This effect could be due to (1) modification of the properties of the transducing sensory cell, (2) changes in the synapse between sensory cell and MGI/LGI, (3) more complex modification of the wiring diagrams, or (4) some combination of the above.

We have obtained some support for point (3) by examining the crossed inhibitory pathway in these specimens (Fig. 6). As in the deafferented preparations, this pathway was enhanced. Thus the relative contributions of excitation and inhibition to MGI and LGI responses are altered by this experimental paradigm. Inhibition was again more predominant in treated than in control neurons. However, the enhanced inhibitory pathway did not account entirely for the lowered responsiveness of MGI and LGI since covering of the control cercus, thereby removing the crossed inhibitory pathway, led to a higher but still subnormal level of sensitivity. Thus other changes must have come about as a result of the deprivation regime.

The list of possibilities by which deprivation-induced changes could come about is the same for all nervous systems. We will continue to test the possibilities in this arthropod nervous system. By elucidating the mechanism for changes in the arthropod nervous system, we hope to provide evidence for the mechanisms by which changes induced by deprivation occur in other nervous systems.

Conclusion

We began by attempting to alter the neural pathways in an insect nervous system through excess use. Utilizing this procedure, we had only modest success in altering the response properties of the giant INs. However, when we deprived these neurons of normal sensory input, we obtained very large effects. In retrospect, we should have guessed that this would be the case. Most of the positive results in altering developing vertebrate nervous systems have been obtained when sensory input or neural activity was restricted. It may be that neural pathways in general are capable of developing maximum signaling ability if provided even modest sensory input. This could account for the difficulty in obtaining "better" responses by excess use as well as the ease with which the nervous system can be altered by deprivation.

In summary, we have examined an invertebrate nervous system and found that certain sensory pathways can be altered by varying the levels of stimulation which these pathways receive during development. Thus the characteristic properties of the adult arthropod nervous system may not be accounted for by genetic factors alone. Rather, they may depend on normal nervous activity during development. How do these results fit with other evidence showing that the arthropod nervous system is relatively inflexible during development? Clearly the arthropod nervous system is to a large extent "hard-wired"; this seems to be especially true for the motor side of the nervous system. It may be that neural programs for locomotion are at the extreme end of the ''inflexibility'' continuum, while sensory systems are more sensitive to use and disuse for normal development or maintenance.

ACKNOWLEDGMENTS

This work was supported by NIH Research Grant 1 RO1 NS10825-01A1 from NINDS and NSF Research Grant BNS 75-2354.

30

Trophic Interactions of Crustacean Neurons

George D. Bittner

Why Study Trophic Interactions in Invertebrates?

Most of the research discussed in this volume elucidates the neuronal basis of behavior with emphasis on the bioelectric properties and synaptic interactions of crustacean or insect neurons. However, invertebrate neurons (and vertebrate neurons) are also involved in another set of functionally important interactions which are not directly involved with the neuronal control of behavior on a second-to-second basis but which alter behavior on a long-term basis by altering the metabolic state of neurons or effector organs; that is, the various parts of a neuron (axon, dendrites, terminal regions, etc.) interact trophically with each other and with adjacent glial, presynaptic, and postsynaptic elements (Guth, 1968, 1969; Bittner, 1973a).

The relatively larger size and smaller number of neurons in crustaceans and other invertebrates have often made them desirable for studying basic neuronal bioelectrical properties such as axonal conduction and synaptic transmission. These characteristics can also be advantageous for studies of trophic interactions. For example, a researcher who looks for changes in a uniquely identifiable cell with a specific lesion has an easier task than one who looks for changes among vast numbers of essentially indistinguishable cells, all of which may not have received the same lesion or treatment. In addition to their large size, some crustacean neurons have other properties which make them advantageous for studying trophic interactions. For example, the long-term survival of severed crustacean motor axons makes it easier to distinguish between muscular atrophy due to lack of neuronal activity and atrophy due to lack of neuronal trophic substances (Bittner, 1973a,b; Boone and Bittner, 1974). The long-term survival of severed motor and medial giant axons in crayfish also enables one to study trophic interactions among axons, glia, and pre- or postsynaptic cells in a preparation in which one is almost certainly examining the transfer of substances important to the survival of the severed axons (Bittner et al., 1974; Bittner and Nitzberg, 1975; Bittner and Mann, 1976; Meyer and Bittner, 1977a,b).

Data on the general nature and cellular mechanisms of bioelectric phenomena in invertebrate neurons would have had much less impact if such phenomena had

George D. Bittner • Department of Zoology, University of Texas, Austin, Texas 78712.

been found to be very different in different organisms. However, throughout the entire animal kingdom, it appears that there has been a rather conservative evolution of basic neuronal properties such as the mechanisms for axonal conduction of spikes and synaptic transmission by release of transmitter substances or electrotonic gap junctions. Reasoning along these same lines, it seems likely to me that there has also been a conservative evolution of many basic cellular mechanisms which provide for trophic interactions in neurons. Hence not only will data on the nature and cellular mechanisms of trophic phenomena be technically easier to obtain using invertebrate preparations, but also the results obtained will apply to most neurons in other organisms. If this reasoning is valid, then current data from crayfish showing that intact and severed lateral giant axons normally exchange proteins and possibly other substances at sites of electronic contact (Meyer, 1973; Bittner *et al.*, 1974; Hermann *et al.*, 1975; Meyer and Bittner, 1977*a,b*) imply that a significant amount of inter- cellular exchange of high molecular weight proteins or other trophic substances may occur at electronic junctions in many organisms. In fact, the possibility for in- creased trophic interactions rather than an increased spread of electrical activity may be the primary reason for the formation of weak electrotonic synapses which loosely couple many invertebrate (Wiens and Gerstein, 1975) and vertebrate (Bennett, 1972) neurons. Similarly, the exchange of substances between crayfish motor axons or medial giant axons and surrounding tissues following axonotomy may well prove to be an extreme example of a general phenomenon observable to a lesser degree in most vertebrate and invertebrate tissues.

In this chapter, I would like to discuss my present view of the nature of trophic interactions in the peripheral and central nervous systems of crayfish. In addition to presenting data relating to these interactions at the cellular level, I will attempt to indicate how these phenomena are adaptively important to the entire organism.

Survival of Sensory and Motor Axons in Singly Cut Limb Nerves

The classical studies of Ramon y Cajal showed that severed distal* stumps of vertebrate nerve axons morphologically degenerate within 3–7 days after lesioning. The distal stumps of crustacean peripheral sensory axons which innervate tactile hairs also undergo morphological and physiological degeneration within 5–14 days (Bittner, 1973*a*; Nordlander and Singer, 1973). However, the distal stumps of

---

*In referring to singly or doubly cut nerve axons, the axonal segment connected to its original cell body will be called the "proximal segment," whereas the axonal segment separated from its cell body but connected to its postsynaptic structures will be called the "distal segment." In doubly cut nerve axons, that segment disconnected from both its cell body and all pre- or postsynaptic structures will be termed an "isolated segment." The terms "central" and "peripheral" or "anterior" and "posterior" will be used only in reference to the relationship of an axonal segment to the central nervous system (CNS). These distinctions are very important in arthropods; for example, the *peripheral* portion of a singly cut limb nerve contains the *distal* segments of motor axons whose cell bodies are located in ganglia of the ventral nerve cord and the *proximal* segments of sensory axons whose cell bodies are located just beneath the exoskeleton. Similarly, the *anterior* portion of a severed abdominal connective contains the *proximal* segments of the medial giant axons and the *distal* segments of the (septate) lateral giant axons.

motor axons innervating muscles in the peripheral limbs of crayfish and other crustaceans often remain physiologically active and morphologically intact for 100–250 days after being severed from their cell bodies (Hoy et al., 1967; Nordlander and Singer, 1972; Atwood et al., 1973; Bittner, 1973a; Bittner and Johnson, 1974; Kennedy and Bittner, 1974).

The peripheral nerve trunk entering the most proximal segment of the cheliped or walking legs of crayfish contains many tens of thousands of nerve axons (Sutherland and Nummermacher, 1968), of which about 25 are motor axons (Bittner, unpublished). Motor axons usually have larger diameters (15–60 μm) than sensory axons (0.1–20 μm), are clustered in characteristic groupings (Fig. 1A), and are surrounded by three to ten layers of glial cytoplasmic processes interposed between extracellular layers of collagen fibrils (Fig. 1B,F). Sensory axons are usually surrounded by one or two layers of glial cytoplasm and collagen fibrils (Fig. 1B,C).

Within 7 days after lesioning, the glial layer surrounding the distal segments of singly cut sensory axons may hypertrophy slightly. By 14 days, the distal segments of most sensory axons have completely lysed. Remnants of sensory axons are often found in the cytoplasm of glial cells which show many signs of active phagocytosis of degenerating sensory axons (Bittner, 1973a; Nordlander and Singer, 1973). These morphological data are in general agreement with physiological data showing that severed sensory axons are unable to conduct action potentials within 5–10 days after lesioning (Bittner and Johnson, 1974) and with biochemical data showing that sensory axons in lobsters lose their ability to synthesize acetylcholine (Barker et al., 1972) within 14 days after lesioning.

Morphological studies show that singly cut motor axons undergo relatively few ultrastructural changes for many months after lesioning (Nordlander and Singer, 1972; Bittner, 1973a; Kennedy and Bittner, 1974). However, the surrounding glial cells often undergo hypertrophy and hyperplasia resulting in an increase in the number and thickness of the sheathing layers (Fig. 1E,F). Our present data indicate that this glial reaction is detectable within 24–48 hr around those portions of the proximal and distal stumps of severed motor axons that are within a few millimeters of the lesion site. Within 15–30 days, the glial reaction is usually noticeable for 10–20 mm distal to the lesion site. At longer time periods, the glial reaction is often noticeable over the entire length of the severed distal stump. The glial reaction is particularly visible in the adaxonal layer (Nordlander and Singer, 1972) (Fig. 1E).

Singly cut motor axons release detectable amounts of neurotransmitter at each nerve impulse when the distal stumps are chronically stimulated at 20–50 Hz for 1–5 hr each day over a 30–60 day period (Bittner, 1973a, and personal observations). However, these opener terminals release reduced amounts of neurotransmitter 7–10 days after lesioning. With further passage of time, severed terminals tend to release fewer and fewer transmitter quanta than normal at 1 Hz or 10 Hz stimulation, although it is possible to evoke the release of a few quanta for 100–350 days after lesioning (Hoy et al., 1967; Bittner and Johnson, 1974; Velez and Bittner, personal observations).

The data presented in the preceeding paragraphs contradict the hypothesis that the perikaryon is *the* trophic center for all nerve axons. Rather, the data suggest that

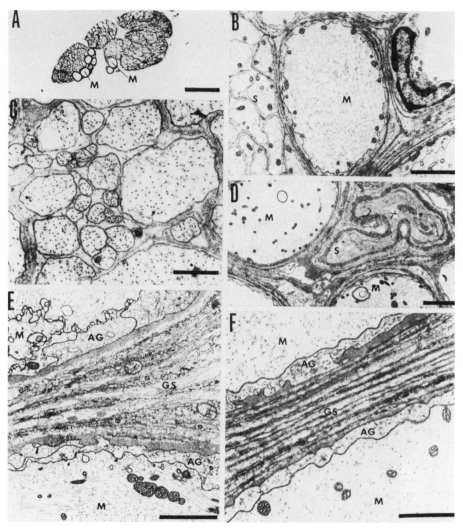

Fig. 1. Motor and sensory axons taken from normal (A,B), isolated (C,D), or singly cut (E,F) nerve trunks in the peripheral limbs of the crayfish *Procambarus clarkii*. A: Cross-section of a normal crayfish peripheral nerve in the carpodite segment showing eight motor (M) axons and many sensory axons. Calibration line: $100\,\mu$m. B: Ultramicrograph of motor (M) and sensory (S) nerve axons in an unoperated peripheral nerve. An adaxonal layer of glial cytoplasm completely surrounds all motor axons. Calibration line: 4 μm. C: Ultramicrograph of sensory axons 1 week after transplantation of a peripheral nerve segment. The adaxonal layer of glial cytoplasm is not always continuous around sensory axons. Calibration line: 1 μm. D: Motor (M) and sensory (S) axons 2 weeks after transplantation. Calibration line: 10 μm. E: Cross-section through the distal stumps of two adjacent motor (M) axons severed 34 days previously. AG, Adaxonal glial cytoplasm; GS, glial sheath. Calibration line: 1.0 μm. F: Cross-section through two adjacent motor (M) axons in a control peripheral nerve. Calibration line: 0.5 μm.

glial sheath cells may provide substances which allow severed motor axons to function at a subnormal level for many months. It is, therefore, interesting to note that glial cells transfer greater amounts of peroxidase to severed than to control motor axons (Nordlander *et al.*, 1975).

Survival of Isolated Segments of Limb Nerves

Motor axons in long (3 cm) and short (0.3 cm) segments of isolated crayfish peripheral nerves transplanted to the abdomen survive morphologically intact for 20–30 days, whereas sensory axons degenerate within 7–14 days (Bittner and Nitzberg, 1975; Bittner and Mann, 1976) (Fig. 1C). The observation that the rate and pattern of degeneration of sensory axons in these transplanted segments (Fig. 1C,D) is the same as singly cut axons left *in situ* suggests that transplantation *per se* does not produce more rapid degeneration. This interpretation is supported by more recent experiments showing that doubly cut sensory axons left *in situ* degenerate in 7–14 days, whereas motor axons in the same segments degenerate within 35 days (Mann and Bittner, personal observations). As in singly cut peripheral nerves, glial cells phagocytize isolated sensory axons, whereas glial cells around isolated motor axons undergo hypertrophy and hyperplasia at 7–14 days after lesioning (Bittner and Mann, 1976). Glial cells do phagocytize motor axons after 20–25 days.

These data suggest that the long-term survival of motor axons depends not only on the nature of the glial reaction but also on the presence of intact synaptic contacts, since isolated segments lacking synaptic contacts have a shorter survival time than singly cut segments. These data also suggest that the nature of the glial reaction may, in part, account for the difference in survival times between isolated sensory and isolated motor axons. Furthermore, degeneration of the motor axons in an isolated segment is associated with a change in the nature of the glial reaction from a nutritive to a phagocytic role.

Trophic Dependencies of Opener Muscle Fibers

As discussed above, motor axons probably receive trophic inputs from muscle fibers. Our results also suggest that immobilized, tenotomized, decentralized,* and denervated crayfish opener muscles, in turn, receive trophic substances from motor axons as long as the neuromuscular synapses remain functionally competent.

*I will use the term "decentralized" to refer to muscles with severed motor axons that remain morphologically and functionally intact. Conversely, I will use the term "denervated" to refer to muscles with degenerated motor axons. This distinction is important since neuronal lesions often leave crustacean muscles decentralized for 100–250 days, during which time trophic substances may be spontaneously released from motor synapses which can be shown to remain functional. Although they are quite capable of conducting action potentials, these decentralized motor axons are electrically quiescent as long as they remain severed from their CNS cell body (Bittner, 1973a; Bittner and Johnson, 1974).

The morphological arrangement of opener muscle fibers on a single central tendon is most advantageous because it enables one to decentralize all or a selected set of muscle fibers without directly damaging any muscle fiber, to tenotomize all or part of the entire muscle with or without decentralization, and to immobilize the opener muscle in the fully open or the fully closed position. Furthermore, the long-term survival of the single excitor and inhibitor motor axons which innervate the opener allows one to decentralize this muscle without denervation. Our previously published results (Atwood *et al.*, 1973; Bittner, 1973*a,b*; Boone and Bittner, 1974) showed the following:

1. Immobilization in the fully open or fully closed position for up to 10 months does not produce atrophy of opener muscle fibers. These data suggest that the ability to generate tension isotonically is not important to the maintenance of normal fiber morphology since immobilization essentially prevents fiber shortening.

2. Decentralization procedures which leave a long piece of distal axon produce few detectable changes in opener fiber morphology, input resistance, or resting potential for up to 250 days (Fig. 2A). However, once the nerve terminals degenerate, then we observe muscle atrophy associated with severe disruptions of actin filaments, myosin filaments, and Z bands (Fig. 2B). The lack of atrophy for up to 250 days after decentralization with long distal stumps suggests that membrane electrical activity or tension development does not play a major role in maintaining normal muscle morphology. The muscle atrophy associated with disruption of muscle ultrastructure after denervation suggests that the opener fibers are dependent on neurotrophic substances which can be released without the generation of action potentials in decentralized motor axons. However, if the decentralization procedure leaves a very short (<3 mm) segment of motor axon, then the nerve terminals may degenerate within 3–4 weeks, and the denervated fibers show severe disruptions in fiber ultrastructure within 3–5 weeks. This latter result helps rule out the possibility that the fiber atrophy associated with long-stump decentralization is due to a disuse phenomenon. All these results are consistent with the hypothesis that opener fibers are trophically dependent on substances released from functionally competent synapses.

3. Tenotomized muscle fibers show decreases in fiber diameter within about 15 days and, with time, show further decreases in fiber diameter as long as the tendon remains cut. (Tenotomy initially causes opener fibers to shorten to a resting length which is 10–35% shorter than the shortest length which they normally attain when the muscle is placed in the fully open position. The resting length of tenotomized fibers continues to shorten with time as

---

Fig. 2. A: Longitudinal sectional through nerve terminal and opener muscle fiber decentralized 34 days previously. Z, Z band; SV, synaptic vesicles. Inset: Cross-section through same muscle fiber showing normal arrangement of thick and thin filaments. Calibration line: 1μm; 0.5μm for inset. B: Longitudinal section through opener muscle fiber denervated 364 days previously. Calibration line: 1μm.

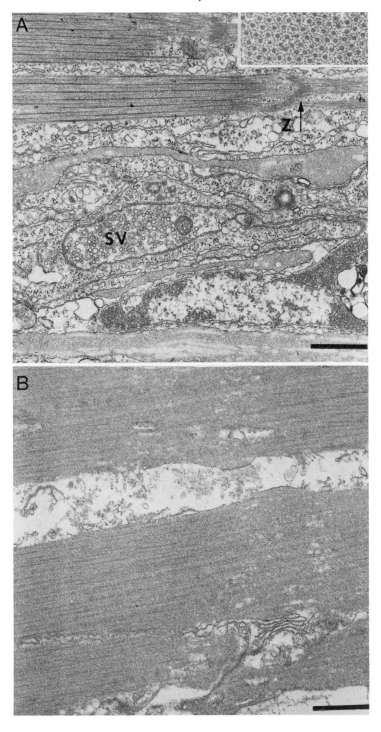

long as the tendon does not reattach to the exoskeleton.) Since tenotomy results in greater shortening of opener fibers than that which occurs in the fully open position, the maintenance of normal fiber morphology seems to require that the muscle retain a minimum resting length or passive tension. The observation that increase in the amount of atrophy with maintained tenotomy is roughly correlated with a progressive decrease in resting length is in agreement with this hypothesis. One alternate hypothesis, that atrophy results from an inability of opener fibers to develop much active tension, is strongly contradicted by the observation that long-stump decentralized fibers do not atrophy for many months even though these fibers never actively contract.

All these data imply that the normal morphology of crayfish opener muscles is heavily dependent on the release of neurotrophic substances from motor neuron (MN) terminals and on the maintenance of a minimum resting length but not on use and disuse of the muscle mass. In contrast, the rate of atrophy seen in mammalian twitch muscles following immobilization, denervation, or tenotomy is dependent on the pattern of muscle activity (Lømo and Rosenthal, 1972; Bittner, 1973a). Hence in mammalian muscles it has been rather difficult to separate the possible existence of a neural trophic factor from the effects of muscle activity. It has been easier to identify a neural trophic effect in crayfish opener muscles because decentralized muscles having long distal nerve stumps do not atrophy for many months, whereas decentralized muscles having short distal nerve stumps rapidly degenerate.

More recent ultrastructural data obtained in collaboration with Harold Atwood (Toronto) indicate that the opener muscles have an increased number of glycogen deposits at 15–50 days after tenotomy. After about 50 days, tenotomized muscles often show an abnormal morphology similar to that seen in denervated muscles, i.e., disruption of Z bands and disorganization of thick and thin filaments. Opener nerve terminals on tenotomized muscles usually remain ultrastructurally normal for 40–60 days. After this time, many terminals appear abnormal and some terminals are almost completely degenerated.

For the first 60–80 days, terminals on tenotomized opener muscles show rather little change in their ability to release transmitter (Velez and Bittner, personal observations) compared to normal terminals at 1 or 10 Hz stimulation (Bittner, 1968a,b; Atwood and Bittner, 1971). After 60–80 days, terminals on tenotomized muscles show a progressive decrease in their ability to release transmitter. In fact, the release of transmitter after long-term tenotomy is very similar to that seen after long-term decentralization; that is, junctional potentials (jp's) tend to be very small and cannot be recorded in some muscle fibers even though adjacent fibers show small jp's when the excitor nerve is stimulated at 10/sec. Preliminary results also show that the excitor nerve axon continues to conduct action potentials to all tenotomized opener muscles and that terminals of this same excitor axon on the more proximal, nontenotomized opener or stretcher muscles continue to release transmitter normally.

These results are all consistent with our hypothesis that MN axons and muscle fibers mutually exchange trophic substances across intact synapses. For the first 30 days, short-term tenotomization and short-stump denervation appear to produce muscle atrophy by different mechanisms (extreme reduction of resting length vs. loss of neurotrophic substance) which have different ultrastructural signs (glycogen deposits vs. disruption of ultrastructural organization). However, tenotomy of a muscle fiber eventually appears to have an effect on the functioning of its nerve terminals, suggesting that this postsynaptic structure may supply trophic substances important for axonal maintenance in an otherwise intact neuron. This effect on the functioning of excitor nerve terminals by tenotomization, in turn, is associated with changes in muscle fiber ultrastructure similar to those seen in denervated fibers.

Relevance of Neuronal Trophic Interactions to Regeneration of Motor and Sensory Axons

The different trophic interactions and responses to autotomy of severed motor and sensory axons help determine their regeneration mechanisms. As discussed previously, the perikaryon seems to be the primary trophic source for maintenance of sensory axons, since distal stumps of severed sensory axons degenerate within a few weeks' time. Compared to crustacean sensory axons, the perikaryon seems less important to the trophic maintenance of severed motor axons which appear to receive a significant input from glial cells and postsynaptic muscle fibers. Without these additional sources for trophic substances, severed distal stumps of motor axons might not remain morphologically intact and physiologically active for many months. Without long-term survival, it would be impossible for rather slowly growing processes arising from the original proximal stump (Bittner and Johnson, 1974) to activate or fuse with the severed distal stump.

The evidence that motor axons *can* regenerate by this rather unusual mechanism of morphological fusion (or electrotonic activation) of a severed distal stump with outgrowing proximal processes is now rather substantial:

1. Function returns simultaneously to all fibers of the opener and stretcher muscles, even though these muscles are located in different limb segments and receive their *sole* excitatory innervation by different branches of the same MN (Hoy *et al.*, 1967).
2. At no time during the recovery of reflex function can supernumerary junctional potentials be recorded from decentralized or recently reconnected opener or stretcher muscles, even though the distal stump remains functional at all times (Hoy *et al.*, 1967).
3. Regeneration of a motor axon within 20–50 days after lesioning is associated with the appearance of small axonal processes (satellite axons) which penetrate the glial sheaths so as to lie beside the original, severed distal stump for 0.5–1.5 cm distal to the lesion site (Nordlander and Singer,

1972; Bittner, 1973a; Kennedy and Bittner, 1974). These satellite axons are not found to extend to the more peripheral portions of the regenerated axon (Kennedy and Bittner, 1974).

4. There is no ultrastructural evidence for degeneration of motor axonal stumps in muscles that have recently reconnected (Bittner, 1973a; Kennedy and Bittner, 1974).

This "fusion" mechanism for regeneration may, in fact, be rather widespread among several invertebrate phyla since similar phenomena have now been reported for regenerating motor axons in other decapod crustaceans (Bittner and Johnson, 1974) and in the CNS of annelids (Frank et al., 1975; Birse and Bittner, 1976).

The most obvious advantage of regeneration by morphological or physiological fusion compared to regeneration by outgrowth is that fusion shortens regeneration time and eliminates the necessity for re-forming a new synaptic apparatus. Fusion has also been associated with precise reconnection specificity in both crustacean motor axons (Hoy et al., 1967; Bittner and Johnson, 1974) and annelid CNS axons (Frank et al., 1975; Birse and Bittner, 1976), perhaps because regenerating axons need grow only a few millimeters before contacting their "target" (a surviving distal stump). Conversely, when peripheral motor axons in a crayfish are first prevented from regrowing for many months and then allowed to regenerate after many of the original distal stumps have degenerated, these motor axons are capable of growing out fine processes to the peripheral muscle masses and forming new synapses. These synapses may now be made on inappropriate muscles (Bittner, 1973a; Bittner and Johnson, 1974; Kennedy and Bittner, 1974) and do not have the transmitter-release characteristics of the original axons (Bittner, personal observations). Consequently, another major adaptive advantage of distal stump survival may be to ensure precise connection specificity in an organism with very few MNs.

However, fusion obviously is not an absolute prerequisite for high regeneration specificity in crayfish, since regenerating sensory axons re-form appropriate synaptic connections which reestablish reflex arcs on opener and closer motor axons located in CNS ganglia. For example, stimulation of the hairs on the dorsal surface of the dactylopodite results in excitation of the opener excitor and inhibition of the closer excitor in normal limbs (Wilson and Davis, 1965) and in limbs with regenerated sensory and motor axons (Bittner and Johnson, 1974).

In fact, consideration of the effects of limb loss by autotomy or other means leads to the prediction that fusion would be a maladaptive regeneration mechanism for sensory axons. The cell bodies of most sensory axons are located in the limb itself and hence new cell bodies must differentiate and grow out new axons in the regenerating limb. Since the number of sensory axons in a regenerating limb is much smaller than the number in the original limb (Bittner, personal observations), it seems likely that none of the original axons would have appropriate CNS connections for any of the newly differentiated axons. Hence fusion would always lead to inappropriate CNS connections of sensory axons after limb loss. Furthermore, since the diameter of regenerating sensory axons after limb loss is much less than the diameter of the original sensory axons (Bittner, personal observations), fusion of a small outgrowing axon with a larger surviving stump would greatly reduce the safety factor for spike transmission.

Given these data, it seems adaptively correct that sensory axons regenerate by outgrowth and re-formation of CNS synapses after limb loss. This mechanism for regeneration after loss of a limb may well determine the response to axonotomy following a peripheral nerve cut. Given that sensory axons *do* regenerate by an outgrowth mechanism, it seems appropriate that the rate of growth from the proximal stump of peripheral sensory axons (1–2 mm/day) is greater than that of motor axons (0.05–0.33 mm/day: Bittner and Johnson, 1974), the rate of degeneration of the severed distal stump is more rapid, and the major source of trophic input is the perikaryon. We have also noted that the loss of a limb by autotomy or other means is associated with damage to nerve and muscle tissue and that this damage acts to increase molt frequency (Bittner and Kopanda, 1973). This effect has obvious adaptive significance since the rate at which the limb regenerates is dependent on molting frequency (Bliss, 1960).

Trophic Interactions and Regeneration of Motor Axons Innervating Abdominal Muscles

The "curious" nature of trophic interactions and regeneration of crayfish MNs is very evident in the abdominal flexor and extensor muscles. Hoy (1969, 1973) has reported that severed distal stumps of superficial flexor MNs (SFs) or deep flexor MNs (DFs) remain functionally intact for at least 40 or 120 days, respectively (degeneration was not followed to conclusion). The severed stumps of DFs continued to release transmitter normally for about 100 days. After 120 days, nongiant MNs often produced much smaller (≤ 1 mV) jp's than normal (5–10 mV) at 105 Hz stimulation. Regeneration seemed to occur rather rapidly to the deep flexor muscles after cutting or crushing of the motor axons in the ventral nerve cord (VNC) anterior to the exit of the third root. Regeneration occurred less rapidly in SFs, especially after cutting of the VNC, but appeared to return by fusion of an SF motor axon and its surviving distal stump after crusing of the motor axons in the VNC. Usually, regeneration seemed to occur by fusion of DFs after cutting or pinching of the peripheral roots or after cutting of *one* VNC connective, although several cases of reinnervation by outgrowth were seen after complete transection of DFs by cutting of the VNC above and below the exit of the third root. The original DF distal stumps continued to produce jp's after reinnervation by outgrowth had occurred; that is, regenerating motor axons did not render other motor axons nonfunctional, as reported for vertebrates (Mark *et al.,* 1972; *cf.* Scott, 1975; Hoy, 1973, did not determine if any of the original MNs reinnervated the DF muscle).

Samuel Velez and I have reexamined the response of SFs to axonotomy. Our physiological tests indicate that these MNs regenerate by a fusion mechanism if we pinch SF axons in the third abdominal root distal to the point where it exits from the VNC; that is, function is restored simultaneously to all decentralized superficial flexor muscle fibers within 20–40 days after lesioning. However, we have not yet detected regeneration of any SF axons after cutting the peripheral root at any point between its exit from the VNC and the most proximal SF fiber. In fact, the proximal portion of the severed root is almost totally reabsorbed into the VNC. Conversely, all superficial flexor muscle fibers are reinnervated within 120 days after cutting of the SF axons in the peripheral root distal to the most proximal superficial flexor muscle fiber so that the proximal nerve stump retains a point of mechanical attachment to the superficial flexor muscle (we do not yet know whether reinnervation occurs by fusion or outgrowth). In other words, regenerative success for severed crustacean SFs is, in part, determined by the type of lesion (cutting, pinching, etc.) and the lesion site.

Using similar physiological tests, Dr. Thomas Hamilton and I have shown that *pinching* superficial extensor MNs (SEs) between the lateral and medial heads of the superficial extensor muscle usually leads to regeneration by fusion within 20–30 days. Conversely, if the SE motor axons are *cut* at this same site, regeneration occurs by outgrowth. In all cases, the most recently formed synapses on more distal superficial extensor muscle fibers produce more normal-sized jp's (Hamilton and Bittner, 1976).

Simultaneous intracellular recordings from superficial extensor muscle fibers distal and proximal to the cut always show a 1:1 correspondence in jp's produced in both sets of muscle fibers. Similarly, simultaneous extracellular recordings of nerve action potentials recorded distal to the cut always show a 1:1 correspondence to action potentials recorded from the proximal stump. Hence we are rather certain that the original motor axons reinnervate the superficial extensor muscle by outgrowth and re-formation of synapses. However, we do not yet know if each SF or SE motor axon reinnervates its original set of muscle fibers (cell-to-cell specificity). Furthermore, since each MN innervates each superficial flexor muscle fiber in a very precise fashion with respect to the pattern of release of transmitter from its nerve terminals (Velez, 1974), we are also examining if reinnervation restores the "subcellular" specificity of synaptic connections.

Severed SE stumps continue to produce jp's for up to 120 days, whether or not reinnervation occurs. Unlike the data previously reported for SF and DF synapses (Hoy, 1969, 1973), careful analysis of transmitter release from severed SE axons shows a decrease in jp amplitude within the first 10 days after lesioning, particularly for those SE axons which normally release many quanta during low-frequency (<10 Hz) stimulation; that is, after the first 10 days, all decentralized axons produce rather small (<2 mV) jp's during low-frequency stimulation. This decrease is similar to that found in decentalized opener axons within the first 10 days after lesioning (Velez and Bittner, personal observations). As in the case of decentralized opener axons, we observe further decreases in SE axon jp amplitude after the first 10 days. We suspect that this decrease in jp amplitude in SE axons is presynaptic in origin since, in some fibers, stimulation of surviving distal stumps produces small jp's, whereas stimulation of axons apparently regenerated for some time produces normal-sized jp's in the same fiber (Hamilton and Bittner, 1976).

All these data show that singly cut abdominal motor axons continue to function for many months, perhaps because they receive trophic substances from surrounding glial cells and from postsynaptic muscle cells. This interpretation is similar to that postulated for singly cut motor axons which innervate limb muscles. Furthermore, decentralized superficial flexor and extensor abdominal muscles maintain normal fiber diameters (Bittner and Traut, 1977; Hamilton and Bittner, 1976; Velez and Bittner, personal observations), as do decentralized limb muscles. Unlike limb muscles, decentralized superficial flexor fibers develop an ability to generate graded membrane responses within 70 days after short-stump decentralization (Velez and Bittner, personal observations; normal superficial flexor fibers do not generate active membrane responses). These data suggest that the trophic dependencies of various physiological properties of SF muscle fibers are not the same. Crayfish opener muscles (Bittner, 1973a; Boone and Bittner, 1974) and vertebrate muscles (Guth, 1968) have also been reported to have different trophic dependencies for different fiber properties.

Trophic Interactions and Regeneration of Stretch Receptor Neurons

The peripheral nerve root (second abdominal) which contains SE motor axons also contains the axons of two stretch receptors (SRs) having cell bodies located in the periphery. The cell bodies of these SR neurons have dendrites which attach to specialized receptor muscles (RM) that lie just medial to the medial head of the superficial extensor muscle. A constant stretch given to both RM muscles produces a tonic discharge in the tonic SR (SR_1) which attaches to the tonic RM_1 and a phasic discharge in the phasic SR_2 which attaches to the phasic RM_2. The SR_1 neuron activates SE_2 (Fields, 1966; Fields et al., 1967) with a latency of about 35 msec at 20°C. Electron micrographs from control animals show that the SR sensory axons and the SE motor axons are ultrastructurally very similar; i.e., SR axons are generally larger and have thicker glial sheaths than do peripheral sensory axons in the limbs (Hamilton and Bittner, 1976).

For the first 20 days after lesioning, SE_2 could be reliably activated with a delay of 35 msec by stimulating the central stump of the second root containing the severed distal process of SR_1 (Hamilton and Bittner, 1976). From 21 to 40 days, the reflex became more difficult to elicit. In all but one animal (tested at 32 days) out of 27 tested between 0 and 40 days, the latency of the reflex remained constant. After 40 days, the reflex was not present in any of 29 animals tested. Several animals (4/13) regenerated the tonic SR axon within 70 days after pinching of the peripheral nerve root. No animal (out of over 60 tested) regenerated an SR axon within 250 days after cutting of the peripheral nerve root between the two heads of the superficial extensor muscle. The proximal stumps of severed SR axons remained functional in all cases. Electron micrographs from the peripheral or central stumps of the nerves sampled at various times after lesioning showed that the severed distal stumps of both SE motor axons and SR sensory axons had much glial thickening and remained intact for at least 150 days.

As in the case of neurons having cell bodies located in the CNS such as motor axons and medial giant axons (see below), the survival of severed SR axons is associated with a thickening of the glial sheath. Similarly, regeneration of SR axons occurs by fusion, if regeneration can be induced at all (as discussed in a later section, medial giant axons of the CNS show no regenerative ability). In fact, Kennedy (1975) has noted that, unlike most peripheral sensory cells, SRs have multiple processes and nonspiking dendrites and are differentiated early in development. Our data given above, and our data that SR cell bodies remain constant in number during ontogeny and do not regenerate if ablated, agree with his observation that these SR cells resemble the central type in all aspects save cell body location. These observations all suggest that SRs may be CNS neurons which migrate to the periphery in early development.

Responses of CNS Axons to Axonotomy

The ventral nerve cord (VNC) of the crayfish consists of a chain of ganglia containing neuronal cell bodies joined by connectives having nerve axons and glia but lacking nerve cell bodies. The VNC contains two pair of easily identifiable giant cells (Fig. 3), the medial and lateral giant axons. Each connective also contains many nongiant axons having a cell body in some other ganglion.

Although we have seen abortive outgrowths from the stumps of one or two lateral giant axons after cutting of the VNC (Bittner et al., 1974), we have never observed successful regeneration of any lateral or medial giant axon even 200 days after pinching of an axonal segment for only 100–500 μm of its length (Ballinger and Bittner, personal observations). Hoy (1969) and Wine (1973) also make no mention of successful regeneration for any severed CNS giant axons. Non giant CNS axons can regenerate (Hoy, 1969; Bittner et al., 1974), but this ability appears to be rather limited compared to that of most sensory and motor axons.

Even though these animals apparently have little or no ability to regenerate CNS axons, crayfish can survive for many months in community tanks after the VNC has been severed. During this time, the severed distal stumps of many giant and nongiant neurons are able to function so as to continue to mediate locally generated reflexes. For example, I have observed that stimulation of tactile hairs on the telson can still generate the escape response mediated by lateral giant (Wiersma, 1961b; Krasne, 1969) and/or nongiant (Schrameck, 1970; Larimer et al., 1971; Wine and Krasne, 1972) neurons which had been severed from their cell bodies for some months. Several female crayfish with transected VNCs have even mated and successfully hatched one or more sets of eggs. In other words, it appears that adaptations for very-long-term survival of severed distal stumps (see below) allow certain CNS neurons to continue to mediate many important reflexes and hence to

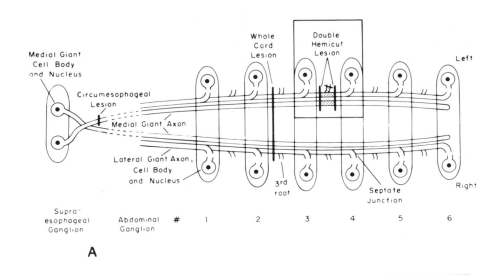

A

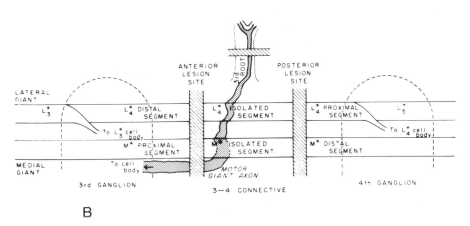

B

Fig. 3. A: Diagram of the anatomical arrangement of the cell bodies of the medial and lateral giant axons with respect to the supraesophageal and abdominal ganglia of the crayfish ventral nerve cord. The lateral giant axons arise from cell bodies located in the contralateral half of each abdominal ganglion. The stippled areas indicate the isolated axonal segments for the double hemicut operation; the dark bars indicate the location of some experimental lesions. B: Schematic enlargement of boxed area in A to illustrate the anatomical relationships among the various segments of the giant axons following a double hemicut on the left (asterisk) side of the VNC. Diagonal bars indicate the location of the anterior and posterior lesions on the left side of the VNC and the lesion on the left third root of the third abdominal ganglion. All three cuts were made in each double hemicut operation. L_3^*, L_4^*, and L_5^* are the left lateral giant axons whose cell bodies are located on the right sides of the third, fourth, and fifth abdominal ganglia, respectively. M^* represents the left medial giant axon. The third motor giant axon shown in light gray has its cell body in the third abdominal ganglion and sends an axonal process which forms an electrotonic contact with the medial giant axon in the 3–4 connective. The motor giant axon then exits in the third root of the third ganglion to innervate the fast flexor muscles of the third abdominal segment. From Meyer and Bittner (1976a).

compensate for a relative lack of regenerative capability. In fact, the medial and lateral giants probably provide the most advantageous preparation to study trophic mechanisms responsible for long-term axonal survival because of their large size, differential response to axonotomy, and lack of regenerative ability.

Trophic Interactions of Medial Giant Axons

Each medial giant axon has its cell body in the supraesophageal ganglion and makes synapses with various cells in the neuropil of each ganglion. This axon also makes electrotonic synapses with the motor giant axon to the deep flexor muscles in each abdominal ganglion (Wiersma, 1961b; Zucker, 1972c; Mittenthal and Wine, 1973).

If a medial giant axon is severed in the abdomen, the distal stump continues to conduct action potentials for up to 200 days. The conduction velocity of these action potentials remains normal for about 50 days and then decreases from 50 to 200 days after lesioning as axonal diameter decreases (Wine, 1973). This decrease in axonal diameter proceeds in a proximal–distal sequence (Meyer and Bittner, 1977a,b) so that by 270–360 days the severed axon is much smaller than normal, except for its most distal portion in the sixth abdominal ganglion (Bittner et al., 1974). The severed medial giants also continue to activate abdominal MNs for at least 3 weeks. These data all suggest that singly cut segments of medial giant axons remain rather functionally and morphologically normal for 20–50 days and then gradually become nonfunctional over the next 150 days.

Within 20–30 days after lesioning, the glial sheaths around medial giant axons usually have an increased thickness for 0.5–1.0 cm distal to the lesion site (Meyer and Bittner, 1977a; Templeton and Bittner, personal observations). By 270–360 days, this glial reaction usually extends over the entire length of the distal segment. At any time after lesioning, significant glial thickening usually occurs for only 2–5 mm anterior to the cut (Bittner et al., 1974). If only one medial giant is severed by cutting one circumesophageal connective, glial hypertrophy usually occurs only around the severed axon and not around an adjacent, intact medial giant in the same animal (Templeton and Bittner, personal observations). These morphological data suggest that, as in the case of motor and SR axons, a progressive glial response may be important for the continued survival of severed medial axons.

When intact nerve cords are incubated (pulsed) for 1 hr in [³H]leucine and then rinsed (chased) for an additional hour in unlabeled saline before preparation for autoradiography, the glial sheath around the medial giants is heavily labeled but the axoplasm of the medial giant does not contain much more label than noncellular background areas (Fig. 4A). If the cord is pulsed for 1 hr and then "chased" for 8 hr in oxygenated van Hareveld's saline containing unlabeled leucine, more and more label appears with time in the axoplasm of the medial giant (Fig. 4C). These results suggest that [³H]leucine is rapidly incorporated into protein in the glial sheaths and then the labeled protein is more slowly transferred to the medial giant axon.

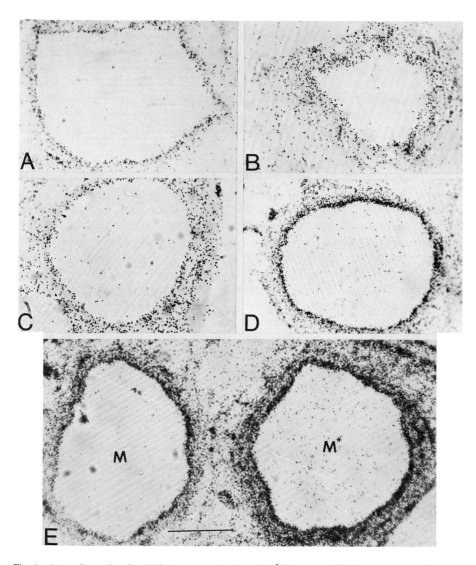

Fig. 4. Autoradiographs of medial giant axons incubated in [³H]leucine. A,B: Paired segments of control (A) and experimental (B) medial axons from 3–4 connectives incubated (pulsed) for 1 hr in [³H]leucine and then chased for 1 hr in oxygenated saline containing unlabeled leucine. The experimental axon (B) had been severed in the 2–3 connective 33 days prior to sampling. C,D: Paired segments of control (C) and experimental (D) medial giant axons from 3–4 connectives incubated for 1 hr in [³H]leucine and then chased for 8 hr in oxygenated saline containing unlabeled leucine. The experimental axon (D) had been severed in the 2–3 connective 33 days prior to sampling. E: Intact (M) and lesioned (M*) medial giant axons from an animal in which the left (asterisk) axon was cut in the circumesophageal connective 55 days prior to sampling. Sections taken from the 3–4 abdominal connective which was pulsed for 1 hr in [³H]leucine and then chased for 8 hr in cold, unlabeled saline. Calibration line: 50 μm for A–D, 40 μm for E. From Meyer and Bittner (1977b).

After 1 hr incubation in [³H]leucine, grain counts from many autoradiographs indicate that the glial sheaths of medial giant axons severed for 1 month incorporate about 2 times more [³H]leucine than do the sheaths around control axons (Fig. 4A,B; the severed axonal segments were sampled about 1 cm distal to the lesion site and showed little morphological thickening of the glial sheath at this time and distance). Quantitative analysis of autoradiographs also shows that axoplasm of severed medial giant axons has about 4 times more label density than do the axoplasm of control axons while the sheath around severed axons has about 2 times more label density than does the sheath around control axons (Fig. 4C,D). Adjacent, nonlesioned segments of lateral giant axons show no significant increase in the labeling density of the axoplasm or sheath (Meyer and Bittner, 1977b). To further ensure that these differences are not due to some nonspecific response to injury, only one medial giant axon was selectively severed by cutting one circumesophageal connective (Meyer and Bittner, 1977b). We then examined the labeling density of the sheath and axoplasm of both the intact and severed axons in the 3–4 abdominal connective (about 4–6 cm distal to the lesion site). At 1 month, we detected no obvious differences in axonal diameter, sheath thickness, or labeling density between intact and severed axons in the same animal. After 2 months, the sheath around the severed axon seemed to be somewhat thickened and had an increased grain density compared to the intact axon (Fig. 4E). All these data suggest that the glia surrounding severed axons incorporate more label and transfer it at a greater rate compared to glia around nonsevered medial axons.

However, when medial giant axons in one connective are isolated not only from their cell bodies but also from all synaptic contacts (Fig. 3, double hemicut lesion), the isolated axonal segments show more rapid decreases in axonal diameter between 7 and 43 days than do singly cut axons. The glial thickening around the isolated segment (Fig. 5) increases with time from 7 to 43 days compared to that of sham-operated medials on the contralateral side of the cord. These histological data are similar to those reported for doubly cut motor axons and suggest that the glia are able to provide some but not all of the substances required for maintenance of severed medial giant axons (Meyer and Bittner, 1977a).

Trophic Interactions of Lateral Giant Axons

In contrast to the unicellular medial giants, the lateral giant neurons of crayfish are multicellular axons composed of a series of axonal segments joined together by septate, electrotonic junctions. Each axonal segment is connected by a small neurite to a cell body on the contralateral side of its ganglion of origin. This neurite expands into the large axonal process which makes an electrotonic (gap) junction with a homologous process in the next most posterior ganglion (see Fig. 3). Each lateral giant axon then extends rostrally to the nextmost anterior ganglion where a similar electrotonic synapse is formed. Therefore, transection of a lateral giant axon in an abdominal connective severs the anterior half from its original cell body but leaves

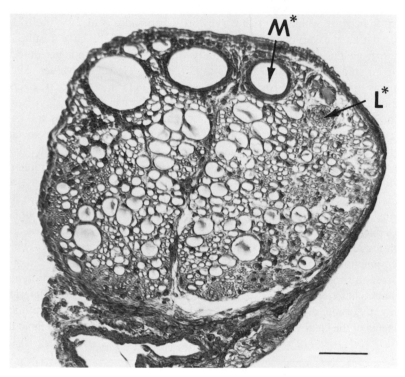

Fig. 5. Cross-section through a 3–4 connective which received a double hemicut lesion on its left side 31 days prior to fixation. Note that the left medial giant axon (M*) is still intact but that the left lateral giant has completely degenerated. Calibration line: 100 μm. From Meyer and Bittner (1976a).

the posterior half in contact with its original cell body. Both the anterior and the posterior halves of the severed lateral giant are in contact with other intact, lateral giant axons across a septate junction (Fig. 3).

Our previous data (Bittner, 1973a; Bittner et al., 1974) showed that the anterior (distal) half and the posterior (proximal) half of a lesioned lateral axon either could degenerate within 1–3 weeks or could survive for over 1 year. We observed all possible combinations of anterior and posterior survival or degeneration. The percentage of severed axonal segments which degenerated increased somewhat with time. Adjacent (nonlesioned) segments of the severed lateral giant axon usually had no degenerative changes, although the intact segment of the lateral giant axon posterior to the lesioned segment had a slight tendency to degenerate. The glial sheaths around either half of severed lateral segments or around adjacent, nonsevered segments demonstrated very little (if any) increase in thickness.

These results suggested to us that severed lateral axons were not very dependent on the cells of the glial sheath and that the anterior portion of a lesioned axon might survive because a rostral–caudal transport mechanism transferred proteins across septate junctions (a rostral–caudal transport of labeled proteins had been reported to occur in whole crayfish nerve cords: Fernandez *et al.*, 1970, 1971). We speculated that the survival of the posterior segment might have resulted from diffusion from the cell body by a rostrally directed transport not yet detected in whole-cord studies of Fernandez *et al.* (1970, 1971). However, Meyer (1973 and Fig. 6) has not yet found a rostral component of axoplasmic transport, even upon double-dose injection of the most posterior abdominal ganglion.

The axolemmas of two normal lateral segments are separated by a 0.5–2 μm space containing glial cell cytoplasm and connective tissue except for specialized areas 1–5 μm in diameter where the two cell membranes are separated by only 20–40 Å (Hama, 1961) (Fig. 8A). At these sites of close apposition (gap junctions), the cytoplasm of the two lateral giants may be in communication via porelike channels (Pappas *et al.*, 1971). Clear vesicles of 400–800 Å diameter are usually associated with both sides of the membrane at the gap junctions, although these vesicles may also be found elsewhere along the apposed membranes. Cross-sections through the region of overlap between two lateral giant axons usually show at least one gap junction and one or more sites of vesicle accumulation.

Given this morphological description, we might hypothesize that proteins pass from a more anterior segment to a more posterior segment of a normal lateral giant axon by diffusion across the porelike channels or by exocytotic–pinocytotic movements of the clear vesicles in both axonal segments. Although we have not yet

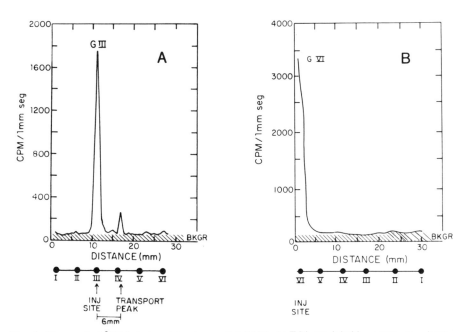

Fig. 6. Transport of ³H-labeled proteins in crayfish VNC. A: TCA-precipitable counts per minute in 1-mm segments of a crayfish VNC 1 week after injection of 0.3 μl of [³H]leucine (10 μCi/μl) into the third abdominal ganglion. B: TCA-precipitable counts per minute in 1-mm segments of a crayfish VNC 1 week after injection of 0.3 μl of [³H]leucine (20 μCi/μl) into the sixth abdominal ganglion. INJ, Injection site: BKGR, background activity. (From Meyer, 1973.)

performed autoradiographic experiments to determine if proteins continue to be transported from an intact (anterior) to a lesioned distal (posterior) stump, we do know that such severed distal segments of lateral giant axons can survive for over 1 year and that the surrounding glial cells show little reaction to severing. Hence the long-term survival of a severed distal segment may be due to rostral–caudal transport across septate junctions, and the interruption of this transport may account for the degeneration of the proximal segment of a severed lateral giant immediately posterior to the cut. The interruption of this transport may also account for the increased rate of degeneration of intact lateral segments in more posterior ganglia (Bittner *et al.*, 1974).

It is therefore interesting to note that these septate junctions in intact neurons are permeable to substances of at least 500 molecular weight (Payton *et al.*, 1969). Furthermore, Meyer (1973) has shown that if [³H]leucine is injected into the third abdominal ganglion, much more label is transported by a lateral giant axon (which has its cell body in that ganglion) than by a medial giant axon (which has its cell body in a much more anterior ganglion) (see Fig. 3). The label in the lateral giant axons is transported *caudally* at about 1 mm/day and the labeled proteins easily appear to pass septate junctions (Fig. 7). Similar results were obtained by Hermann

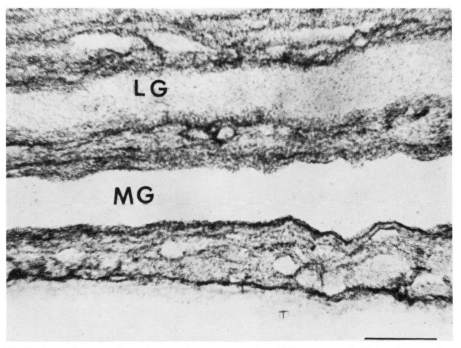

Fig. 7. Autoradiograph of lateral giant (LG) and medial giant (MG) axons sampled in longitudal section at the 3–4 connective 5 days after injection of [³H]leucine into the third abdominal ganglion. The label seen in the LG axon was presumably incorporated into protein in the lateral giant cell body in the third ganglion. The label then had to pass the septate junction in the third ganglion to reach the 3–4 connective. Calibration line: 100 μm. From Meyer (1973).

et al. (1975) after iontophoresis of [³H]glycine into the lateral giant axon. This *rostral-to-caudal* direction of transport for lateral giant axons is rather unexpected on anatomical grounds because the lateral giant neuron in each segment sends its axonal process in a *caudal-to-rostral* direction.

However, an increase in coupling resistance occurs within 30 min after damaging a lateral giant segment (Asada and Bennett, 1971). This increase in coupling resistance is associated with an increased separation of the junctional membranes and a loss of the gap junctions (Pappas *et al.,* 1971). Unless reversed with time, such a response would seem to impede the passage of substances from the anterior to the severed posterior segment. However, it is not necessary that large proteins should move from one cell segment to the next via the same mechanism used by the small ions responsible for electrotonic coupling. It seems quite possible that large numbers of small ions might diffuse down the channels of the gap junctions. Conversely, it seems possible that large proteins might be too large to diffuse in these channels; such proteins might be transported across septate junctions by the vesicles.

In light of these speculations, we (Ballinger and Bittner, personal observations) have noted that within a few days after severing, the apposing membranes of an intact and severed segment are indeed more separated. Clear vesicles of 400–800 Å are found in abundance, but gap junctions are very difficult or impossible to find (Fig. 8). Even after 170 days, the axolemma of an intact lateral giant immediately anterior to a severed segment may become very convoluted and many vesicles may be present in the cytoplasm, but no gap junctions are evident. These data are in agreement with the hypothesis that proteins may be moving from intact to severed segments via the action of these vesicles.

Several lines of evidence seem to rule out an alternate hypothesis that severed lateral segments are maintained by the cells of the surrounding sheath. First, unlike severed segments of medial giant axons, the sheaths around surviving, severed lateral segments show very little (if any) glial hypertrophy when sampled at various times and distances from the lesion site (Bittner *et al.,* 1974; Meyer and Bittner, 1977a). Second, unlike medial giant axons, isolated segments of lateral giant axons usually degenerate within 7 days after being severed from their cell bodies and from all pre- or postsynaptic contacts (Meyer and Bittner, 1977a) (Fig. 5).

Fig. 8. Section through septate junction between two intact lateral axons (A) and between a severed (*) and an intact lateral axon (B). A: Cross-sections through septate junctions in control animals normally have one or two gap junctions (arrow) where the membranes of the two apposing cells are separated by 20–40 Å. Vesicles (V) are found in the cytoplasm of both cells at these sites of close apposition. Vesicles may also be found where the axonal membranes are more widely separated by a glial sheath (GS). Insets show a gap junction in frontal section and an area of vesicle accumulation in cross-section. B: Septate junction between an intact lateral giant and the distal segment of a lateral giant severed 67 days previously. No typical gap junctions were seen in this or other cross-sections. Insert shows an area of close apposition between the severed segment (*) and a profile of unknown origin. Vesicles are present in the cytoplasm of both sides of these apposing membranes. Calibration line: 0.5 μm for A; 0.1 μm for B; 1.0 μm for insets in A and B.

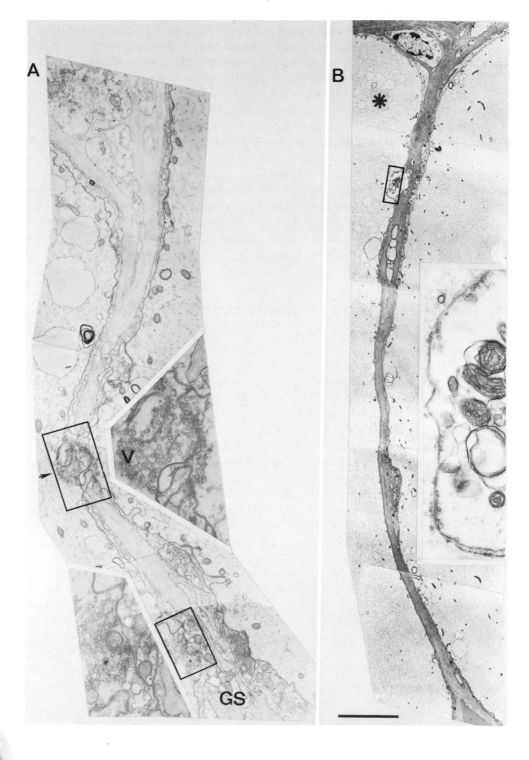

In summary, our morphological and biochemical data indicate that medial and lateral giant axons receive significant amounts of proteins (and possibly other substances) from adjacent neurons, glial cells, and the cell body. Upon separation from the cell body, the glial cells around the distal segment of a medial giant axon more rapidly incorporate amino acids into proteins which are then transferred at a greater rate to the severed axon. Conversely, the glia around severed lateral giant axons do not increase the rate of uptake or the rate of transfer of label. Rather, the severed distal segment of a lateral giant axon would seem to depend primarily on substances transferred from intact neurons across septate junctions. This transfer may be mediated by endocytotic and pinocytotic movements of vesicles in the vicinity of the apposed membranes. Although the mechanisms for distal stump survival may differ between lateral and medial giant axons, the end result is the same for both neurons; that is, severed axonal segments which are incapable of regeneration can nevertheless survive for many months and can continue to mediate reflex actions critical to survival and reproduction.

General Significance of Trophic Interactions in Crustacean Neurons

It has been known for many years that vertebrate or insect axons degenerate within a few days when isolated from the cell body and that regeneration then occurs via outgrowth from the surviving proximal stump. The discovery of slow (Weiss and Hiscoe, 1948) and fast (Ochs, 1972) axoplasmic transport helped explain how substances synthesized in the perikaryon could reach remote portions of the cell. These data led to the conclusion that the cell body was a major trophic center for the nerve axon. However, these data have often been interpreted to say that the cell body is *the* trophic center for the entire neuron and that each neuron is, metabolically speaking, a rather separate entity. This dogma is reinforced by the observation that neurons communicate by specialized means in which neurotransmitters or ionic currents seem to have their primary effect on surface membranes.

Within the last decade, a few iconoclasts have suggested that the cell body is not the *only* trophic source for the nerve axon. For example, Singer and Salpeter (1966) and Singer and Green (1968) have published suggestive evidence that proteins and RNA, respectively, may be transferred from Schwann cells to vertebrate axons. Lasek *et al.* (1973, 1974) have collected data from giant axons in a squid and a polychaete worm suggesting that these axons receive proteins from cells of the glial sheath. Our own data (Meyer and Bittner, 1977b) from medial and lateral giant axons also strongly suggest that these axons receive proteins from surrounding sheath cells. Furthermore, our data show that the rate of exchange of proteins from glia to medial giant axons is increased in segments isolated from their cell body. Finally, morphological data from severed motor, medial giant, and SR axons show that long-term axonal survival is associated with hypertrophy of the glial sheath.*

However, as illustrated by the survival of singly cut distal segments of lateral giant axons, the perikaryon and surrounding glial cells are not the only sources of trophic substances. Severed lateral giant segments almost certainly receive inputs from adjacent neurons with which they make electrotonic connections. The shorter survival times of isolated segments of motor and medial giant axons compared to the survival times of singly cut segments of comparable length also suggest that these neurons receive trophic substances across intact synapses. In fact, our data from denervated, decentralized, and tenotomized opener muscles suggest that the metabolic states of crustacean MNs and muscle fibers are mutually affected by substances transferred in both directions across intact, conventional synapses. While the amount or rate of exchange of substances among nerve, muscle, and glial cells may be quantitatively much greater in certain crustacean neurons compared to most vertebrate neurons, I suspect that qualitatively similar exchanges occur by the same cellular mechanisms in most vertebrate and other invertebrate nervous tissue. In fact, the most obvious means of communication between cells in near contact would be by mutual exchange of chemical substances, and there is no *a priori* reason to believe that neuronal tissue should differ from other tissues in this regard.

The long-term survival of severed crustacean axons really should be viewed in the broader context of cell biology as opposed to the more narrow context of neuronal trophic interactions, since enucleated pieces of cytoplasm are known to survive for long times in other eukaryotes. For example, if the stalk and umbrella of the alga *Acetabularia* are severed from the nucleated rhizoid, these cytoplasmic processes may survive morphologically intact for some 90–120 days. The mechanism responsible for stalk survival is almost certainly long-lasting messenger RNA which directs protein synthesis on ribosomes in the severed stalk (see Goss, 1969, or Harris, 1970, for reviews). As a second example of cytoplasmic survival, one might note that mammalian red blood cells may survive for 90–150 days after the nucleus is extruded. However, unlike *Acetabularia* or crayfish axonal segments, mammalian RBCs do not seem to be very active metabolically (they contain no mitochondria and very small amounts of mRNA). Unlike mammalian RBCs or crayfish axonal segments, *Acetabularia* is a single-celled organism in which trophic substances could hardly come from other somatic cells. Consequently, severed crustacean axons present the only known system to date in Metazoa in which enucleated pieces of cytoplasm survive for a very long time in a very active metabolic state (Bittner, 1973a). Data obtained from these axons on the nature of their trophic interactions and the biochemical basis for their long-term survival should therefore be of interest to cell biologists as well as to neurobiologists.

---

*As yet, we have few data on other mechanisms such as a very slow turnover of axonal proteins or axonal protein synthetic capability that might help explain long-term axonal survival. We might note, however, that we have not yet seen any rough endoplasmic reticulum or free ribosomes in any normal or severed crustacean axon. This observation is in agreement with that of Lasek *et al.* (1973, 1974), who find no evidence for protein synthetic capability in other invertebrate axons.

Finally, it should be remembered that crustaceans have not evolved these extreme examples of trophic interactions to provide employment for a few eclectic neurobiologists. In fact, the curious combinations of degeneration, regeneration, and trophic interactions in different crustacean neurons appear to have much adaptive value. For example, the trophic inputs from glial and muscular tissue are associated with the long-term survival of severed peripheral motor axons. That long-term survival, in turn, is associated with regeneration by morphological or electrotonic fusion which is highly specific and very rapid, even though processes may grow out rather slowly from the severed proximal stump. Long-term survival of severed CNS giant axons is associated with their continued participation in reflex pathways, even though regeneration may never occur (long-term survival without reconnection would be a maladaptive response for severed peripheral motor neurons since nonregenerated motor stumps cannot participate in a reflex pathway). Conversely, the short-term axonal survival of severed peripheral sensory neurons (excluding SR neurons) seems quite appropriate given their regenerative responses following limb autotomy.

31

Some Perspectives on Comparative Neurophysiology

Theodore Holmes Bullock

Introduction

Climbing a steep trail, with eyes on the footing, makes it hard to see far ahead or behind, but during the moments on a mountaintop it is easy to gain perspective. This symposium, ranging as it has from retrospective examination of peaks of past achievement to progress reports on the ascent of new peaks, has truly been a mountaintop experience.

Wiersma's Latest Triumphs

We have been reminded of the remarkable assignment of a visual memory to the periphery, the receptor layer of the retina (Wiersma and Hirsh, 1975b); of the first discovery of space-constant visual units (Wiersma and Yanagisawa, 1971); of the first evidence that a circadian clock can be localized in the eyestalks of crayfish (Aréchiga and Wiersma, 1969b); of the introduction of the term ''command neurons'' (Wiersma, 1962), building on Wiersma's earlier demonstrations of ''pushbutton reflexes'' (Wiersma, 1952b; he has likened them to birthday telegrams in which a single code number releases a specific complex output that may be spoken or even sung!); of the key example, significant in the history of central rhythms, provided by the swimmeret control system (Wiersma and Ikeda, 1964)— to mention some of the nearer peaks.

The Middle Years of Wiersma's Work

To go back a little further, I remember the first demonstration that collisions of impulses, having arisen in more proximal and more distal spike initiation sites in the same neuron, are normal (Wiersma and Hughes, 1961), clearly proving that recep-

Theodore Holmes Bullock • Department of Neuroscience, University of California, San Diego, California 92037.

tive processes (sometimes, although inadvisedly, called "dendrites") are not only near the soma but also far from it.

I remember well the first public announcement of higher-order visual neurons with complex criteria for firing, recorded in the optic ganglion of lobsters long before reports of such units by Maturana, Lettvin, McCulloch and Pitts, or Hubel and Wiesel (read at a symposium by Waterman and Wiersma, 1956; published by Waterman *et al.*, 1961; Waterman and Wiersma, 1963; *et seq.*).

I recall vividly, but with a strange feeling in retrospect, the catalogs (Wiersma, 1958) of 160 identified sensory neurons and afferent interneurons (INs), and (Wiersma and Hughes, 1961) of another 75 in the crayfish central nervous system. While the elegance of these findings was well appreciated at the time, little did most of us realize that they presaged the great boom in identified cells, still nearly 10 years away. Even when, in 1957, Wiersma estimated a surprisingly modest neuronal count in a crayfish CNS (94,722 neurons exclusive of optic lobes), we did not extrapolate from his list of known, consistent afferent INs. We failed to link these data with his earlier, already classic demonstration of consistent motor units (Marmont and Wiersma, 1938; Wiersma, 1941) and to anticipate that identifiable neurons would be found to be so abundant, here as well as in many other types of animals.

These were not the only instances in which Wiersma seems now to have been prescient. In 1952, he clearly ascribed habituation to a presynaptic site. In 1950, with Adams, he showed the dramatic sensitivity on the part of some junctions to the temporal pattern of presynaptic impulses, and the insensitivity on the part of others. In 1949, only 2 years after he had moved into the CNS from a previous concentration on neuromuscular relations, Wiersma gave us a still-unsurpassed example of spatial summation of four adjacent synapses from four different presynaptic sources onto the same postsynaptic unit and described the critical time relations for summation. The importance of such cases is not always that they tell how a particular behavior normally happens. In this instance, each presynaptic giant fiber is normally quite adequate to fire the postsynaptic motor neuron (MN) and summation can be studied only in the experimentally depressed state. Neurophysiology has extensively depended on such pathological preparations as models of more general interest.

Wiersma's Early Work

The peaks of achievement in his first decade of publication stand out above the foothills today even more than they did then. In 1942, he and Novitski demonstrated the antagonistic extrinsic acceleration and inhibition of the neurogenic heart in the crayfish. I appreciated this because I had already tried, unsuccessfully, to make a cardiac ganglion preparation in the lobster and only learned how years later, at the hands of Maynard (1955). Wiersma and van Harreveld (1938a) demonstrated heterosynaptic facilitation and its postsynaptic locus in the crayfish leg abductors.

The discovery by Marmont and Wiersma (1938) of a second type of inhibition of muscle contraction, what they called "supplemented inhibition" in contrast to "simple inhibition" (later designated α and β inhibition, respectively, by Katz, 1949), clearly established what we know today as presynaptic inhibition. Indeed, the direct, facilitating, and impulse-timing-specific inhibition of skeletal muscle demonstrated by Marmont and Wiersma (1938) put inhibition "on the map," as Florey has said.

The discovery of "slow" and "fast" postjunctional responses in the same muscle fiber, depending on the presynaptic fiber stimulated (van Harreveld and Wiersma, 1936), not only gave a functional meaning to the polyneuronal innervation these authors had described earlier but also clearly disproved the universality of the all-or-none law.

Of course, the full significance of these findings was not appreciated at once. I well recall the incredulity of an audience at Yale in 1941 when I reviewed Wiersma and van Harreveld's work. But, as so often in comparative physiology, the seemingly bizarre mechanisms found in an unfamiliar group of animals turned out to be widespread and main-line.

The Future

As we look back at the way we came, the peaks are clear, and Kees Wiersma is responsible for a truly remarkable proportion of them. Looking ahead, the mist obscures the peaks but gives us glimpses of the trails that wind up several of them. Let us attempt the difficult task of gaining perspective by looking ahead as well as back. I confine myself to a selection of directions, glimpsed during the papers of this meeting, that appear to lead to promising heights.

A discovery of Wiersma's that has the ring of importance, although it is far from clear just what the full significance will be, was the result of a series of studies over many years on the mechanoreceptors in the elastic strand sense organs across leg joints. In opener and closer movement detectors, Wiersma et al. (1970) found firing in a temporal distribution they called "skip-type discharge" in which the interspike intervals are multiples, up to ten or more, of the interval at saturation (the interval histogram has upward of ten uniformly spaced peaks). Wood (1975) found this pattern of discharge also in a new class of position receptor. The suggestion is made that the receptor has a rhythmic spontaneous change in membrane potential or excitability. The situation has basic similarities to the so-called probability coders among the tuberous electroreceptors of some gymnotoid electric fish (Eigenmannia, Apteronotus), in which mean frequency is graded by alteration of the probability of firing at a fixed period (Hagiwara et al., 1965; Bullock and Chichibu, 1965) and this period is due to active ringing of the excitability cycle in the receptor (Viancour, 1976). It remains to be determined whether in crayfish there is a useful pattern in the sequence of intervals; Chichibu and I found a weak but statistically significant departure from randomness, toward runs. These observations also raise questions about tuning the receptor. How plastic is the characteristic period? In the gymnotoids named, many receptors are matched in period to the preferred (centrally paced) electric organ discharge frequency of the individual fish.

One direction came to mind, perhaps because of the juxtaposition of electron microscopy and electrophysiology in several papers. The speculation seems worth considering that there can be electrical transmission without so much as a gap junction. This possibility is suggested by both anatomical and physiological hints. Microscopists have several times failed to find expected gap junctions. Functionally, it is only a small extrapolation from the wide diversity of the tightness of electrotonic coupling known, to suggest that there may be a widespread form of such interaction that does not depend on structural specializations by present electron microscopic criteria, and is therefore perhaps less discrete and localized than familiar gap junctions. This would in turn encourage speculation about feeble but effective influences over wide areas of unspecialized proximity.

Some discussions here reminded me of the concept now supported for certain vertebrate smooth muscle that the transmitter released by nerve endings is believed to act over a radius of tens of micrometers. Is it not worth speculating that arthropod skeletal muscle can be under similarly diffuse transmitter control? This would seem to be disproved by the elegant localization of sensitivity, for example, by the Takeuchis. But, as in vertebrate smooth muscle, there might be a variety of types of muscle with a spectrum of forms of nervous control.

The increasing number of demonstrated instances of neurons that work without all-or-none impulses leads me to restate a speculation of long standing: my guess has been that a substantial proportion of neurons work without firing and that another large fraction that *can* fire function much of the time without impulses, even transmitting signals to other neurons by graded, decrementing events.

This and others of my examples point up a special feature of comparative neurophysiology—its dependence on extrapolation from a few instances. Neurons have the greatest variety of all cell types, and the number of examples we can study is small. We have to generalize by a large extrapolation—but how differently we do it, "conservatives" and "radicals"! Can we really tell which is the safer bet, that the familiar examples are representative of the population of cell types, or that the known examples, like the usual spiking neuron, are not necessarily representative?

I would inject the incidental recommendation that temperature be manipulated as a parameter in studies on the incidence of nonspiking. If it can be shown that over a significant range the temperature does not change the ability to fire, it would strengthen the assertion that such neurons work without impulses. Cole (1968) points out that the sharpness of the all-or-none threshold of a squid axon model is markedly reduced by higher temperatures and the probability of an intermediate response to a "threshold" stimulus is greatly increased.

I would also urge renewed efforts to find a function for the retinula axons of the *Limulus* eye—shown by Waterman and Wiersma (1954) not to carry impulses under photic stimuli known to cause influential receptor potentials in the retinula somas.

Are the axons transporting important materials, either centrally or peripherally? Are they conducting an effective electrotonic contribution to the subretinal plexus that mediates lateral inhibition? Are there environmental conditions under which they conduct spikes? Most importantly, are there many other axons elsewhere that behave in the same way?

This leads to a related proposition, questioning the usual tacit assumption that neurons either fire or do not fire impulses. In spite of evidence against the universality of the all-or-none law going back to van Harreveld and Wiersma (1936) and before, as well as more recently, it is commonly forgotten that abortive spikes and graded responses up to and including overshooting local potentials have been recorded many times (Hodgkin, 1938; Bullock, 1948; Bullock and Turner, 1950; Lorente de Nó and Condouris, 1959; Grundfest, 1962, 1967; Cole, 1968; Bryant and Decima, 1976). My summary of the evidence is that events intermediate between all-or-none spikes and subthreshold graded potentials, of all sizes, are not unphysiological or rare but happen to an important degree normally, and especially in some types of neurons.

The papers at this meeting illustrating the power and tractability of arthropod material for studies of development bring to mind the following desideratum. Although not universally accepted, the notion persists that in vertebrates there can exist repressed synapses (Mark, 1974), i.e., synapses held in an ineffective state by the operation of neighboring junctions but ready when derepressed, as by the silencing of those neighbors, to become effective in a few hours. This idea is so potentially significant that a serious effort to test it in invertebrate material, developing or regenerating, is worthwhile.

One more suggestion may be put forward, encouraged by the discussions at the symposium, within and between sessions. May there not be a general difference between arthropods and vertebrates in the character and basis of the ongoing cerebral electrical activity? Could it be that relatively less spread of coherent slow potential activity occurs in arthropod cerebral ganglia compared to lower vertebrate brains of the same size? This is one possible explanation of the usually relatively feeble component of the power spectrum of ongoing extracellular activity below 50 Hz in arthropods compared to the vertebrate brain, where the maximum power is typically below 15 Hz. Measuring the degree of cross-correlation at each frequency and as a function of distance between electrodes appears a more feasible and perhaps better way of estimating the degree of synchrony between cells than intracellular, multichannel recording from many independent sample sets of neurons. Such measurements have not been made, and I anticipate a wide range of variation, depending on state and locus in each species. Nevertheless, it should be a significant descriptor of a population property of organized masses of neurons, and it may turn up another dynamic contrast between major groups of animals that could add insight into the underlying basis of ongoing activity.

Perspective, even from the vantage point of a mountaintop such as this symposium, is limited when we look into the light and mist as we are looking ahead today. One is likely to be influenced by wishes and the power of suggestion. However, this may not be all bad. I am one who believes that these subjective elements are undesirable only when we pretend they are not there or think we are above them. It is a high compliment to Kees Wiersma and the symposium—both organizer and participants—that I have felt such high-voltage ''vibes,'' such a sense of history in the making as well as being reviewed. Salute to our ''forward-looking seeing unit,'' C. A. G. Wiersma!

References

Abbott, B. C., and Parnas, I., 1965, Electrical and mechanical responses in deep abdominal extensor muscles of crayfish and lobster, *J. Gen. Physiol.* **48**:919–931.

Alexandrowicz, J. S., 1951, Muscle receptor organs in the abdomen of *Homarus vulgaris* and *Palinurus vulgaris*, *Q. J. Microsc. Sci.* **92**:163–199.

Alexandrowicz, J. S., 1958, Further observations on proprioceptors in crustacea and a hypothesis about their function, *J. Mar. Biol. Assoc. U.K.* **37**:379–396.

Alexandrowicz, J. S., 1967, Receptor organs in the coxal region of *Palinurus vulgaris*, *J. Mar. Biol. Assoc. U.K.* **47**:415–432.

Alexandrowicz, J. S., 1972, The comparative anatomy of leg proprioceptors in some decapod crustacea, *J. Mar. Biol. Assoc. U.K.* **52**:605–634.

Alexandrowicz, J. S., and Whitear, M., 1957, Receptor elements in the coxal region of decapoda crustacea, *J. Mar. Biol. Assoc. U.K.* **36**:603–628.

Allen, E. J., 1894, Studies on the nervous system of crustacea. I. Some nerve elements of the embryonic lobster, *Q. J. Microsc. Sci.* **36**:461–482.

Alnaes, E., and Rahamimoff, R., 1975, One the role of mitochondria in transmitter release from motor nerve terminals, *J. Physiol. (London)* **248**:285–306.

Altman, J. S., 1975, Changes in the flight motor pattern during development of the Australian plague locust, *Chortoicetes terminifera*, *J. Comp. Physiol.* **97**:127–142.

Altman, J. S., and Tyrer, M. N., 1974, Insect flight as a system for the study of the development of neuronal connections, in: *Experimental Analysis of Insect Behavior* (L. Barton-Browne, ed.), pp. 159–179, Springer-Verlag, New York.

Alving, B. O., 1968, Spontaneous activity in isolated somata of *Aplysia* pacemaker neurons, *J. Gen. Physiol.* **51**:29–45.

Anderson, C. R., Cull-Candy, S. G., and Miledi, R., 1976, Glutamate and quisqualate noise in voltage-clamped locust muscle fibres, *Nature (London)* **261**:151–153.

Anderson, D. T., 1972, The development of hemimetabolous insects, in: *Developmental Systems: Insects*, Vol. I (S. J. Counce and C. H. Waddington, eds.), Academic Press, New York.

Angaut Petit, D., and Clarac, F., 1976, A study of a temporal relationship between two excitatory motor discharges in the crayfish, *Brain Res.* **104**:166.

Angaut-Petit, D., Clarac, F., and Vedel, J. P., 1974, Excitatory and inhibitory innervation of a crustacean muscle associated with a sensory organ, *Brain Res.* **70**:148–152.

Anwyl, R., and Usherwood, P. N. R., 1974a, Voltage-clamp studies of the glutamate response at the insect neuromuscular junction, *J. Physiol. (London)* **242**:86–87.

Anwyl, R., and Usherwood, P. N. R., 1974b, Voltage-clamp studies of the glutamate synapse, *Nature (London)* **252**:591–593.

Anwyl, R., and Usherwood, P. N. R., 1975, The ionic permeability changes caused by the excitatory transmitter at the insect neuromuscular junction, *J. Physiol. (London)* **249**:24–25.

Aréchiga, H., 1974, Circadian rhythm of sensory input in the crayfish, in: *The Neurosciences: Third Study Program* (F. O. Schmitt, ed.), pp. 517–523, M.I.T. Press.

Aréchiga, H., and Atkinson, R. J. A., 1975, The eye and some effects of light on locomotor activity in *Nephrops norvegicus*, *Mar. Biol.* **32**:63–76.

Aréchiga, H., and Mena, F., 1975, Circadian variations of hormonal content in the nervous system of the crayfish, *Comp. Biochem. Physiol.* **52A**:581–584.

Aréchiga, H., and Wiersma, C. A. G., 1969*a,* The effect of motor activity on the reactivity of single visual units in the crayfish, *J. Neurobiol.* **1:**53–69.

Aréchiga, H., and Wiersma, C. A. G., 1969*b,* Circadian rhythm of responsiveness in crayfish visual units, *J. Neurobiol.* **1:**71–85.

Aréchiga, H., and Yanagisawa, K., 1973, Inhibition of visual units of the crayfish, *Vision Res.* **13:**731–744.

Aréchiga, H., Fuentes, B., and Barrera, B., 1973, Circadian rhythm of responsiveness in the visual system of the crayfish, in: *Neurobiology of Invertebrates* (J. Sálanki, ed.), pp. 403–421, Publishing house of the Hungarian Academy of Sciences, Budapest.

Aréchiga, H., Fuentes-Pardo, F., and Barrera-Mera, B., 1974, Influence of retinal shielding pigments on light sensitivity in the crayfish, *Acta Physiol. Lat.* **24:**601–611.

Aréchiga, H., Huberman, A., and Naylor, E., 1974, Humoral modulation of circadian neural activity in *Carcinus maenas* (L.), *Proc. R. Soc. London Ser. B* **187:**299–313.

Aréchiga, H., Barrera-Mera, B., and Fuentes-Pardo, B., 1975, Habituation of mechanoreceptive interneurons in the crayfish, *J. Neurobiol.* **6:**131–144.

Arshavsky, Y. I., Berkinblit, M. G., Fukson, O. I., Gelfand, I. M., and Orlovsky, G. N., 1972, Origin of modulation of neurones of the ventral spinocerebellar tract during locomotion, *Brain Res.* **13:**276–279.

Asada, Y., and Bennett, M. V. L., 1971, Experimental alteration of coupling resistance at an electrotonic synapse, *J. Cell Biol.* **49:**159–172.

Asanuma, H., and Sakata, H., 1967, Functional organization of a cortical efferent system examined with focal depth stimulation in cats, *J. Neurophysiol.* **30:**35–54.

Atwood, H. C., and Wiersma, C. A. G., 1967, Command interneurons in the crayfish central nervous system, *J. Exp. Biol.* **46:**249–261.

Atwood, H. L., 1963, Differences in muscle fibre properties as a factor in "fast" and "slow" contraction in *Carcinus, Comp. Biochem. Physiol.* **10:**17–31.

Atwood, H. L., 1965, Excitation and inhibition in crab muscle fibres, *Comp. Biochem. Physiol.* **16:**409–426.

Atwood, H. L., 1967*a,* Crustacean neuromuscular mechanisms, *Am. Zool.* **7:**527–551.

Atwood, H. L., 1967*b,* Variation in physiological properties of crustacean motor synapses, *Nature (London)* **215:**57–58.

Atwood, H. L., 1973*a,* Crustacean motor units, in: *Control of Posture and Locomotion* (R. B. Stein, K. G. Pearson, R. S. Smith, and J. B. Redford, eds.), pp. 87–104, Plenum Press, New York.

Atwood, H. L., 1973*b,* An attempt to account for the diversity of crustacean muscle, *Am. Zool.* **13:**357–378.

Atwood, H. L., 1974, Crustacean motor units, in: *Control of Posture and Locomotion* (R. B. Stein, K. B. Pearson, R. S. Smith, and J. B. Redford, ed.), pp. 87–104, Plenum Press, New York.

Atwood, H. L., 1976, Organization and synaptic physiology of crustacean neuromuscular systems, *Prog. Neurobiol.,* in press.

Atwood, H. L., and Bittner, G. D., 1971, Matching of excitatory and inhibitory inputs to crustacean muscle fibres, *J. Neurophysiol.* **34:**157–170.

Atwood, H. L., and Hoyle, G., 1965, A further study of the paradox phenomenon of crustacean muscle, *J. Physiol. (London)* **181:**225–234.

Atwood, H. L., and Johnston, H. S., 1968, Neuromuscular synapses of a crab motor axon, *J. Exp. Zool.* **167:**457–470.

Atwood, H. L., and Jones, A., 1967, Presynaptic inhibition in crustacean muscle: *Axo-axonal synapse, Experientia* **23:**1036–1038.

Atwood, H. L., and Kwan, I., 1976, Development of synapses in crayfish opener muscle, *J. Neurobiol.,* **7:**289–312.

Atwood, H. L., and Lang, F., 1973, Differential responses of crab neuromuscular synapses to cesium ion, *J. Gen. Physiol.* **61:**747–766.

Atwood, H. L., and Morin, W. A., 1970, Neuromuscular and axo-axonal synapses of the crayfish opener muscle, *J. Ultrastruct. Res.* **32:**351–369.

Atwood, H. L., and Parnas, I., 1968, Synaptic transmission in crustacean muscles with dual motor innervation, *Comp. Biochem. Physiol.* **27**:381–404.

Atwood, H. L., and Pomeranz, B., 1974, Crustacean motor neuron connections traced by backfilling for electron microscopy, *J. Cell Biol.* **63**:329–334.

Atwood, H. L., and Wiersma, C. A. G., 1967, Command interneurons in the crayfish central nervous system, *J. Exp. Biol.* **46**:249–261.

Atwood, H. L., Hoyle, G., and Smyth, T., 1965, Electrical and mechanical responses of single innervated crab-muscle fibres, *J. Physiol. (London)* **180**:449–482.

Atwood, H. L., Parnas, I., and Wiersma, C. A. G., 1967, Inhibition in crustacean phasic neuromuscular systems, *Comp. Biochem. Physiol.* **20**:163–177.

Atwood, H. L., Lang, F., and Morin, W. A., 1972, Synaptic vesicles: Selective depletion in crayfish excitatory and inhibitory axons, *Science* **176**:1353–1355.

Atwood, H. L., Govind, C. K., and Bittner, G. D., 1973, Ultrastructure of nerve terminals and muscle fibres in denervated crayfish muscle, *Z. Zellforsch. Mikrosk. Anat.* **146**:155–165.

Atwood, H. L., Swenarchuk, L. E., and Gruenwald, C. R., 1975, Long-term synaptic facilitation during sodium accumulation in nerve terminals, *Brain Res.* **100**:198–204.

Auber, J., 1960, Observations sur l'innervation motrice des muscles des insectes, *Z. Zellforsch. Mikrosk. Anat.* **51**:705–724.

Autrum, H. J., and von Zwehl, V., 1962, Zur spektralen Empfindlichkeit einzelner Sehzellen der Drohne (*Apis Mellifica* O.), *Z. Vgl. Physiol.* **46**:8–12.

Ayers, J., 1976, Neuronal control of locomotion in the lobster *Homarus americanus*, Ph.D. thesis, University of California, Santa-Cruz.

Ayers, J. L., and Davis, W. J., 1977, Neuronal control of locomotion in the lobster, *Homanis americanus*. II. The organization of joint reflexes, *J. Comp. Physiol.* **A115**:18–46.

Baker, P. F., Blaustein, M. P., Hodgkin, A. L., and Steinhardt, R. A., 1969, The influence of calcium on sodium efflux in squid axons, *J. Physiol. (London)* **200**:431–458.

Balnave, R. J., and Gage, P. W., 1974, On facilitation of transmitter release at the toad neuromuscular junction, *J. Physiol. (London)* **239**:657–675.

Barber, V. C., Evans, E. M., and Land, M. F., 1967, The fine structure of the eye of the mollusc *Pecten maximus*, *Z. Zellforsch. Mikrosk. Anat.* **76**:295–312.

Barker, D. L., Herbert, E., Hildebrand, J. G., and Kravitz, E. A., 1972, Acetylcholine and lobster sensory neurones, *J. Physiol. (London)* **226**:205–229.

Barker, J. L., and Gainer, H., 1975, Studies on bursting pacemaker potential activity in molluscan neurons. I. Membrane properties and ionic contributions, *Brain Res.* **84**:461–477.

Barlow, H. B., 1961, Possible principles underlying the transformations of sensory messages, in: *Sensory Communication* (W. A. Rosenblith, ed.), M.I.T. Press, Cambridge, Mass.

Barnes, W. J. P., and Horridge, G. A., 1969, Interaction of the movements of the two eyecups in the crab *Carcinus*, *J. Exp. Biol.* **50**:651–672.

Barnes, W. J. P., Spirito, C. P., and Evoy, W. H., 1972, Nervous control of walking in the Crab *Cardisoma quanhumi*. II. Role of resistance reflexes in walking, *Z. Vgl. Physiol.* **76**:16–32.

Barrett, E. F., and Stevens, C. F., 1972, The kinetics of transmitter release at the frog neuromuscular junction, *J. Physiol. (London)* **227**:691–708.

Barrett, J. N., 1975, Motoneuron dendrites: Role in synaptic integration, *Fed. Proc.* **34**:1398–1407.

Barth, G., 1934, Untersuchungen über Myochordotonal organe bei dekapoden crustacean, *Z. Wiss. Zool. Abt. A* **145**:576–624.

Bate, C. M., 1976*a*, Embryogenesis of an insect nervous system. I. A map of the thoracic and abdominal neuroblasts in *Locusta migratoria*, *J. Embryol. Exp. Morphol.* **35**:107–123.

Bate, C. M., 1976*b*, Pioneer neurons in an insect embryo, *Nature (London)* **260**:54–55.

Baylor, E. R., 1959, Is polarized light a valuable navigation aid to invertebrates? in: *International Oceanographic Congress* (M. Sears, ed.), pp. 178–180, A.A.A.S., Washington, D.C.

Baylor, E. R., and Kennedy, D., 1958, Evidence against a polarizing analyzer in the bee eye, *Anat. Rec.* **132**:411 (abst.).

Baylor, E. R., and Smith, F. E., 1953, The orientation of Cladocera to polarized light, *Am. Nat.* **87:**97–101.

Baylor, E. R., and Smith, F. E., 1958, Extra-ocular polarization analysis in the honey bee, *Anat. Rec.* **132:**411–412 (abst.).

Behrendt, R., 1940, Untersuchung über die Wirkungen erblichen und nichterblichen Fehlens bzw. Nichtgebrauchs der Flügel auf die Flugmuskulatur von *Drosophila melanogaster*, *Z. Wiss. Zool. Abt. A* **152:**129–158.

Bennett, M. R., and Florin, T., 1974, A statistical analysis of the release of acetylcholine at newly formed synapses in striated muscle, *J. Physiol. (London)* **238:**93–107.

Bennett, M. R., and Pettigrew, A. G., 1975, The formation of synapses in amphibian striated muscle during development, *J. Physiol. (London)* **252:**203–239.

Bennett, M. R., Florin, T., and Hall, R., 1975, The effect of calcium ions on the binomial statistic parameters which control acetylcholine release at synapses in striated muscle, *J. Physiol. (London)* **247:**429–446.

Bennett, M. R., Florin, T., and Pettigrew, A. G., 1976, The effect of calcium ions on the binomial statistic parameters that control acetylcholine release at preganglionic nerve terminals, *J. Physiol. (London)*, **257:**597–620.

Bennett, M. V. L., 1972, A comparison of electrically and chemically mediated transmission, in: *Structure and Function of Synapses* (G. D. Pappas and D. P. Purpura, eds.), pp. 221–256, Rowen Press, New York.

Bennett-Clark, H. C., 1975, The energetics of the jump of the locust *Schistocerca gregaria*, *J. Exp. Biol.* **63:**53–83.

Bennitt, R., 1932, Diurnal rhythm in the proximal cells of the crayfish retina, *Physiol. Zool.* **5:**65–69.

Bentley, D. R., 1969*a*, Intracellular activity in cricket neurons during the generation of behavior patterns, *J. Insect Physiol.* **15:**677–699.

Bentley, D. R., 1969*b*, Intracellular activity in cricket neurons during generation of song patterns, *Z. Vgl. Physiol.* **62:**267–283.

Bentley, D. R., 1971, Genetic control of an insect neuronal network, *Science* **174:**1139–1141.

Bentley, D. R., 1975, Single-gene cricket mutants: Effects on behavior, sensilla, sensory neurons and identified interneurons, *Science* **187:**760–764.

Bentley, D. R., and Hoy, R. R., 1970, Post-embryonic development of adult motor patterns in crickets: A neural analysis, *Science* **170:**1409–1411.

Bentley, D. R., and Hoy, R. R., 1972, Genetic control of the neuronal network generating cricket song patterns, *Anim. Behav.* **20:**478–492.

Bentley, D. R., and Hoy, R. R., 1974, The neurobiology of cricket song, *Sci. Am.* **231(2):**34–42.

Berànek, R., and Miller, P. L., 1968, The action of iontophoretically applied glutamate on insect muscle fibres, *J. Exp. Biol.* **49:**83–93.

Bern, H., and Hagedorn, I., 1965, Neurosecretion, in: *Structure and Function In the Nervous Systems of Invertebrates*, Vol. 1 (T. Bullock and A. Horridge, eds.), Chapter 6, Freeman, San Francisco.

Bernhard, C. G., 1966, *The Functional Organization of the Compound Eye*, 591 pp., Pergamon Press, Oxford.

Bethe, A., 1897*a*, Das Nervensystem von *Carcinus maenas*. Ein anatomisch-physiologischer Versuch. I. Theil, I. Mittheil, *Arch. Mikrosk. Anat. Entwicklungsmech.* **50:**460–546.

Bethe, A., 1897*b*, Das Centralnervensystem von *Carcinus maenas*. Ein anatomisch-physiologischer Versuch. I. Theil, II. Mittheil, *Arch. Mikrosk. Anat. Entwicklungsmech.* **50:**589–639.

Betz, W. J., 1970, Depression of transmitter release at the neuromuscular junction of the frog, *J. Physiol. (London)* **206:**629–644.

Biedermann, W., 1887, Beiträge zur allgeneinen Neven- und Muskel-physiologie. XX. Über die Innervation der Krebsschere, *S. B. Akad. Wiss. Wien. Abt. 3* **95:**7–40.

Biedermann, W., 1888, Zur Kenntniss der Nerven und Nervenendigungen in den guergestreiften Muskeln der Wirbellosen, *Sitzungsber. Akad. Wiss. Wien Math. Naturwiss. Kl. Abt.* **96:**8–39.

Biedermann, W., 1889, Beitrage zur allgemeinen Nerven- und Musdel-physiologie, 21. Mittheilung.

Ueber die Innervation der Krebsschere, *Sitzungsber. Adad. Wiss. Wien Math. Naturwiss. Kl. Abt.* **97:**49–82.

Biersma, D. G. M., Stavenga, D. G., and Kuiper, J. W., 1975, Organization of visual axes in the compound eye of the fly *Musca domestica* L. and behavioral consequences, *J. Comp. Physiol.* **102:**305–320.

Bigelow, R. S., 1960, Interspecific hybrids and speciation in the genus *Acheta* (Orthoptera; Gryllidae), *Can. J. Zool.* **38:**509–524.

Birks, R. I., 1963, The role of sodium ions in the metabolism of acetylcholine, *Can. J. Biochem.* **41:**2573–2597.

Birks, R. I., and Cohen, M. W., 1968*a*, The action of sodium pump inhibitors on neuromuscular transmission, *Proc. R. Soc. London Ser. B* **170:**381–399.

Birks, R. I., and Cohen, M. W., 1968*b*, The influence of internal sodium on the behavior of motor nerve endings, *Proc. R. Soc. London Ser. B* **170:**401–421.

Birse, S., and Bittner, G. D., 1976, Regeneration of giant axons in earthworms, *Brain Res.* **113:**575–581.

Bischof, H. J., 1975, Club-shaped hairs in cerci of cricket *Gryllus domesticus* acting as gravity receptors, *J. Comp. Physiol.* **98:**277–288.

Bittner, G. D., 1968*a*, Differentiation of nerve terminals in the crayfish opener muscle and its functional significance, *J. Gen. Physiol.* **51:**731–758.

Bittner, G. D., 1968*b*, The differentiation of crayfish muscle fibres during development, *J. Exp. Zool.* **167:**439–456.

Bittner, G. D., 1973*a*, Degeneration and regeneration in crustacean neuromuscular systems, *Am. Zool.* **13:**379–408.

Bittner, G. D., 1973*b*, Trophic dependence of fiber diameter in a crustacean muscle, *Exp. Neurol.* **41:**38–53.

Bittner, G. D., and Harrison, J., 1970, A reconsideration of the Poisson hypothesis for transmitter release at the crayfish neuromuscular junction, *J. Gen. Physiol.* **51:**731–758.

Bittner, G. D., and Johnson, A., 1974, Degeneration and regeneration in crustacean peripheral nerves, *J. Comp. Physiol.* **89:**1–21.

Bittner, G. D., and Kopanda, R., 1973, Factors influencing molting in the crayfish *Procambarus clarkii*, *J. Exp. Zool* **186:**7–17.

Bittner, G. D., and Mann, D. W., 1977, Differential survival of isolated portions of crayfish axons, *Cell Tissue Res.* **169:**301–311.

Bittner, G. D., and Nitzberg, M., 1975, Degeneration of sensory and motor axons in transplanted segments of a crustacean peripheral nerve, *J. Neurocytol.* **4:**7–21.

Bittner, G. D., and Sewell, V. L., 1976, Facilitation at crayfish neuromuscular junctions, *J. Comp. Physiol.* **109:**287 308.

Bittner, G. D., and Traut, D. L., 1977, Growth of crustacean muscles, *J. Comp. Physiol.* (in press).

Bittner, G. D., Ballinger, M. L., and Larimer, J. L., 1974, Crayfish CNS: Minimal degenerative-regenerative changes after lesioning, *J. Exp. Zool.* **189:**13–36.

Blakemore, C., 1974, Developmental factors in the formation of feature extracting neurons, in: *The Neurosciences. Third Study Program* (F. O. Schmitt and F. G. Worden, eds.), pp. 105–113, M.I.T. Press, Cambridge, Mass.

Blakemore, C., and Cooper, G., 1970, Development of the brain depends on the visual environment, *Nature (London)* **228:**477–478.

Blaschko, H., Cattell, M., and Kahn, J. L., 1931, On the nature of the two types of response in the neuromuscular system of the crustacean claw, *J. Physiol. (London)* **73:**25–35.

Bliss, D., 1960, Autotomy and regeneration, in: *The Physiology of Crustacea* (T. H. Waterman, ed.), pp. 561–590, Academic Press, New York.

Boistel, J., and Fatt, P., 1958, Membrane permeability change during inhibitory transmitter action in crustacean muscle, *J. Physiol. (London)* **144:**176–191.

Boone, L. P., and Bittner, G. D., 1974, Morphological and physiological measures of trophic dependence in a crustacean muscle, *J. Comp. Physiol.* **89:**123–144.

Bowerman, R. F., and Larimer, J. L., 1974a, Command fibres in the circumesophageal connectives of crayfish. I. Tonic fibres, *J. Exp. Biol.* **60:**95–117.

Bowerman, R. F., and Larimer, J. L., 1974b, Command fibres in the circumesophageal connectives of crayfish. II. Phasic fibres, *J. Exp. Biol.* **60:**119–134.

Bowerman, R. F., and Larimer, J. L., 1976, Command neurons in crustaceans, *Comp. Biochem. Physiol.* **54A:**1–5.

Bracho, H., and Orkand, R. K., 1970, Effect of calcium on excitatory neuromuscular transmission in the crayfish, *J. Physiol. (London)* **206:**61–72.

Branisteanu, D. D., Miyamoto, M. D., and Volle, R. L., 1976, Effects of physiologic alterations on binomial transmitter release at magnesium-depressed neuromuscular junctions, *J. Physiol. (London)* **254:**19–37.

Brenner, H. R., 1972, Evidence for peripheral inhibition in an arachnid muscle, *J. Comp. Physiol.* **80:**227–231.

Brodal, A., 1969, *Neurological Anatomy in Relation to Clinical Medicine,* 2nd ed., Oxford University Press, London.

Brodwick, M. S., and Junge, D., 1973, Post-stimulus hyperpolarization and slow potassium conductance increase in *Aplysia* giant neurone, *J. Physiol. (London)* **233:**249–270.

Brown, B. E., 1967, Neuromuscular transmitter substance in insect visceral muscle, *Science* **155:**595–597.

Brown, M. C., and Stein, R. B., 1966, Quantitative studies on the slowly adapting stretch receptor of the crayfish, *Kybernetik* **3:**175–185.

Brown, T. G., 1911, The intrinsic factors in the act of progression in the mammal, *Proc. R. Soc. London Ser. B* **84:**308–319.

Brown, T. G., 1914, On the nature of the fundamental activity of the nervous centres, together with an analysis of the conditioning of rhythmic activity in progression, and a theory of the evolution of function in the nervous system, *J. Physiol. (London)* **48:**18–46.

Brown, T. H., Perkel, D. N., and Feldman, M. W., 1976, Evoked neurotransmitter release: Statistical effects of nonuniformity and nonstationarity, *Proc. Natl. Acad. Sci. USA* **73:**2913–2917.

Bruner, J., and Kennedy, D., 1970, Habituation: Occurrence at a neuromuscular junction, *Science* **169:**92–94.

Bryan, J. S., and Krasne, F. B., 1977a, Protection from habituation of the crayfish lateral giant fiber escape response, *J. Physiol.,* in press.

Bryan, J. S., and Krasne, F. B., 1977b, Presynaptic inhibition: The mechanism of protection from habituation of the crayfish lateral giant fiber escape response, *J. Physiol.,* in press.

Bryant, H., and Decima, E., 1976, Graded action potentials in *Aplysia* neurons, *Soc. Neurosci. (abst.).*

Bullock, T. H., 1948, Properties of a single synapse in the stellate ganglion of squid, *J. Neurophysiol.* **11:**343–364.

Bullock, T. H., 1969, The reliability of neurons, *J. Gen. Physiol.* **55:**565–584.

Bullock, T. H., 1974, Comparisons between vertebrates and invertebrates in nervous organization, in: *The Neurosciences. Third Study Program* (F. O. Schmitt and F. G. Worden, eds.), pp. 343–346, M.I.T. Press, Cambridge, Mass.

Bullock, T. H., 1975, Are we learning what actually goes on when the brain recognizes and controls? *J. Exp. Zool.* **194:**13–34.

Bullock, T. H., and Chichibu, S., 1965, Further analysis of sensory coding in electroreceptors of electric fish, *Proc. Natl. Acad. Sci. USA* **54:**422–429.

Bullock, T. H., and Horridge, G. A., 1965, *Structure and Function in the Nervous Systems of Invertebrates,* Vol. I, 798 pp., Vol. II, 1719 pp., Freeman, San Francisco.

Bullock, T. H., and Turner, R. S., 1950, Events associated with conduction failure in nerve fibres, *J. Cell. Comp. Physiol.* **36:**59–82.

Burke, R. E., Levine, D. N., Zajac, F. E., Tsairis, P., and Engel, W. K., 1971, Mammalian motor units: Physiological histochemical correlation in three types in cat gastrocnemius, *Science* **174:**709–712.

Burke, R. E., Rymer, W. Z., and Walsh, J. V., Jr., 1974, Functional specialization in the motor unit population of cat medial gastrocnemius muscle, in: *Control of Posture and Locomotion* (R. B. Stein, K. G. Pearson, R. S. Smith, and J. B. Redford, eds.), pp. 29–44, Plenum Press, New York.

Burke, W., 1954, An organ for proprioception and vibration sense in *Carcinus maenas, J. Exp. Biol.* **31:**127–138.

Burrows, M., 1973*a,* The role of delayed excitation in the co-ordination of some metathoracic flight motoneurons of a locust, *J. Comp. Physiol.* **83:**135–164.

Burrows, M., 1973*b,* The morphology of an elevator and a depressor motoneuron of the hindwing of a locust, *J. Comp. Physiol.* **83:**165–178.

Burrows, M., 1973*c,* Physiological and morphological properties of the metathoracic common inhibitory neuron of the locust, *J. Comp. Physiol.* **82:**59–78.

Burrows, M., 1974, Modes of activation of motoneurons controlling ventilatory movements of the locust abdomen, *Philos. Trans. R. Soc. London Ser. B* **269:**29–48.

Burrows, M., 1975*a,* Integration by motor neurons in the central nervous system of insects, in: *Simple Nervous Systems* (P. N. R. Usherwood and D. R. Newth, eds.), pp. 345–379, Crane-Russak, London.

Burrows, M., 1975*b,* Monosynaptic connexions between wing stretch receptors and flight motor neurons of the locust, *J. Exp. Biol.* **62:**189–219.

Burrows, M., 1975*c,* Co-ordinating interneurones of the locust which convey two patterns of motor commands. Their connexions with ventilatory motoneurones, *J. Exp. Biol.* **63:**735–754.

Burrows, M., 1976, Neural control of flight in the locust, in: *Neural Control of Locomotion* (R. H. Herman, S. Grillner, P. S. G. Stein, and D. G. Stuart, eds.), pp. 419–438, Plenum Press, New York.

Burrows, M., and Horridge, G. A., 1968*a,* The action of the eyecup muscles of the crab, *Carcinus,* during optokinetic movements, *J. Exp. Biol.* **49:**223–250.

Burrows, M., and Horridge, G. A., 1968*b,* Motoneurone discharges to the eyecup muscles of the crab, *Carcinus, J. Exp. Biol.* **49:**251–267.

Burrows, M., and Horridge, G. A., 1968*c,* Eyecup withdrawal in the crab, *Carcinus,* and its interaction with the optokinetic response, *J. Exp. Biol.* **49:**285–297.

Burrows, M., and Horridge, G. A., 1974, The organization of inputs to motoneurons of the locust metathoracic leg, *Philos. Trans. R. Soc. London Ser. B* **269:**49–94.

Burrows, M., and Hoyle, G., 1973*a,* Neural mechanisms underlying behavior in the locust *Schistocerca gregaria.* III. Topography of limb motor neurons in the metathoracic ganglion, *J. Neurobiol.* **4:**167–186.

Burrows, M., and Hoyle, H., 1973*b,* The mechanism of rapid running in the ghost crab, *Ocypode ceratophthalma, J. Exp. Biol.* **58:**327–349.

Burrows, M., and Rowell, C. H. F., 1973, Connections between descending visual interneurons and metathoracic motoneurons in the locust, *J. Comp. Physiol.* **85:**221–234.

Burrows, M., and Siegler, M. V. S., 1976, Transmission without spikes between locust interneurones and motoneurones, *Nature (London)* **262:**222–224.

Burtt, E. T., and Catton, W. T., 1954, Visual perception of movement in the locust, *J. Physiol. (London)* **125:**566–580.

Burtt, E. T., and Catton, W. T., 1962, A diffraction theory of insect vision. I. An experimental investigation of visual acuity and image formation in the compound eyes of three species of insects, *Proc. R. Soc. London Ser. B* **157:**53–82.

Burtt, E. T., and Catton, W. T., 1966, Perception by locust of rotated pattern, *Science* **151:**224.

Burtt, E. T., and Catton, W. T., 1969, Resolution of the locust eye measured by rotation of radial striped patterns, *Proc. R. Soc. London Ser. B* **173:**513–529.

Burtt, E. T., Catton, W. T., and Cosens, D. J., 1963, Correlation between visual threshold and potential changes during light and dark adaptation in the locust eye, *J. Physiol. (London)* **170:**57–58.

Bush, B. M. H., 1962*a,* Peripheral reflex inhibition in the claw of the crab *Carcinus maenas* (L.), *J. Exp. Biol.* **39:**71–88.

Bush, B. M. H., 1962b, Proprioceptive reflexes in the legs of *Carcinus maenas* (L.), *J. Exp. Biol.* **39:**89–105.

Bush, B. M. H., 1963, A comparative study of certain limb reflexes in decapod crustaceans, *Comp. Biochem. Physiol.* **10:**273–290.

Bush, B. M. H., 1965a, Proprioception by chordotonal organs in the mero-carpopodite and carpo-propodite joints of *Carcinus maenas* legs, *Comp. Biochem. Physiol.* **14:**185–199.

Bush, B. M. H., 1965b, Proprioception by the coxo-basal chordotonal organ, CB, in legs of the crab *Carcinus maenas, J. Exp. Biol.* **42:**285–297.

Bush, B. M. H., 1975c, Leg reflexes from chordotonal organs in the crab, *Carcinus maenas, Comp. Biochem. Physiol.* **15:**567–587.

Bush, B. M. H., 1976, Non-impulsive thoracic-coxal receptors in crustaceans, in: *Structure and Function of Proprioceptors in the Invertebrates* (P. J. Mill, ed.), Chapter 3, Chapman and Hall, London.

Bush, B. M. H., and Cannone, A. J., 1973, A stretch reflex in crabs evoked by muscle receptor potentials in non-impulsive afferents, *J. Physiol. (London)* **232:**95–97.

Bush, B. M. H., and Cannone, A. J., 1974, A positive feed-back reflex to a crustacean muscle receptor, *J. Physiol. (London)* **236:**37–39.

Bush, B. M. H., and Clarac, F., 1975, Intersegmental reflex excitation of leg muscles and myochordotonal efferents in decapod crustacea, *J. Physiol. (London)* **246:**58–60.

Bush, B. M. H., and Godden, D. H., 1974, Tension changes underlying receptor potentials in non-impulsive crab muscle receptors, *J. Physiol. (London)* **242:**80–82.

Bush, B. M. H., and Roberts, A., 1968, Resistance reflexes from a crab muscle receptor without impulses, *Nature (London)* **218:**1171–1173.

Bush, B. M. H., and Roberts, A., 1971, Coxal muscle receptors in the crab: The receptor potentials of S and T fibres in response to ramp stretches, *J. Exp. Biol.* **55:**813–832.

Bush, B. M. H., Wiersma, C. A. G., and Waterman, T. H., 1964, Efferent mechanoreceptive responses in the optic nerve of the crab *Podophthalmus, J. Cell. Comp. Physiol.* **64:**327–346.

Bush, B. M. H., Godden, D. H., and Cannone, A. J., 1975, Efferent gain control in a non-impulsive muscle receptor, *Proc. Aust. Physiol. Pharmacol. Soc.* **6:**32–33.

Bush, B. M. H., Godden, D. H., and Macdonald, G. A., 1975a, A simple and inexpensive servo system for the control of length or tension of small muscles or stretch receptors, *J. Physiol. (London)* **245:**1–3.

Bush, B. M. H., Godden, D. H., and Macdonald, G. A., 1975b, Voltage clamping of non-impulsive afferents of the crab thoracic-coxal muscle receptor, *J. Physiol. (London)* **245:**3–5.

Calabrese, R. L., and Kennedy, D., 1974, Multiple sites of spike initiation in a single dendritic system, *Brain Res.* **82:**316–321.

Callec, J. J., Guillet, J. C., Pichon, Y., and Boistel, J., 1971, Further studies on synaptic transmission in insects. II. Relations between sensory information and its synaptic integration at the level of a single giant axon in the cockroach, *J. Exp. Biol.* **55:**123–150.

Camhi, J. M., 1970a, Yaw correcting postural changes in locusts, *J. Exp. Biol.* **52:**519–531.

Camhi, J. M., 1970b, Sensory control of abdomen posture in flying locusts, *J. Exp. Biol.* **52:**533–537.

Camhi, J. M., 1971, Flight orientation in locusts, *Sci. Am.* **225(2):**74–81.

Camhi, J. M., 1976, Influence of non-rhythmic sensory inputs on locomotory outputs in arthropods, in: *Neural Control of Locomotion* (R. H. Herman, S. Grillner, P. S. G. Stein, and D. G. Stuart, eds.), Plenum Press, New York.

Camougis, G., 1960, Visual responses in crayfish. I. Recoding shock responses to light with remote electrodes, *J. Cell. Comp. Physiol.* **55:**189–194.

Camougis, G., 1964, Visual responses in crayfish. II. Central transmission and integration, *J. Cell. Comp. Physiol.* **63:**339–352.

Camougis, G., and Kasprzak, H., 1966, Visual responses in crayfish. III. Further studies on transmission through the brain, *J. Cell. Physiol.* **67:**45–52.

Cannone, A. J., 1974, Analysis of a crab stretch reflex mediated by non-impulsive muscle receptor afferents, Ph.D. thesis, University of Bristol, U.K.

Carafoli, E., 1973, The transport of calcium by mitochondria: Problems and perspectives, *Biochimie* **55:**755–762.

Carlson, J. G., 1961, The grasshopper neuroblast culture technique and its value in radiobiological studies, *Ann. N.Y. Acad. Sci.* **95:**932–941.

Chalazonitis, N., 1963, The effect of changes in pCO$_2$ and pO$_2$ on rhythmic potentials from giant neurones, *Ann. N. Y. Acad. Sci.* **109:**451–479.

Chase, R., 1975, The electrophysiology of transduction, retinal interaction and axonal conduction in invertebrate photoreceptors, *Comp. Biochem. Physiol.* **52A:**571–576.

Chernetski, K. E., 1964, Sympathetic enhancement of peripheral sensory input in the frog, *J. Neurophysiol.* **27:**493–515.

Christensen, B. N., and Martin, A. R., 1970, Estimates of probability of transmitter release at the mammalian neuromuscular junction, *J. Physiol. (London)* **210:**933–945.

Cisne, J. L., 1974, Trilobites and the origin of arthropods, *Science* **186:**13–18.

Clarac, F., 1968a, Proprioceptor anatomy of the ischio-meropodite region in legs of the crab *Carcinus mediterraneus* C., *Z. Vgl. Physiol.* **61:**203–223.

Clarac, F., 1968b, Proprioception by the ischio-meropodite region in leges of the crab *Carcinus mediterraneus* C., *Z. Vgl. Physiol.* **61:**224–245.

Clarac, F., 1970, Fonctions proprioceptives au niveau de la région basi-ischio-meropodite chez *Astacus leptodactylus*, *Z. Vgl. Physiol.* **68:**1–24.

Clarac, F., 1976, Crustacean cuticular stress detectors, in: *Structure and Function of Proprioceptors in the Invertebrates* (P. J. Mill, ed.), Chapter 7, Chapman and Hall, London.

Clarac, F., 1977, Motor co-ordination in crustacean limbs, in: *Identified Neurons and Behavior of Arthropods* (G. Hoyle, ed.), Plenum Press, New York.

Clarac, F., and Coulmance, M., 1971, La marche latérale du crabe (*Carcinus*): Coordination des mouvements articulaires et régulation proprioceptive, *Z. Vgl. Physiol.* **73:**408–438.

Clarac, F., and Dando, M. R., 1973, Tension receptor reflexes in the walking legs of the crab *Cancer pagurus*, *Nature (London)* **423:**94–95.

Clarac, F., and Masson, C., 1969, Anatomie comparée des propriocepteurs de la région basi-ischio-méropodite chez certains Crustacés décapodes, *Z. Vgl. Physiol.* **65:**242–273.

Clarac, F., and Vedel, J. P., 1971, Etude des relations fonctionnelles entre le muscle fléchisseur accessoire et les organes sensoriels chordotonaux et myochordotonaux des appendices locomoteurs de la langouste *Palinurus vulgaris*, *Z. Vgl. Physiol.* **72:**386–410.

Clarac, F., and Wales, W., 1970, Contrôle sensoriel des muscles élévateurs au cours de la marche et del'autotomie chez certains Crustacés décapodes, *C. R. Acad. Sci.* **271:**2163–2166.

Clarac, F., Wales, W., and Laverack, M. S., 1971, Stress detection at the autotomy plane in the Decapod crustacea. II. The function of receptors associated with the cuticle of the basi-ischipodite, *Z. Vgl. Physiol.* **73:**383–407.

Clark, L. B., 1935, The visual acuity of the fiddler crab *Uca pugnax*, *J. Gen. Physiol.* **19:**311–319.

Cochran, D. M., 1935, The skeletal musculature of the blue crab *Callinectes sapidus Rathbun*, *Smithson. Misc. Publ.* **92:**1–76.

Cochrane, D. G., Rees, D., and Usherwood, P. N. R., 1968, Changes in structural, physiological and pharmacological properties of insect excitatory nerve–muscle synapses after motor nerve section, *Nature (London)* **218:**589–591.

Cochrane, D. G., Elder, H. Y., and Usherwood, P. N. R., 1972, Physiology and ultrastructure of phasic and tonic skeletal muscle fibres in the locust *Schistocerca gregaria*, *J. Cell Sci.* **10:**419–441.

Cohen, M. J., 1963, The crustacean myochordotonal organ as a proprioceptive system, *Comp. Biochem. Physiol.* **8:**223–243.

Cohen, M. J., 1965, The dual role of sensory system: Detection and setting central excitability, *Cold Spring Harbor Symp. Quant. Biol.* **30:**587–599.

Cohen, M. J., 1970, A comparison of invertebrate and vertebrate central neurons, in: *The Neurosciences: Second Study Program* (F. O. Schmitt, ed.), pp. 798–812, Rockefeller University Press, New York.

Cohen, M. J., and Jacklet, J. W., 1967, The functional organization of motor neurons in an insect ganglion, *Philos. Trans. R. Soc. London Ser. B* **252**:561–572.

Cole, K. S., 1968, *Membranes, Ions and Impulses,* 569 pp., University of California Press, Berkeley.

Constantine-Paton, M., and Capranica, R. R., 1975, Central projection of optic tract from translocated eyes in the leopard frog *Rana pipiens, Science* **189**:480–482.

Cooke, I. M., 1966, The sites of action of pericardial organ extract and 5-hydroxytryptamine in the decapod crustacean heart, *Am. Zool.* **6**:107–121.

Cooke, J. D., and Quastel, D. M. J., 1973, Cumulative and persistent effects of nerve terminal depolarization on transmitter release, *J. Physiol. (London)* **228**:407–434.

Cosens, D. J., 1966, Visual sensitivity in light- and dark-adapted compound eye of the desert locust, *J. Insect Physiol.* **12**:871–890.

Couteaux, R., and Pécot-Dechavassine, M., 1974, Les zones specialisées des membranes présynaptiques, *C. R. Seances Acad. Sci.* **278**:291–293.

Crawford, A. C., and McBurney, R. N., 1976, On the elementary conductance event produced by L-glutamate and quanta of the natural transmitter at the neuromuscular junctions of *Maia squinado, J. Physiol. (London)* **258**:205–226.

Crozier, W. J., and Wolf, E., 1939, The flicker response contour for the crayfish. II. Retinal pigment and the theory of the asymmetry of the curve, *Biol. Bull.* **77**:126–134.

Cull-Candy, S. G., and Usherwood, P. N. R., 1973, Two populations of L-glutamate receptors on locust muscle fibres, *Nature (London) New Biol.* **246**:62–64.

Dagan, D., and Parnas, I., 1970, Giant fibre and small fibre pathways involved in the evasive response of the cockroach, *Periplaneta americana, J. Exp. Biol.* **52**:313–324.

Daumer, K., Jander, R., and Waterman, T. H., 1963, Orientation of the ghost-crab *Ocypode* in polarized light, *Z. Vgl. Physiol.* **47**:56–76.

Davis, H., 1961, Some principles of sensory receptor action, *Physiol. Rev.* **41**:391–416.

Davis, W. J., 1968*a,* Quantitative analysis of swimmeret beating in the lobster, *J. Exp. Biol.* **48**:643–662.

Davis, W. J., 1968*b,* The neuromuscular basis of lobster swimmeret beating, *J. Exp. Zool.* **168**:363–378.

Davis, W. J., 1968*c,* Lobster righting responses and their neural control, *Proc. R. Soc. London Ser. B* **170**:435–456.

Davis, W. J., 1969, The neural control of swimmeret beating in the lobster, *J. Exp. Biol.* **50**:99–118.

Davis, W. J., 1970, Motoneuron morphology and synaptic contacts: Determination by intracellular dye injection, *Science* **168**:1358–1360.

Davis, W. J., 1971, Functional significance of motor neuron size and soma position in swimmeret system of the lobster, *J. Neurophysiol.* **34**:274–288.

Davis, W. J., 1973*a,* Development of locomotor patterns in the absence of peripheral sense organs and muscles, *Proc. Natl. Acad. Sci. USA* **70**:954–958.

Davis, W. J., 1973*b,* Neuronal organization and ontogeny in the lobster swimmeret system, in: *Control of Posture and Locomotion* (R. B. Stein, K. G. Pearson, R. S. Smith, and J. B. Redford, eds.), pp. 437–455, Plenum Press, New York.

Davis, W. J., 1976, Organizational concepts in the central motor networks of invertebrates, in: *Neural Control of Locomotion* (R. H. Herman, S. Grillner, P. S. G. Stein, and D. G. Stuart, eds.), Plenum Press, New York.

Davis, W. J., and Ayers, J. L., 1972, Locomotion: Control by positive-feedback optokinetic responses, *Science* **177**:183–185.

Davis, W. J., and Davis, K. B., 1973, Ontogeny of a simple locomotor system: Role of the periphery in specifying the development of the central nervous system, *Am. Zool.* **13**:409–425.

Davis, W. J., and Kennedy, D., 1972*a,* Command interneurons controlling swimmeret movements in the lobster. I. Types of effects on motoneurons, *J. Neurophysiol.* **35**:1–12.

Davis, W. J., and Kennedy, D., 1972*b,* Command interneurons controlling swimmeret movements in the lobster. II. Interaction of effects on motoneurons, *J. Neurophysiol.* **35**:13–19.

Davis, W. J., and Kennedy, D., 1972*c,* Command interneurons controlling swimmeret movements in the lobster. III. Temporal relationships among bursts in different motoneurons, *J. Neurophysiol.* **35:**20–29.

Davis, W. J., Siegler, M. V. S., and Mpitsos, G. J., 1973, Distributed neuronal oscillators and efference copy in the feeding system of *Pleurobranchaea, J. Neurophysiol.* **36:**258–274.

Davis, W. J., Mpitsos, G. J., Siegler, M. V. S., Pinneo, J. M., and Davis, K. B., 1974, Neuronal substrates of behavioral hierarchies and associative learning in the mollusc *Pleurobranchaea, Am. Zool.* **14:**1037–1050.

Debaisieux, P., 1944, Les yeux des Crustacés, *Cellule* **50:**9–122.

De Bruin, G. H. P., and Crisp, D. J., 1957, The influence of pigment migration on vision of higher crustacea, *J. Exp. Biol.* **34:**447–463.

del Castillo, J., and Katz, B., 1954, Quantal components of the end-plate potential, *J. Physiol. (London)* **124:**560–573.

del Portillo, J., 1936, Beziehungen zwischen den Öffnungswinkel der Ommatidien: Krummung and Gestalt der Insektenaugen und ihrer funktionellen Aufgabe, *Z. Vgl. Physiol.* **23:**100–145.

Dembowski, J., 1913, Über den Bau der Augen von *Ocypoda ceratophthalma Fabr., Zool. Jahrb. Abt. Anat. Ontog. Tiere* **36:**513–524.

Dennis, M. J., and Miledi, R., 1974, Characteristics of transmitter release at regenerating frog neuromuscular junctions, *J. Physiol. (London)* **239:**571–594.

Diamond, J., 1971, The Mauthner cell, in: *Fish Physiology,* Vol. 5 (W. S. Hoar and D. J. Randall, eds.), pp. 265–346, Academic Press, New York.

Dickerson, R. E., 1971, The structure of cytochrome *c* and the rates of molecular evolution, *J. Mol. Evol.* **1:**26–45.

Dijkgraaf, S., 1955, Die Augenstielbewegungen der Languste *Palinurus vulgaris, Experientia* **11:**329–330.

Dijkgraaf, S., 1956*a,* Über die kompensatorischen Augenstielbewegungen bei Brachyuren, *Publ. Staz. Zool. Napoli* **28:**341–358.

Dijkgraaf, S., 1956*b,* Structure and function of the statocysts of crabs, *Experientia* **12:**394–396.

Dodge, F. A., Jr., and Rahamimoff, R., 1967, Co-operative action of calcium ions in transmitter release at the neuromuscular junction, *J. Physiol. (London)* **193:**419–432.

Dorai Raj, B. S., 1964, Diversity of crab muscle fibers innervated by a single motor axon, *J. Cell. Comp. Physiol.* **64:**41–54.

Dorsett, D. A., Willows, A. O. D., and Hoyle, G., 1969, Centrally generated nerve impulse sequences determining swimming behavior in *Tritonia, Nature (London)* **224:**711–712.

Dorsett, D. A., Willows, A. O. D., and Hoyle, G., 1973, The neuronal basis of behavior in *Tritonia.* IV. The central origin of a fixed action pattern demonstrated in the isolated brain, *J. Neurobiol.* **4:**287–300.

Dresden, D., and Nijenhuis, E. D., 1958, Fiber analysis of the nerves of the second thoracic leg in *Periplaneta americana, Proc. K. Ned. Akad.* **61:**213–233.

Dreyer, F., Peper, K., Akert, K., Sandri, C., and Moor, H., 1973, Ultrastructure of the "active zone" in the frog neuromuscular junction, *Brain Res.* **62:**373–380.

Dudel, J., 1963, Presynaptic inhibition of the excitatory nerve terminal in the neuromuscular junction of the crayfish, *Pfluegers Arch.* **277:**537–557.

Dudel, J., 1965*a,* Potential changes in the crayfish motor nerve terminal during repetitive stimulation, *Pfluegers. Arch.* **282:**323–337.

Dudel, J., 1965*b,* The mechanism of presynaptic inhibition at the crayfish neuromuscular junction, *Pfluegers Arch.* **284:**66–80.

Dudel, J., 1971, The effect of polarizing current on action potential and transmitter release in crayfish motor nerve terminals, *Pfluegers Arch.* **324:**227–248.

Dudel, J., 1973, Recording of action potentials and polarization of a single crayfish motor axon through a sucrose-gap capillary suction electrode, *Pfluegers Arch.* **338:**187–199.

Dudel, J., 1975*a,* Potentiation and desensitization after glutamate induced postsynaptic currents at the crayfish neuromuscular junction, *Pfluegers Arch.* **356:**317–327.

Dudel, J., 1975*b,* Kinetics of postsynaptic action of glutamate pulses applied iontophoretically through high resistance micropipettes, *Pfluegers Arch.* **356:**329–346.

Dudel, J., and Kuffler, S. W., 1961a, The quantal nature of transmission and spontaneous miniature potentials at the crayfish neuromuscular junction, *J. Physiol. (London)* **155:**514–529.

Dudel, J., and Kuffler, S. W., 1961b, Mechanism of facilitation at the crayfish neuromuscular junction, *J. Physiol. (London)* **155:**530–542.

Dudel, J., and Kuffler, S. W., 1961c, Presynaptic inhibition at the crayfish neuromuscular junction, *J. Physiol. (London)* **155:**543–562.

Durand, J. B., 1956, Neurosecretory cell types and their secretory activity in the crayfish, *Biol. Bull.* **111:**62–76.

Duysens, J., and Pearson, K. G., 1976a, The role of cutaneous afferents from the distal hindlimb in the regulation of the step cycle of thalamic cats, *Exp. Brain Res.* **24:**245–255.

Duysens, J., and Pearson, K. G., 1976b, A possible role for large cutaneous fibers in cat locomotion, in: *Neural Control of Locomotion* (R. H. Herman, S. Grillner, P. S. G. Stein, and D. G. Stuart, eds.), Plenum Press, New York.

Eccles, J. C., Eccles, R. M., and Magni, F., 1961, Central inhibitory actions attributable to presynaptic depolarization produced by muscle afferent volleys, *J. Physiol. (London)* **159:**147–166.

Eckert, B., 1959, Über das Zussamenwirken des erregenden und des hemmenden Neurons des M. abductor des Krebsschere beim Ablauf von Reflexen des myotatischen Typus, *Z. Vgl. Physiol.* **41:**500–526.

Eckert, H. E. A., 1972, Optomotor response of the housefly *Musca* as a function of long spatial wavelengths, *Annu. Rep. Div. Eng. Appl. Sci.,* California Institute of Technology, Item 246.

Eckert, H. E. A., 1973, Optomotorische Untersuchungen am visuellen System der Stubenfliege *Musca domestica* L., *Kybernetik* **14:**1–23.

Edelman, G. M., 1974, The problem of molecular recognition by a selective system, in: *Studies in the Philosophy of Biology* (F. J. Ayala and T. Dobzhansky, eds.), pp. 45–56, Macmillan, New York.

Edgerton, V. R., Grillner, S., Sjostrom, A., and Zangger, P., 1976, Central generation of locomotion in vertebrates, in: *Neural Control of Locomotion* (R. H. Herman, S. Grillner, P. S. G. Stein, and D. G. Stuart, eds.), Plenum Press, New York.

Edwards, J. S., 1967, Some questions for the insect nervous system, in: *Insects and Physiology* (J. Treherne and J. W. L. Beament, eds.), pp. 165–174, Oliver and Boyd, Edinburgh.

Edwards, J. S., and Palka, J., 1974, The cerci and abdominal giant fibers of the house cricket *Acheta domesticus*. I. Anatomy and physiology of normal adults, *Proc. R. Soc. London B* **185:**83–103.

Edwards, J. S., and Palka, J., 1976, Neural generation and regeneration in insects, in: *Simple Networks and Behavior* (J. Fentress, ed.), Sinauer Associates, Cambridge, Mass.

Edwards, J. S., and Sahota, T. S., 1967, Regeneration of a sensory system: The formation of central connections by normal and transplanted cerci of the house cricket *Acheta domesticus, J. Exp. Zool.* **166:**387–396.

Egger, M. D., and Wyman, R. J., 1969, A reappraisal of reflex stepping in the cat, *J. Physiol. (London)* **202:**501–516.

Eguchi, E., 1964, The structure of rhabdom and action potentials of single retinula cells in crayfish, Ph.D. thesis, Kyushu University, Japan.

Eguchi, E., 1965, Rhabdom structure and receptor potentials in single crayfish retinular cells, *J. Cell. Comp. Physiol.* **66:**411–430.

Eguchi, E., and Waterman, T. H., 1966, Fine structure patterns in crustacean rhabdoms, in: *The Functional Organization of the Compound Eye* (C. G. Bernhard, ed.), pp. 105–124, Pergamon Press, Oxford.

Eguchi, E., and Waterman, T. H., 1967, Changes in retinal fine structure induced in the crab *Libinia* by light and dark adaptation, *Z. Zellforsch. Microsk. Anat.* **79:**209–229.

Eguchi, E., and Waterman, T. H., 1968, Cellular basis for polarized light perception in the spider crab *Libinia, Z. Zellforsch. Microsk. Anat.* **84:**87–101.

Eguchi, E., and Waterman, T. H., 1973, Orthogonal microvillus pattern in the eighth rhabdomere of the rock crab *Grapsus, Z. Zellforsch. Mikrosk. Anat.* **137:**145–157.

Eguchi, E., Waterman, T. H., and Akiyama, J., 1973, Localization of the violet and yellow receptor cells in the crayfish retinula, *J. Gen. Physiol.* **62:**355–374.

Elmqvist, D., and Quastel, D. M. J., 1965, A quantitative study of end-plate potentials in isolated human muscle, *J. Physiol. (London)* **178**:505–529.

Elofsson, R., and Odselius, R., 1975, The anostracan rhabdom and the basement membrane. An ultrastructural study of the *Artemia* compound eye *Crustacea, Acta Zool.* **56**:141–153.

Elsner, N., 1970, Kommandofasern im Zentralnervensystem der Heuschrecke *Gastrimargus africanus* (Oedipodinae), *Zool. Anz.* **33**:456.

Elsner, N., 1975, Neuroethology of sound production in gomphocerine grasshoppers (Orthoptera: Acrididae). II. Neuromuscular activity underlying stridulation, *J. Comp. Physiol.* **97**:291–322.

Emson, P. C., Bush, B. M. H., and Joseph, M. H., 1976, Transmitter metabolizing enzymes and free amino acid levels in sensory and motor nerves and ganglia of the shore crab *Carcinus maenas, J. Neurochem.* **26**:779–783.

Engberg, I., and Lundberg, A., 1969, An electromyographic analysis of muscular activity in the hindlimb of the cat during unrestrained locomotion, *Acta Physiol. Scand.* **75**:614–630.

Evans, P. D., Talamo, B. R., and Kravitz, E. A., 1975, Octopamine neurons: Morphology, release of octopamine and possible physiological role, *Brain Res.* **90**:340–347.

Evarts, E. V., 1971, Central control of movements, *Neurosci. Res. Bull.* **9**:1–170.

Evarts, E. V., Bizzi, E., Burke, R. E., DeLong, M., and Thach, W. T., Jr., 1971, Central control of movement, *Neurosci. Res. Bull.* **9**:1–170.

Evoy, W. H., and Beranek, R., 1972, Pharmacological localization of excitatory and inhibitory synaptic regions in crayfish slow abdominal flexor muscle fibers, *Comp. Gen. Pharmacol.* **3**:178–186.

Evoy, W. H., and Cohen, M. J., 1969, Sensory and motor interactions in the locomotor reflexes of crabs, *J. Exp. Biol.* **51**:151–169.

Evoy, W. H., and Cohen, M. J., 1971, Central and peripheral control of Arthropod movements, *Adv. Comp. Physiol. Biochem.* **4**:225–266.

Evoy, W. H., and Fourtner, C. R., 1973a, Crustacean walking, in: *Control of Posture and Locomotion* (R. B. Stein, K. G. Pearson, R. S. Smith, and J. B. Redford, eds.), pp. 477–493, Plenum Press, New York.

Evoy, W. H., and Fourtner, C. R., 1973b, Nervous control of walking in the crab *Cardisoma guanhumi.* III. Proprioceptive influences on intra- and inter-segmental coordination, *J. Comp. Physiol.* **83**:303–318.

Evoy, W. H., and Kennedy, D., 1967, The central nervous organization underlying control of antagonistic muscles in the crayfish. I. Types of command fibres, *J. Exp. Zool.* **165**:223–238.

Evoy, W. H., Kennedy, D., and Wilson, D. M., 1967, discharge patterns of neurons supplying tonic abdominal flexor muscles in the crayfish, *J. Exp. Biol.* **46**:393–411.

Ewing, A. W., 1969, The genetic basis of sound production in *Drosophila pseudoobscura* and *D. persimilis, Anim. Behav.* **17**:555–560.

Exner, S., 1891, *Die Physiologie der facettirten Augen von krebsen und Insecten,* Franz Deuticke, Leipzig.

Eyzaguirre, C., and Kuffler, S. W., 1955, Processes of excitation in the dendrites and in the soma of single isolated sensory nerve cells of the lobster and crayfish, *J. Gen. Physiol.* **39**:87–119.

Faeder, I. R., and Salpeter, M. M., 1970, Glutamate uptake by a stimulated insect nerve–muscle preparation, *J. Cell Biol.* **46**:300–307.

Farley, R. D., and Case, J. F., 1968, Sensory modulation of ventilative pacemaker output in the cockroach, *Periplaneta americana, J. Insect Physiol.* **14**:591–601.

Farley, R. D., Case, J. F., and Roeder, K. D., 1967, Pacemaker for tracheal ventilation in the cockroach, *Periplaneta americana* L., *J. Insect Physiol.* **13**:1713–1728.

Fatt, P., and Katz, B., 1953a, The effect of inhibitory nerve impulses on a crustacean muscle fibre, *J. Physiol. (London)* **121**:374–388.

Fatt, P., and Katz, B., 1953b, Distributed "end-plate" potentials of crustacean muscle fibres, *J. Exp. Biol.* **30**:433–439.

Fatt, P., and Katz, B., 1953c, The electrical properties of crustacean muscle fibres, *J. Physiol. (London)* **120**:171–204.

Fay, R. R., 1973, Multisensory interaction in control of eye-stalk rotation response in the crayfish *Procambarus clarkii, J. Comp. Physiol. Psychol.* **84**:527–533.

Fay, R. R., 1975, Dynamic properties of the compensatory eyestalk rotation response of the crayfish *Procambarus clarkii, Comp. Biochem. Physiol.* **51A,** 101–103.

Feldman, A. G., and Orlovsky, G. N., 1975, Activity of interneurons mediating reciprocal Ia inhibition during locomotion, *Brain Res.* **84:**181–194.

Fernandez, H. L., Huneeus, F. C., and Davison, P. F., 1970, Studies on the mechanism of axoplasmic transport in the crayfish cord, *J. Neurobiol.* **1:**395–409.

Fernandez, H. L., Burton, P. R., and Samson, F. E., 1971, Axoplasmic transport in the crayfish nerve cord, *J. Cell Biol.* **51:**176–197.

Fernandez, J. H., Soledad, M., and Fernandez, G., 1974, Morphological evidence for an experimentally induced synaptic field, *Nature (London)* **251:**428–430.

Fernlund, P., 1971, Chromactivating hormones of *Pandalus borealis;* isolation and purification of a light-adapting hormone, *Biochim. Biophys. Acta.* **237:**519–529.

Feynman, R. R., Leighton, R. B., and Sands, M., 1971, *The Feynman Lectures on Physics,* Vol. 1, Addison-Wesley, Reading, Mass.

Field, L. H., 1974, Sensory and reflex physiology underlying cheliped flexion behavior in hermit crabs, *J. Comp. Physiol.* **92:**397–414.

Field, L. H., and Larimer, J. L., 1975, Cardioregulatory system of crayfish: The role of circumesophageal interneurons, *J. Exp. Biol.* **62:**531–543.

Fields, H. L., 1966, Proprioceptive control of posutre in the crayfish abdomen, *J. Exp. Biol.* **44:**455–468.

Fields, H. L., 1976, Crustacean abdominal and thoracic MRO's, in: *Structure and Function of Proprioceptors in the Invertebrates* (P. J. Mill, ed.), Chapter 2, Chapman and Hall, London.

Fields, H. L., Evoy, W. H., and Kennedy, D., 1967, Reflex role played by efferent control of an invertebrate stretch receptor, *J. Neurophysiol.* **30:**859–874.

Finlayson, L. H., 1968, Proprioceptors in the invertebrates, *Symp. Zool. Soc. London* **23:**217–249.

Finlayson, L. H., 1976, Abdominal and thoracic receptors in insects, centipedes and scorpions, in: *Structure and Function of Proprioceptors in the Invertebrates* (P. J. Mill, ed.), pp. 153–211, Chapman and Hall, London.

Finlayson, L. H., and Lowenstein, O., 1958, The structure and function of abdominal stretch receptors in insects, *Proc. R. Soc. London Ser B* **148:**433–449.

Florey, E., 1973, Acetylcholine as sensory transmitter in Crustacea, *J. Comp. Physiol.* **83:**1–16.

Florey, E., 1975, The integrative capacity of chemical transmission at arthropod neuromuscular synapses, in: *"Simple" Nervous Systems* (P. N. R. Usherwood and D. R. Newth, eds.), pp. 323–344, Edward Arnold, London.

Florey, E., and Chapman, D. D., 1961, The non-identity of the transmitter substance of crustacean inhibitory neurons and gamma-aminobutyric acid, *Comp. Biochem. Physiol.* **3:**92–98.

Florey, E., and Hoyle, G., 1961, Neuromuscular synaptic activity in the crab, in: *Nervous Inhibition* (E. Florey, ed.), pp. 105–110, Pergamon, Oxford.

Florey, E., and Hoyle, G., 1976, The effects of temperature on nerve–muscle systems of the Hawaiian ghost crab, *Ocypode ceratophthalma* Pallas, *J. Comp. Physiol.* **110:**51–67.

Florey, E., and Rathmayer, W., 1972, Excitation of crustacean muscle by inhibitory neurons and GABA, *Pfluegers Arch.* **336:**359–362.

Florkin, M., 1975, Biochemical evolution in animals, *Comp. Biochem.* **29(B):**79–229.

Forssberg, H., and Grillner, S., 1973, The locomotion of the acute spinal cat injected with clonidine i.v., *Brain Res.* **50:**184–186.

Forssberg, H., Grillner, S., and Rossignol, S., 1975, Phase dependent reflex reversal during walking in chronic spinal cats, *Brain Res.* **85:**103–107.

Forssberg, H., Grillner, S., Rossignol, S., and Wallen, P., 1976, Phasic control of reflexes during locomotion in vertebrates, in: *Neural Control of Locomotion* (R. H. Herman, S. Grillner, P. S. G. Stein, and D. G. Stuart, eds.), Plenum Press, New York.

Fourtner, C., 1976, The central nervous system control of insect walking, in: *Neural Control of Locomotion* (R. H. Herman, S. Grillner, P. S. G. Stein, and D. G. Stuart, eds.), Plenum Press, New York.

Fourtner, C. R., and Evoy, W. H., 1973, Nervous control of walking in the crab *Cardiosoma guanhumi*. IV. Effects of myochordotonal organ ablation, *J. Comp. Physiol.* **83:**319–329.

Fraenkel-Conrat, H., 1933, Die Innervation der Krebsschere, *Z. Vgl. Physiol.* **19:**38–46.

Frank, E., 1973, Matching of facilitation at the neuromuscular junction of the lobster: A possible case for influence of muscle on nerve, *J. Physiol. (London)* **233:**635–658.

Frank, E., 1974, The sensitivity to glutamate of denervated muscles of the crayfish, *J. Physiol. (London)* **242:**371–382.

Frank, E., Jansen, J. K. S., and Rinvek, E., 1975, A multisomatic axon in the central nervous system of the leech, *J. Comp. Neurol.* **159:**1–14.

Frank, K., and Fuortes, M. G. F., 1957, Presynaptic and postsynaptic inhibition of monosynaptic reflexes, *Fed. Proc.* **16:**39–40.

Frantsevich, L. I., Mokrushov, P. A., Yushina, L. A., and Suprunovich, A. W., 1971, Role of the optomotor reaction of *Geotrupes* (Coleoptera Scarabaeidae) under natural conditions, *Vestn. Zool.* **2:**71–75.

Fraser, P. J., and Sandeman, D. C., 1975, Effects of angular and linear accelerations on semicircular canal interneurons of the crab *Scylla serrata*, *J. Comp. Physiol.* **96:**205–221.

Friesen, W. O., 1975, Antifacilitation and facilitation in the cardiac ganglion of the spiny lobster *Panulirus interruptus*, *J. Comp. Physiol.* **101:**207–224.

Fröhlich, F. W., 1907, Die Analyse der an der Krebsschere auftretenden Hemmungen, *Z. Allg. Physiol.* **7:**393–443.

Fulton, B. B., 1933, Inheritance of song in hybrids of two subspecies of *Nemobius fasciatus* (Orthoptera), *Ann. Entomol. Soc. Am.* **26:**368–376.

Furshpan, E. J., and Potter, D. D., 1959, Transmission at the giant motor synapses of the crayfish, *J. Physiol. (London)* **145:**289–325.

Gage, P. W., and Hubbard, J. I., 1966, An investigation of the post-tetanic potentiation of end-plate potentials at a mammalian neuromuscular junction, *J. Physiol. (London)* **184:**353–375.

Gainer, H., Reuben, J. P., and Grundfest, H., 1967, The augmentation of postsynaptic potentials in crustacean muscle fibers by cesium: A presynaptic mechanism, *Comp. Biochem. Physiol.* **20:**877–900.

Gambarian, P. P., Orlovsky, G. N., Protopopova, T. Y., Serverin, F. V., and Shik, M. L., 1971, The activity of muscles during different gaits and adaptive changes of moving organs in family Felidae: Morphology and ecology of vertebrates, *Proc. Inst. Zool. Acad. Sci. USSR* **48:**220–239.

Geduldig, D., and Junge, D., 1968, Sodium and calcium components of action potentials in the *Aplysia* giant neurone, *J. Physiol. (London)* **199:**347–365.

Geisler, M., 1961, Untersuchungen zur Tagesperiodik des Mistkäfers *Geotrupes silvaticus* Panz, *Z. Tierpsychol.* **18:**389–420.

Gerstein, G. L., and Perkel, D. H., 1972, Mutual temporal relationships among neuronal spike trains, *Biophys. J.* **12:**453–475.

Getting, P. A., 1974, Modification of neuron properties by electrotonic synapses. I. Input resistance, time constant and integration, *J. Neurophysiol.* **37:**846–857.

Getting, P. A., 1975, *Tritonia* swimming: Triggering of a fixed action pattern, *Brain Res.* **96:**128–133.

Getting, P. A., and Willows, A. O. D., 1974, Modification of neuron properties by electrotonic synapses. II. Burst formation by electrotonic synapses, *J. Neurophysiol.* **37:**858–868.

Gettrup, E., 1962, Thoracic proprioceptors in the flight system of locusts, *Nature (London)* **193:**498–499.

Gettrup, E., 1966, Sensory regulation of wing twisting in locusts, *J. Exp. Biol.* **44:**1–16.

Gewecke, M., 1974, The antennae of insects of air-current sense organs and their relationship to the control of flight, in: *Experimental Analysis of Insect Behaviour* (L. Barton-Brown, ed.), pp. 100–113, Springer-Verlag, Berlin.

Gilhousen, H. C., 1927, The use of vision and the antennae in the learning of crayfish, *Univ. Calif. Berkeley Publ. Physiol.* **7:**73–89.

Gillary, H. L., and Kennedy, D., 1969a, Pattern generation in a crustacean motoneuron, *J. Neurophysiol.* **32:**595–606.

Gillary, H. L., and Kennedy, D., 1969b, Neuromuscular effects of impulse pattern in a crustacean motoneuron, *J. Meurophysiol.* **32:**607–612.

Gillette, H. R., and Davis, W. J., 1975, Control of feeding behavior by the metacerebral giant neuron of *Pleurobranchaea, Neurosci. Abst.* **1:**571 (abst.).

Gillette, R., and Davis, W. J., 1977a, The role of the metacerebral giant neuron in the feeding behavior of *Pleurobranchaea, J. Comp. Physiol.* **A116:**129–159.

Gillette, R., and Davis, W. J., 1977b, The role of the ventral white cell of the buccal ganglion of *Pleurobranchaea* in the control of feeding behavior, in preparation.

Gillette, R., and Davis, W. J., 1977c, The role of the paracerebral command neurons in the control of feeding behavior of *Pleurobranchaea,* in preparation.

Gillette, R., and Pomeranz, B., 1973, Neuron geometry and circuitry via the electron microscope: Intracellular staining with osmiophilic polymer, *Science* **182:**1256–1257.

Gillette, R., Kovac, M. P., and Davis, W. J., 1976, Command neurons receive synaptic feedback from the motor networks they excite, submitted.

Glantz, R. M., 1968, Light adaptation in the photoreceptor of the crayfish, *Vision Res.* **8:**1407–1421.

Glantz, R. M., 1971, Peripheral versus central adaptation in the crustacean visual system, *J. Neurophysiol.* **34:**485–492.

Glantz, R. M., 1973a, Spatial integration in the crustacean visual system: Peripheral and central sources of non-linear summation, *Visual Res.* **13:**1801–1814.

Glantz, R. M., 1973b, Five classes of visual interneurons in the optic nerve of the hermit crab, *J. Neurobiol.* **4:**301–319.

Glantz, R. M., 1974a, The visually evoked defense reflex of the crayfish: Habituation, facilitation and the influence of picrotoxin, *J. Neurobiol.* **5:**263–280.

Glantz, R. M., 1974b, Habituation of the motion detectors of the crayfish optic nerve: Their relationship to the visually evoked defense reflex, *J. Neurobiol.* **5:**489–510.

Glantz, R. M., 1974c, Defense reflex and motion detector responsiveness to approaching targets: The motion detector trigger to the defense reflex pathway, *J. Comp. Physiol.* **95:**297–314.

Glegg, G. L., 1969, *The Design of Design,* 93 pp., Cambridge University Press, Cambridge.

Gola, M., 1977, Electrical properties of bursting pacemakers neurones, in press.

Goldsmith, T. H., 1975a, Photoreceptor processes: Some problems and perspectives, *J. Exp. Zool.* **194:**89–102.

Goldsmith, T. H., 1975b, The polarization sensitivity—dichroic absorption paradox in arthropod photo-receptors, in: *Photoreceptor Optics* (A. W. Snyder and R. Menzel, eds.), pp. 392–409, Springer-Verlag, New York.

Goldsmith, T. H., and Bernard, G. D., 1974, The visual system of insects, in: *The Physiology of Insects,* Vol. 2, 2nd ed. (M. Rockstein, ed.), pp. 165–272, Academic Press, New York.

Goodman, C. S., 1976, Constancy and uniqueness in a large population of small interneurons, *Science* **193:**502–504.

Goodman, L. J., 1965, The role of certain optomotor reactions in regulating stability in the rolling plane during flight in the desert locust, *Schistocerca gregaria, J. Exp. Biol.* **42:**385–407.

Gordon, W. H., and Larimer, J. L., 1975, Neural coupling mechanisms for reflexive and circadian movements, *Neurosci. Abst.* **1:**582.

Gordon, W. H., Larimer, J. L., and Page, T. L., 1977, Circumesophageal interneurons required for reflexive and circadian locomotor behaviors in crayfish, *J. Comp. Physiol.* in preparation.

Goslow, G. E., Jr., Reinking, R. M., and Stuart, D. G., 1973, The cat step cycles: Limb joint angles and muscle lengths during unrestrained locomotion, *J. Morphol.* **141:**1–41.

Goss, R., 1969, *Principals of Regeneration,* Academic Press, New York.

Götz, K. G., 1964, Optomotorische Untersuchung des visuellen Systems einiger Augenmutanten der Fruchtfliege *Drosophila, Kybernetik* **2:**77–92.

Govind, C. K., Atwood, H. L., and Lang, F., 1973, Synaptic differentiation in a regenerating crab-limb muscle, *Proc. Natl. Acad. Sci. USA* **70:**822–826.

Govind, C. K., Atwood, H. L., and Lang, F., 1974, Sarcomere length increases in developing crusta-cean muscle, *J. Exp. Zool.* **189:**395–400.

Graubard, K., 1975, Voltage attenuation within *Aplysia* neurons: The effect of branching pattern, *Brain Res.* **88**:325–332.

Gray, J., 1968, *Animal Locomotion,* 479 pp., Weidenfeld and Nicolson, London.

Gregory, G. E., 1974, Neuroanatomy of the mesothoracic ganglion of the cockroach *Periplaneta americana* L. I. The roots of peripheral nerves, *Philos. Trans. R. Soc. London Ser. B* **267**:421–465.

Gregory, G. E., 1977, Neuroanatomy of the mesothoracic ganglion of the cockroach *Periplaneta americana* L. II. Neuron cell body groups, in preparation.

Gribakin, F. C., 1975, Functional morphology of the compound eye of the bee, in: *The Compound Eye and Vision of Insects* (G. A. Horridge, ed.), pp. 154–176, Clarendon Press, Oxford.

Grillner, S., 1974, On the generation of locomotion in the spinal dogfish, *Exp. Brain Res.* **20**:459–470.

Grillner, S., 1975, Locomotion in vertebrates: Central mechanisms and reflex interaction, *Physiol. Rev.* **55**:247–304.

Grillner, S., 1976, Some aspects on the descending control of the spinal circuits generating locomotor movements, in *Neural Control of Locomotion* (R. H. Herman, S. Grillner, P. S. G. Stein, and D. G. Stuart, eds.), Plenum Press, New York.

Grillner, S., and Kashin, S. M., 1976, On the generation and performance of swimming in fishes, in: *Neural Control of Locomotion* (R. H. Herman, S. Grillner, P. S. G. Stein, and D. G. Stuart, eds.), Plenum Press, New York.

Grillner, S., and Shik, M. L., 1973, On the descending control of the lumbosacral spinal cord from the "mesencephalic locomotor region," *Acta Physiol. Scand.* **87**:320–333.

Grillner, S., and Zangger, P., 1974, Locomotor movements generated by the deafferented spinal cord, *Acta Physiol. Scand.* **91**:38–39A.

Grillner, S., and Zangger, P., 1975, How detailed is the central pattern generator for locomotion? *Brain Res.* **88**:367–371.

Grundfest, H., 1962, Ionic transport across neural and non-neural membranes, in: *Properties of Membrane and Diseases of the Nervous System* (M. Yahr, ed.), pp. 71–101, Springer, New York.

Grundfest, H., 1967, Comparative physiology of electric organs of elasmobranch fishes, in: *Sharks, Skates and Rays* (P. W. Gilbert, R. F. Mathewson, and D. P. Rall, eds.), John Hopkins Press, Baltimore.

Grundler, O. J., 1974, Elektronmikroskopische Untersuchungen am Auge der Honigbiene *Apis mellifica* L.: Untersuchungen zur Morphologie und Anordnung der neun Retinulazellen in Ommatidien verscheidener Augenbereiche und zur Perzeption linear polarisierten Lichtes, *Cytobiologie* **9**:203–220.

Guth, L., 1968, "Trophic" influences of nerve on muscle, *Physiol. Rev.* **48**:645–687.

Guth, L., 1969, "Trophic" effects of vertebrate neurons, *Neurosci. Res. Prog.* **7**:1–73.

Gurfinkel, V. S., and Shik, M. L., 1973, The control of posture and locomotion, in: *Motor Control* (A. A. Gydikov, T. T. Tankov, and Kosarov, P. M., eds), pp. 217–234, Plenum Press, New York.

Gymer, A., and Edwards, J. S., 1967, the development of the insect nervous system. I. An analysis of postembryonic growth in the terminal ganglion of *Acheta domesticus, J. Morphol.* **123**:191–197.

Hafner, G. S., 1973, The neural organization of the lamina ganglionaris in the crayfish: A Golgi study, *J. Comp. Neurol.* **152**:255–280.

Hafner, G. S., 1974, The ultrastructure of retinula cell endings in the compound eye of the crayfish, *J. Neurocytol.* **3**:295–311.

Hagins, W. A., and Liebman, P. A., 1962, Light induced pigment migration in the squid retina, *Biol. Bull.* **123**:498.

Hagiwara, S., 1958, Synaptic potential in the motor giant axon of the crayfish, *J. Gen. Physiol.* **41**:1119–1128.

Hagiwara, S., 1961, Nervous activities of the heart in crustacea, *Ergeb. Biol.* **24**:287–311.

Hagiwara, S., and Takahashi, K., 1967, Surface density of calcium ions and calcium spikes in the barnacle muscle fiber membrane, *J. Gen. Physiol.* **50**:583–601.

Hagiwara, S., Szabo, T., and Enger, P. S., 1965, Electroreceptor mechanisms in a high frequency weakly electric fish. *Sternarchus albifrons, J. Neurophysiol.* **28**:784–799.

Hajek, I., Chari, N., Bass, A., and Gutmann, E., 1973, Differences in contractile and some biochemical properties between fast and slow abdominal muscles of the crayfish, *Physiol. Bohemoslov.* **22:**603–612.

Halbertsma, J. M., Miller, S., and van der Meche, F. G. A., 1976, Basic "programs" for the phasing of flexion and extension movements of the limbs during locomotion, in:*Neural Control of Locomotion* (R. H. Herman, S. Grillner, P. S. G. Stein, and D. G. Stuart, eds.), Plenum Press, New York.

Hama, K., 1961, Some observations on the fine structure of the giant fibres of the crayfish *Cambarus virilus* and *Cambarus clarkii* with special reference to the submicroscopic organization of the synapses, *Anat. Rec.* **141:**275–293.

Hamilton, T., and Bittner, G. D., 1977, Trophic interactions and regenerative capabilities of motor axons, receptor muscles, and muscle receptor organs in crayfish, in preparation.

Hammond, A., 1879, On the thoras of the blow fly *Musca vornitoria, J. Linn. Soc.* **15:**9–31.

Hanström, B., 1927, Über die Frage ob funktionell verscheidene, zappen- und stabchenartige Sehzellen im Komplexauge der Arthropoden vorkommen, *Z. Vgl. Physiol.* **6:**566–597.

Harri, M., and Florey, E., 1977, The effects of temperature on a neuromuscular system of the crayfish *Astacus leptodactylus, J. Comp. Physiol.* **117:**47–61.

Harris, H., 1970, *Nucleus and Cytoplasm,* Clarenden Press, Oxford.

Harrison, R. G., 1935, The origin and development of the nervous system studied by the methods of experimental embryology: The Croonian Lecture *Proc. R. Soc. London Ser.* B **118:**155–196.

Hartline, D. K., 1967, Impulse identification and axon mapping of the nine neurons in the cardiac ganglion of the lobster *Homarus americanus, J. Exp. Biol.* **47:**327–340.

Hartline, D. K., and Maynard, D. M., 1975, Motor patterns in the stomatogastric ganglion of the lobster *Palinurus argus, J. Exp. Biol.* **62:**405–420.

Hartman, B., and Boettiger, E. G., 1967, The functional organization of the propus-dactylus organ in *Cancer irroratus* Say, *Comp. Biochem. Physiol.* **22:**651–663.

Hatt, H., 1974, Desensitization to the action of γ-aminobutyric acid (GABA) in crayfish: Different effects in the two muscles of the propodite, in: *Proceedings of the Twenty-sixth International Congress of Physiological Science* (abst.).

Hatt, H., and Smith, D. O., 1976a, Synaptic depression related to presynaptic axon conduction block, *J. Physiol. (London)* **259:**367–393.

Hatt, H., and Smith, D. O., 1976b, Nonuniform probabilities of quantal release at the crayfish neuromuscular junction, *J. Physiol. (London)* **259:**395–604.

Hays, D., and Goldsmith, T. H., 1969, Microspectrophotometry of the visual pigment of the spider crab *Libinia emarginata, Z. Vgl. Physiol.* **65:**218–232.

Heitler, W. J., 1974, The locust jump. Specialization of the metathoracic femoral-tibial joint, *J. Comp. Physiol.* **89:**93–104.

Heitler, W. J., and Burrows, M., 1977, The locust jump. I. The motor programme, *J. Exp. Biol.* **66:**203–220.

Heitler, W. J., Goodman, C. S., and Rowell, C. H. F., 1977, The effects of temperature on the threshold of identified neurons in the locust, *J. Comp. Physiol.* **117:**163–182.

Henneman, E., Somjen, G., and Carpenter, D., 1965a, Functional significance of cell size in spinal motoneurons, *J. Neurophysiol.* **28:**560–580.

Henneman, E., Somjen, G., and Carpenter, D., 1965b, Excitability and inhibitability of motoneurons of different sizes, *J. Neurophysiol.* **28:**599–620.

Herman, R. H., Grillner, S., Stein, P. S. G., and Stuart, D. G. (eds.), 1976, *Neural Control of Locomotion,* Plenum Press, New York.

Hermann, A., Rieske, E., Kreutzberg, G. W., and Lux, H. D., 1975, TGransjunctional flux of radioactive precursors across e.ectrotonic synapses between lateral giant axons of the crayfish, *Brain Res.* **95:**125–131.

Hertweck, H., 1931, Anatomie und Variabilität des Nervensystems und der Sinnesorgane von *Drosophila melanogaster* (Meigen), *Z. Wiss. Zool. Abt. A* **139:**559–663.

Heuser, J. E., and Reese, T. S., 1973, Evidence for recycling of synaptic vesicle membrane during transmitter release at the frog neuromuscular junction, *J. Cell Biol.* **57:**315–344.

Hibbard, E., 1965, Orientation and directed growth of cell axons from duplicated vestibular nerve roots, *Exp. Neurol.* **13:**289–301.

Highstein, S. M., and Bennett, M. V. L., 1975, Fatigue and recovery of transmission at the Mauthner fiber–giant fiber synapse of the hatchetfish, *Brain Res.* **98:**229–242.

Hill, D. K., 1968, Tension due to interaction between the sliding filaments in resting striated muscle: The effect of stimulation, *J. Physiol. (London)* **199:**637–684.

Hironaka, T., 1975, Excitatory potentials induced by stimulation of the inhibitory axon at the crustacean neuromuscular junction, *Jpn. J. Physiol.* **25:**79–91.

Hirsch, H. V. B., and Spinelli, D. N., 1970, Visual experience modifies distribution of horizontally and vertically oriented receptive fields in cuts, *Science* **168:**869–971.

Hirsh, R., and Wiersma, C. A. G., 1977, The effect of the spacing of background elements upon optomotor memory responses in the Hi crab: The influence of adding or deleting features during darkness, *J. Exp. Biol.,* **66:**33–46.

Hobbs, H. H., and Barr, T. C., 1960, The origins and affinities of the troglobitic crayfishes of North America (Decapoda, Astacidae). I. The genus *Cambarus, Am. Midl. Nat.* **64:**12–33.

Hobbs, H. H., and Barr, T. C., 1972, Origins and affinities of the troglobitic crayfishes of North American (Decapoda: Astacidae). II. Genus *Orconectes, Smithson. Contrib. Zool.* **105:**84.

Hobbs, H. H., and Means, D., 1971, Two new troglobitic crayfishes (Decapoda, Astacidae) from Florida, *Proc. Biol. Soc. Wash.* **84:**393–410.

Hochachka, P. W., and Mustafa, T., 1972, Invertebrate facultative anaerobiosis, *Science* **178:**1056–1060.

Hodgkin, A. L., 1938, The subthreshold potentials in a crustacean nerve fibre, *Proc. R. Soc. London Ser. B* **126:**247–285.

Hodgkin, A. L., 1948, The local electric changes associated with repetitive action in a non-medullated axon, *J. Physiol.* **107:**165–181.

Hodgkiss, J., 1976, Transmitter release from locust motoneurones, Ph.D. thesis, University of Glasgow.

Hoffmann, P., 1914, Über die doppelte Innervation der Krebsmuskeln: Zugleich ein Beitrag zur Kenntnis nervöser Hemmungen, *Z. Biol.* **63:**411–422. (Cited by Wiersma, 1961).

Hofmann, W. P., 1976, The morphology of depressor and remotor motoneurons in *Procambarus clarkii*, M.S. thesis, University of Miami.

Höglund, G., 1966, Pigment migration, light screening and receptor sensitivity in the compound eye of nocturnal Lepidoptera, *Acta Physiol. Scand.* **6a:**1–56 (Suppl. 282).

Holtzman, E., Freeman, A. R., and Kashner, L. A., 1971, Stimulation-dependent alterations in peroxidase uptake at lobster neuromuscular junctions, *Science* **173:**733–736.

Horn, G., and Rowell, C. H. F., 1968, Medium and long-term changes in the behavior of visual neurones in the tritocerebrum of locusts, *J. Exp. Biol.* **49:**143–169.

Horridge, G. A., 1965, Arthropoda: Receptors for light, and optic lobe, in: *Structure and Function in the Nervous Systems of Invertebrates* (T. H. Bullock and G. A. Horridge, eds.), pp. 1063–1113, Freeman, San Francisco.

Horridge, G. A., 1966*a,* Optokinetic memory in the crab *Carcinus, J. Exp. Biol.* **44:**233–245.

Horridge, G. A., 1966*b,* Perception of edges versus areas by the crab *Carcinus, J. Exp. Biol.* **44:**247 254.

Horridge, G. A., 1966*c,* Optokinetic memory in the locust, *J. Exp. Biol.* **44:**255–261.

Horridge, G. A., 1966*d,* Optokinetic response of the crab *Carcinus,* to a single moving light, *J. Exp. Biol.* **44:**263–274.

Horridge, G. A., 1966*e,* Direct response of the crab *Carcinus,* to the movement of the sun, *J. Exp. Biol.* **44:**275–283.

Horridge, G. A., 1966*f,* Adaptation and other phenomena in the optokinetic response of the crab *Carcinus, J. Exp. Biol.* **44:**285–295.

Horridge, G. A., 1966*g,* The retina of the locust, in: *The Functional Organization of the Compound Eye* (C. G. Bernhard, ed.), pp. 513–541, Pergamon Press, Oxford.

Horridge, G. A., 1968, Reception and integration in the compound eye, Chapter 9, pp. 145–173; Arthropod ventral cord, Chapter 7, pp. 108–126, in: *Interneurons,* Freeman, San Francisco.

Horridge, G. A., 1969*a*, The interpretation of behavior in terms of interneurons, in: *The Interneuron* (M. A. B. Brazier, ed.), pp. 1–20, University of California Press.

Horridge, G. A., 1969*b*, The eye of the firefly *Photuris, Proc. R. Soc. London Ser. B* **171**:445–463.

Horridge, G. A., 1972, Further observations on the clear zone eye of *Ephestia, Proc. R. Soc. London Ser. B* **181**:157–173.

Horridge, G. A., 1975*a*, Optical mechanism of clear zone eyes, in: *The Compound Eye and Vision of Insects* (G. A. Horridge, ed.), pp. 255–298, Oxford University Press, Oxford.

Horridge, G. A., 1975*b*, Arthropod receptor optics, in: *Photoreceptor Optics* (A. W. Snyder and R. Menzel, eds.), pp. 459–478, Springer-Verlag, New York.

Horridge, G. A., 1975*c*, *The Compound Eye and Vision of Insects,* 595 pp., Clarendon Press, Oxford.

Horridge, G. A., and Burrows, M., 1968*a*, Tonic and phasic systems in parallel in the eyecup responses of the crab, *Carcinus, J. Exp. Biol.* **49**:269–284.

Horridge, G. A., and Burrows, M., 1968*b*, The onset of the fast phase in the optokinetic response of the crab *Carcinus, J. Exp. Biol.* **49**:299–313.

Horridge, G. A., and Burrows, M., 1968*c*, Efferent copy and voluntary eyecup movement in the crab *Carcinus, J. Exp. Biol.* **49**:315–324.

Horridge, G. A., and Giddings, C., 1971, The ommatidium of the termite *Mastotermes darwiniensis, Tissue Cell.* **3**:463–476.

Horridge, G. A., and Henderson, I., 1976, The ommatidium of the lacewing *Chrysopa* (Neuroptera), *Proc. R. Soc. London Ser. B* **192**:259–271.

Horridge, G. A., and Meinertzhagen, I. A., 1970, The exact neural projection of the visual fields upon the first and second ganglia of the insect eye, *Z. Vgl. Physiol.* **66**:369–378.

Horridge, G. A., and Mimura, K., 1975, Fly photoreceptors. I. Physical separation of two visual pigments in *Calliphora* retinula cells 1–6, *Proc. R. Soc. London Ser. B* **190**:211–224.

Horridge, G. A., and Sandeman, D. C., 1964, Nervous control of optokinetic responses in the crab *Carcinus, Proc. R. Soc. London Ser. B* **167**:216–246.

Horridge, G. A., and Shepheard, P. R. B., 1966, Perception of movement by the crab, *Nature (London)* **209**:267–269.

Horridge, G. A., Giddings, C., and Stange, G., 1972, The superposition eye of skipper butterflies, *Proc. R. Soc. London Ser. B* **182**:457–495.

Horridge, G. A., Mimura, K., and Tsukahara, Y., 1975, Fly photoreceptors. II. Spectral and polarized light sensitivity in the drone fly *Eristalis, Proc. R. Soc. London Ser. B* **190**:225–237.

Horridge, G. A., Mimura, K., and Hardie, R. C., 1976, Fly photoreceptors. III. Angular sensitivity as a function of wavelength and the limits of resolution, *Proc. R. Soc. London Ser. B* **144**:151–177.

Houk, J. C., 1972, The phylogency of muscular control configurations, in: *Biocybernetics IV* (V. E. B. Gustav, ed.), pp. 125–144, Fischer Verlag, Jena.

Hoy, R. R., 1969, Degeneration and regeneration in abdominal flexor motor neurons in the crayfish, *J. Exp. Zool.* **172**:219–232.

Hoy, R. R., 1973, The curious nature of degeneration and regeneration in motor neurons and central connectives of the crayfish, in: *Developmental Neurobiology of Arthropods* (D. Young, ed.), Cambridge University Press, Cambridge.

Hoy, R. R., Bittner, G. D., and Kennedy, D., 1967, Regeneration in crustacean motoneurons: Evidence for axonal fusion, *Science* **156**:251–252.

Hoyle, G., 1955, The anatomy and innervation of locust skeletal muscle, *Proc. R. Soc. London Ser. B* **143**:281–292.

Hoyle, G., 1957, The nervous control of insect muscle, in: *Recent Advances in Invertebrate Physiology* (B. T. Scheer, ed.), pp. 73–97, University of Oregon Press, Corvallis, Ore.

Hoyle, G., 1960, The action of carbon dioxide gas on an insect spiracular muscle, *J. Insect Physiol.* **4**:63–79.

Hoyle, G., 1961, Functional contracture in a spiracular muscle, *J. Ins. Physiol.* **7**:305–314.

Hoyle, G., 1964, Exploration of neuronal mechanisms and underlying behavior in insects, in: *Neural Theory and Modelling* (R. F. Reiss, ed.), pp. 346–375, Stanford University Press, California.

Hoyle, G., 1966, Functioning of the inhibitory conditioning axon innervating insect muscles, *J. Exp. Biol.* **44:**429–453.

Hoyle, G., 1968, Resting tension, "negative" contraction and "break" contraction in specialized crustacean muscle fibers, *J. Exp. Zool.* **167:**551–566.

Hoyle, G., 1970, Cellular mechanisms underlying behavior—Neuroethology, *Adv. Insect Physiol.* **7:**349–444.

Hoyle, G., 1973, Correlated physiological and ultrastructural studies on specialized muscles. III. Fine structure of the power-stroke muscle of the swimming leg of *Portunus sanguinolentus, J. Exp. Zool.* **185:**97–110.

Hoyle, G., 1974, A function for neurons (DUM) neurosecretory on skeletal muscle of insects, *J. Exp. Zool.* **189:**401–406.

Hoyle, G., 1975a, Identified neurons and the future of neuroethology, *J. Exp. Zool.* **194:**51–74.

Hoyle, G., 1975b, Evidence that insect dorsal unpaired median (DUM) neurons are octopaminergic, *J. Exp. Zool.* **193:**425–431.

Hoyle, G., and Barker, D. L., 1975, Synthesis of octopamine by insect dorsal median unpaired neurons, *J. Exp. Zool.* **193:**433–439.

Hoyle, G., and Burrows, M., 1973a, Neural mechanisms underlying behavior in the locust *Schistocerca gregaria.* I. Physiology of identified neurons in the metathoracic ganglion, *J. Neurobiol.* **4:**3–41.

Hoyle, G., and Burrows, M., 1973b, Neural mechanisms underlying behavior in the locust *Schistocerca gregaria.* II. Integrative activity in metathoracic neurons, *J. Neurobiol.* **4:**43–67.

Hoyle, G., and Burrows, M., 1973c, Correlated physiological and ultrastructural studies on specialized muscles. IIIa. Neuromuscular physiology of the power-stroke muscle of the swimming leg of *Portunus sanguinolentus, J. Exp. Zool.* **185:**83–96.

Hoyle, G., and O'Shea, M., 1974, Intrinsic rhythmic contractions in insect skeletal muscle, *J. Exp. Zool.* **189:**407–412.

Hoyle, G., and Wiersma, C. A. G., 1958a, Excitation at neuromuscular junctions in crustacea, *J. Physiol. (London)* **143:**403–425.

Hoyle, G., and Wiersma, C. A. G., 1958b, Inhibition at neuromuscular junctions in crustacea, *J. Physiol. (London)* **143:**426–440.

Hoyle, G., and Wiersma, C. A. G., 1958c, Coupling of membrane potential to contraction in crustacean muscles, *J. Physiol. (London)* **143:**441–453.

Hoyle, G., Dagan, D., Moberly, B., and Colquhoun, W., 1974, Dorsal unpaired median insect neurons make neurosecretory endings on skeletal muscle, *J. Exp. Zool.* **187:**159–165.

Hubbard, J., 1970, Mechanism of transmitter release, *Prog. Biophys. Mol. Biol.* **21:**35–124.

Hubbard, J. I., Llinas, R., and Quastel, D. M. J., 1969, in: *Electrophysiological Analysis of Synaptic Transmission,* pp. 66–68, Williams and Wilkins, Baltimore.

Huber, F., 1960a, Untersuchungen zur nervösen Atmungsregulation der Orthopteren (Saltatoria: Gryllidae), *Z. Vgl. Physiol.* **43:**359–391.

Huber, F., 1960b, Untersuchungen uber die Funktion des Zentralnervensystems und insbesondere des Gehirnes bei der Fortbewegung und der Lauterzeugung der Grillen, *Z. Vgl. Physiol.* **44:**60–132.

Huber, F., 1974, Neural integration (central nervous system), in: *The Physiology of Insecta* Vol. 4, 2nd ed. (M. Rockstein, ed.), pp. 3–100, Academic Press, New York.

Hughes, A. F. W., 1968, *Aspects of Neural Ontogeny,* Logos Press, New York.

Hughes, G. M., 1965, Neuronal pathways in the insect central nervous system, in: *The Physiology of the Insect Central Nervous System* (J. E. Treherne and J. W. L., Beament, eds.), pp. 74–112, Academic Press, New York.

Hughes, G. M., and Mill, P. J., 1966, Patterns of ventilation in dragonfly larvae, *J. Exp. Biol.* **44:**314–333.

Hughes, G. M., and Wiersma, C. A. G., 1960a, Neuronal pathways and synaptic connections in the abdominal cord in the crayfish, *J. Exp. Biol.* **37:**291–307.

Hughes, G. M., and Wiersma, C. A. G., 1960b, The coordination of swimmeret movements in the crayfish *Procambarus clarkii, J. Exp. Biol.* **37:**657–670.

Hunt, R. K., and Jacobson, M., 1974, Neuronal specificity revisited, *Curr. Top. Dev. Biol.* **8:**203–259.

Ikeda, K., 1965, The electrical activity of the longitudinal muscle of the fly, *Musca domestica, Proc. Int. Union Physiol. Sci.* **6:**286.

Ikeda, K., 1974, Patterned motor activities released by anesthetics, *Proc. Int. Union Physiol. Sci.* **11:**160.

Ikeda, K., and Kaplan, W. D., 1970, Patterned neural activity of a mutant *Drosophila melanogaster, Proc. Natl. Acad. Sci. USA* **66:**765–772.

Ikeda, K., and Kaplan, W. D., 1974, Neurophysiological genetics in *Drosophila melanogaster, Am. Zool.* **14:**1055–1066.

Ikeda, K., and Wiersma, C. A. G., 1964, Autogenic rhythmicity in the abdominal ganglia of the crayfish: The control of swimmeret movements, *Comp. Biochem. Physiol.* **12:**107–115.

Ikeda, K., Tsuruhara, T., and Hori, N., 1975, Motor innervation of the dorsal longitudinal flight muscle of *Drosophila melanogaster, Am. Zool.* **15:**789.

Iles, J. F., 1972, Structure and synaptic activation of the fast coxal depressor motoneurone of the cockroach, *Periplaneta americana, J. Exp. Biol.* **56:**647–656.

Iles, J. F., and Mulloney, B., 1971, Procion yellow staining of cockroach motorneurons without the use of microelectrodes, *Brain Res.* **30:**397–400.

Jack, J. J. B., Noble, D., and Tsien, R. W., 1975, in: *Electric Current Flow in Excitable Cells,* pp. 59–66. Oxford University Press, Oxford.

Jacobson, M., 1970, *Developmental Neurobiology,* 465 pp., Holt, New York.

Jahromi, S. S., and Atwood, H. L., 1974, Three-dimensional ultrastructure of the crayfish neuromuscular apparatus, *J. Cell biol.* **63:**599–613.

Jander, R., 1963, Grundleistungen der Licht- und Schwereorientierung von Insekten, *Z. Vgl. Physiol.* **47:**381–430.

Jander, R., and Waterman, T. H., 1960, Sensory discrimination between polarized light and light intensity patterns by arthropods, *J. Cell. Comp. Physiol.* **56:**137–160.

Jander, R., Daumer, K., and Waterman, T. H., 1963, Polarized light orientation by two Hawaiian decapod cephalopods, *Z. Vgl. Physiol.* **46:**383–394.

Jankowska, E., and Roberts, W. J., 1972, Synaptic actions of single interneurons mediating reciprocal Ia inhibition of motoneurones, *J. Physiol. (London)* **222:**623–642.

Jankowska, E., Jukes, M. G. M., Lund, S., and Lundberg, A., 1967a, The effect of DOPA on the spinal cord. 5. Reciprocal organization of pathways transmitting excitatory action to alpha motoneurones of flexors and extensors, *Acta Physiol. Scand.* **70,** 369–388.

Jankowska, E., Jukes, M. G. M., Lund, S., and Lundberg, A., 1967b, The effect of DOPA on the spinal cord. 6. Half-centre organization of interneurones transmitting effects from the flexor reflex afferents, *Acta Physiol. Scand.* **70:**389–402.

Jensen, M., 1956, Biology and physics of locust flight. III. The aerodynamics of locust flight, *Philos. Trans. R. Soc. London Ser. B* **239:**511–552

Johansson, A. S., 1957, The nervous system of the milkweed bug, *Oncopeltus fasciatus* (Dallas) (Heteroptera, Lygaeidae), *Trans. Am. Entomol. Soc.* **83:**119–183.

John, E. R., 1972, Switchboard versus statistical theories of learning and memory, *Science* **177:**850–864.

Johnson, E. W., and Wernig, A., 1971, The binomial nature of transmitter release at the crayfish neuromuscular junction, *J. Physiol. (London)* **218:**757–767.

Johnson, G. E., 1924, Giant nerve fibers in crustaceans with special reference to *Cambarus* and *Palaemontes, J. Comp. Neurol.* **36:**323–373.

Jordan, L. M., and Steeves, J. D., 1976, Chemical lesioning of the spinal noradrenaline pathway: Effects on locomotion in the cat, in: *Neural Control of Locomotion* (R. H. Herman, S. Grillner, P. S. G. Stein, and D. G. Stuart, eds.), Plenum Press, New York.

Junge, D., and Stephans, C. L., 1973, Cyclic variation of potassium conductance in a burst-generating neurone in *Aplysia, J. Physiol. (London)* **235:**155–181.

Kaiser, W., 1975, The relationship between visual movement detection and colour vision in insects, in:

The Compound Eye and Vision of Insects (G. A., Horridge, ed.), pp. 359–377, Oxford University Press, Oxford.

Kaiser, W., and Liske, E., 1974, Die optomotorischen Reaktionen von fixiert fliegenden Bienen bei Reizung mit Spektrallichtern, *J. Comp. Physiol.* **89**:391–408.

Kalmring, K., 1975*a*, The afferent auditory pathway in the ventral card of *Locusta migratoria* (Acrididae). I. Synaptic connectivity and information processing among the auditory neurons of the ventral cord, *J. Comp. Physiol.* **104**:103–142.

Kalmring, K., 1975*b*, The afferent auditory pathway in the ventral cord of *Locusta migratoria* (Acrididae). II. Responses of the auditory ventral cord neurons to natural sounds, *J. Comp. Physiol.* **104**:143–160.

Kalmus, H., 1938, Das Aktogram des Flusskrebses und seine Beeinflussung durch Organextrakte, *Z. Vgl. Physiol.* **25**:798–802.

Kandel, E. R., 1974, An invertebrate system for the cellular analysis of simple behavior, in: *The Neurosciences: Third Study Program* (F. O. Schmitt and F. G. Worden, eds.), pp. 347–370, M.I.T. Press, Cambridge, Mass.

Kandel, E. R., Castellucci, V., Pinsker, H., and Kupfermann, I., 1970, The role of synaptic plasticity in the short-term modification of behaviour, in: *Short-Term Changes in Neural Activity and Behaviour* (G. Horn and R. A. Hinde, eds.), pp. 281–322, Cambridge University Press, London.

Kanellis, A., 1952, Anlagenplan und Regulationserscheinungen in der Keimanlage des Eies von *Gryllus domesticus, Wilhelm Roux Arch. Entwicklungsmech. Org.* **145**:417–461.

Kao, C. Y., 1960, Postsynaptic electrogenesis in septate giant axons. II. Comparison of medial and lateral giant axons of crayfish, *J. Neurophysiol.* **23**:618–635.

Kashin, S. M., Feldman, A. G., and Orlovsky, G. N., 1974, Locomotion of fish evoked by electrical stimulation of the brain, *Brain Res.* **82**:41–45.

Kater, S. B., 1974, Feeding in *Helisoma trivolvis:* The morphological and physiological bases of a fixed action pattern, *Am. Zool.* **14**:1017–1036.

Kater, S. B., Nicholson, C., and Davis, W. J., 1973, Intracellular dye injection techniques, in: *Intracellular Staining Techniques in Neurobiology* (S. B. Kater and C. Nicholson eds.), pp. 307–325, Springer-Verlag, New York.

Katz, B., 1936, Neuromuscular transmission in crabs, *J. Physiol. (London)* **87**:199–221.

Katz, B., 1949, Neuro-muscular transmission in invertebrates, *Biol. Rev.* **24**:1–20.

Katz, B., 1966, *Nerve Muscle and Synapse,* 193 pp., McGraw-Hill, New York.

Katz, B., and Kuffler, S. W., 1946, Excitation of the nerve-muscle system in crustacea, *Proc. R. Soc. London Ser. B* **133**:374–389.

Katz, B., and Miledi, R., 1965, Propagation of electric activity in motor nerve terminals, *Proc. R. Soc. London Ser. B* **161**:453 482.

Katz, B., and Miledi, R., 1967*a*, Tetrodotoxin and neuromuscular transmission, *Proc. R. Soc. London Ser. B* **167**:8–22.

Katz, B., and Miledi, R., 1967*b*, The release of acetylcholine from nerve endings by graded electric pulses, *Proc. R. Soc. London Ser. B* **167**:23–38.

Katz, B., and Miledi, R., 1967*c*, A study of synaptic transmission in the absense of nerve impulses, *J. Physiol. (London)* **192**:407–436.

Katz, B., and Miledi, R., 1968, The role of calcium in neuromuscular facilitation, *J. Physiol. (London)* **195**:481–492.

Katz, B., and Miledi, R., 1969, Tetrodotoxin-resistant electric activity in presynaptic terminals, *J. Physiol. (London)* **203**:459–487.

Katz, B., and Thesleff, S., 1957, A study of the "desensitization" produced by acetylcholine at the motor end-plate, *J. Physiol. (London)* **138**:63–80.

Kendig, J. J., 1968, Motor neuron coupling in locust flight, *J. Exp. Biol.* **48**:389–404.

Kennedy, D., 1963, Physiology of photoreceptor neurons in the abdominal nerve cord of the crayfish, *J. Gen Physiol.* **46**:551–572.

Kennedy, D., 1968, Input and output connections of single arthropod neurons, in: *Physiological and*

Biochemical Aspects of Nervous Integration (F. D. Carlson, ed.), pp. 285–306. Prentice-Hall, Englewood Cliffs, N. J.

Kennedy, D., 1969, The control of output by central neurons, in: *The Interneuron* (M. A. B. Brazier, ed.), pp. 21–36, University of California Press, Los Angeles.

Kennedy, D., 1973, Control of motor output, in: *Control of Posture and Locomotion* (R. B. Stein, K. G. Pearson, R. S. Smith, and J. B. Redford, eds.), pp. 429–436, Plenum Press, New York.

Kennedy, D., 1974, Connections among neurons of different types in crustacean nervous systems, in: *The Neurosciences: Third Study Program* (F. O. Schmitt and F. G. Worden, eds.), pp. 379–388, M.I.T. Press, Cambridge, Mass.

Kennedy, D., 1975, Comparative strategies in the investigation of neural networks, *J. Exp. Zool.* **194:**35–50.

Kennedy, D., and Bittner, G. D., 1974, Ultrastructural correlates of motor nerve regeneration in crayfish, *Cell. Tissue Res.* **148:**97–110.

Kennedy, D., and Davis, W. J., 1977, The organization of invertebrate motor systems, in: *Handbook of Physiology,* Vol. 2: *Neurophysiology,* 2nd ed. (E. R. Kandel, ed.), American Physiological Society, Bethesda, Md.

Kennedy, D., and Evoy, W. H., 1966, The distribution of pre- and postsynaptic inhibition at crustacean neuromusclar junctions, *J. Gen. Physiol.* **49:**457–468.

Kennedy, D., and Mellon, DeF., 1964, Synaptic activation and receptive fields in crayfish interneurons, *Comp. Biochem. Physiol.* **13:**275–300.

Kennedy, D., and Takeda, K., 1965*a*, Reflex control of abdominal flexor muscles in the crayfish. I. The twitch system, *J. Exp. Biol.* **43:**211–227.

Kennedy, D., and Takeda, K., 1965*b*, The reflex control of abdominal flexor muscles in the crayfish. II. The tonic system, *J. Exp. Biol.* **43:**229–246.

Kennedy, D., Evoy, W. H., and Fields, H. L., 1965, The unit basis of some crustacean reflexes, *Symp. Soc. Exp. Biol.* **20:**75–109.

Kennedy, D., Evoy, W. H., and Hanawalt, J. T., 1966, Release of coordinated behavior in crayfish by single central neurons, *Science* **154:**917–919.

Kennedy, D., Evoy, W. H., Dane, B., and Hanawalt, J. T., 1967, The central nervous organization underlying control of antagonistic muscles in the crayfish. II. Coding of position by command fibers, *J. Exp. Zool.* **165:**239–248.

Kennedy, D., Selverston, A. I., and Remler, M. P., 1969, Analysis of restricted neural networks, *Science* **164:**1488–1496.

Kennedy, D., Calabrese, R. L., and Wine, J. J., 1974, Presynaptic inhibition: Primary afferent depolarization in crayfish neurons, *Science* **186:**451–454.

Kerkut, G. A., and Walker, R. J., 1966, The effect of L-glutamate, acetylcholine, and gamma-aminobutyric acid on the miniature end-plate potentials and contractures of the coxal muscles of the cockroach, *Periplaneta americana, Comp. Biochem. Physiol.* **17:**435–454.

Kerkut, G. A., Shapira, A., and Walker, R. J., 1965, The effect of acetylcholine, glutamic acid and GABA on the contractions of the perfused cockroach leg, *Comp. Biochem. Physiol.* **16:**37–48.

Kernell, D., 1966, Input resistance, electrical excitability and size of ventral horn cells in the cat spinal cord, *Science* **152:**1637–1640.

Kien, J., 1974, Sensory integration in the locust optomotor system. I. Behavioural analysis, *Vision Res.* **14:**245–254.

Kien, J., 1975, Neuronal mechanisms subserving directional selectivity in the locust optomotor system, *J. Comp. Physiol.* **102:**337–355.

King, D. G., 1976, Organization of crustacean neuropil: Synapses of identified motor neurons in lobster stomatogastric ganglion, Ph.D. thesis, University of California, San Diego.

Kirschfeld, K., 1972, The visual system of *Musca:* Studies on optics, structure and function, in: *Information Processing in the Visual Systems of Arthropods* (R. Wehner, ed.), pp. 61–74, Springer-Verlag, New York.

Kirschfeld, K., 1973*a,* Das neurale Superpositionsauge, in: *Fortschritt d. Zoologie* Vol. 21 (M. Lindauer, ed.), pp. 229–257, Gustav Fischer, Stuttgart.

Kirschfeld, K., 1973*b*, Optomotorische Reaktionen der Biene auf bewegte Polarisations-Muster, *Z. Naturforsch.* **28**:329–338.

Kirschfeld, K., and Snyder, A. W., 1975, Waveguide mode effects, birefringence and dichroism in fly photoreceptors, in: *Photoreceptor Optics* (A. W. Snyder and R. Menzel, eds.), pp. 56–77, Springer-Verlag, New York.

Kleinholz, L. H., 1949, Responses of the proximal retinal pigment of the isolated crustacean eyestalk to light and to darkness, *Proc. Natl. Acad. Sci. USA* **35**:215–218.

Kleinholz, L. H., 1966, Hormonal regulation of retinal pigment migration in crustaceans, in: *The Functional Organization of the Compound Eye* (C. G. Bernhard, ed.), pp. 89–101, Pergamon Press, London.

Kling, U., and Szekely, G., 1968, Stimulation of rhythmic nervous activities. I. Function of networks with cyclic inhibitions, *Kybernetik* **5**:89–103.

Koester, J., Mayeri, E., Liebeswar, G., and Kandel, E. R., 1974, Neural control of circulation in *Aplysia*. II. Interneurons, *J. Neurophysiol.* **37**:476–496.

Konopka, R. J., and Benzer, S., 1971, Clock mutants of *Drosophila melanogaster, Proc. Natl. Acad. Sci. USA* **68**:2112–2116.

Kramer, A. P., 1976, New motor coordinating interneurons used by giant and nongiant escape systems in the crayfish, *Procambarus clarkii, Neurosci. Abst.* **2**:459.

Krasne, F., 1969, Excitation and habituation of the crayfish escape reflex: The depolarizing response in lateral giant fibres of the isolated abdomen, *J. Exp. Biol.* **50**:29–46.

Krasne, F. B., 1976, Invertebrate systems as a means of gaining insight into the nature of learning and memory, in: *Neural Mechanisms of Learning and Memory* (M. R. Rosenzweig and E. L. Ennnett, eds.), pp. 401–429, M.I.T. Press, Cambridge, Mass.

Krasne, F. B., and Bryan, J., 1973, Habituation: Regulation via presynaptic inhibition, *Science* **182**:582–584.

Krasne, F. B., and Roberts, A., 1967, Habituation of the crayfish escape response during release from inhibiton induced by picrotoxin, *Nature (London)* **215**:769–770.

Krasne, F. B., and Wine, J. J., 1975, Extrinsic modulation of crayfish escape behavior, *J. Exp. Biol.* **63**:433–450.

Krasne, F. B., and Woodsmall, K. S., 1969, Waning of the crayfish escape response as a result of repeated stimulation, *Anim. Behav.* **17**:416–424.

Krauhs, J. M., and Mirolli, M., 1975, Morphological changes associated with stretch in a mechano-receptor, *J. Neurocytol.* **4**:231–246.

Kravitz, E. A., Kuffer, S. W., Potter, D. D., and Van Gelder, W. M., 1963*a*, Gamma-amino butyric acid and other blocking compounds in crustacea. II. Peripheral nervous system, *J. Neurophysiol.* **26**:729–738.

Kravitz, E. A., Kuffler, S. W., and Potter, D. D., 1963*b*, Gamma-aminobutyric acid and other blocking compounds in crustacea. III. Their relative concentrations in separated motor and inhibitory axons, *J. Neurophysiol.* **26**:739–751.

Kravitz, E. A., Molinoff, P. B., and Hall, Z. W., 1967, A comparison of the enzymes and substrates of gamma-aminobutyric acid metabolism in lobster excitatory and inhibitory axons, *Proc. Natl. Acad. Sci. USA* **54**:778–782.

Kravitz, E. A., Batelle, B.-A., Evans, P. D., Talamo, B. R., and Wallace, B. G., 1976, Octopamine neurones in lobsters, *Soc. Neurosci. Symp.* **1**:67–81.

Krebs, W., 1972, The fine structure of the retinula of the compound eye of *Astacus fluviatilis, Z. Zellforsch. Mikrosk. Anat.* **133**:399–414.

Kriebel, M. E., and Gross, C. E., 1974, Multimodal distribution of frog miniature endplate potentials in adult, denervated, and tadpole leg muscle, *J. Gen. Physiol.* **64**:85–103.

Kristan, W. B., Jr., Stent, G. S., and Ort, C. A., 1974, Neuronal control of swimming in the medicinal leech. III. Impulse patterns of motor neurons, *J. Comp. Physiol.* **94A**:155–176.

Krnjevic, K., and Miledi, R., 1959, Presynaptic failure of neuromuscular propagation in rats, *J. Physiol (London)* **149**:1–22.

Kuffler, S. W., and Katz, B., 1946, Inhibition at the nerve-muscle junction in crustacea, *J. Neurophysiol.* **9**:337–346.

Kulagin, A. S., and Shik, M. L., 1970, Interaction of symmetrical limbs during controlled locomotion, *Biophysics* **11**:879–886.

Kuno, M., Turkanis, S. A., and Weakley, J. N., i971, Correlation between nerve terminal size and transmitter release at the neuromuscular junction of the frog, *J. Physiol. (London)* **213**:545–556.

Kunze, P., 1963, Der Einfluss der Grosse bewegter Felder auf den optokinetischen Augenstielnystagmus der Winker-Krabbe, *Ergeb. Biol.* **26**:55–62.

Kunze, P., 1964, Eyestalk reactions of the ghost crab *Ocypode,* in: *Neural Theory and Modelling* (R. F. Reiss, ed.), pp. 293–305, Stanford University Press, Stanford, Calif.

Kunze, P., 1967, Histologische Untersuchungen zum Bau des Auges von *Ocypode cursor* (Brachyura), *Z. Zellforsch. Mikrosk. Anat.* **82**:466–478.

Kunze, P., 1972, Comparative studies of arthropod superposition eyes, *Z. Vgl. Physiol.* **76**:347–357.

Kunze, P., and Boschek, C. G., 1968, Elektronenmikroskopische Untersuchung zur Form der achten Retinulazelle bei *Ocypode, Z. Naturforsch.* **23**:568b–569b.

Kusano, K., and Grundfest, H., 1965, Circus reexcitation as a cause of repetitive activity in crayfish lateral giant axons, *J. Cell. Comp. Physiol.* **65**:325–336.

Kusano, K., and Landau, E. M., 1975, Depression and recovery of transmission at the squid giant synapse, *J. Physiol. (London)* **245**:13–32.

Kutsch, W., 1968, Neuromuskuläre Aktivität bei verschiedenen Verhaltensweisen von drei Grillenarten, Ph.D. thesis, University of Köln, German Federal Republic.

Kutsch, W., 1971, The development of the flight pattern in the desert locust, *Schistocerca gregaria, Z. Vgl. Physiol.* **74**:156–168.

Kutsch, W., 1974, The development of the flight pattern in locusts, in: *Experimental Analysis of Insect Behaviour* (L. Barton Browne, ed.), pp. 149–158, Springer-Verlag, New York.

Labhart, T., 1974, Behavioural analysis of light intensity discrimination and spectral sensitivity in the honey bee, *Apis mellifera, J. Comp. Physiol.* **95**:203–216.

Labhart, T., and Wiersma, C. A. G., 1976, Habituation and inhibition in a class of visual interneurons of the rock lobster, *Panulirus interruptus, Comp. Biochem. Physiol.* **55A**:219–224.

Lang, F., and Atwood, H. L., 1973, Crustacean neuromuscular mechanisms: Functional morphology of nerve terminals and the mechanism of facilitation, *Am. Zool.* **13**, 337–355.

Larimer, J. L., 1964, Sensory-induced modifications of ventilation and heart rate in crayfish, *Comp. Biochem. Physiol.* **12**:25–36.

Larimer, J. L., 1976, Command interneurons and locomotor behavior in crustaceans, in: *Neural Control of Locomotion* (R. Herman, S. Grillner, P. S. G. Stein, and D. G. Stuart, eds.), Plenum Press, New York.

Larimer, J. L., and Eggleston, A. C., 1971, Motor programs for abdominal positioning in crayfish, *Z. Vgl. Physiol.* **74**:388–402.

Larimer, J. L., and Kennedy, D., 1969, Innervation patterns of fast and slow muscle in the uropods of crayfish, *J. Exp. Biol.* **51**:119–133.

Larimer, J. L., Trevino, D. L., and Ashby, E. A., 1966, A comparison of spectral sensititives of caudal photoreceptors of epigeal and cavernicolous crayfish, *Comp. Biochem. Physiol.* **19**:409–415.

Larimer, J. L., Eggleston, A. C., Masukawa, L. M., and Kennedy, D., 1971, The different connections and motor outputs of lateral and medial giant fibres in the crayfish, *J. Exp. Biol.* **54**:391–402.

Lasek, R. L., Dabrowski, C., and Nordlander, R., 1973, Analysis of RNA from invertebrate giant axons, *Nature (London)* **136**:162–165.

Lasek, R. L., Gainer, H., and Przybylski, R. J., 1974, Transfer of newly synthetized proteins from Schwann cells to the squid giant axon, *Proc. Natl. Acad. Sci. USA* **71**:1188–1192.

Laughlin, S. B., 1975, The function of the lamina ganglionaris, in: *The Compound Eye and Vision in Insects* (G. A. Horridge, ed.), Clarendon Press, Oxford.

Laverack, M. S., 1962, Responses of cuticular sense organs of the lobster *Homarus vulgaris* (Crustacea). II. Hair-fan organs as pressure receptors, Comp. Biochem. Physiol. **6**:137–145.

Lea, T., and Usherwood, P. N. R., 1970, Increased chloride permeability of insect muscle fibres on exposure to ibotenic acid, *J. Physiol. (London)* **211:**32P.

Lea, T., and Usherwood, P. N. R., 1973*a*, Effect of ibotenic acid on chloride permeability of insect muscle fibres, *Comp. Gen. Pharmacol.* **4:**351–363.

Lea, T. J., and Usherwood, P. N. R., 1973*b*, The site of action of ibotenic acid and the identification of two populations of glutamate receptors on insect muscle fibres, *Comp. Gen. Pharmacol.* **4:**333–350.

Leggett, L. M. W., 1976, Polarized light-sensitive interneurones in a swimming crab, *Nature* **262:**709–711.

Lennard, P. R., 1975, Neural control of swimming in the turtle, Ph.D. thesis, Washington University, St. Louis.

Lennard, P. R., and Stein, P. S. G., 1974, Control of swimming in the turtle by electrical stimulation of the spinal cord, *Proceedings of the 4th Annual Meeting of the Society of Neurosciences,* p. 303.

Lennard, P. R., and Stein, P. S. G., 1977, Swimming movements elicited by electrical stimulation of the turtle spinal cord. I. The low spinal and the intact preparations, *J. Neurophysiol.,* in press.

Leroy, Y., 1966, Signaux acoustiques, comportement et sytematique de quelque éspèces de Gryllides (Orthoptéres, Ensiferes), *Bull. Biol. Fr. Belg.* **100:**63–134.

Lettvin, J. Y., Maturana, H. R., McCulloch, W. S., and Pitts, W. H., 1959, What the frog's eye tells the frog's brain, *Proc. Inst. Radio Eng.* **47:**1940–1951.

Levine, J. D., and Hughes, M., 1973, Stereotaxic map of the muscle fibers in the indirect flight muscles of *Drosophila melanogaster, J. Morphol.* **140:**153–158.

Leveine, J. D., and Wyman, R. J., 1973, Neurophysiology of flight in wild-type and mutant *Drosophila, Proc. Natl. Acad. Sci. USA* **70:**1050–1054.

Lewis, G. M., Miller, P. L., and Mills, P. S., 1973, Neuromuscular mechanisms of abdominal lpumping in the locust, *J. Exp. Biol.* **59:**149–168.

Liley, A. W., and North, K. A. K., 1953, An electrical investigation of effects of repetitive stimulation on mammalian neuromuscular junction, *J. Neurophysiol.* **16:**509–527.

Linder, T. M., 1973, Calcium and facilitation at two classes of crustacean neuromuscular synapses, *J. Gen. Physiol.* **61:**56–73.

Linder, T. M., 1974, The accumulative properties of facilitation at crayfish neuromuscular synapses, *J. Physiol. (London)* **238:**223–234.

Lømo, T., and Rosenthal, J., 1972, Control of acetylcholine sensitivity by muscle activity in the rat, *J. Physiol. (London)* **221:**493–513.

LoPresti, V., Macagno, E. R., and Levinthal, C., 1973, Structure and development of neuronal connections in isogenic organisms: Cellular interactions in the development of the optic lamina of *Daphnia, Proc. Natl. Acad. Sci. USA* **70:**433–437.

Lorente de Nó, R., and Condouris, G. A., 1959, Decremental conduction in peripheral nerve: Integration of stimuli in the neuron, *Proc. Natl. Acad. Sci. USA* **45:**592–617.

Lowenstein, O., and Finlayson, L. H., 1960, The response of the abdominal stretch receptor of an insect to phasic stimulation, *Comp. Biochem. Physiol.* **1:**56–61.

Lucas, K., 1907, The analysis of complex excitable tissue by their response to electric currents of short duration, *J. Physiol. (London)* **35:**310–331.

Lucas, K., 1917, On summation of propagated disturbances in the claw of *Astacus* and on the double neuro-muscular system of the abductor, *J. Physiol. (London)* **51:**1–35.

Ludolph, C., Pagnanelli, D., and Mote, M. I., 1973, Neural control of migration of proximal screening pigment by retinular cells of the swimming crab, *Callinectes sapidus, Biol. Bull.* **145:**159–170.

Luks, C., 1883, Über die Brustmuskulatur der Insecten, Jena, *Z. Naturwiss.* **16:**529–552.

Lundberg, A., 1969, Reflex control of stepping, *The Nansen Memorial Lecture V,* pp. 1–42, Universitetsforlaget, Oslo.

Macagno, E. R., Lopresti, V., and Levinthal, C., 1973, Structure and development of neuronal connection in isogenic organisms: Variations and similarities in the optic system of *Daphnia magna, Proc. Natl. Acad. Sci. USA* **70:**57–61.

MacMillan, D. L., 1975, A physiological analysis of walking in the american lobster, *Homarus americanus, Philos. Trans. R. Soc. London Ser. B* **270**:1–59.

MacMillan, D. L., 1976, Arthropod tension receptors, in: *Structure and Function of Proprioceptors in the Invertebrates* (P. J. Mill, ed.), Chapter 10, Chapman and Hall, London.

MacMillan, D. L., and Dando, M. R., 1972, Tension receptors on the apodemes of muscles in the walking legs of the crab, *Cancer magister, Mar. Behav. Physiol.* **1**:185–208.

Magleby, K. L., 1973*a*, The effect of repetitive stimulation on transmitter release at the frog neuromuscular junction, *J. Physiol. (London)* **234**:327–352.

Magleby, K. L., 1973*b*, The effect of tetanic and post-tetanic potentiation on facilitation of transmitter release at the frog neuromuscular junction, *J. Physiol. (London)* **234**:353–371.

Magleby, K. L., and Zengel, J. E., 1975*a*, A dual effect of repetitive stimulation on post-tetanic potentiation of transmitter release at the frog neuromuscular junction, *J. Physiol. (London)* **245**:163–182.

Magleby, K. L., and Zengel, J. E., 1975*b*, A quantitative description of tetanic and post-tetanic potentiation of transmitter release at the frog neuromuscular junction, *J. Physiol. (London)* **245**:183–208.

Malzacher, P., 1968, Die Embryogenese des Gehirnes paurometaboler Insekten: Untersuchungen an *Carausius morosus* und *Periplaneta americana, Z. Morph. Oekol. Tiere.* **62**:103–161.

Mangold, E., 1905, Untersuchungen über die Endigungen der Nerven in den guergestreiften Muskeln der Arthropoden, *Z. Allg. Physiol.* **5**:135–205.

Manton, S. M., 1969*a*, Introduction to classification of Arthropoda, in: *Treatise on Invertebrate Paleontology,* Vol. 1 (R. C. Moore, ed.), pp. R3-R15, Part R (Arthropoda 4), University of Kansas Press, Lawrence, Ks.

Manton, S. M., 1969*b*, Evolution and affinities of Onychophora, Myriapoda, Hexapoda and Crustacea, in: *treatise on Invertebrate Paleontology,* Vol. 1 (R. C. Moore, ed.), pp. R15–R56, Part R (Arthropoda 4), University of Kansas Press, Lawrence, Ks.

Manton, S. M., 1973, Arthropod phylogeny—A modern synthesis, *J. Zool. Soc. (London)* **171**:111–130.

Marcu, O., 1929, Nervenendigungen an den Muskefasern von Insekten, *Anat. Anz.* **67**:369–380.

Marder, E., 1974, Acetylcholine as an excitatory neuromuscular transmitter in the stomatogastric system of the lobster, *Nature (London)* **251**:730–731.

Mark, R., 1974, *Memory and Nerve Cell Connections,* pp. 85–88, Oxford University Press, New York.

Mark, R. F., Marotte, L. R., and Mart, P. E., 1972, The mechanism of selective reinnervation of fish eye muscles. IV. Identification of repressed synapses, *Brain Res.* **46**:149–157.

Markert, C. L., 1975, *Isozymes I: Molecular structure,* 879 pp., *Isozymes II: Physiological Function,* 912 pp., *Isozymes III: Developmental Biology,* 1056 pp., *Isozymes IV: Genetics and Evolution,* pp. 978, Academic Press, New York.

Marler, P., and Tamura, M., 1964, Culturally transmitted patterns of vocal behavior in sparrows, *Science* **146**:1483–1486.

Marmont, G., and Wiersma, C. A. G., 1938, On the mechanism of inhibition and excitation of crayfish muscle, *J. Physiol. (London)* **93**:173–193.

Martin, A. R., 1955, A further study of the statistical composition of the end-plate potential, *J. Physiol. (London)* **130**:114–122.

Martin, A. R., 1976, Effect of membrane capacitance on nonlinear summation of synaptic potentials, *J. Theoret. Biol.* **59**:179–187.

Mathers, D. A., and Usherwood, P. N. R., 1976, Concanavalin A blocks desensitization of glutamate receptors on insect muscle fibres, *Nature (London)* **259**:409–411.

Matsumoto, S. G., and Murphy, R. K., 1977, Sensory deprivation during development decreases the responsiveness of cricket giant interneurones, *J. Physiol.* **268**:533–548.

Matthews, P. B. C., 1972, *Mammalian Muscle Receptors and Their Central Actions,* Edward Arnold, London.

Maturana, H. R., Lettvin, J. Y., McCulloch, W. S., and Pitts, W. H., 1960, Anatomy and physiology of vision in the frog *Rana pipiens, J. Gen. Physiol. Suppl.* **43**:129–175.

Maynard, D. M., 1955, Direct inhibition in the lobster cardiac ganglion, Ph.D. thesis, University of California, Los Angeles.

Maynard, D. M., 1966, Integration in crustacean ganglia, *Symp. Soc. Exp. Biol.* **20**:111–149.

Maynard, D. M., 1972, Simpler networks, *Ann. N.Y. Acad. Sci.* **193**:59–72.

Maynard, D. M., and Cohen, M. J., 1965, The function of a heteromorph antennule in a spiny lobster, *Panulirus argus, J. Exp. Biol.* **43**:55–78.

Maynard, D. M., and Dingle, H., 1963, An effect of eyestalk ablation on antennular function in the spiny lobster, *Panulirus argus, Z. Vgl. Physiol.* **46**:515–540.

Maynard, D. M., and Selverston, A. I., 1975, Organization of the stomatogastric ganglion of the spiny lobster. IV. The pyloric system, *J. Comp. Physiol.* **100**:161–182.

Maynard, D. M., and Walton, K., 1975, Effects of maintained depolarization of presynaptic neurons on inhibitory transmission in lobster neuropil, *J. Comp. Physiol.* **97**:215–243.

Mayrat, A., 1956, Oeil, centres optiques et glandes endocrines de *Praunus flexuosus* (O. F. Muller) (Crustacés Mysidacés), *Arch. Zool. Exp. Gen.* **93**:319–366.

Mayrat, A., 1962, Premier résultats d'une étude au microscope électronique des yeux des Crustacés, *C. R. Acad. Sci. Paris* **255**:766–768.

McKinlay, R. G., and Usherwood, P. N. R., 1973, The role of the synaptic vesicles in transmission at the insect nerve–muscle junction, *Life Sci.* **13**:1051–1056.

McLachlan, E. M., 1975a, An analysis of the release of acetylcholine from preganglionic nerve terminals, *J. Physiol. (London)* **245**:447–466.

McLachlan, E. M., 1975b, Changes in statistical release parameters during prolonged stimulation of preganglionic nerve terminals, *J. Physiol. (London)* **253**:477–491.

McLean, M. R., and Edwards, J. S., 1977, Target discrimination in regenerating insect sensory nerve, *J. Embryol. Exp. Morphol.*, in press.

Meech, R. W., and Standen, N. B., 1975, Potassium activation in *Helix aspersa* under voltage clamp: A component mediated by calcium influx, *J. Physiol. (London)* **249**:211–239.

Melamed, J., and Trujillo-Cenóz, O., 1968, The fine structure of the central cells in the ommatidia of Dipterans, *J. Ultrastruct. Res.* **21**:313–334.

Mellon, DeF., 1977a, Retention of oculomotor reflexes in visually-deprived cave-dwelling crayfish, *Brain Res.*, in press.

Mellon, DeF., 1977b, The anatomy and motor nerve distribution of the eye muscles in the crayfish, *J. Comp. Physiol.*, in press.

Mellon, DeF., and Lorton, E. D., 1977, Reflex actions of the functional divisions in the crayfish oculomotor system, *J. Comp. Physiol.*, in press.

Mellon, DeF., Tufty, R. M., and Lorton, E. D., 1976, Analysis of spatial constancy of oculomotor neurons in the crayfish, *Brain Res.* **109**:587–594.

Mendelson, M., 1971, Oscillator neurons in crustacean ganglia, *Science* **171**:1170–1173.

Mendenhall, B., and Murphey, R. K., 1974, The morphology of cricket giant interneurons, *J. Neurobiol.* **5**:565–580.

Menzel, R., 1973, Spectral response of moving detecting and "sustaining" fibres in the optic lobe of the bee, *J. Comp. Physiol.* **82**:135–150.

Menzel, R., 1974, Spectral sensitivity of monopolar cells in the bee lamina, *J. Comp. Physiol.* **93**:337–346.

Menzel, R., 1975a, Polarization sensitivity in insect eyes with fused rhabdoms, in: *Photoreceptor Optics* (A. W. Snyder and R. Menzel, eds.), pp. 372–387, Springer-Verlag, New York.

Menzel, R., 1975b, Colour receptors in insects, in: *The Compound Eye and Vision of Insects* (G. A. Horridge), pp. 121–153, Oxford University Press, New York.

Menzel, R., and Blakers, M., 1975, Functional organization of an insect ommatidium with fused rhabdom, *Cytobiologie* **2**:279–298.

Menzel, R., and Snyder, A. W., 1974, Polarized light detection in the bee, *Apis mellifera, J. Comp. Physiol.* **88**:247–270.

Menzel, R., and Snyder, A. W., 1975, Introduction to photoreceptor optics—an overview, in: *Photoreceptor Optics* (A. W. Snyder and R. Menzel, eds.), pp. 1–37, Springer-Verlag, New York.

Meyer, M. R., 1973, Unidirectional slow transport in axons of crayfish ventral nerve cord, *Am. Zool.* **13**:216A.

Meyer, M. R., and Bittner, G. D., 1977a, Histological evidence for trophic dependencies of crayfish giant axons, *Brain Res.,* in press.

Meyer, M. R., and Bittner, G. D., 1977b, Biochemical evidence for trophic dependencies of crayfish giant axons, *Brain Res.,* in press.

Meyer-Rochow, V. B., 1971, A crustacean-like organization of insect rhabdoms, *Cytobiologie* **4:**241–249.

Meyer-Rochow, V. B., 1974, The dioptric system in beetle compound eyes, in: *The Compound Eye and Vision of Insects* (G. A. Horridge, ed.), pp. 299–313, Clarendon Press, Oxford.

Meyer-Rochow, V. B., 1975, Larval and adult eye of the western rock lobster *Panulirus longipes, Cell Tissue Res.* **162:**439–457.

Meyer-Rochow, V. B., and Horridge, G. A., 1975, The eye of *Anoplognathus* (Coleoptera, Scarabaeidae), *Proc. R. Soc. London Ser. B* **188:**1–30.

Mihályi, F., 1935, Untersuchungen über Anatomie und Mechanik der Flügorgane an der Stubenfliege, *Ung. Biol. Forsch.* **1:**106–119.

Miledi, R., 1973, Transmitter release induced by injection of calcium ions into nerve terminal, *Proc. R. Soc. London Ser. B* **183:**421–425.

Miledi, R., and Thies, R., 1971, Tetanic and post-tetanic rise in frequency of miniature end-plate potentials in low-calcium solutions, *J. Physiol. (London)* **212:**245–257.

Mill, P. J., 1963, Neural activity in the abdominal nervous system of aeschnid nymphs, *Comp. Biochem. Physiol.* **8:**83–98.

Mill, P. J., 1964, The structure of the abdominal nervous system of Aeschnid nymphs, *J. Comp. Neurol.* **122:**157–171.

Mill, P. J., 1965, An anatomical study of the abdominal nervous and muscular system of dragonfly (Aeschnidae) nymphs, *Proc. Zool. Soc.* **145:**57–73.

Mill, P. J., 1970, Neural patterns associated with ventilatory movements in dragonfly larvae, *J. Exp. Biol.* **52:**167–175.

Mill, P. J., 1972, *Respiration in the Invertebrates,* pp. 212, Macmillan, London.

Mill, P. J., 1974, Respiration: Aquatic insects, in: *The Physiology of Insecta,* Vol. 6, 2nd ed. (M. Rockstein, ed.), pp. 403–467, Academic Press, New York.

Mill, P. J., 1976, Chordotonal organs of crustacean appendages, in: *Structure and Function of Proprioceptors in the Invertebrates* (P. J. Mill, ed.), Chapter 6, Chapman and Hall, London.

Mill, P. J., and Hughes, C. M., 1966, The nervous centrol of ventilation in dragonfly larvae, *J. Exp. Biol.* **44:**297–316.

Mill, P. J., and Lowe, D. A., 1971a, Ultrastructure of the respiratory and non-respiratory muscles of the larvae of a dragonfly, *J. Insect Physiol.* **17:**1947–1960.

Mill, P. J., and Lowe, D. A., 1971b, Transduction processes of movement and position sensitive cells in a crustacean limb proprioceptor, *Nature (London)* **229:**206–208.

Mill, P. J., and Lowe, D. A., 1973, The fine structure of the PD proprioceptor of *Cancer pagurus.* I. The receptor strand and the movement sensitive cells, *Proc. R. Soc. London Ser. B* **184:**179–197.

Mill, P. J., and Pickard, R. S., 1972a, A review of the types of ventilation and their neural control in aeshnid larvae, *Odonatologica* **1:**41–50.

Mill, P. J., and Pickard, R. S., 1972b, Anal valve movement and normal ventilation in aeshnid dragonfly larvae, *J. Exp. Biol.* **56:**537–543.

Mill, P. J., and Pickard, R. S., 1975, Jet-propulsion in anisopteran dragonfly larvae, *J. Comp. Physiol.* **97:**324–338.

Miller, J. P., 1975, Neuropil recording in the lobster stomatogastric ganglion, *Neurosci. Abst.* **1:**579.

Miller, P. L., 1960a, Respiration in the desert locust. I. The control of ventilation, *J. Exp. Biol.* **37:**224–236.

Miller, P. L., 1960b, Respiration in the desert locust. III. Ventilation and the spiracles during flight, *J. Exp. Biol.* **37:**264–278.

Miller, P. L., 1962, Spiracle control in adult dragonflies (Odonata), *J. Exp. Biol.* **39:**513–535.

Miller, P. L., 1964, Factors altering spiracle control in adult dragonflies: Hypoxia and temperature, *J. Exp. Biol.* **41:**345–357.

Miller, P. L., 1965, The central nervous control of respiratory movements, in: *The Physiology of the Insect Central Nervous System* (J. E. Treherne and J. W. L. Beament, eds.), pp. 141–155, Academic Press, New York.

Miller, P. L., 1967, The derivation of the motor command to the spiracles of the locust, *J. Exp. Biol.* **46**:349–371.

Miller, P. L., 1969, Inhibitory nerves to insect spiracles, *Nature (London)* **221**:171–173.

Miller, P. L., 1971, Rhythmic activity in the insect nervous system: Thoracic ventilation in non-flying beetles, *J. Insect Physiol.* **17**:395–405.

Miller, P. L., 1973, Spatial and temporal changes in the coupling of cockroach spiracles to ventilation, *J. Exp. Biol.* **59**:137–148.

Miller, P. L., 1974a, Respiration: Aerial gas transport, in: *The Physiology of Insecta,* 2nd ed. (M. Rockstein, ed.), Academic Press, New York.

Miller, P. L., 1974b, The neural basis of behaviour, in: *Insect Neurobiology* (J. E. Treherne, ed.), pp. 359–430, North-Holland, Amsterdam.

Miller, S., and van der Burg, J., 1973, The function of long propriospinal pathway in the coordination of quadrupedal stepping the cat, in: *Control of Posture and Locomotion* (R. B. Stein, K. B. Pearson, R. S. Smith, and J. B. Redford, eds.), pp. 561–577, Plenum Press, New York.

Minkiewiez, R., 1907, Amylase experimentale de l'instinct de déguisement chez les Brochyures Oxyrhynches, *Arch. Zool. Exp. Gen.* **7**:37–67.

Mittenthal, J. E., and Wine, J. J., 1973, Connectivity patterns of crayfish giant interneurons: Visualization of synaptic regions with cobalt dye, *Science* **179**:182–184.

Mirolli, M., 1974, Evidence for a metabolically dependent electronic process contributing to the resting potential of a crustacean stretch receptor, *Physiologist* **17**:289.

Miyamoto, M. D., 1975, Binomial analysis of quantal transmitter release at glycerol treated frog neuromuscular junctions, *J. Physiol. (London)* **250**:121–142.

Moody, C., 1970, Aproximally directed intersegmental reflex in a walking leg of the crayfish, *Am. Zool.* **10**:501.

Möss, D., 1971, Sinnesorgene im Bereich des Flügels der Feldgrille (*Gryllus campestris* L.) und ihre Biudetung für die Kontrolle der Singbewegung und die Einstellunge der Flugellage, *Z. Vergl. Physiol.* **73**:53–83.

Moulins, M., 1976, Ultrastructure of chordotonal organs, in: *Structure and Function of Proprioceptors in the Invertebrates* (P. J. Mill, ed.), Chapman and Hall, London.

Müller, J., 1835, On the peculiar properties of nerves, in: *Handbuch der Physiologie des Menschen für Vorlesungen,* Vol. 1, Book 3, Section 4, 2nd ed., Coblene.

Mulloney, B., 1970, Organization of flight motor neurons, *J. Neurophysiol.* **33**:86–95.

Mulloney, B. M., and Selverston, A. I., 1974a, Organization of the stomatogastric ganglion of the spiny lobster, *J. Comp. Physiol.* **91**:1–32.

Mulloney, B. M., and Selverston, A. I., 1974b, Organization of the stomatogastric ganglion in the spiny lobster. III. Coordination of the two subsets of the gastric system, *J. Comp. Physiol.* **91**:53–78.

Munk, O., 1966, Ocular anatomy of some deep-sea teleosts, *Dana-Rep. Carlsberg Found.* **70**:1–62.

Munz, F. W., and McFarland, W. N., 1973, The significance of spectral position in the rhodopsins of tropical marine fishes, *Vision Res.* **13**:1829–1874.

Murphey, R. K., 1973, Characterization of an insect neuron which cannot be visualized *in situ,* in: *Intracellular Staining in Neurobiology* (S. B. Kater and C. Nicholson eds.), pp. 135–150, Springer-Verlag, New York.

Murphey, R. K., and Matsumoto, S. G., 1976, Experience modifies the plastic properties of identified neurons, *Science* **191**:564–566.

Murphey, R. K., Matsumoto, S. G., and Levine, R. B., 1975, Habituation and its modification by experience in cricket giant interneurons, *Soc. Neurosci. Abst.*

Murphey, R. K., Mendenhall, B., Palka, J., and Edwards, J. S., 1975, Deafferentation slows the growth of specific dendrites of identified giant interneurons, *J. Comp. Neurol.* **159**:407–418.

Murphey, R. K., Matsumoto, S. G., and Mendenhall, B., 1976, Recovery from deafferentation by cricket interneurons after reinnervation by their peripheral field, *J. Comp. Neurol.* **169**:335–347.

Myers, T., and Fisk, F. W., 1962, Breathing movements of the cuban burrowing cockroach, *Ohio J. Sci.* **62**:253–257.

Myers, T., and Retzlaff, E., 1963, Localization and action of the respiratory centre of the cuban burrowing cockroach, *J. Insect. Physiol.* **9**:607–611.

Nässel, D. R., 1975, The organization of the lamina ganglionaris of the prawn, *Pandalus borealis* (Kröyer), *Cell Tissue Res.* **163**:445–464.

Nässel, D. R., 1976, The retina and retinal projection on the lamina ganglionaris of the crayfish *Pacifastacus leniusculus* (Dana), *J. Comp. Neurol.* **167**:341–360.

Nastuk, W. L., 1967, Activation and inactivation of muscle post junctional receptors of frog skeletal muscle, *J. Gen. Physiol.* **56**:218–249.

Neder, R., 1959, Allometrisches Wachstum von Hirnteilen be drei verschieden grossen Schabenarten, *Zool. Jahrb. Abt. Anat. Ontog. Tiere* **77**:411–464.

Nelson, R., Lützow, A. V., Kolb, H., and Gouras, P., 1975, Horizontal cells in cat retina with independent dendritic systems, *Science* **189**:137–139.

Nemanic, P., 1975, Fine structure of the compound eye of *Porcellis scaber* in light and dark adaption, *Tissue Cell* **7**:453–468.

Nordlander, R. H., and Singer, M., 1972, Electron microscopy of severed motor fibres in the crayfish, *Z. Zellforsch. Mikrosk. Anat.* **126**:157–181.

Nordlander, R. H., and Singer, M., 1973, Degeneration and regeneration of severed crayfish sensory fibers: An ultrastructural study, *J. Comp. Neurol.* **152**:175–192.

Nordlander, R. H., and Singer, M., 1976, Synaptoid profiles in regenerating crustacean peripheral nerves, *Cell Tissue Res.* **166**:445–461.

Nordlander, R. H., Masnyi, J. A., and Singer, M., 1975, Distribution of ultrastructural tracers in crustacean axons, *J. Comp. Neurol.* **161**:499–514.

Northrop, R. B., 1974, Information processing in the insect compound eye, in: *The Compound Eye and Vision in Insects* (G. A. Horridge, ed.), pp. 378–408, Clarendon Press, Oxford.

Nunnemacher, R. F., 1966, The fine structure of optic tracts of Decapoda, in: *The functional Organization of the Compound Eye* (C. G. Bernhard, ed.), pp. 363–375, Pergamon Press, London.

Nunnemacher, R. F., Camougis, G., and McAlear, J. H., 1962, The fine structure of the crayfish nervous system, *Proc. Vth Int. Congr. Electron Microsc.* **2**:N-11.

Ochs, S., 1972, Fast transport of materials in mammalian nerve fibers, *Science* **176**:252–260.

Ohly, K. P., 1975, The neurons of the first synaptic region of the optic neuropil of the firefly *Phausis splendidula* L. (Coleoptera), *Cell Tissue Res.* **158**:89–109.

Onodera, K., and Takeuchi, A., 1975, Ionic mechanism of the excitatory synaptic membrane of the crayfish neuromuscular junction, *J. Physiol. (London)* **252**:295–318.

Orchard, I., 1975, Structure and properties of the abdominal chordotoral organ in the stick insect *Carausius morosus* and the cockroach *(Blaberus discoidalis)*, *J. Insect Physiol.* **21**:1491–1500.

Orkand, R. K., 1962a, The relation between membrane potential and contraction in single crayfish muscle fibres, *J. Physiol. (London)* **161**:143–159.

Orkand, R. K., 1962b, Chemical inhibition of contraction in directly stimulated crayfish muscle fibres, *J. Physiol. (London)* **164**:103–115.

Orlovsky, G. N., 1970, The activity of reticulo spinal neurones during locomotion, *Biofizika* **15**:728–737.

Orlovsky, G. N., 1972, The effect of different descending systems on flexor and extensor activity during locomotion, *Brain Res.* **40**:359–371.

Ort, C. A., Kristan, W. B., Jr., and Stent, G. S., 1974, Neuronal control of swimming in the medicinal leech. II. Identification and connections of motor neurons, *J. Comp. Physiol.* **94A**:121–154.

Ortiz, C. L., 1972, Crayfish neuromuscular junction: Facilitation with constant nerve terminal potential, *Experientia* **28**:1035–1036.

Ortiz, C. L., and Bracho, H., 1972, Effect of reduced calcium on excitatory transmitter release at the crayfish neuromuscular junction, *Comp. Biochem. Physiol.* **41A**:805–812.

Osborne, M. P., 1975, The ultrastructure of nerve-muscle synapses, in: *Insect Muscle* (P. N. R. Usherwood, ed.), pp. 151–205, Academic Press, New York.

Osborne, M. P., Finlayson, L. H., and Rice, M. J., 1971, Neurosecretory endings associated with striated muscles in three insects (*Schistocera, Carausius,* and *Phormia*) and a frog (*Rana*), *Z. Zellforsch. Mikrosk. Anat.* **116:**391–404.

O'Shea, M., 1975, Two sites of axonal spike initiation in a bimodal interneuron, *Brain Res.* **96:**93–98.

O'Shea, M., and Rowell, C. H. F., 1975*a*, Protection from habituation by lateral inhibition, *Nature (London)* **254:**53–55.

O'Shea, M., and Rowell, C. H. F., 1975*b*, A spike-transmitting electrical synapse between visual interneurones in the locust movement detector system, *J. Comp. Physiol.* **97:**143–158.

O'Shea, M., and Rowell, C. H. F., 1976, The neuronal basis of a sensory analyser, the acridid movement detector system. II. Response decrement, convergence, the nature of the excitatory afferents to the LGMD, *J. Exp. Biol.* **65:**289–308.

O'Shea, M., and Williams, J. L. D., 1974, The anatomy and output connection of a locust visual interneurone; the lobular giant movement detector (LGMD) neurone, *J. Comp. Physiol.* **91:**257–266.

O'Shea, M., Rowell, C. H. F., and Williams, J. L. D., 1974, The anatomy of a locust visual interneurone: The descending contralateral movement detector, *J. Exp. Biol.* **60:**1–12.

Otsuka, M., Iversen, L. L., Hall, I. W., and Kravitz, E. A., 1966, Release of gamma-aminobutyric acid from inhibitory nerves of lobster, *Proc. Natl. Acad. Sci. USA* **56:**1110–1115.

Otsuka, M., Kravitz, E. A., and Potter, D. D., 1967, Physiological and chemical architecture of a lobster ganglion with particular reference to gamma-aminobutyrate and glutamate, *J. Neurophysiol.* **30:**725–752.

Pabst, H., 1965, Electrophysiologische Untersuchungen des Streckrezeptors am Flügelgelenk der Wanderheuschrecke *Locusta migratoria, Z. Vgl. Physiol.* **50:**498–541.

Pabst, H., and Schwartzkopff, J., 1962, Zur Leistung der Flügelgelenk von *Locusta migratoria, Z. Vgl. Physiol.* **45:**396–404.

Page, C. H., 1975, Command fiber control of crayfish abdominal movement. II. Generic differences in the extension reflexes of *Orconectes* and *Procambarus, J. Comp. Physiol.* **102:**77–84.

Page, C. H., and Sokolove, P. G., 1972, Crayfish muscle receptor organ: Role in regulation of postural flexion, *Science* **175:**647–650.

Page, T. L., and Larimer, J. L., 1972, Entrainment of the circadian locomotor activity rhythm in crayfish: The role of the eyes and caudal photoreceptor, *J. Comp. Physiol.* **78:**107–120.

Page, T. L., and Larimer, J. L., 1975*a*, Neural control of circadian rhythmicity in the crayfish. I. The locomotor activity rhythm, *J. Comp. Physiol.* **97:**59–80.

Page, T. L., and Larimer, J. L., 1975*b*, Neural control of circadian rhythmicity in the crayfish. II. The ERG amplitude rhythm, *J. Comp. Physiol.* **97:**81–96.

Page, T. L., and Larimer, J. L., 1976, Extraretinal photoreception in entrainment of crustacean circadian rhythms, *J. Photochem. Photobiol.* **23:**245–251.

Palka, J., 1965, Diffraction and visual activity in insects, *Science* **149:**551–553.

Palka, J., 1967*a*, An inhibitory process influencing visual responses in a fibre of the ventral nerve cord of locusts, *J. Insect Physiol.* **13:**235–248.

Palka, J., 1967*b*, Head movement inhibits locust visual units response to target movement, *Am. Zool.* **7:**728.

Palka, J., 1969, Discrimination between movements of eye and object by visual interneurones of crickets, *J. Exp. Biol.* **50:**723–732.

Palka, J., and Edwards, J. S., 1974, The cerci and abdominal giant fibres of the house cricket, *Acheta domesticus.* II. Regeneration and effects of chronic deprivation, *Proc. R. Soc. London* **185:**105–121.

Palka, J., and Pinter, R. B., 1975, Theoretical and experimental analysis of visual activity in insects, in: *The Compound Eye and Vision in Insects* (G. A. Horridge, ed.), pp. 321–337, Oxford University Press, New York.

Palka, J., and Schubiger, M., 1975, Central connections of receptors on rotated and exchanged cerci of crickets, *Proc. Natl. Acad. Sci. USA* **72:**966–973.

Panov, A. A., 1960, the structure of the insect brain during successive stages of postembryonic development. III. Optic lobes, *Entomol. Rev.* **39:**55–68.

Panov, A. A., 1966, Correlations in the ontogenetic development of the central nervous system in the house cricket, *Gryllus domesticus* L. and the mole cricket, *Gryllotalpa gryllotalpa* L. (Orthoptera, Grylloidea), *Entomol. Rev.* **45:**179–185.

Pantin, C. F. A., 1934, On the excitation of crustacean muscle, *J. Exp. Biol.* **11:**11–27.

Pappas, G. D., Asada, Y., and Bennett, M. V. L., 1971, Morphological correlates of increased coupling resistance at an electrotonic synapse, *J. Cell Biol.* **49:**173–178.

Parker, G. H., 1891, The compound eye in crustaceans, *Bull. Mus. Comp. Zool. Harv. Univ.* **21:**45–140.

Parker, G. H., 1895, The retina and optic ganglia in decapods especially in *Astacus, Mitt. Zool. Sta. Neapel.* **12:**1–73.

Parker, G. H., 1932, The movements of the retinal pigment, *Ergeb. Biol.* **9:**239–291.

Parnas, I., 1972, Differential block at high frequency of branches of a single axon innervating two muscles, *J. Neurophysiol.* **35:**903–914.

Parnas, I., and Atwood, H. L., 1966, Phasic and tonic neuromuscular systems in the abdominal extensor muscles of the crayfish and rock lobster, *Comp. Biochem. Physiol.* **18:**701–723.

Parnas, I., and Dagan, D., 1971, Functional organisations of giant axons in the central nervous systems of insects: New aspects, *Adv. Insect Physiol.* **8:**95–144.

Parnas, I., and Grossman, Y., 1973, Presynaptic inhibition in the phallic neuro-muscular system of the cockroach, *Periplaneta americana, J. Comp. Physiol.* **82:**23–32.

Parnas, I., Abbott, B. C., Shapiro, B., and Lang, F., 1968, Neuromuscular system of *Limulus* leg closer muscle, *Comp. Biochem. Physiol.* **26:**467–478.

Parnas, I., Spira, M. E., Werman, R., and Bergmann, F., 1969, Nonhomogeneous conduction in giant axons of the nerve cord of *Periplaneta americana, J. Exp. Biol.* **50:**635–649.

Parnas, I., Rahamimoff, R., and Sarne, Y., 1975, Tonic release of transmitter at the neuromuscular junction of the crab, *J. Physiol. (London)* **250:**275–286.

Parrack, D. W., 1964, Stepping sequences in the crayfish, Ph.D. dissertation, University of Illinois, Urbana, Ill.

Paul, D. H., 1972, Decremental conduction over "giant" afferent processes in an arthropod, *Science* **176:**680–682.

Payton, B. W., Bennett, M. V. L., and Pappas, G. D., 1969, Permeability and structure of junctional membranes at an electrotonic synapse, *Science* **166:**1641–1643.

Peabody, E. B., 1939, Pigmentary responses in the isopod, Idothea, *J. Exp. Zool.* **82:**47–83.

Pearson, K. G., 1972, Central programming and reflex control of walking in the cockroach, *J. Exp. Biol.* **56:**173–193.

Pearson, K. G., 1973, Function of peripheral inhibitory axons in insects, *Am. Zool.* **13:**321–330.

Pearson, K. G., 1976, Nerve cells without action potentials, in: *Simpler Networks* (J. Fentress, ed.), Sinauer Associates, Cambridge, Mass.

Pearson, K. G., and Bergman, S. J., 1969, Common inhibitory motor neurons in insects, *J. Exp. Biol.* **50:**445–471.

Pearson, K. G., and Duysens, J., 1976, Reflex control of stepping in cockroach and cat, in: *Neural Control of Locomotion* (R. H. Herman, S. Grillner, P. S. G. Stein, and D. G. Stuart, eds.), Plenum Press, New York.

Pearson, K. G., and Fourtner, C. R., 1973, Identification of the somata of common inhibitory motor neurons in the metathoracic ganglion of the cockroach, *Can. J. Zool.* **51:**859–866.

Pearson, K. G., and Fourtner, C. R., 1975, Nonspiking interneurons in walking system of the cockroach, *J. Neurophysiol.* **38:**33–52.

Pearson, K. G., and Iles, J. F., 1970, Discharge patterns of coxal levator and depressor motoneurones of the cockroach, *Periplaneta americana, J. Exp. Biol.* **52:**139–165.

Pearson, K. G., and Iles, J. F., 1971, Innervation of coxal depressor muscles in the cockroach, *Periplaneta americana, J. Exp. Biol.* **54:**215–232.

Pearson, K. G., and Iles, J. F., 1973, Nervous mechanisms underlying intersegmental co-ordination of leg movements during walking in the cockroach, *J. Exp. Biol.* **58:**725–744.

Pearson, K. G., Fourtner, C. R., and Wong, R. K., 1973, Nervous control of walking in the cockroach, in: *Control of Posture and Locomotion* (R. B. Stein, K. B. Pearson, R. S. Smith, and J. B. Redford, eds.) pp. 495–514, Plenum Press, New York.

Pearson, K. G., Wong, R. K. S., and Fourtner, C. R., 1976, Connections between hair plate afferents and motoneurons in the cockroach leg, *J. Exp. Biol.* **64:**251–266.

Perdeck, A. C., 1958, The isolating value of specific song pattern in two sibling species of grasshoppers (*Chorthippus brunneus* Thumb. and *C. biguttulus* L.), *Behaviour* **12:**1–75.

Perkel, D. H., and Mulloney, B., 1974, Motor pattern production in reciprocally inhibitory neurons exhibiting postinhibitory rebound, *Science* **185:**181–183.

Perkel, D. M., Gerstein, G. L., and Moore, G. P., 1967, Neuronal spike trains and stochastic point processes. II. Simultaneous spike trains, *Biophys. J.* **7:**419–440.

Pickard, R. S., and Mill, P. J., 1972, Ventilatory muscle activity in intact preparations of aeshnid dragonfly larvae, *J. Exp. Biol.* **56:**527–536.

Pickard, R. S., and Mill, P. J., 1974a, Ventilatory movements of the abdomen and branchial apparatus in dragonfly larvae (Odonata: Anisoptera), *J. Zool. (London)* **174:**23–40.

Pickard, R. S., and Mill, P. J., 1974b, The effects of carbon dioxide and oxygen on respiratory dorso-ventral muscle activity during normal ventilation in *Anax imperator* Leach (Anisoptera: Aeshnidae), *Odonatologica* **3:**249–255.

Pickard, R. S., and Mill, P. J., 1975, Ventilatory muscle activity in restrained and free-swimming dragonfly larvae (Odonata: Anisoptera), *J. Comp. Physiol.* **96:**37–52.

Pitman, R. M., Tweedle, C. D., and Cohen, M. J., 1972, Branching of central neurons, Intracellular cobalt injection for light and electron microscopy, *Science* **176:**412–414.

Pittendrigh, C., 1960, Circadian rhythms and the circadian organization of living systems, *Cold Spring Harbor Symp. Quant. Biol.* **25:**159–184.

Pollard, T. G., and Larimer, J. L., 1977, Circadian rhythmicity of heart rate in crayfish, *J. Comp. Physiol.*, in preparation.

Poodry, C. A., and Schneiderman, H. A., 1970, The ultrastructure of the developing leg of *Drosophila melanogaster, Wilhelm Roux Arch Entwicklungsmech. Org.* **166:**1–44.

Pringle, J. W. S., 1939, The motor mechanism of the insect leg, *J. Exp. Biol.* **16:**220–231.

Prosser, C. L., 1934, Action potentials in the nervous system of the crayfish. II. Responses to illumination of the eye and caudal ganglion, *J. Cell. Comp. Physiol.* **4:**363–377.

Rahamimoff, R., 1968, A dual effect of calcium ions on neuromuscular facilitation, *J. Physiol. (London)* **195:**471–480.

Rakic, P., 1975, Local circuit neurons, *Neurosci. Res. Prog. Bull.* **13(3):**291–446.

Rall, W., 1964, Theoretical significance of dendritic trees for neuronal input–output relations, in: *Neural Theory and Modelling* (R. F. Reiss, ed.), pp. 73–97, Stanford University Press, Stanford, Calif.

Rall, W., 1967, Distinguishing theoretical synaptic potentials computed for different soma–dendritic distributions of synaptic input, *J. Neurophysiol.* **30:**1138–1168.

Rathmayer, W., and Florey, E., 1974a, Different time courses of post- and pre-synaptic inhibition at crab neuromuscular junctions, *Proceedings Twenty-Sixth Congress of Physiological Science* (abst.).

Rathmayer, W., and Florey, E., 1974b, Presynaptic inhibition of long duration at crab neuromuscular junctions, *Pfluegers Arch.* **348:**77–81.

Rees, D., 1974, The spontaneous release of transmitter from insect nerve terminals as predicted by the negative binomial theorem, *J. Physiol. (London)* **236:**129–142.

Rees, D., and Usherwood, P. N. R., 1972a, Effects of denervation on the ultrastructure of insect muscle, *J. Cell Sci.* **10:**667–682.

Rees, D., and Usherwood, P. N. R., 1972b, Fine structure of normal and degenerating motor axons and nerve–muscle synapses in the locust, *Schistocerca gregaria, Comp. Biochem. Physiol.* **43A:**83–101.

Rehbein, H. G., Kalmring, K., and Römer, H., 1974, Structure and function of acoustic neurons in the thoracic ventral nerve cord of *Locusta migratoria* (Acrididae), *J. Comp. Physiol.* **95:**263–280.

Relyea, K., and Sutton, B., 1975, A new troglobitic crayfish of the genus *Procambarus* from Florida (Decapoda: Astacidae), *Tulane Stud. Zool. Bot.* **19:**8–16.

Remler, M., Selverston, A., and Kennedy, D., 1968, Lateral giant fibers of crayfish: Location of somata by dye injection, Science **162**:281–283.

Rensing, L., and Bogenschütz, H., 1966, Vorzugsrichtungen von *Corixa punctata* Illig. in polarisiertem Licht, *Zool. Jahrb. Abt. Allg. Zool. Physiol.* **72**:123–135.

Retzius, G., 1890, Zur Kenntniss des Nervensystems der Crustaceen, *Biol. Untersuch. N.F.* **1**:1–50.

Reuben, J. P., 1960, Electronic connections between lobster muscle fibres, *Biol. Bull.* **119**:334.

Rheinlaender, J., 1975, Transmission of acoustic information at three neuronal levels in the auditory system of *Decticus verrucivorus* (Tettigoniidae, Orthoptera), *J. Comp. Physiol.* **97**:1–53.

Ribi, W. A., 1974, Neuron in the first synaptic region of the bee, *Apis mellifera, Cell. Tissue Res.* **148**:277–286.

Richet, C., 1879, Contribution a la physiologie des centres nerveux et des muscles de l'ecrevisse, *Arch. Physiol. Nor. Pathol.* **6**:262–294, 522–576.

Richet, C., 1882, *Physiologie des Muscles et des Nerfs* (Wiersma, 1961), 924 pp., Balliere, Paris.

Ripley, S. H., and Wiersma, C. A. G., 1953, The effect of spaced stimulation of excitatory and inhibitory axons of the crayfish, *Physiol. Comp. Oecol.* **3**:1–17.

Ripley, S. H., Bush, B. M. H., and Roberts, A., 1968, Crab muscle receptor which responds without impulses, *Nature (London)* **218**:1170–1171.

Ritter, W., 1911, A flying apparatus of the blow-fly, a contribution to the morphology and physiology of the organs of flight in insects, *Smithson. Misc. Collect.* **56:12**:1–77.

Roaf, H. E., and Sherrington, C. S., 1910, Further remarks on the spinal mammalian preparation, *Q. J. Exp. Physiol.* **3**:209–211.

Roberts, A., 1968*a*, Recurrent inhibition in the giant-fibre system of the crayfish and its effect on the excitability of the escape response, *J. Exp. Biol.* **48**:545–567.

Roberts, A., 1968*b*, Some features of the central co-ordination of a fast movement in the crayfish, *J. Exp. Biol.* **49**:645–656.

Roberts, A., and Bush, B. M. H., 1971, Coxal muscle receptors in the crab: The receptor current and some properties of the receptor nerve fibres, *J. Exp. Biol.* **54**:515–524.

Robinson, J., 1976, Estimation of parameters for a model of transmitter release at synapses, *Biometrics* **32**:61–68.

Roonwall, M. L., 1937, Studies on the embryology of the African migratory locust, *Locusta migratoria migratorioides, Philos. Trans. R. Soc. London Ser. B* **227**:175–244.

Rosenthal, J., 1969, Post-tetanic potentiation at the neuromuscular junction of the frog, *J. Physiol. (London)* **203**:121–134.

Rovainen, C. M., 1967, Physiological and anatomical studies on large neurons of the central nervous system of the sea lamprey (*Petromyzon marinus*). I. Muller and Mauthner cells, *J. Neurophysiol.* **30**:1000–1023.

Rovainen, C. M., 1974, Respiratory motoneurons in lampreys, *J. Comp. Physiol.* **94**:57–68.

Rowell, C. H. F., 1971*a*, The orthopteran descending movement detector (DMD) neurones: A characterisation and review, *Z. Vgl. Physiol.* **73**:167–194.

Rowell, C. H. F., 1971*b*, Variable responsiveness of a visual interneurone in the free-moving locust, and its relation to behavior and arousal, *J. Exp. Biol.* **55**:727–747.

Rowell, C. H. F., 1971*c*, Antennal cleaning, arousal and visual interneurone responsiveness in a locust, *J. Exp. Biol.* **55**:749–761.

Rowell, C. H. F., 1974, Boredom and attention in a cell in the locust visual system, in: *Experimental Analysis of Insect Behavior* (L. Barton Browne, ed.), pp. 87–99, Springer-Verlag, New York.

Rowell, C. H. F., 1976, Small system neurophysiology and the study of plasticity, in: *Neural Mechanisms of Learning and Memory* (M. Rozenzweig and E. Bennett, eds.), M.I.T. Press, Cambridge, Mass.

Rowell, C. H. F., and Horn, G., 1967, Response characterization of neurones in an insect brain, *Nature (London)* **216**:702–703.

Rowell, C. H. F., and Horn, G., 1968, Dishabituation and arousal in the response of single nerve cells in an insect brain, *J. Exp. Biol.* **49**:171–187.

Rowell, C. H. F., and O'Shea, M., 1977a, The neuronal basis of a sensory analyser, the acridid movement detector system. I. Effects of simple incremental and decremental stimuli in light and dark adapted animals, *J. Exp. Biol.* **65:**273–288.

Rowell, C. H. F., and O'Shea, M., 1977b, The neuronal basis of a sensory analyser, and acridid movement detector system. III. Control of response amplitude by tonic lateral inhibition, *J. Exp. Biol.* **65:**617–626.

Rowell, C. H. F., O'Shea, M., and Williams, J. L. D., 1977, The neuronal basis of a sensory analyser, the acridid movement detector system. IV. The preference for small field stimuli, *J. Exp. Biol.* **68:**157–185.

Russell, D. F., 1976, Rhythmic excitatory inputs to the lobster stomatogastric ganglion, *Brain Res.* **101:**582–588.

Rutherford, D. J., and Horridge, G. A., 1965, The rhabdom of the lobster eye, *Q. J. Microsc. Sci.* **106:**119–130.

Sandeman, D. C., 1964, Functional distinction between oculomotor and optic nerves in *Carcinus* (Crustacea), *Nature (London)* **201:**302–303.

Sandeman, D. C., 1967, Excitation and inhibition of the reflex eye withdrawal of the crab, *Carcinus, J. Exp. Biol.* **46:**475–485.

Sandeman, D. C., 1968, A sensitive position measuring device for biological systems, *Comp. Biochem. Physiol.* **24:**635–638.

Sandeman, D. C., 1969a, The site of synaptic activity and impulse initiation in an identified motoneuron in the crab brain, *J. Exp. Biol.* **50:**771–784.

Sandeman, D. C., 1969b, Integrative properties of a reflex motoneuron in the brain of the crab, *Carcinus maenas, Z. Vgl. Physiol.* **64:**450–464.

Sandeman, D. C., 1971, The excitation and electrical coupling of four identified motoneurons in the brain of the Australian mud crab, *Scylla serrata, Z. Vgl. Physiol.* **72:**111–130.

Sandeman, D. C., and Luff, S. E., 1974, Regeneration of the antennules in the Australian freshwater crayfish, *Cherax destructor, J. Neurobiol.* **5:**475–488.

Sandeman, D. C., and Okajima, A., 1972, Statocyst-induced eye movements in the crab *Scylla serrata.* I. The sensory input from the statocysts, *J. Exp. Biol.* **57:**187–204.

Sandeman, D. C., and Okajima, A., 1973a, Statocyst-induced eye movements in the crab *Scylla serrata.* II. The responses of the eye muscles, *J. Exp. Biol.* **58:**197–212.

Sandeman, D. C., and Okajima, A., 1973b, Statocyst-induced eye movements in the crab *Scylla serrata.* III. The anatomical projections of sensory and motor neurones and the responses of the motor neurons, *J. Exp. Biol.* **59:**17–38.

Sandeman, D. C., Erber, J., and Kien, J., 1975, Optokinetic eye movements in the crab *Carcinus maenas.* I. Eye torque, *J. Comp. Physiol.* **101:**243–258.

Sandeman, D. C., Kien, J., and Erber, J., 1975, Optokinetic eye movements in the crab *Carcinus maenas.* II. Responses of optokinetic interneurons, *J. Comp. Physiol.* **101:**259–274.

Sanes, J., and Hildebrand, J., 1975, Nerves in the antennae of pupal *Manduca sexta* Johanssen (Lepidoptera; Sphingidae), *Wilhelm. Roux Arch. Enlwicklungemech. Org.* **178:**71–78.

Sbrenna, G., 1971, Postembryonic growth of the ventral cord in *Schistocerca gregaria* Forst (Orthoptera: Acrididae), *Boll. Zool.* **38:**49–74.

Scharrer, B., 1968, Neurosecretion. XIV. Ultrastructural study in sites of release of neurosecretory material in blattarian insects, *Z. Zellforsch. Mikrosk. Anat.* **89:**1–16.

Scheer, B. T., 1957, *Recent Advances in Invertebrate Physiology,* pp. 304, University of Oregon Publications, Eugene, Ore.

Schiff, H., and Gervasio, A., 1969, Functional morphology of the *Squilla* retina, *Pubbl. Stm. Zool. Napoli* **37:**610–629.

Schiller, P. H., and Stryker, M., 1972, Single-unit recording and stimulation in superior colliculus of the alert rhesus monkey, *J. Neurophysiol.* **35:**915–924.

Schlieper, C., 1927, Farbensinn der Tiere und optomotorische Reaktionen, *Z. Vgl. Physiol.* **6:**453–472.

Schmidt, K., and Gnatzy, W., 1972, Die Feinstruktur der Sinneshaare auf den Cerci von *Gryllus bimaculatus* Deg. (Saltatoria, Gryllidae). III. Die Kurzen Borstenhaare, *Z. Zellforsch. Mikrosk. Anat.* **126**:206–222.

Schmidt, R. F., 1971, Presynaptic inhibition in the vertebrate central nervous system, *Ergeb. Physiol. Biol. Chem. Exp. Pharmakol.* **63**:20–101.

Scholl, G., 1969, Die Embryonalentwicklung des Kophes und Prothorax von *Carausius morosus* Br. (Insecta, Phasmatida), *Z. Morphol.* **65**:1–142.

Schöne, H., 1961, Complex behavior, in: *The Physiology of Crustacea,* Vol. 2 (T. H. Waterman, ed.), pp. 465–520, Academic Press, New York.

Schrameck, J. E., 1970, Crayfish swimming: Alternating motor output and giant fiber activity, *Science* **169**:698–700.

Schreuder, J. B., and de Wilde, J., 1952, Analysis of the dyspnoeic action of carbon dioxide in the cockroach (*Periplaneta americana* L.), *Physiol. Comp. Oecol.* **2**:355–361.

Scott, S., 1975, Persistence of foreign innervation on reinnervated extraoccular muscle, *Science* **189**:644–646.

Segaar, A., 1929, Über die Funktion der nervösen Zentren bei Crustaceen, *Z. Vgl. Physiol.* **10**:120–226.

Segundo, J. P., Perkel, D. H., Wyman, H., Hegstad, H., and Moore, G. P., 1968, Input–output relations in computer simulated nerve cells, *Kybernetik* **4**:157–171.

Selverston, A. I., 1974, Structural and functional basis of motor pattern generation in the stomatogastric ganglion of the lobster, *Am. Zool.* **14**:957–972.

Selverston, A. I., 1976, Neuronal mechanism for rhythmic motor pattern generation in a simple system, in: *Neural Control of Locomotion* (R. H. Herman, S. Grillner, P. S. G. Stein, and D. G. Stuart, eds.), Plenum Press, New York.

Selverston, A. I., and Mulloney, B. M., 1974*a*, Organization of the stomatogastric ganglion of the spiny lobster. II. Neurons driving the medial tooth, *J. Comp. Physiol.* **91**:33–51.

Selverston, A. I., and Mulloney, B. M., 1974*b*, Synaptic and structural analysis of a small neural system, in: *The Neurosciences: Third Study Program* (F. O. Schmitt and F. G. Worden, eds.), pp. 389–396, M.I.T. Press, Cambridge, Mass.

Selverston, A. I., and Remler, M. P., 1972, Neural geometry and activation of crayfish fast flexor motoneurons, *J. Neurophysiol.* **35**:797–814.

Selverston, A. I., Russell, D. F., Miller, J. P., and King, D. G., 1976, The stomatogastric nervous system: Structure and function of a small neural network, *Prog. Neurobiol.* **6**:1–75.

Shafiq, 1964, An electron microscopical study of the innervation and sarcoplasmic reticulum of the fibrillar flight muscle of *Drosophila melanogaster, Q. J. Microsc. Sci.* **105**:1–6.

Shaw, K. C., 1968, An analysis of the phonoresponse of males of the true katydid, *Pterophylla camellifolia* (Fabricius) (Orthoptera: Tettigoniidae), *Behaviour* **31**:203–260.

Shaw, S. R., 1969*a,* Sense-cell structure and interspecies comparisons of polarized light absorption in arthropod compound eyes, *Vision Res.* **9**:1031–1040.

Shaw, S. R., 1969*b,* Optics of arthropod compound eye, *Science* **165**:88–89.

Shaw, S. R., 1972, Decremental conduction of the visual signal in barnacle lateral eye, *J. Physiol. (London)* **220**:145–175.

Shelton, R. G. J., and Laverack, M. S., 1968, Observations on a redescribed crustacean cuticular sense organ, *Comp. Biochem. Physiol.* **25**:1049–1059.

Shepheard, P. R. B., 1966, Optokinetic memory and the perception of movement by the crab *Carcinus,* in: *Functional Organisation of the Compound Eye* (G. G. Bernard, ed.), pp. 543–557, Pergamon Press, Oxford.

Shepherd, G. M., 1972, The neuron doctrine: A revision of functional concepts, *Yale J. Biol. Med.* **45**:584–599.

Shepherd, G. M., 1974, *The Synaptic Organization of the Brain,* 364 pp., Oxford University Press, New York.

Sherman, R. G., and Atwood, H. L., 1971*a,* Structure and neuromuscular physiology of a newly discovered muscle in the walking legs of the lobster *Homarus americanus, J. Exp. Zool.* **176**:461–474.

Sherman, R. G., and Atwood, H. L., 1971*b*, Synaptic facilitation: Long term neuromuscular facilitation in crustaceans, *Science* **171:**1248–1250.

Sherman, R. C., and Atwood, H. L., 1972, Correlated electrophysiological and ultrastructural studies of a crustacean motor unit, *J. Gen. Physiol.* **59:**586–615.

Sherrington, C. S., 1910, Flexion-reflex of the limb, crossed extension reflex, and reflex stepping and standing, *J. Physiol. (London)* **40:**28–121.

Shik, M. L., and Orlovsky, G. N., 1976, Neurophysiology of loco motor automatism, *Physiol. Rev.* **56:**465–501.

Shik, M. L., Severin, F. V., and Orlovsky, G. N., 1966, Control of walking and running by means of electrical stimulation of the midbrain, *Biophysics* **11:**756–765.

Sidman, R. L., 1974, Cell–cell recognition in the developing central nervous system, in: *The Neurosciences: Third Study Program* (F. O. Schmitt and F. G. Worden, eds.), pp. 743–758, Rockefeller University Press, New York.

Siegler, M. V. S., Mpitsos, G. J., and Davis, W. J., 1974, Motor organization and generation of rhythmic feeding output in the buccal ganglion of *Pleurobranchaea, J. Neurophysiol.* **37:**1173–1196.

Silvey, G. E., and Sandeman, D. C., 1976*a*, Integration between statocyst sensory neurons and oculomotor neurons in the crab *Scylla serrata*. I. Horizontal compensatory eye movements, *J. Comp. Physiol.* **108:**35–43.

Silvey, G. E., and Sandeman, D. C., 1976*b*, Integration between statocyst sensory neurons and oculomotor neurons in the crab *Scylla serrata*. III. The sensory to motor synapse, *J. Comp. Physiol.* **108:**53–65.

Silvey, G. E., and Sandeman, D. C., 1976*c*, Integration between statocyst sensory neurons and oculomotor neurons in the crab *Scylla serrata*. IV. Integration, phase lags and conjugate eye movements, *J. Comp. Physiol.,* **108:**67–73.

Silvey, G. E., Dunn, P. A., and Sandeman, D. C., 1976, Integration between statocyst sensory neurons and oculomotor neurons in the rat *Scylla serrata*. II. The thread hair sensory receptors, *J. Comp. Physiol.* **108:**45–52.

Singer, M., and Green, M. R., 1968, Autoradiographic studies of urdine incorporation in peripheral nerve of the newt, *Triturus, J. Morphol.* **124:**321–344.

Singer, M., and Salpeter, M. M., 1966, The transport of ^{3}H-1-histidine through the Schwann and myelin sheath into the axon of peripheral nerves, *J. Morphol.* **120:**281–316.

Smith, D. O., 1972, Central nervous control of presynaptic inhibition in the crayfish claw, *J. Neurophysiol.* **35:**333–343.

Smith, D. O., 1973, Central nervous control of excitatory and inhibitory neruons of opener muscle of the crayfish claw, *J. Neurophysiol.* **37:**108–118.

Smith, D. O., 1974*a*, Central nervous control of excitatory and inhibitory neurons of opener muscle of the crayfish claw, *J. Neurophysiol.* **37:**108–118.

Smith, D. O., 1974*b*, Autogenic production of paired impulses by the opener excitor neuron of the crayfish claw, *Brain Res.* **70:**356–360.

Smith, D. O., 1975, Temporal characteristics of efferent neuron discharge during muscle contraction in the crayfish claw, *J. Comp. Physiol.* **96A:**273–283.

Smith, D. S., 1960, Innervation of the fibrillar flight muscle of an insect, *Tenebrio molitor* (Coleoptera), *J. Biophys. Biochem. Cytol.* **8:**447–466.

Smith, F. E., and Baylor, E. R., 1960, Bees, *Daphnia* and polarized light, *Ecology* **41:**360–363.

Sneath, P. H. A., and Sokal, R. R., 1973, *Numerical Taxonomy,* 573 pp., Freeman, San Francisco.

Snodgrass, R. E., 1929, The thoracic mechanism of a grasshopper and its antecedents, *Smithson. Misc. Collect.* **82(2):**1–111.

Snyder, A. W., 1975, Optical properties of invertebrate photoreceptors, in: *The Compound Eye and Vision of Insects* (G. A. Horridge, ed.), pp. 179–235, Clarendon Press, Oxford.

Snyder, A. W., 1977, Acuity of compound eyes. Physical limitations and design, *J. Comp. Physiol.* **A116:**161–182.

Snyder, A. W., and McIntyre, P., 1975, Polarization sensitivity of twisted fused rhabdoms, in: *Photo-receptor Optics* (A. W. Snyder and R. Menzel, eds.), pp. 388–391, Springer-Verlag, New York.

Snyder, A. W., and Menzel, R., eds., 1975, *Photoreceptor Optics*, 523 pp., Springer-Verlag, New York.

Sokolove, P. G., 1973, Crayfish stretch receptor and motor unit behavior during abdominal extension, *J. Comp. Physiol.* **84**:251–266.

Sommer, E., and Wehner, R., 1975, The retina-lamina-projection in the visual system of the bee, *Apis mellifera, Cell. Tissue Res.* **163**:45–61.

Somero, G., 1975, Temperature as a selective factor in protein evolution: The adaptational strategy of "compromise," *J. Exp. Zool.* **194**:175–188.

Souček, B., 1971, Complete model for the statistical composition of the end-plate potential, *J. Theoret. Biol.* **30**:631–645.

Spirito, C. P., 1970, Reflex control of the opener and stretcher muscles in the cheliped of the fiddler crab, *Uca pugnax, Z. Vgl. Physiol.* **68**:211–228.

Spirito, C. P., Evoy, W. H., and Barnes, W. J. P., 1972, Nervous control of walking in the crab, *Cardisoma guanhumi.* I. Characteristics of resistance reflexes, *Z. Vgl. Physiol.* **76**:1–15.

Stein, P. S. G., 1971, Intersegmental coordination of swimmeret motoneuron activity in crayfish, *J. Neurophysiol.* **34**:310–318.

Stein, P. S. G., 1974, The neural control of interappendage phase during locomotion, *Am. Zool.* **14**:1003–1016.

Stein, P. S. G., 1976, Mechanisms of interlimb coordination, in: *Neural Control of Locomotion* (R. H. Herman, S. Grillner, P. S. G. Stein, and D. G. Stuart, eds.), Plenum Press, New York.

Stein, P. S. G., 1977, Swimming movements elicited by electrical stimulation of the turtle spinal cord. II. The high spinal preparation, submitted for publication.

Stein, R. B., 1974, Peripheral control of movement, *Physiol. Rev.* **54**:215–243.

Stein, R. B., Pearson, K. G., Smith, R. S., and Redford, J. B., 1973, *Control of Posture and Locomotion,* 635 pp., Plenum Press, New York.

Steinacker, T., 1975, Proprioceptive feedback in the oculomotor system of the crab, *Brain Res.* **89**:353–357.

Stephens, C. L., 1973, Relative contribution of synaptic and non-synaptic influences to response decrements in a postsynaptic neurone, *J. Exp. Biol.* **59**:315–321.

Stinnakre, J., and Tauc, L., 1973, Calcium influx in active *Aplysia* neurones detected by injected aequorin, *Nature (London) New Biol.* **242**:113–115.

Stocker, R., Edwards, J. S., Palka, J., and Schubiger, G., 1976, Projection of sensory neurons from a homeotic mutant appendage, *Antennapedia* in *Drosophila melanogaster, Dev. Biol.* **52**:210–220.

Strausfeld, B. J., 1976, *Atlas of an Insect Brain,* 214 pp., Springer-verlag, New York.

Stretton, A. O. W., and Kravitz, E. A., 1968, Neuronal geometry; Determination with a technique of intracellular dye injection, *Science* **162**:132–134.

Strumwasser, F., 1968, Membrane and intracellular mechanism governing intracellular activity in neurons, in: *Physiological and Biochemical Aspects of Nervous Integration* (F. D. Carlson, ed.), pp. 329–341, Prentice-Hall, Englewood Cliffs, N.J.

Suga, N., and Katsuki, Y., 1962, Vision in insects in terms of electrical activities of the descending nerve fibre, *Nature (London)* **194**:658–660.

Sutherland, N. S., 1968, Shape discrimination and receptive fields, *Nature (London)* **197**:118–122.

Sutherland, R. M., and Nunnemacher, R. F., 1968, Microanatomy of crayfish thoracic cord and roots, *J. Comp. Neurol.* **132**:499–518.

Suzuki, D. T., Grigliatti, T., and Williamson, R., 1971, Temperature-sensitive mutations in *Drosophila melanogaster.* VII. A mutation (para^{ts}) causing reversible adult paralysis, *Proc. Natl. Acad. Sci. USA* **68**:890–893.

Swenarchuk, L. E., and Atwood, H. L., 1975, Long-term synaptic facilitation with minimal calcium entry, *Brain Res.* **100**:205–208.

Szekeley, G., 1968, Development of limb movements: Embryological, physiological and model studies, in: *Ciba Found. Symposium: Growth of the Nervous System* (G. E. W. Wolstenholme and M. O'Connor, eds.), pp. 431–444, Churchill, London.

Szekeley, G., Czeh, G., and Voros, G., 1969, The activity pattern of limb muscles in freely moving and deafferented newts, *Exp. Brain Res.* **9:**53–62.

Takeda, K., and Kennedy, D., 1964, Soma potentials and modes of activation of crayfish motoneurons, *J. Cell. Comp. Physiol.* **64:**165–182.

Takeda, K., and Kennedy, D., 1965, The mechanism of discharge pattern formation in crustacean interneurons, *J. Gen Physiol.* **48:**435–453.

Takeuchi, A., and Onodera, K., 1973, Reversal potentials of the excitatory transmitter and L-glutamate at the crayfish neuromuscular junction, *Nature (London) New Biol.* **242:**124–126.

Takeuchi, A., and Takeuchi, N., 1964, The effect on crayfish muscle of iontophoretically applied glutamate, *J. Physiol. (London)* **170:**296–317.

Takeuchi, A., and Takeuchi, N., 1965, Localized action of gama-aminobutyric acid on the crayfish muscle, *J. Physiol. (London)* **177:**225–238.

Takeuchi, A., and Takeuchi, N., 1966a, A study of the inhibitory action of _-aminobutyric acid on the neuromuscular transmission in the crayfish, *J. Physiol. (London)* **183:**418–432.

Takeuchi, A., and Takeuchi, N., 1966b, On the permeability of the presynaptic terminal of the crayfish neuromuscular junction during synaptic inhibition and the action of γ-aminobutyric acid, *J. Physiol. (London)* **183:**433–449.

Takeuchi, A., and Takeuchi, N., 1967, Anion permability of the inhibitory post-synaptic membrane of the crayfish neuromuscular junction, *J. Physiol. (London)* **191:**575–590.

Takeuchi, A., and Takeuchi, N., 1969, A study of the action of picrotoxin on the inhibitory neuromuscular junction of the crayfish, *J. Physiol. (London)* **205:**377–391.

Takeuchi, A., and Takeuchi, N., 1971a, Anion interaction at the inhibitory post-synaptic membrane of the crayfish neuromuscular junction, *J. Physiol. (London)* **212:**337–351.

Takeuchi, A., and Takeuchi, N., 1971b, Variations in the permeability properties of the inhibitory post-synaptic membrane of the crayfish neuromuscular function when activated by different concentrations of GABA, *J. Physiol. (London)* **217:**341–358.

Takeuchi, A., and Takeuchi, N., 1972, Actions of transmitter substances on the neuromuscular junctions of vertebrates and invertebrates, *Adv. Biophys.* **3:**45–95.

Taraskevich, P. S., 1971, Reversal potentials of L-glutamate and the excitatory transmitter at the neuromuscular junction of the crayfish, *Biochim. Biophys. Acta* **241:**700–704.

Taraskevich, P. S., 1975, Dual effect of L-glutamate on excitatory post junctional membranes of crayfish muscle, *J. Gen. Physiol.* **65:**677–691.

Tatton, W. G., and Sokolove, P. G., 1975, Analysis of postural motoneuron activity in crayfish abdomen. II. Coordination by excitatory and inhibitory connections between motoneurons, *J. Neurophysiol.* **38:**332–346.

Täuber, U., 1974, Analyse des Polarisationszustandes des aus dem Rhabdomer austretenden Lichtes, *J. Comp. Physiol.* **95A:**169–183.

Taylor, R. C., 1970, Environmental factors which control the sensitivity of a single crayfish interneuron, *Comp. Biochem. Physiol.* **33:**911–921.

Tcalc, E. W., 1949, *The Insect World of D. Henri Fabre,* 19 pp., Dodd, Mead, New York.

ten Cate, J., 1930, Sur Physiologie des ZNS der Einsiedler Krebse, *Arch. Neerl. Physiol.* **15:**242–252.

Terzuolo, C. A., and Knox, C. K., 1971, Static and dynamic behaviour of the stretch receptor organ of Crustacea, in: *Handbook of Sensory Physiology,* Vol. 1: *Principles of Receptor Physiology* (W. R. Loewenstein, ed.), Chapter 16, Springer-Verlag, Berlin.

Thies, R. E., 1965, Neuromuscular depression and the apparent depletion of transmitter in mammalian muscle, *J. Neurophysiol.* **28:**427–442.

Tiegs, O. W., 1955, The flight muscles of insects—their anatomy and histology: With some observations on the structure of striated muscle in general, *Philos. Trans. R. Soc. London* **656:**221–348.

Tonner, F., 1936, Mechanik und Koordination der Atem-und Schwimmbewegung bei Libellenlarven, *Z. Wiss. Zool. Abt. A* **147:**433–454.

Treistman, S. N., and Remler, M. P., 1974, Antifacilitating and simple following responses in a single motoneuron, *J. Neurobiol.* **5**:581–584.

Treistman, S. N., and Remler, M. P., 1975, Extensor motoneurons of crayfish abdomen, *J. Comp. Physiol.* **100A**:85–100.

Trujillo-Cenóz, O., 1965, Some aspects of the structural organization of the intermediate retina of dipterans, *J. Ultrastruct. Res.* **13**:1–33.

Tuurala, O., and Lehtinen, A., 1971, Über die Einwirkung von Licht und Dunkel auf die Feinstruktur der Lichtsinneszellen der Assel *Oniscus asellus* L. 2. Microvilli und multivesikuläre Körper nach starker Belichtung, *Ann. Acad. Sci. Fenn. Ser. A4* **177**:1–8.

Tyndall, J., 1888, *The Sky,* published in *The Forum* for February 1888, and republished in *The Fragments of Science,* 9th ed., Longmans, Green, London, 1902.

Tyrer, N. M., and Altman, J. S., 1974, Motor and sensory flight neurones in a locust demonstrated using cobalt chloride, *J. Comp. Neurol.* **157**:117–138.

Umminger, B. L., 1969, Polarotaxis in copepods. III. A light contrast reaction in *Diaptomus shoshone* Forbes, *Crustaceana* **16**:202–204.

Usherwood, P. N. R., 1961, Spontaneous miniature potentials from insect muscle fibres, *Nature (london)* **191**:814–815.

Usherwood, P. N. R., 1963a, Spontaneous miniature potentials from insect muscle fibres, *J. Physiol. (London)* **169**:149–150.

Usherwood, P. N. R., 1963b, Response of insect muscle to denervation. II. Changes in neuromuscular transmission, *J. Insect Physiol.* **9**:811–825.

Usherwood, P. N. R., 1967, Insect neuromuscular mechanisms, *Am. Zool.* **7**:553–582.

Usherwood, P. N. R., 1968, A critical study of the evidence for peripheral inhibitory axons in insects, *J. Exp. Biol.* **49**:201–222.

Usherwood, P. N. R., 1969, Glutamate sensitivity of denervated insect muscle fibres, *Nature (London)* **223**:411–413.

Usherwood, P. N. R., 1972, Transmitter release from insect excitatory motor nerve terminals, *J. Physiol. (London)* **227**:527–551.

Usherwood, P. N. R., 1973, Release of transmitter from degenerating locust motoneurones, *J. Exp. Biol.* **59**:1–16.

Usherwood, P. N. R., 1974, Nerve–muscle transmission, in: *Insect Neurobiology* (J. E. Treherne), pp. 245–305, North-Holland, Amsterdam.

Usherwood, P. N. R., 1976, Transmitter release from insect motoneurons, in: *Perspectives in Experimental Biology,* Vol. 1 (P. Spencer Davies, ed.), pp. 353–360, Pergamon Press, New York.

Usherwood, P. N. R., and Cull-Candy, S. G., 1974, Distribution of glutamate sensitivity on insect muscle fibres, *Neuropharmacology* **13**:455–461.

Usherwood, P. N. R., and Cull-Candy, S. G., 1975, *Insect Muscle* (P. N. R. Usherwood, ed.), pp. 207–280, Academic Press, London, New York.

Usherwood, P. N. R., and Grundfest, H., 1964, Inhibitory postsynaptic potentials in grasshopper muscle, *Science* **143**:817–818.

Usherwood, P. N. R., and Grundfest, H., 1965, Peripheral inhibition in skeletal muscles of insects, *J. Neurophysiol.* **28**:497–518.

Usherwood, P. N. R., and Machili, P., 1966, Chemical transmission at the insect excitatory neuromuscular synapse, *Nature (London)* **210**:634–636.

Usherwood, P. N. R., and Machili, P., 1968, Pharmacological properties of excitatory neuromuscular synapses in the locust, *J. Exp. Biol.* **49**:341–361.

Usherwood, P. N. R., and Rees, D., 1972, Quantitative studies of the spatial distribution of synaptic vesicles within normal and degenerating motor axons of the locust, *Schistocerca gregaria, Comp. Biochem. Physiol.* **43A**:103–118.

Usherwood, P. N. R., and Wood, M. R., 1972, Structure and physiology of denervated and reinnervated cockroach muscle, *J. Physiol. (London)* **230P**:1–2.

Uvarov, B., 1966, *Grasshoppers and Locusts: A Handbook of General Acridology,* Vol. 1, Cambridge University Press, Cambridge.

van der Glas, H. W., 1975, Polarization induced colour patterns: A model of the perception of the polarized skylight by insects. I. Tests in choice experiments with running honey bees, *Apis mellifera, Neth. J. Zool.* **25**:476–505.

Van Harreveld, A., and Mendelson, M., 1959, Glutamate-induced contractions in crustacean muscle, *J. Cell. Comp. Physiol.* **54**:85–94.

Van Harreveld, A., and Wiersma, C. A. G., 1936, The double motor innervation of the abductor muscle in the claw of the crayfish, *J. Physiol. (London)* **88**:78–99.

Van Harreveld, A., and Wiersma, C. A. G., 1937, The triple innervation of crayfish muscle and its function in contraction and inhibition, *J. Exp. Biol.* **14**:448–461.

Van Harreveld, A., and Wiersma, C. A. G., 1939, The function of the quintuple innervation of a crustacean muscle, *J. Exp. Biol.* **16**:121–133.

van Ruiten, T. M., and Sprey, T. E., 1974, The ultrastructure of the developing leg disk of *Calliphora erythrocephala, Z. Zellforsch. Mikrosk. Anat.* **143**:373–400.

Vater, G., 1961, Vergleichende Untersuchungen über die Morphologie des Nervensystems der Dipteran, *Z. Wiss. Zool. Abt. A* **167**:137–196.

Vedel, J. P., and Clarac, F., 1975, Neurophysiological study of the antennal motor patterns in the rock lobster *Palinurus vulgaris.* II. Motoneuronal discharge patterns during passive and active flagellum movements. *J. Comp. Physiol.* **102**:223–235.

Vedel, J. P., Angaut-Petit, D., and Clarac, F., 1975, Reflex modulations of motoneurone activity in the leg of the crayfish *Astacus leptodactylus, J. Exp. Biol.* **63**:551–567.

Vedel, J. P., Clarac, F., and Bush, B. M. H., 1975, Coordination motrice proximo-distale au niveau des appendices locomoteurs de la langouste, *C. R. Acad. Sci. Ser. D* **281**:723–726.

Velez, S. J., 1974, A study in the specificity of neuromuscular connections, Ph.D. thesis, Yale University.

Velez, S. J., and Wyman, R. J., 1976a, A "gradient directed" neural projection. I. Synaptic connectivity, unpublished manuscript.

Velez, S. J., and Wyman, R. J., 1976b, A "gradient directed" neural projection. II. Nerve–muscle matching, unpublished manuscript.

Vere-Jones, D., 1966, Simple stochastic models for the release of quanta of transmitter from a nerve terminal, *Aust. J. Statist.* **8**:53–63.

Viancour, T. A., 1976, Neuronal response autorhymicity associated with non-mechanical frequency filtering in the electrosense system of *Eigenmannia virescens, Society for Neuroscience 6th Annual Meeting, Toronto Program and Abstracts,* p. 335.

von Buddenbrock, W., and Friedrich, H., 1933, Neue Beobachtungen Über die kompensatorischen Augenbewegungen und den Farbensinn der Taschkrabben (*Carcinus maenas*), *Z. Vgl. Physiol.* **19**:747–761.

von Frisch, K., 1948, Gelöste und ungelöste Rätsel der Bienensprache, *Naturwissenschaften* **35**:38–43.

von Helversen, O., 1972, Zur spektralen Unterschiedsempfindlichkeit der Honigbiene, *J. Comp. Physiol.* **80**:439–472.

von Helversen, O., and Edrich, W., 1974, Der Polarisationsempfänger im Bienenauge: Ein Ultraviolettrezeptor, *J. Comp. Physiol.* **94**:33–47.

von Helversen, D., and von Helversen, O., 1975, Genetic approach to acoustic communication system of grasshoppers. I. Song pattern of interspecific hybrids between *Chorthippus biguttulus* and *C. mollis, J. Comp. Physiol.* **104**:273–300.

Wachmann, E., and Schröer, W. D., 1975, Zur Morphologie des Dorsal- und Ventralauges des Taumelkäfers *Gyrinus substriatus* (Steph.) (Coleoptera, Gyrinidae), *Zoomorphology* **82**:43–61.

Walcott, B., 1971a, Cell movement on light adaptation in the retina of *Lethocerus* (Belostomatidae, Hemiptera), *Z. Vgl. Physiol.* **74**:1–16.

Walcott, B., 1971b, Unit studies on receptor movement on the retina of *Lethocerus* (Belostomatidae, Hemiptera), *Z. Vgl. Physiol.* **74**:17–25.

Walcott, B., 1974, Unit studies on light adaptation in the retina of the crayfish *Cherax destructor, J. Comp. Physiol.* **94**:207–218.

Walcott, B., and Burrows, M., 1969, The ultrastructure and physiology of the abdominal air-guide retractor muscles in the giant water bug, *Lethocerus, J. Insect Physiol.* **15**:1855–1872.

Wales, W., Clarac, F., Dando, M. R., and Laverack, M. S., 1970, Innervation of the receptors present at the various joints of the pereiopods and third maxilliped of *Homarus gammarus* (L.) and other macruran decapods (Crustacea), *Z. Vgl. Physiol.* **68**:345–384.

Wales, W., Clarac, F., and Laverack, M. S. 1971, Stress detection at the autotomy plane in the decapod crustacea. I. Comparative anatomy of the receptors of the basi-ischiopodite region, *Z. Vgl. Physiol.* **73**:357–382.

Wall, P. D., 1958, Excitability changes in afferent fibre terminations and their relation to slow potentials, *J. Physiol. (London)* **142**:1–21.

Waloff, Z., 1960, Some notes on the desert locust and on its occurrence at sea, *Mar. Obs.* **30**:40–45.

Walther, C., and Usherwood, P. N. R., 1972, Characterization of the glutamate receptors at the locust excitatory neuromuscular junction, *Verh. Dtsch. Zool. Ges.* **65**:309–312.

Warshaw, H. S., and Hartline, D. K., 1974, A network model of the pyloric rhythm in the lobster stomatogastric ganglion, *Fourth Meeting of the Society of Neuroscience* pp. 467 (abst.).

Warshaw, H. S., and Hartline, D. K., 1976, Simulation of network activity in stomatogastric ganglion of the spiny lobster, *Panulirus, Brain Res.* **110**:259–272.

Washio, H. M., and Inouye, S. T., 1975, The mode of spontaneous transmitter release at the insect neuromuscular junction, *Can. J. Physiol. Pharmacol.* **53**:679–682.

Watanabe, A., Obara, S., and Akiyama, T., 1967, Pacemaker potentials for the periodic burst discharge in the heart ganglion of a stomatopod, *Squilla oratoria, J. Gen. Physiol.* **50**:839–862.

Waterman, T. H., 1941, A comparative study of the effects of ions on whole nerve and isolated single nerve fiber preparations of crustacean neuromuscular systems, *J. Cell. Comp. Physiol.* **18**:109–128.

Waterman, T. H., 1943, Crustacean neuromuscular transmission, Ph.D. thesis, Harvard University.

Waterman, T. H., 1954a, Polarization patterns in submarine illumination, *Science* **120**:927–932.

Waterman, T. H., 1954b, Directional sensitivity of single ommatidia in the compound eye of *Limulus, Proc. Nat. Acad. Sci.* **40**:252–257.

Waterman, T. H., 1954c, Polarized light and angle of stimulus incidence in the compound eye of *Limulus, Proc. Nat. Acad. Sci.* **40**:258–262.

Waterman, T. H., 1960, An analysis of spatial orientation, *Erg. Biol.* **26**:98–117.

Waterman, T. H., 1961a, Comparative physiology, in: *The Physiology of Crustacea,* Vol. II (T. H. Waterman, ed.), pp. 521–593, Academic Press, New York.

Waterman, T. H., 1961b, Light sensitivity and vision, in: *The Physiology of Crustacea,* Vol. II (T. H. Waterman, ed.), pp. 1–64, Academic Press, New York.

Waterman, T. H., 1961c, Submarine polarized light and the spatial orientation of animals, *Abst. 10th Pacific Science Cong.* 162–163.

Waterman, T. H., 1972, Visual direction finding by fishes, in: *Animal Orientation and Navigation* (S. R. Galler, K. Schmidt-Koenig, G. J. Jacobs, and R. E. Belleville, eds.), pp. 437–456, N.A.S.A., Washington.

Waterman, T. H., 1973, Responses to polarized light: Animals, in: *Biology Data Book* (P. L. Altman and D. S. Dittmer, eds.), pp. 1272–1289 F.A.S.E.B., Bethesda, Md.

Waterman, T. H., 1974, Underwater light and the orientation of animals, in: *Optical Aspects of Oceanography* (N. G. Jerlov and E. Steemann Nielsen, eds.), pp. 415–443, Academic Press, London and New York.

Waterman, T. H., 1975a, Natural polarized light and e-vector discrimination by vertebrates, in: *Light as an Ecological Factor, II* (R. Bainbridge and G. C. Evans, eds.), British Ecological Society, Cambridge.

Waterman, T. H., 1975b, The optics of polarization sensitivity, in: *The Optics of Polarization Sensitivity* (A. W. Snyder and R. Menzel, eds.), pp. 339–371, Springer-Verlag, New York.

Waterman, T. H., 1975c, Expectation and achievement in comparative physiology, *J. Exp. Zool.* **194**:309–344.

Waterman, T. H., and Fernández, H. R., 1970, E-vector wavelength discrimination by retinular cells of the crayfish *Procambarus, Z. Vergl. Physiol.* **68**:154–174.

Waterman, T. H., Fernández, H. R., and Goldsmith, T. H., 1969, Dichroism of photosensitive pigment in rhabdoms of the crayfish *Orconectes, J. Gen. Physiol.* **54**:415–432.

Waterman, T. H., and Forward, R. B., Jr., 1970, Field evidence for polarized light sensitivity in the fish *Zenarchopterus, Nature* **228**:85–87.

Waterman, T. H., and Horch, K. W., 1966, Mechanism of polarized light perception, *Science* **154**:467–475.

Waterman, T. H., and Wiersma, C. A. G., 1954, The functional relation between retinal cells and optic nerve in *Limulus, J. Exp. Zool.* **126**:59–86.

Waterman, T. H., and Wiersma, C. A. G., 1963, Electrical responses in decapod crustacean visual systems, *J. Cell. Comp. Physiol.* **61**:1–16.

Waterman, T. H., Wiersma, C. A. G. and Bush, B. M. H. 1961 Impulse traffic in the optic nerve of decapod Crustacea, *Science* **134**:1435.

Waterman, T. H., Wiersma, C. A. G., and Bush, B. M. H., 1964, Afferent visual responses in the optic nerve of the crab, *Podophthalmus, J. Cell. Comp. Physiol.* **63**:135–155.

Weber, T., 1972, Stabilisierung des Flugrhythmus durch "Erfahrung" bei der Feldgrille, *Naturwissenschaften* **59**:366.

Wehner, R., 1972, *Information Processing in the Visual Systems of Arthropods*, 334 pp., Springer-Verlag, New York.

Wehner, R., 1975*a,* Pattern recognition, in: *The Compound Eye and Vision of Insects* (G. A. Horridge, ed.), pp. 75–113, Oxford University Press, Oxford.

Wehner, R., 1975*b,* In search of pattern recognition concepts in insects, in: *Biokybernetic IV* (H. Drieschen and P. Dettmar, eds.), 231 pp., Fischer, Jena.

Weinreich, D., 1971, Ionic mechanism of post-tetanic potentiation at the neuromuscular junction of the frog, *J. Physiol. (London)* **212**:431–446.

Weis-Fogh, T., 1956, Biology and physics of locust flight. II. Flight performance of the desert locust *Schistocerca gregaria. Philos. Trans. R. Soc. London Ser. B* **239**:459–510.

Weiss, P., and Hiscoe, H. B., 1948, Experiments on the mechanism of nerve growth, *J. Exp. Zool.* **107**:315–395.

Welsh, J. H., 1939, The action of eye-stalk extracts on retinal pigment migration in the crayfish, *Cambarus bartoni, Biol. Bull.* **77**:119–125.

Welsh, J. H., 1961, Neurohumors and neurosecretion, in: *The Physiology of Crustacea,* Vol. 2 (T. Waterman, ed.), Chapter 8, Academic Press, New York.

Welsh, J. H., and Chace, F. A., Jr., 1937, Eyes of deep sea crustaceans, II. Acanthephyridae, *Biol. Bull.* **72**:57–74.

Wendler, G., 1966, The co-ordination of walking movements in arthropods, *Symp. Soc. Exp. Biol.* **20**:229–249.

Wendler, G., 1972, Einflusserzwungener Flügelbewegungen auf das motorische Flugmuster von Heuschrecken, *Naturwissenschaften* **59**:220.

Wendler, G., 1974, The influence of proprioceptive feedback on locust flight co-ordination, *J. Comp. Physiol.* **88**:173–200.

Wernig, A., 1972*a,* The effects of calcium and magnesium on statistical release parameters at the crayfish neuromuscular junction, *J. Physiol. (London)* **226**:761–768.

Wernig, A., 1972*b,* Changes in statistical parameters during facilitation at the crayfish neuromuscular junction, *J. Physiol. (London)* **226**:751–759.

Wernig, A., 1975, Estimates of statistical release parameters from crayfish and frog neuromuscular junctions, *J. Physiol. (London)* **244**:207–221.

Wetzel, M. C., and Stuart, D. G., 1976, Emsemble characteristics of cat locomotion and its neural control, *Prog. Neurobiol.* **7**:1–98.

Whedon, A. D., 1919, The comparative physiology and possible adaptations of the abdomen in the Odonata, *Trans. Am. Entomol. Soc. (Philadelphia)* **44**:373–437.

Whitear, M., 1962, The fine structure of crustacean proprioceptors. I. The chordotonal organs in the legs of the shore crab, *Carcinus maenas, Philos. Trans. R. Soc. London Ser. B* **245**:291–324.

Whitear, M., 1965, The fine structure of crustacean proprioceptors. II. The thoracico-coxal organs in *Carcinus, Pagurus,* and *Astacus, Philos. Trans. R. Soc. London Ser. B* **248**:437–456.

Wiens, T. J., and Atwood, H. L., 1975, Dual inhibitory control in crab leg muscles, *J. Comp. Physiol.* **99**:211–230.

Wiens, T. J., and Gerstein, G. L., 1975, Cross connections among crayfish claw efferents, *J. Neurophysiol.* **38**:909–921.

Wiens, T. J., and Gerstein, G. L., 1976, Reflex pathways of the crayfish claw, *J. Comp. Physiol.* **107**:309–326.

Wiersma, C. A. G., 1933, Vergleichende Untersuchungen uber das periphere Nerven-muskelsystem von Crustaceen, *A. Vgl. Physiol.* **19**:349–385.

Wiersma, C. A. G., 1938, Function of the giant fibers of the central nervous system of the crayfish, *Proc. Soc. Exp. Biol. Med.* **38**:661–662.

Wiersma, C. A. G., 1941, The inhibitory nerve supply of the leg muscles of different decapod crustaceans, *J. Comp. Neurol.* **74**:63–79.

Wiersma, C. A. G., 1947*a,* Giant nerve fiber system of the crayfish: A contribution to comparative physiology of synapse, *J. Neurophysiol.* **10**:23–38.

Wiersma, C. A. G., 1947*b,* On the motor nerve supply of some segmented muscles of the crayfish, *Arch. Neerl. Physiol.* **28**:413–418.

Wiersma, C. A. G., 1949, Synaptic facilitation in the crayfish, *J. Neurophysiol.* **4**:267–275.

Wiersma, C. A. G., 1951, A bifunctional sigle motor axon system of a crustacean muscle, *J. Exp. Biol.* **28**:13–21.

Wiersma, C. A. G., 1952*a,* The neuron soma: Neurons of arthropods, *Cold Spring Harbor Symp. Quant. Biol.* **17**:155–163.

Wiersma, C. A. G., 1952*b,* Repetitive discharges of motor fibers caused by a single impulse in giant fibers of the crayfish, *J. Cell. Comp. Physiol.* **40**:399–419.

Wiersma, C. A. G., 1958, On the functional connections of single units in the central nervous system of the crayfish, *Procambarus clarkii* Girard, *J. Comp. Neurol.* **110**:421–472.

Wiersma, C. A. G., 1959, Movement receptors in decapod crustacea, *J. Mar. Biol. Assoc. U.K.* **38**:143–152.

Wiersma, C. A. G., 1961*a,* The neuromuscular system, in: *The Physiology of Crustacea,* Vol. 2 (T. H. Waterman, ed.), pp. 191–240, Academic Press, New York.

Wiersma, C. A. G., 1961*b,* Reflexes and the central nervous system, in: *The Physiology of Crustacea,* Vol. 2 (T. H. Waterman, ed.), pp. 241–279, Academic Press, New York.

Wiersma, C. A. G., 1962, The organization of the arthropod central nervous system, *Am. Zool.* **2**:67–68.

Wiersma, C. A. G., 1966, Integration in the visual pathway of Crustacea, in: *Nervous and Hormonal Mechanisms of Integration (Symp. Soc. Exp. Biol. 20),* Cambridge University Press, Cambridge.

Wiersma, C. A. G., 1967, Visual central processing in Crustaceans, in: *Invertebrate Nervous Systems* (C. A. G. Wiersma, ed.), University of Chicago Press, Chicago.

Wiersma, C. A. G., 1969, Regulative mechanisms for the discharge of specific interneurons, in: *The Interneuron (UCLA Forum Med. Sci. II)* (M. A. B. Brazier, ed.), pp. 113–129, University of California Press, Los Angeles.

Wiersma, C. A. G., 1970, Neuronal components of the optic nerve of the crab, *Carcinus maenas, Proc. K. Ned. Akad. Wet.* **73**:25–34.

Wiersma, C. A. G., 1974, Behavior of neurons, in: *The Neurosciences: Third Study Program* (F. O. Schmitt, ed.), pp. 419–443, M.I.T. Press, Cambridge, Mass.

Wiersma, C. A. G., 1976, Central processing of proprioceptive information, in: *Structure and Function of Proprioceptors in the Invertebrates* (P. J. Mill, ed.), Chapter 16, Chapman and Hall, London.

Wiersma, C. A. G., and Adams, R. T., 1950, The influence of nerve impulse sequence of the contractions of different crustacean muscles, *Physiol. Comp. Oecol.* **2**:20–33.

Wiersma, C. A. G., and Boettiger, E. G., 1959, Unidirectional movement fibres from a proprioceptive organ of the crab, *Carcinus maenas, J. Exp. Biol.* **36**:102–112.

Wiersma, C. A. G., and Bush, B. M. H., 1963, Functional neural connections between the thoracic and abdominal cords of the crayfish, *Procambarus clarkii* (Girard), *J. Comp. Neurol.* **121**:207–235.

Wiersma, C. A. G., and Ellis, C. H., 1942, A comparative study of peripheral inhibition in decapod crustaceans, *J. Exp. Biol.* **18:**223–236.

Wiersma, C. A. G., and Fiore, L., 1971*a*, Factors regulating the discharge frequency in optomotor fibers of *Carcinus maenas*, *J. Exp. Biol.* **54:**497–506.

Wiersma, C. A. G., and Fiore, L., 1971*b*, Unidirectional rotation neurons in the optomotor system of the crab, *Carcinus*, *J. Exp. Biol.* **54:**507–514.

Wiersma, C. A. G., and Helfer, R. G., 1941, The effect of peripheral inhibition on the muscle action potentials of the crab, *Physiol. Zool.* **14:**296–304.

Wiersma, C. A. G., and Hirsh, R., 1974, Memory evoked optomotor responses in crustaceans, *J. Neurobiol.* **5:**213–230.

Wiersma, C. A. G., and Hirsh, R., 1975*a*, Contrast induced zones as the basis of optomotor memory in the crab *Pachygrapsus*, *J. Comp. Physiol.* **102:**173–188.

Wiersma, C. A. G., and Hirsh, R., 1975*b*, On the organisation of memory in the optomotor systems of the crab, *Pachygrapsus crassipes*, *J. Neurobiol.* **6:**115–123.

Wiersma, C. A. G., and Hughes, G. M., 1961, On the functional anatomy of neuronal units in the abdominal cord of the crayfish, *Procambarus clarkii* (Girard), *J. Comp. Neurol.* **116:**209–228.

Wiersma, C. A. G., and Ikeda, K., 1964, Interneurons commanding swimmeret movements in the crayfish, *Procambarus clarkii* (Girard), *Comp. Biochem. Physiol.* **12:**509–525.

Wiersma, C. A. G., and Mill, P. J., 1965, Descending neuronal units in the commissure of the crayfish central nervous system; and the integration of visual, tactile and proprioceptive stimuli, *J. Comp. Neurol.* **125:**67–94.

Wiersma, C. A. G., and Novitski, 1974, The mechanism of the nervous regulation of the crayfish heart, *J. Exp. Biol.* **19:**255–265.

Wiersma, C. A. G., and Oberjat, T., 1968, The selective responsiveness of various crayfish oculomotor fibers to sensory stimuli, *Comp. Biochem. Physiol.* **26:**1–16.

Wiersma, C. A. G., and Ripley, S. H., 1952, Innervation patterns of crustacean limbs, *Physiol. Comp. Oecol.* **2:**391–405.

Wiersma, C. A. G., and Schalleck, W., 1947, Potentials from motor roots of the crustacean central nervous system, *J. Neurophysiol.* **10:**323–329.

Wiersma, C. A. G., and Schalleck, W., 1948, Influence of drugs on response of a crustacean synapse to preganglionic stimulation, *J. Neurophysiol.* **11:**491–496.

Wiersma, C. A. G., and Turner, R. S., 1950, The interaction between the synapses of a single motor fiber *J. Gen. Physiol.* **34:**137–145.

Wiersma, C. A. G., and van Harreveld, A., 1936, The double motor innervation of a crayfish muscle, *Proc. Natl. Acad. Sci. USA* **22:**190–191.

Wiersma, C. A. G., and van Harreveld, A., 1938*a*, A comparative study of the double motor innervation in marine crustaceans, *J. Exp. Biol.* **15:**18–31.

Wiersma, C. A. G., and van Harreveld, A., 1938*b*, The influence of the frequency of stimulation on the slow and the fast contraction in crustacean muscle, *Physiol. Zool.* **11:**75–81.

Wiersma, C. A. G., and Yamaguchi, T., 1966, The neuronal components of the optic nerve of the crayfish as studied by single unit analysis, *J. Comp. Neurol.* **128:**333–358.

Wiersma, C. A. G., and Yamaguchi, T., 1967*a*, Integration of visual stimuli by the crayfish central nervous system, *J. Exp. Biol.* **47:**409–431.

Wiersma, C. A. G., and Yamaguchi, T., 1967*b*, The integration of visual stimuli in the rock lobster, *Vision Res.* **7:**197–204.

Wiersma, C. A. G., and Yanagisawa, K., 1971, On types of interneurons responding to visual stimulation present in the optic nerve of the rock lobster, *Panulirus interruptus*, *J. Neurobiol.* **2:**291–304.

Wiersma, C. A. G., and York, B., 1972, Properties of the seeing fibers in the rock lobster: Field structure habituation, attention and distraction, *Vision Res.* **12:**627–640.

Wiersma, C. A. G., and Zawadski, B., 1948, On the relation between ions and peripheral inhibition in crustacean muscles, *J. Cell. Comp. Physiol.* **32:**101–103.

Wiersma, C. A. G., van der Mark, F., and Fiore, L., 1970, On the firing patterns of "movement" receptors of the elastic organs of the crab *Carcinus*, *Comp. Biochem. Physiol.* **34:**833–840.

Wiersma, C. A. G., Bush, B. M. H., and Waterman, T. H., 1964, Efferent visual responses of contralateral origin in the optic nerve of the crab, *Podophthalmus, J. Cell. Comp. Physiol.* **64:**309–326.

Wiersma, C. A. G., Furshpan, E., and Florey, E., 1953, Physiological and pharmacological observations on muscle receptor organs of the crayfish, *Cambarus clarkii* Girard, *J. Exp. Biol.* **30:**136–150.

Wiese, K., 1976, Mechanoreceptors for near-field water displacements in crayfish, *J. Neurophysiol.,* in press.

Wiese, K., Calabrese, R. L., and Kennedy, D., 1976, Integration of directional mechanosensory input by crayfish interneurons, *J. Neurophysiol.,* in press.

Wiesel, T. N., and Hubel, D. H., 1963, Single-cell responses in striate cortex of kittens deprived of vision in one eye, *J. Neurophysiol.* **26:**1003–1017.

Wilkens, J. L., Wilkens, L. A., and McMahon, B. R., 1974, Central control of cardiac and scaphognathite pacemakers in the crab, *Cancer magister, J. Comp. Physiol.* **90:**89–104.

Wilkens, L. A., and Larimer, J. L., 1972, The CNS photoreceptor of crayfish: Morphology and synaptic activity, *J. Comp. Physiol.* **80:**389–407.

Wilkens, L. A., and Larimer, J. L., 1973, Sensory interneurons: Some observations concerning the physiology and related structural significance of two cells in the crayfish brain, *Tissue Cell* **5:**393–400.

Wilkens, L. A., and Larimer, J. L., 1977, Photosensitivity in the sixth abdominal ganglion of decapod crustaceans: A comparative study, *J. Comp. Physiol.,* in press.

Wilkens, L. A., and Wolfe, G. E., 1974, A new electrode design for *en passant* recording, stimulation and intracellular dye infusion, *Comp. Biochem. Physiol.* **48:**217–220.

Williams, C. M., and Williams, M. V., 1943, The flight muscles of *Drosophila repleta, J. Morphol.* **72:**589–599.

Williams, J. D., and Bowen, J. M., 1974, Effects of quantal unit latency on statistics of Poisson and binomial neurotransmitter release mechanism, *J. Theoret. Biol.* **43:**151–165.

Willows, A. O. D., 1976, Command neurons in the mollusk *Tritonia,* in: *neural Control of Locomotion* (R. H. Herman, S. Grillner, P. S. G. Stein, and D. G. Stuart, eds.), Plenum Press, New York.

Willows, A. O. D., and Hoyle, G., 1969, Neuronal network triggering a fixed action pattern, *Science* **166:**1549–1551.

Willows, A. O. D., Dorsett, D. A., and Hoyle, G., 1973*a,* The neuronal basis of behavior in *Tritonia.* III. Neuronal mechanism of a fixed action pattern, *J. Neurobiol.* **4:**255–285.

Willows, A. O. D., Getting, P. A., and Thompson, S., 1973*b,* Bursting mechanisms in molluscan locomotion, in: *Control of Posture and Locomotion* (R. B. Stein, K. G. Pearson, R. S. Smith, and J. B. Redford, eds.), pp. 457–475, Plenum Press, New York.

Wilson, A. H., and Sherman, R. G., 1975, Mapping of neuron somata in the thoracic nerve cord of the lobster using cobalt chloride, *Comp. Biochem. Physiol.* **50A:**47–50.

Wilson, D. M., 1961, The central nervous control of flight in a locust, *J. Exp. Biol.* **38:**471–490.

Wilson, D. M., 1962, Bifunctional muscles in the thorax of grasshoppers, *J. Exp. Biol.* **39:**669–677.

Wilson, D. M., 1965, The nervous co-ordination of insect locomotion, in: *The Physiology of the Insect Central Nervous System* (J. E. Treherne and J. W. L. Beament, eds.), pp. 125–140, Academic Press, New York.

Wilson, D. M., 1966*a,* Central nervous mechanisms for the generation of rhythmic behavior in arthropods, *Symp. Soc. Exp. Biol.* **20:**199–228.

Wilson, D. M., 1966*b,* Insect walking, *Annu. Rev. Entomol.* **11:**103–122.

Wilson, D. M., 1967, An approach to the problem of control of rhythmic behavior, in: *Invertebrate Nervous Systems* (C. A. G. Wiersma, ed.), pp. 219–229, University of Chicago Press, Chicago.

Wilson, D. M., 1968*a,* The flight control system of a locust, *Sci. Am.* **218(5):**83–90.

Wilson, D. M., 1968*b,* Inherent asymetry and reflex modulation of the locust flight pattern, *J. Exp. Biol.* **48:**631–641.

Wilson, D. M., 1968*c,* The nervous control of insect flight and related behavior, *Adv. Insect Physiol.* **5:**289–338.

Wilson, D. M., 1972, Genetic and sensory mechanisms for locomotion and orientation in animals, *Am. Sci.* **69:**358–365.

Wilson, D. M., and Davis, W. J., 1965, Nerve impulse patterns and reflex control in the crayfish claw motor system, *J. Exp. Biol.* **43:**193–210.

Wilson, D. M., and Gettrup, E., 1963, A stretch reflex controlling wing-beat frequency in grasshoppers, *J. Exp. Biol.* **40:**171–185.

Wilson, D. M., and Larimer, J. L., 1968, The catch property of ordinary muscle, *Proc. Natl. Acad. Sci. USA* **61:**909–916.

Wilson, D. M., and Waldron, I., 1968, Models for the generation of the motor output pattern in flying locusts, *Proc. IEEE* **56:**1058–1064.

Wilson, D. M., and Weis-Fogh, T., 1962, Patterned activity of co-ordinated motor units, studied in flying locusts, *J. Exp. Biol.* **39:**643–667.

Wilson, D. M., and Wyman, R. J., 1965, Motor output patterns during random and rhythmic stimulation of locust thoracic ganglia, *Biophys. J.* **5:**121–143.

Wilson, D. M., Smith, D. O., and Dempster, P., 1970, Length and tension hysteresis during sinusoidal and step function stimulation of arthropod muscle, *Am. J. Physiol.* **218:**916–922.

Wine, J. J., 1971, Escape reflex circuit in crayfish: Interganglionic interneurons activated by the giant command neurons, *Biol. Bull.* **141:**408.

Wine, J. J., 1972, Slowly developing hyperreflexia in the crayfish abdomen following nerve cord transection, *Abst. Soc. Neurosci. 2nd Mtg.,* p. 190.

Wine, J. J., 1973, Invertebrate central neurons: Orthograde degeneration and retrograde changes after axonotomy, *Exp. Neurol.* **38:**157–169.

Wine, J. J., 1977, Neuronal organization of crayfish escape behavior: Inhibition of the giant motoneuron via a disynaptic pathway from other motoneurons, *J. Neurophysiol.* **40:**1078–1097.

Wine, J. J., and Krasne, F. B., 1972, The organization of escape behavior in the crayfish, *J. Exp. Biol.* **56:**1–18.

Wine, J. J., and Mistick, D. C., 1977, Temporal organization of crayfish escape behavior: Delayed recruitment of peripheral inhibition, *J. Neurophysiol.* **40:**904–925.

Wine, J. J., Gauthier, R., and Mittenthal, J. E., 1974, Electrophysiological analysis of input to a multimodal command interneuron, *Abst. Soc. Neurosci. 4th Mtg.,* p. 481.

Wine, J. J., Mittenthal, J. E., and Kennedy, D., 1974, The structure of tonic flexor motoneurons in crayfish abdominal ganglia, *J. Comp. Physiol.* **93:**315–335.

Wine, J. J., Krasne, F. B., and Chen, L., 1975, Habituation and inhibition of the crayfish lateral giant fibre escape response, *J. Exp. Biol.* **62:**771–782.

Wong, R. K. S., and Pearson, K. G., 1976, Properties of the trochanteral hair plate and its function in the control of walking in the cockroach, *J. Exp. Biol.* **64:**233–249.

Wood, J., 1975, Activity recorded from the propodite dactylopodite organ of *Pachygrapsus crassipes* at rest and at constant speeds of movement, *Comp. Biochem. Physiol.* **50A:**765–769.

Woodcock, A. E. R., and Goldsmith, T. H., 1973, Differential wavelength sensitivity in the receptive fields of sustaining fibers in the optic tract of the crayfish *Procambarus, J. Comp. Physiol.* **87:**247–257.

Wright, E. B., and Adelman, W. J., 1954, Accommodation in three single motor axons of the crayfish claw, *J. Cell. Comp. Physiol.* **43:**119–132.

Wyse, G. A., 1972, Intracellular and extracellular motor neuron activity underlying rhythmic respiration in *Limulus, J. Comp. Physiol.* **81:**259–276.

Yamaguchi, T., 1967, Effects of eye motion and body position on crayfish movement fibers, in: *Invertebrate Nervous Systems* (C. A. G. Wiersma, ed.), pp. 285–288, University of Chicago Press, Chicago.

Yamaguchi, T., Katagiri, Y., and Ochi, K., 1976, Polarized light responses from retina cells and sustaining fibers of the mantis shrimp, *Biol. J. Okayama Univ.* **17:**61–66.

Young, D., 1969, The motor neurons of the mesothoracic ganglion of *Periplaneta americana, J. Insect. Physiol.* **15:**1175–1180.

Young, D., 1972, Specific re-innervation of limbs transplanted between segments in the cockroach, *Periplaneta americana, J. Exp. Biol.* **57**:305–316

Young, R. E., 1975, Neuromuscular control of ventilation in crab *Carcinus maenas, J. Comp. Physiol.* **100A**:1–37.

Younkin, S. G.; 1974, An analysis of the role of calcium in facilitation at the frog neuromuscular junction, *J. Physiol. (London)* **237**:1–14.

York, B., and Wiersma, C. A. G., 1975, Visual processing in the rock lobster, *Prog. Neurobiol.* **5**:127–166.

Zachar, J., Zacharova, D., Kuncova, M. J., and Hencek, M., 1964, The effect of γ-aminobutyric acid on the potassium and chloride conductances of the muscle membrane of the crayfish (in Russian), *Abst. Xth Physiol. Congr. USSR in Jerevan,* Vol. II, Part 1, p. 311.

Zawarzin, A., 1924a, Über die histologische Beschaffenheit des unpaaren ventralen Nervs der Insekten, *Z. Wiss. Zool. Abt. A* **122**:97–115.

Zawarzin, A., 1924b, Zur Morphologie der Nervenzentren. Das Bauchmark der Insekten. Ein Beitrag zur vergleichenden Histologie, *Z. Wiss. Zool. Abt. A* **122**:323–424.

Zucker, R. S., 1972a, Crayfish escape behavior and central synapses. I. Neural circuit exciting lateral giant fiber, *J. Neurophysiol.* **35**:599–620.

Zucker, R. S., 1972b, Crayfish escape behavior and central synapses. II. Physiological mechanisms underlying behavioral habituation, *J. Neurophysiol.* **35**:621–637.

Zucker, R. S., 1972c, Crayfish escape behavior and central synapses. III. Electrical junctions and dendrite spikes in fast flexor motorneurons, *J. Neurophysiol.* **35**:638–651.

Zucker, R. S., 1973, Changes in the statistics of transmitter release during facilitation, *J. Physiol. (London)* **229**:787–810.

Zucker, R. S., 1974a, Crayfish neuromuscular facilitation activated by constant presynaptic action potentials and depolarizing pulses, *J. Physiol. (London)* **241**:69–90.

Zucker, R. S., 1974b, Characteristics of crayfish neuromuscular facilitation and their calcium dependence, *J. Physiol. (London)* **241**:91–110.

Zucker, R. S., 1974c, Excitability changes in crayfish motor neurone terminals, *J. Physiol. (London)* **241**:111–126.

Zucker, R. S., and Bruner, J., 1974, Studies on a long-lasting neuromuscular depression, *Proceedings of the Twenty-sixth International Congress of Physiology (abst.).*

Zucker, R. S., Kennedy, D., and Selverston, A. I., 1971, Neuronal circuit mediating escape responses in crayfish, *Science* **173**:645–650.

Index

*(=) indicates that common name has been used in the text.

589